Prioritization, Delegation, & Management of Care *for the* NCLEX-RN® Exam

Prioritization, Delegation, & Management of Care *for the* NCLEX-RN® Exam

Ray A. Hargrove-Huttel, RN, PhD

Kathryn Cadenhead Colgrove, RN, MS, CNS

F.A. Davis Company • Philadelphia

F. A. Davis Company
1915 Arch Street
Philadelphia, PA 19103
www.fadavis.com

Printed in the United States of America

Last digit indicates print number: 10 9 8 7 6 5 4 3 2

Publisher, Nursing: Robert G. Martone
Director of Content Development: Darlene D. Pedersen
Project Editor: Jacalyn C. Clay
Electronic Project Editor: Sandra A. Glennie
Illustration and Design Manager: Carolyn O'Brien

As new scientific information becomes available through basic and clinical research, recommended treatments and drug therapies undergo changes. The author(s) and publisher have done everything possible to make this book accurate, up to date, and in accord with accepted standards at the time of publication. The author(s), editors, and publisher are not responsible for errors or omissions or for consequences from application of the book, and make no warranty, expressed or implied, in regard to the contents of the book. Any practice described in this book should be applied by the reader in accordance with professional standards of care used in regard to the unique circumstances that may apply in each situation. The reader is advised always to check product information (package inserts) for changes and new information regarding dose and contraindications before administering any drug. Caution is especially urged when using new or infrequently ordered drugs.

Library of Congress Cataloging-in-Publication Data

Library of Congress Cataloging-in-Publication Data

ISBN: 978-0-8036-3313-1

Thank you to all the nursing students, nursing faculty, and nursing colleagues we have had the privilege to work with during our careers. We want to thank Robert Martone for his vision and support, who was there when our writing career started and has been with us every step of the way. Our thanks to computer extraordinaire Glada Norris, who fixes our mistakes, makes the questions look "pretty," and is responsible for making this book possible. Thank you to Kathryn McAfee who codes all the questions, leaving us time to write the questions.

I want to thank all my friends for love, support, and prayers as I battled ovarian cancer this last year. Thanks to aunts, uncles, and cousins, my Los Angeles friends, my Trinity Valley Community College friends, my Texas friends, my Hawaiian friends, and the Lee girls. My thanks to my sisters Gail and Debbie, my nephew Ben, and Paula who brought me home and cared for me. I thank my children Teresa and Aaron for making me want to get up every day and fight the fight. As always, I dedicate this book to my parents, T/Sgt Leo R. Hargrove and Nancy, who made me believe I can do anything. I am an ovarian cancer survivor.

—RAY A. HARGROVE-HUTTEL
(This was Ray's dedication. Ray lost her battle with cancer on December 23, 2012. She is much loved and greatly missed. -Kathy Colgrove)

I would like to dedicate this book to the memory of my mother, Mary Cadenhead, and grandmother, Elsie Rogers. They always told me I could accomplish anything I wanted to accomplish. I would also like to dedicate this book to my husband, Larry, children, Laurie and Todd and Larry Jr. and Mai, and grandchildren, Chris, Ashley, Justin C., Justin A., Connor, Sawyer, and Carson—without their support and patience the book would not have been possible.

—KATHRYN CADENHEAD COLGROVE

Reviewers

Debra Bailey, RN, PhD candidate, FNP, CDE
Associate Professor of Nursing, Department Head Health Sciences
Colorado Mesa University
Grand Junction, Colorado

Patricia A. Bicknell, EdD, APRN, ACNS-BC, CNL
Assistant Professor of Nursing; Track Coordinator for Clinical Nurse Leader (CNL)
La Salle University
Philadelphia, Pennsylvania

Donna Bowles, EdD, MSN, CNE
Associate Professor
Indiana University Southeast
New Albany, Indiana

Diane Cohen, RN, MSN
Professor
MassBay Community College
Framingham, Massachusetts

Diane L. Cooper-McLean, RN, BSN, MSN
Nursing Instructor
Faulkner State Community College
Bay Minette, Alabama

Pamela DeWitt, RN, MN, CNE
Residential Faculty
Phoenix College
Department of Nursing
Phoenix, Arizona

Kathleen Walsh Free, MSN, RN-C, APRN-BC
Clinical Professor
Indiana University Southeast
New Albany, Indiana

Lynn D. Kennedy, MSN, RN
Assistant Professor of Nursing
Francis Marion University
Florence, South Carolina

Maria McCormick, MSN, MS, RN
Faculty
Spencerian College
Louisville, Kentucky

Mary Ann Siciliano McLaughlin, MSN, RN
Faculty, UMDNJ School of Nursing
UMDNJ School of Nursing
Stratford, New Jersey

Elizabeth Murray, PhD, RN, CNE
Assistant Professor
Florida Gulf Coast University School of Nursing
Fort Myers, Florida

L. Jane Rosati, EdD, MSN, RN-BC
Assistant Chair/Program Manager of the ADN Program
Daytona State College
Daytona Beach, Florida

Faye Sigman, PhD
Professor of Nursing
Dyersburg State
Dyersburg, Tennessee

Thomas Worms, RN, MSN
Professor of Nursing
Truman College
Chicago, Illinois

Polly Gerber Zimmermann, RN, MS, MBA, CEN, FAEN
Associate Professor
Harry S Truman College
Chicago, Illinois

Table of Contents

Introduction to Prioritization, Assignment, Delegation, and Management

Each problem that I solved became a rule which served afterwards to solve other problems.

—Rene Descartes

This book is designed to assist the student nurse in nursing school and in taking nursing examinations, particularly the NCLEX-RN® exam for licensure as a registered nurse (RN). *Prioritization, Delegation & Management of Care for the NCLEX-RN® Exam* focuses on aspects of management such as setting priorities for client care, delegating and assigning nursing tasks, and managing clients and staff. It contains practice questions on these topics in a wide variety of nursing arenas, including medical, surgical, critical care, pediatric, geriatric, rehabilitation, home health, and mental health nursing. Answers—and why each possible response is correct or incorrect—are given for all questions.

Management, prioritizing, and delegation questions are some of the most difficult questions for the student and new graduate to answer because there is no reference book in which to find the correct answers. Answers to these types of questions require knowledge of basic scientific principles, standards of care, pathophysiology, and psychosocial behaviors, and leadership qualities and the ability to think critically. It is important to note that the test taker may not always agree with the authors' rationale for the correct answer. It is poor test taking to read rationales for the incorrect answers; the students will remember reading the rationale but not if the rationale was for the correct or incorrect answer.

Many of the answers in this book include tips to help the test taker. Termed "Making Nursing Decisions," these tips provide help for the student in identifying exactly what the question is asking, in analyzing the question, and in determining the correct response.

A Comprehensive Examination with answers and rationales is also included for each field of nursing.

Practice questions and answers and practice examinations are valuable in preparing for an examination, but the test taker should remember that there is no substitute for studying the material.

(For general information on how to prepare for an examination and on the types of questions used in nursing examinations, refer to *Fundamentals Success: A Q&A Review Applying Critical Thinking to Test Taking* by Patricia Nugent, RN, MA, MS, EdD, and Barbara Vitale, RN, MA.)

NCSBN BLUEPRINT FOR QUESTIONS

The National Council of State Boards of Nursing (NCSBN) provides a blueprint that assists nursing faculty in developing test questions for the NCLEX-RN®. Content included in management of care provides and directs nursing care that enhances the care delivery setting to protect clients, family/significant others, and healthcare personnel. Related content includes, but is not limited to, advance directives, advocacy, case management, client rights, collaboration with the interdisciplinary team, delegation, establishing priorities, ethical practice, informed consent, information technology, and performance improvement. Other topics also include legal rights and responsibilities, referrals, resource management, staff education, supervision, confidentiality/information security, and continuity of care. The questions in this book follow this blueprint.

GUIDELINES FOR MAKING A DECISION

Nurses* base their decisions on many different bodies of information in order to arrive at a course of action. Among the basic guidelines to apply in nursing practice—and in answering test questions—are the nursing process and Maslow's Hierarchy of Needs.

The Nursing Process

One of the basic guidelines to apply in nursing practice is the nursing process, which consists of five steps—assessment, nursing diagnosis, planning, intervention, and evaluation—usually completed in a systematic order.

Many questions can be answered based on "assessment." If a priority-setting question asks the test taker which step to implement first, the test taker should look for an answer that would assess for the problem discussed in the stem of the question.

EXAMPLE

> The nurse is caring for a client diagnosed with congestive heart failure who is currently complaining of dyspnea. Which intervention should the nurse implement first?
> 1. Administer furosemide (Lasix), a loop diuretic, IVP.
> 2. Check the client for adventitious lung sounds.
> 3. Ask the respiratory therapist to administer a treatment.
> 4. Notify the healthcare provider.
>
> **Answer: 2**
> Checking for adventitious lung sounds is assessing the client to determine the extent of the client's breathing difficulties causing the dyspnea.

There are numerous words, such as "check," that can be used to indicate assessment. The test taker should not discard an option because the word "assess" or "assessment" is not used. Alternatively, the test taker shouldn't assume that an option is correct merely because the word "assess" is used. The test taker must also be aware that the assessment data must match the problem stated in the stem, regardless of terminology. The nurse must assess for the correct information. If option 2 in the above example said, "Assess urinary output," it would not be a correct option even though it includes the word "assess," since urinary output is not related to heart failure or breathing difficulties. In addition, the test taker should be aware that assessment is not always the correct answer when the question asks which should be done first. Suppose, for example, that the above question had listed option 3 as "Apply oxygen via nasal cannula at 2 LPM." In that case, assessment does not come first. The nurse would first attempt to relieve the client's distress and then assess.

When a question asks what a nurse should do next, the test taker should determine from the information given in the question which steps in the nursing process have been completed and then choose an option that matches the next step in the nursing process.

In this book, the term "nurse," unless otherwise specified, refers to a licensed registered nurse (RN). An RN can assign tasks to an LPN or delegate to unlicensed assistive personnel (UAP), which may be known under other terms such as medical assistant or nurse's aide. An LPN can delegate tasks to UAP. Each state will have specific regulations that govern what duties/tasks can be delegated/assigned to each of these types of personnel.

The term "healthcare provider," as used in this book, refers to a client's primary provider of medical care. It includes physicians (including osteopathic physicians), nurse practitioners (NPs), and physician assistants (PAs). Depending on state regulations, many NPs and some PAs have prescriptive authority at least for some categories of prescribed drugs.

EXAMPLE

> The client diagnosed with peptic ulcer disease has a blood pressure of 88/42, an apical pulse of 132, and respirations are 28. The nurse writes the nursing diagnosis "altered tissue perfusion related to decreased circulatory volume." Which intervention should the nurse implement first?
> 1. Notify the laboratory to draw a type & crossmatch.
> 2. Assess the client's abdomen for tenderness.
> 3. Insert an 18-gauge catheter and infuse lactated Ringer's.
> 4. Check the client's pulse oximeter reading.
>
> **Answer: 3**
> 1. Notifying the laboratory for a type & crossmatch would be an appropriate intervention since the client is showing signs of hypovolemia, but it is not the first intervention because it would not directly support the client's circulatory volume.
> 2. The stem of the question has provided enough assessment data to indicate the client's problem of hypovolemia. Further assessment data are not needed.
> **3. The vital signs indicate hypovolemia, which is a life-threatening emergency that requires the nurse to intervene to support the client's circulatory volume. The nurse can do this by infusing lactated Ringer's.**
> 4. A pulse oximeter reading would not support the client's circulatory volume.

The nurse has assessed the client and formulated a nursing diagnosis. The next step in the nursing process is implementation. The nurse should proceed to a nursing intervention appropriate to the situation.

These types of questions are designed to determine if the test taker can set priorities in client care.

Maslow's Hierarchy of Needs

If the test taker has looked at the question and the nursing process can't help in determining the correct option, then using a tool such as Maslow's Hierarchy of Needs (Fig. 1-1) can assist in choosing the correct answer.

Remember that the bottom of the pyramid—physiological needs—represents the top priority in instituting nursing interventions. If a question asks the test taker to determine which is the priority intervention and a physiological need is listed among the options, then that is the priority. If a physiological need is not listed, safety and security take priority, and so on up the pyramid.

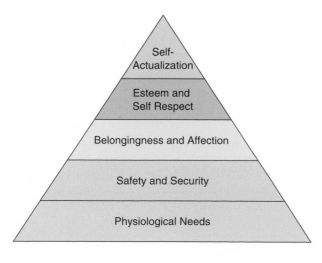

Figure 1-1. Maslow's Hierarchy of Needs.

TYPES OF QUESTIONS

Most of the questions on the NCLEX-RN® are multiple choice. The questions involve prioritizing client care, delegating staff tasks, and managing issues dealing with clients and staff. These questions may include interpreting medication administration records (MARs), knowing when notifying the primary healthcare provider (HCP) is priority, and knowing which tasks can be assigned to a licensed practical nurse (LPN) or unlicensed assistive personnel (UAP) and which must be performed by a registered nurse (RN).

Some questions on the NCLEX-RN® are termed alternate-format questions and including choosing more than one option that correctly answers a question, ranking procedures or actions in correct order, drop-and-drag questions, and fill-in-the-blank questions.

EXAMPLE

> The nurse is assigning tasks to the UAP. Which is an appropriate delegation to the UAP? Select all that apply.
> 1. Check the area around an incisional wound for redness.
> 2. Help a client with an upper limb cast to eat.
> 3. Assist a patient recovering from a hysterectomy to walk to the bathroom.
> 4. Explain to a client being discharged how to empty and clean the colostomy.
> 5. Transport a client with a suspected fractured tibia to the x-ray department.

Prioritizing Questions/Setting Priorities

In test questions that ask the nurse which action to take first, two or more of the options will be appropriate nursing interventions for the situation described. When choosing the correct answer, the test taker must decide which intervention should occur *first* in a sequence of events, or which intervention directly impacts the situation.

With a question that asks which client should the nurse assess first, the test taker should first look at each option and determine if the signs/symptoms the client is exhibiting are normal or expected for the disease process; if so, the nurse does not need to assess that particular client first. Second, if two or more of the options state signs/symptoms that are not normal or expected for the disease process, then the test taker should select the option that has the greatest potential for a poor outcome. Each option should be examined carefully to determine the priority by asking these questions:

- Is the situation life threatening or life altering? *If yes, this client is the highest priority.*
- Is the situation unexpected for the disease process? *If yes, then this client may be priority.*
- Is the data presented abnormal? *If yes, then this client may be priority.*
- Is the situation expected for the disease process and not life threatening? *If yes, then this client may be—but probably is not—priority.*
- Is the situation/data normal? *If yes, this client can be seen last.*

The test taker should try to make a decision pertaining to each option. On pencil-and-paper examinations, it may be helpful to note the decision near the option. On a computerized test, the test taker should make the decision and move on to the next question.

Delegating and Assigning Care

Although each state and province has its own Nursing Practice Acts, there are some general guidelines that apply to all professional nurses.

- When delegating to an unlicensed assistive personnel (UAP), the nurse may not delegate any activity that requires nursing judgment. These include assessing, teaching, evaluating, or administering medications to any client and the care of any unstable client.
- When assigning care to an LPN, the RN can assign the administration of some medications but cannot assign assessing, teaching, or evaluating any client and cannot delegate the care of an unstable client.

Management Decisions

The nurse is frequently called upon to make decisions about staffing, movement of clients from one unit to another, or handling conflicts as they arise. Some general guidelines for answering questions in this area include the following:

- The most experienced nurse gets the most critical client.
- A graduate nurse can take care of any client who is receiving care from a student with supervision.
- The most stable client can move or be discharged; whereas, the most unstable client must move to intensive care unit (ICU) or stay in ICU.

When the nurse must make a decision regarding a conflict in the nursing station, a good rule to follow is to use the chain of command. The primary nurse should confront a peer (another primary nurse) or a subordinate unless the situation is illegal (such as stealing drugs). The primary nurse should use the chain of command in situations that address superiors (a manager or director of nursing); then the nurse should discuss the situation with the next in command above the superior.

PUTTING THE PIECES TOGETHER

The nurse is required to acquire information, analyze the data, and make inferences based on the available information. Sometimes this process is relatively easy and at other times the pieces of information do not seem to fit. This is precisely where critical thinking and nursing judgment must guide in making the decision.

Cardiovascular Management

2

*When you do the common things in life in an uncommon
way, you will command the attention of the world.*

—George Washington Carver

QUESTIONS

1. The nurse on the cardiac unit has received the shift report from the outgoing nurse.
   Which client should the nurse assess first?
   1. The client who has just been brought to the unit from the emergency department
      (ED) with no report of complaints.
   2. The client who received pain medication 30 minutes ago for chest pain that was a
      level 3 on a 1-to-10 pain scale.
   3. The client who had a cardiac catheterization in the morning and has palpable pedal
      pulses bilaterally.
   4. The client who has been turning on the call light frequently and stating her care has
      been neglected.

2. The nurse on the cardiac unit is preparing to administer medications after receiving
   the morning change-of-shift report. Which medication should the nurse administer
   first?
   1. The cardiac glycoside to the client who has an apical pulse of 58.
   2. The loop diuretic to a client with a serum K+ level of 3.2 mEq/L.
   3. The antidysrhythmic to the client in ventricular fibrillation.
   4. The calcium-channel blocker who has a blood pressure of 110/68.

3. Which client should the telemetry nurse assess first after receiving the a.m. shift report?
   1. The client diagnosed with deep vein thrombosis who has an edematous right calf.
   2. The client diagnosed with mitral valve stenosis who has heart palpitations.
   3. The client diagnosed with arterial occlusive disease who has intermittent
      claudication.
   4. The client diagnosed with congestive heart failure who has pink frothy sputum.

4. The charge nurse is making assignments for clients on a cardiac unit. Which client
   should the charge nurse assign to a new graduate nurse?
   1. The 44-year-old client diagnosed with a myocardial infarction.
   2. The 65-year-old client admitted with unstable angina.
   3. The 75-year-old client scheduled for a cardiac catheterization.
   4. The 50-year-old client complaining of chest pain.

5. The charge nurse is making assignments for a 30-bed cardiac unit staffed with three registered nurses (RNs), three licensed practical nurses (LPNs), and three unlicensed assistive personnel (UAPs). Which assignment is most appropriate by the charge nurse?
   1. Assign an RN to perform all sterile procedures.
   2. Assign an LPN to give all IV medications.
   3. Assign an UAP to complete the a.m. care.
   4. Assign an LPN to write the care plans.

6. The nurse on a cardiac unit is discussing a client with the case manager. Which information should the nurse share with the case manager?
   1. Discuss personal information the client shared with the nurse in confidence.
   2. Provide the case manager with any information that is required for continuity of care.
   3. Explain that client confidentiality prevents the nurse from disclosing information.
   4. Ask the case manager to get the client's permission before sharing information.

7. The nurse assesses erratic electrical activity on the telemetry reading while the client is talking to the nurse on the intercom system. Which task should the nurse instruct the UAP to implement?
   1. Call a Code Blue immediately.
   2. Check the client's telemetry leads.
   3. Find the nurse to check the client.
   4. Remove the telemetry monitor.

8. The charge nurse on the cardiac unit has to float a nurse to the emergency department for the shift. Which nurse should be floated to the emergency department?
   1. The nurse who has 4 years of experience on the cardiac unit.
   2. The nurse who just transferred from critical care to the cardiac unit.
   3. The nurse with 1 year of experience on the cardiac unit who has been on a week's sick leave.
   4. The nurse who has worked in the operating room for 2 years and in the cardiac unit for 3 years.

9. The cardiac nurse is preparing to administer one unit of blood to a client. Which interventions should the nurse implement? Rank in order of priority.
   1. Infuse the unit of blood at 20 gtts/min the first 15 minutes.
   2. Check the unit of blood and the client's blood band with another nurse.
   3. Initiate Y-tubing with normal saline via an 18-gauge angiocatheter.
   4. Assess the client's vital signs and lung sounds, and assess for a rash.
   5. Obtain informed consent for the unit of blood from the client.

10. The charge nurse in the cardiac critical care unit is making rounds. Which client should the nurse see first?
    1. The client with coronary artery disease who is complaining that the nurses are being rude and won't answer the call lights.
    2. The client diagnosed with an acute myocardial infarction who has an elevated creatinine phosphokinase-cardiac muscle (CPK-MB) level.
    3. The client diagnosed with atrial fibrillation on an oral anticoagulant who has an International Normalized Ratio (INR) of 2.8.
    4. The client 2 days' postoperative coronary artery bypass who is being transferred to the cardiac unit.

11. The nurse is preparing to administer digoxin 0.25 mg IVP to a client in severe congestive heart failure who is receiving $D_5W/0.9$ NaCL at 25 mL/hr. Rank in order of importance.
    1. Administer the medication over 5 minutes.
    2. Dilute the medication with normal saline.
    3. Draw up the medication in a tuberculin syringe.
    4. Check the client's identification band.
    5. Clamp the primary tubing distal to the port.

12. The client is in the cardiac intensive care unit on dopamine, a vasoconstrictor, and B/P increases to 210/130. Which intervention should the intensive care nurse implement first?
   1. Discontinue the client's vasoconstrictor, dopamine.
   2. Notify the client's healthcare provider.
   3. Administer the vasopressor hydralazine.
   4. Assess the client's neurological status.

13. The charge nurse is making client assignments in the cardiac critical care unit. Which client should be assigned to the most experienced nurse?
   1. The client with acute rheumatic fever carditis who does not want to stay on bed rest.
   2. The client who has the following ABG values: pH, 7.35; PaO_2, 88; $PaCO_2$, 44; HCO_3, 22.
   3. The client who is showing multifocal premature ventricular contractions (PVCs).
   4. The client diagnosed with angina who is scheduled for a cardiac catheterization.

14. The primary cardiac nurse is delegating tasks to the unlicensed assistive personnel (UAP). Which delegation task warrants intervention by the charge nurse of the cardiac unit?
   1. The UAP is instructed to bathe the client who is on telemetry.
   2. The UAP is requested to obtain a bedside glucometer reading.
   3. The UAP is asked to assist with a portable chest x-ray.
   4. The UAP is told to feed a client who is dysphagic.

15. The nurse is administering medications to clients in the cardiac critical care area. Which client should the nurse question administering the medication?
   1. The client receiving a calcium channel blocker (CCB) who is drinking a glass of grapefruit juice.
   2. The client receiving a beta-adrenergic blocker who has an apical heart rate of 62 beats/min.
   3. The client receiving nonsteroidal anti-inflammatory drugs (NSAIDs) who has just finished eating breakfast.
   4. The client receiving an oral anticoagulant who has an International Normalized Ratio (INR) of 2.8.

16. The charge nurse on the cardiac unit is counseling a female staff nurse because the nurse has clocked in late multiple times for the 7:00 a.m. to 7:00 p.m. shift. Which conflict resolution uses the win-win strategy?
   1. The charge nurse terminates the staff nurse as per the hospital policy so that a new nurse can be transferred to the unit.
   2. The charge nurse discovers that the staff nurse is having problems with child care; therefore, the charge nurse allows the staff nurse to work a 9:00 a.m. to 9:00 p.m. shift.
   3. The charge nurse puts the staff nurse on probation with the understanding that the next time the staff nurse is late to work she will be terminated.
   4. The staff nurse asks another staff member to talk to the charge nurse to explain that she is a valuable part of the team.

17. Which client warrants immediate intervention by the nurse?
   1. The client diagnosed with pericarditis who has chest pain with inspiration.
   2. The client diagnosed with mitral valve regurgitation who has thready peripheral pulse.
   3. The client diagnosed with Marfan syndrome who has pectus excavatum.
   4. The client diagnosed with atherosclerosis who has slurred speech and drooling.

18. The UAP working in a long-term care facility notifies the nurse that the client diagnosed with congestive heart failure who is on a low-sodium diet is complaining that the food is inedible. Which intervention should the nurse implement first?
  1. Have the family bring food from home for the client.
  2. Check to see what the client has eaten in the past 24 hours.
  3. Tell the client that a low-sodium diet is an important part of the diagnosis.
  4. Ask the dietician to discuss food preferences with the client.

19. The charge nurse on the cardiac unit is making shift assignments. Which client should be assigned to the most experienced nurse?
  1. The client diagnosed with mitral valve stenosis.
  2. The client diagnosed with asymptomatic sinus bradycardia.
  3. The client diagnosed with fulminant pulmonary edema.
  4. The client diagnosed with acute atrial fibrillation.

20. The evening nurse in a long-term care facility is preparing to administer medications to a client diagnosed with atrial fibrillation. Which medication should the nurse question administering?

Client: Mr. A	Admit Number: 654321		Allergies: Penicillin
Date: Today	Height: 71 inches Weight: 77.27 kg/170 pounds		Diagnosis: Atrial Fibrillation
Medication	0701–1500	1501–2300	2301–0700
Warfarin (Coumadin) 5 mg PO daily		1800 INR: 3.4/today	
Metoclopramide (Reglan) 5 mg PO tid	0900 DN 1300 DN	1800	
Docusate (Colace) PO bid	0900 DN	1800	
Atorvastatin (Lipitor) PO daily		1800	
Nurses Name/Initials	Day Nurse RN/DN	Evening Nurse RN/EN	

  1. Warfarin (Coumadin), an anticoagulant.
  2. Metoclopramide (Reglan), a gastric motility medication.
  3. Docusate (Colace), a stool softener.
  4. Atorvastatin (Lipitor), an antihyperlipidemic.

21. The nurse and the UAP enter the client's room and discover that the client is unresponsive. Which action, according to the American Heart Association (AHA) guidelines, should the nurse assign to the UAP first?
  1. Ask the UAP to check whether the client is asleep.
  2. Tell the UAP to perform cardiac compressions.
  3. Instruct the UAP to get the crash cart.
  4. Request the UAP to put the client in a recumbent position.

22. The elderly client on a cardiac unit has a do not resuscitate (DNR) order written. Which intervention should the nurse implement?
  1. Continue to care for the client's needs as usual.
  2. Place notification of the DNR inside the client's chart.
  3. Refer the client to a hospice organization.
  4. Limit visitors to two at a time, so as not to tire the client.

23. The nurse is initiating discharge teaching to a 68-year-old male client who had quadruple coronary bypass surgery. Which priority question should the nurse ask the client?
    1. "Are you sexually active?"
    2. "Can you still drive your car?"
    3. "Do you have pain medications at home?"
    4. "Do you know when to call your HCP?"

24. The LPN informs the clinic nurse that the client diagnosed with atrial fibrillation has an INR of 4.5. Which intervention should the nurse implement?
    1. Tell the LPN to notify the clinic healthcare provider (HCP).
    2. Instruct the LPN to assess the client for abnormal bleeding.
    3. Obtain a stat electrocardiogram on the client.
    4. Take no action because this INR is within the normal range.

25. The nurse at a disaster site is triaging victims when a woman states, "I am a certified nurse aide. Can I do anything to help?" Which action should the nurse implement?
    1. Request the woman to please leave the area.
    2. Ask the woman to check the injured clients.
    3. Tell the woman to try and keep the victims calm.
    4. Instruct the woman to help the paramedics.

26. The cardiac clinic nurse hears the UAP tell the client, "You have gained over 15 pounds since your last visit." The scale is located in the office area. Which action should the clinic nurse implement?
    1. Tell the UAP in front of the client to not comment on the weight.
    2. Ask the UAP to put the client in the room and take no action.
    3. Explain to the UAP, in private, that this is an inappropriate comment and violates HIPAA.
    4. Report the UAP to the director of nurses of the clinic.

27. The nurse on the cardiac unit is discussing case management with a client who asks, "Why do I need a case manager for my heart disease?" Which statements are most appropriate for the nurse to respond? **Select all that apply.**
    1. "Case management helps contain the costs of your healthcare."
    2. "It will help enhance your quality of life with a chronic illness."
    3. "It decreases the fragmentation of care across many healthcare settings."
    4. "Case management is a form of health insurance for clients with chronic illnesses."
    5. "We try to provide quality care along the healthcare continuum."

28. The client diagnosed with arterial hypertension and has been taking a calcium channel blocker, a loop diuretic, and an ACE inhibitor for 3 years. Which statement by the client would warrant intervention by the nurse?
    1. "I have to go to the bathroom a lot during the morning."
    2. "I get up very slowly when I have been sitting for a while."
    3. "I do not salt my food when I am cooking it but I add it at the table."
    4. "I drink grapefruit juice every morning with my breakfast."

29. The director of nurses in the cardiac clinic is counseling an unlicensed assistive personnel (UAP) in the clinic who returned late from her lunch break seven times in the past 2 weeks. Which conflict resolution uses the win-lose strategy?
    1. The UAP explains she is checking on her ill mother during lunch, and the nurse allows her to take a longer lunch break if she comes in early.
    2. The director of nurses offers the UAP a transfer to the emergency weekend clinic so that she will be off during the week.
    3. The director of nurses terminates the UAP, explaining that all staff must be on time so that the clinic runs smoothly.
    4. The UAP is placed on 1-month probation, and any further occurrences will result in termination from this position.

30. The cardiac clinic nurse has told the female unlicensed assistive personnel (UAP) twice to change the sharps container in the examination room, but it has not been changed. Which action should the nurse implement first?
    1. Tell the UAP to change it immediately.
    2. Ask the UAP why the sharps container has not been changed.
    3. Change the sharps container as per clinic policy.
    4. Document the situation and place a copy of the documentation in the employee file.

31. The wife of a client calls the clinic and tells the nurse her husband is having chest pain but won't go to the hospital. Which action should the nurse implement first?
    1. Instruct the wife to call 911 immediately.
    2. Tell the wife to have the client chew an aspirin.
    3. Ask the wife what the client had to eat recently.
    4. Request the husband talk to the clinic nurse.

32. The home health (HH) nurse received phone messages from the agency secretary. Which client should the nurse phone first?
    1. The client diagnosed with hypertension who is reporting a BP of 148/92.
    2. The client diagnosed with cardiomyopathy who has a pulse oximeter reading of 93%.
    3. The client diagnosed with congestive heart failure who has edematous feet.
    4. The client diagnosed with chronic atrial fibrillation who is having chest pain.

33. The client is diagnosed with end-stage congestive heart failure. The nurse finds the client lying in bed, short of breath, unable to talk, and with buccal cyanosis. Which intervention should the nurse implement first?
    1. Assist the client to a sitting position.
    2. Assess the client's vital signs.
    3. Call 911 for the paramedics.
    4. Auscultate the client's lung sounds.

34. The home health (HH) nurse is visiting a client diagnosed with congestive heart failure. The client has an out-of-hospital do not resuscitate (DNR) order, has stopped breathing, and has no pulse or blood pressure. The client's family is at the bedside. Which intervention should the HH nurse implement first?
    1. Contact the agency's chaplain.
    2. Pronounce the client's death.
    3. Ask the family to leave the bedside.
    4. Call the client's funeral home.

35. The cardiac nurse received laboratory results on the following clients. Which client warrants immediate intervention from the nurse?
    1. The client who has an INR of 2.8.
    2. The client who has a serum potassium level of 3.8 mEq/L.
    3. The client who has a serum digoxin level of 2.6 mg/dL.
    4. The client who has a glycosylated hemoglobin of 6%.

36. The home health (HH) nurse is completing the admission assessment for an obese client diagnosed with a myocardial infarction with comorbid type 1 diabetes and arterial hypertension. Which priority intervention should the nurse implement?
    1. Encourage the client to walk 30 minutes a day.
    2. Request an HH-registered dietician to talk to the client.
    3. Refer the client to a cardiac rehabilitation unit.
    4. Discuss the client's need to lose 1 to 2 pounds a week.

37. The home health (HH) nurse is preparing for the initial visit to a client diagnosed with congestive heart failure. Which intervention should the HH nurse implement first?
    1. Prepare all the needed equipment for the visit.
    2. Call the client to arrange a time for the visit.
    3. Review the client's referral form/pertinent data.
    4. Make the necessary referrals for the client.

38. Which information should the experienced home health (HH) nurse discuss when orienting a new nurse to HH nursing?
1. If the client or family is hostile or obnoxious, call the police.
2. Carry the HH care agency identification in a purse or wallet.
3. Visits can be scheduled at night with permission from the agency.
4. Inform the agency of the times of the client's scheduled visits.

39. The home health (HH) aide tells the HH nurse that the grandson of the client she is caring for asked her out on a date. Which statement is the HH nurse's best response?
1. "I am so excited for you; he seems like a very nice young man."
2. "You should not go out with him as long as she is a client of our agency."
3. "I think you should tell the director of the HH care agency about this date."
4. "You should never date someone you meet while taking care of a client."

40. The cardiac nurse is teaching the client diagnosed with congestive heart failure. Which teaching interventions should the nurse discuss with the client? **Select all that apply.**
1. Notify the healthcare provider (HCP) if the client gains more than 2 lb in one day.
2. Keep the head of the bed elevated when sleeping.
3. Take the loop diuretic once a day before going to sleep.
4. Teach the client which foods are high in sodium and should be avoided.
5. Perform isotonic exercises at least once a day.

41. The nurse is administering medications on a cardiac unit. Which medication should the nurse question administering?
1. Warfarin (Coumadin), an anticoagulant, to a client with a prothrombin time (PT) of 14 and an International Normalized Ratio (INR) of 1.6 mg/dL.
2. Digoxin (Lanoxin), a cardiac glycoside, to a client with a potassium level of 3.3 mEq/L.
3. Atenolol (Tenormin), a beta-blocker, for the client with an aspirate aminotransferase (AST) of 18 U/L.
4. Lisinopril (Zestril), an ACE-inhibitor, for the client with a serum creatinine level of 0.8 mg/dL.

42. The nurse is providing end-of-life care to the client diagnosed with cardiomyopathy who is in hospice. Which priority assessment intervention should the nurse implement?
1. Assess the client's spiritual needs.
2. Assess the client's financial situation.
3. Assess the client's support system.
4. Assess the client's medical diagnosis.

43. The husband of the client diagnosed with infective endocarditis and who has a do not resuscitate (DNR) tells the nurse, "My wife is not breathing." Which intervention should the nurse implement first?
1. Contact the client's healthcare provider (HCP).
2. Notify the Rapid Response Team.
3. Stay with the client and her husband.
4. Instruct the UAP to perform post-mortem care.

44. The hospice nurse is triaging phone calls from clients. Which client should the nurse call first?
1. The client whose family reports the client is not eating.
2. The client who wants to rescind the out-of-hospital DNR.
3. The client whose pain is not being controlled with the current medications.
4. The client whose urinary incontinence has caused a Stage 1 pressure ulcer.

45. The hospice nurse is working with a volunteer. Which task could the nurse delegate to the volunteer?
1. Sit with the client while he or she reminisces about life experiences.
2. Give the client a sponge bath and rub lotion on the bony prominences.
3. Provide spiritual support for the client and family members.
4. Check the home to see that all necessary medical equipment is available.

46. The nurse delegates post-mortem care to the unlicensed assistive personnel (UAP). The UAP tells the nurse she has never performed post-mortem care. Which statement is the best response by the nurse to the UAP?
1. "It can be uncomfortable. I will go with you and show you what to do."
2. "The client is already dead. You cannot hurt him now."
3. "There is nothing to it; it is just a bed bath and change of clothes."
4. "Don't worry. You can skip it this time but you need to learn what to do."

47. The unlicensed assistive personnel (UAP) tells the nurse the client is complaining of chest pain. Which task should the nurse delegate to the UAP?
1. Call the healthcare provider (HCP) and report the client's chest pain.
2. Give a client some acetaminophen (Tylenol) while the nurse checks the client.
3. Get the client's medical records and bring them to the client's room.
4. Notify the client's family of the onset of chest pain.

48. The registered nurse (RN) and licensed practical nurse (LPN) are caring for a group of clients on a cardiac unit. Which nursing task should not be assigned to the LPN?
1. Feed the client who has an IV in both forearms.
2. Assess the client diagnosed with stage IV heart failure.
3. Discharge the client who had a cardiac catheterization.
4. Administer the intravenous piggyback (IVPB) antibiotic ceftriaxone (Rocephin).

49. The hospice nurse is discussing the clients' care with the unlicensed assistive personnel (UAP). Which statement contains the best information about caring for a client with end-stage heart failure who is dying?
1. "Perform as much care for the client as possible to conserve his or her strength."
2. "Do not get too attached to the client because it will hurt when he or she dies."
3. "Be careful not to promise to withhold healthcare information from the team."
4. "The client may want to talk about his or her life, but you should discourage that."

50. The client on telemetry is showing ventricular tachycardia. Which action should the telemetry nurse delegate to the unlicensed assistive personnel (UAP)?
1. Have the UAP call the operator and announce the code.
2. Tell the UAP to answer the other call lights on the unit.
3. Send the UAP to the room to start rescue breaths.
4. Ask the family to step out of the room during the code.

51. The female family member of the client experiencing a cardiac arrest refuses to leave the client's room. Which intervention should the administrative supervisor implement?
1. Stay with the family member and explain what the team is doing.
2. Call hospital security to escort the family member out of the room.
3. Ask the healthcare provider (HCP) whether the family member can stay.
4. Ignore the family member unless she becomes hysterical.

52. The male client presents to the emergency department with a complaint of chest pain but does not have the ability to pay for the services. Which action should the emergency department nurse implement first?
1. Place the client on a telemetry monitor and assess the client.
2. Call an ambulance to transfer the client to a charity hospital.
3. Have the client sign a form agreeing to pay the bill.
4. Ask the client why he chose to come to this hospital.

53. The nurse is caring for clients on a cardiac unit. Which client should the nurse assess first?
1. The client diagnosed with angina who is reporting chest pain.
2. The client diagnosed with CHF who has bilateral 4+ peripheral edema.
3. The client diagnosed with endocarditis who has a temperature of 100°F.
4. The client diagnosed with aortic valve stenosis who has syncope.

54. Which medication should the nurse administer first after receiving the morning shift report?
1. The IVPB antibiotic to the client with endocarditis admitted at 0530 today.
2. The antiplatelet medication to the client who had a myocardial infarction.
3. The coronary vasodilator patch to the client with coronary artery disease.
4. The statin medication to the client diagnosed with atherosclerosis.

55. The nurse in a critical care cardiac unit is administering medications to a client. Which intervention should the nurse implement first?
1. Check the radial pulse before administering digoxin, a cardiac glycoside.
2. Monitor the amiodorone level for the client receiving amiodorone.
3. Obtain the latest PTT results on the client with a heparin drip.
4. Check the liver function panel for the client receiving a dopamine drip.

56. The surgical nurse is admitting a client having heart surgery to the operating room. Which information would require the nurse to call a time-out?
1. The client is drowsy from the preoperative medication and drifts off to sleep.
2. The consent form states mital valve replacement and the client states aortic valve replacement.
3. The chart and client's armband states the client is allergic to the narcotic analgesic morphine.
4. The client states his or her name and birth date as it appears on the chart.

57. The nurse is administering medications at 1800 to a client and uses the following medication administration record (MAR). Which intervention should the nurse implement first?

Client's Name: CC	Account Number: 45678-98		Allergies: NKDA
Diagnosis: Heart Failure	**Weight:** 178 pounds		**Height:** 68 inches
Medication	0701–1500	1501–2300	2301–0700
Digoxin (Lanoxin) 0.125 mg PO daily	0900 DN		
Furosemide (Lasix) 40 mg IVP daily	0900 DN		
Cephalosporin 1800 (Keflex) 500 mg PO every 6 hours	1200 DN	1800	
Warfarin (Coumadin) 5 mg PO daily		1800	
Nurse Name/Initials	Day Nurse RN/DN	Evening Nurse RN/EN	

1. Assess the client's potassium and digoxin levels.
2. Monitor the client's partial thromboplastin level.
3. Check the client's International Normalized Ratio (INR).
4. Verify the client's name and identification (ID) number with the MAR.

58. The nurse is administering medications to clients on a cardiac unit. Which medication should the nurse question administering?
1. The loop-diuretic furosemide (Lasix) to a client who had a 320-mL output in 4 hours.
2. The anticoagulant enoxaparin (Lovenox) to a client who had open-heart surgery.
3. The antiplatelet ticlopidine (Ticlid) to a client being prepared for surgery.
4. The ACE inhibitor captopril (Capoten) to a client who has a B/P of 100/68.

59. The intensive care unit nurse and a UAP are caring for a client who has had a coronary artery bypass graft (CABG). Which nursing task should the nurse assign to the UAP?
    1. Monitor the client's arterial blood gases.
    2. Re-infuse the client's blood using the cell saver.
    3. Assist the client to take a sponge bath.
    4. Change the client's saturated leg dressing.

60. The nurse is preparing to administer two units of PRBCs to a client diagnosed with congestive heart failure (CHF). Which HCP order should the nurse question?
    1. Administer each unit over 2 hours.
    2. Administer the loop diuretic furosemide (Lasix) IVP once.
    3. Restrict the client's fluids to 1000 mL per 24 hours.
    4. Have a complete blood count (CBC) done the following morning.

61. The elderly client on the cardiac unit was found on the floor by the bed. Which information should the nurse document in the client's chart?
    1. Fell. No injuries noted. Incident report completed. HCP notified.
    2. Found on floor. No complaints of pain. Able to move all extremities.
    3. States no one answered call light, so attempted to get up without help.
    4. Got out of bed without assistance and fell by the bedside.

62. The home health (HH) nurse is caring for an elderly client. Which nursing task should the nurse delegate to the HH aide?
    1. Cook and freeze meals for the client.
    2. Assist the client to sit on the front porch.
    3. Take the client for outings to the store.
    4. Monitor the client's mental status.

63. The client admitted to rule out (R/O) a myocardial infarction is complaining of substernal chest pain radiating to the left arm and jaw. Which intervention should the nurse implement first?
    1. Take the client's pulse, respirations, and blood pressure.
    2. Call for a stat electrocardiogram and a troponin level.
    3. Place sublingual nitroglycerin 1/150 g under the tongue.
    4. Notify the HCP that the client has pain.

64. The client on the cardiac unit has a cardiac arrest. Which is the administrative supervisor nurse's first intervention during the code?
    1. Begin to take notes to document the code.
    2. Make sure all the jobs are being done.
    3. Arrange for an intensive care unit bed.
    4. Administer the emergency medications.

65. Which client should the cardiac nurse assess first after receiving the p.m. shift report?
    1. The client who is completing the second unit of PRBCs.
    2. The client who is crying after being informed of a terminal diagnosis.
    3. The client who refused to eat the dietary tray but got food from home.
    4. The client who became short of breath ambulating in the hallway.

66. The nurse is caring for Mr. A.B., a client on a telemetry unit. At 0830 the client complains of chest pain. Which medication should the nurse administer?

Client Name: Mr. A.B.	Account Number: 1122337		Allergies: Meperidine	
Height: 72 inches	Weight in pounds: 202 Weight in kg: 91.82		Date of Birth: 01/05/1945	
Date: Today	Medication	2301–0700	0701–1500	1501–2300
	Morphine Sulfate 2 mg IVP every 1 hour PRN chest pain			
	Oxycodone 7.5/ acetaminophen 325 mg PO every 4 hours PRN pain	0030 NN 0545 NN		
	Maalox 30 mL PO PRN indigestion			
	Nitroglycerin 0.4 mg SL every 5 minutes up to 3 tablets PRN Chest pain			
	Nitroglycerin transdermal cream 1/2 inch		0900 Apply	2100 Remove
Signature/ Initials		Night Nurse RN/NN	Day Nurse RN/DN	

1. Administer 1/2 inch of nitroglycerin transdermally now.
2. Morphine sulfate 2 mg IVP STAT.
3. Oxycodone 7.5 mg/acetaminophen 325 mg PO now.
4. Nitroglycerin 0.4 mg sublingual STAT.

67. The charge nurse on a cardiac unit has received laboratory reports to assess. Which lab report is priority for the charge nurse to assess?

1. Ms. C.T., who is on a heparin drip.

Client Name: C.T.	Account Number: 2233669	Allergies: NKDA
Diagnosis: Deep Vein Thrombosis	Height: 66 inches	Weight in pounds: 132 Weight in kg: 60
	Laboratory Report	
Lab Test	Client Value	Normal Value
aPT	15	10–13 seconds
INR	1.4	2.0–3.0 (therapeutic value)
aPTT	56	25–35 seconds

2. Mr. R.S., who is scheduled for a coronary artery bypass graft (CABG) this morning.

Client Name: R.S.	Account Number: 8855992	Allergies: Sulfa
Diagnosis: Coronary Artery Disease	Height: 73inches	Weight in pounds: 248 Weight in kg: 112.73
	Laboratory Report	
Lab Test	Client Value	Normal Value
aPT	11	10–13 seconds
INR	1.0	2.0–3.0 (therapeutic value)
aPTT	34	25–35 seconds
WBC	5.9	4.5–11.0 (10^3 mm)
RBC	4.9	Male: 4.7–5.1 (10^6 cells/mm)
		Female: 4.2–4.8 (10^6 cells/mm)
Hemoglobin	13.5	Male: 13.2–17.3 g/dL
		Female: 11.7–15.5 g/dL
Hematocrit	44.2	Male: 43%–49%
		Female: 38%–44%
Platelets	292	150–450 (10^3 mm)

3. Ms. T.R., who had a cardiac cauterization 18 hours ago.

Client Name: T.R.	Account Number: 6655774	Allergies: Penicillin
Diagnosis: Chest pain	Height: 62 inches	Weight in pounds: 200 Weight in kg: 90.9
	Laboratory Report	
Lab Test	Client Value	Normal Value
aPT	12	10–13 seconds
INR	1.0	2.0–3.0 (therapeutic value)
aPTT	29	25–35 seconds

4. Mr. J.E., who was admitted to rule out gallbladder disease.

Client Name: J.E.	Account Number: 6251489	Allergies: NKDA
Diagnosis: R/O Gall-bladder Disease	Height: 68 inches	Weight in pounds: 198 Weight in kg: 90
	Laboratory Report	
Lab Test	Client Value	Normal Value
aPT	9.8	10–13 seconds
INR	1.3	2.0–3.0 (therapeutic value)
aPTT	26	25–35 seconds
Platelet	392	150–450 (10^3 mm)

68. The nurse on a medical unit is making rounds after receiving the shift report. Which client should the nurse see first? Rank in order of priority.
    1. The 45-year-old client who complained of having chest pain at midnight last night and received NTG sublingually.
    2. The 62-year-old client who is complaining that no one answered the call light for 2 hours yesterday.
    3. The 29-year-client diagnosed with septicemia who called to request more blankets because of being cold.
    4. The 78-year-old client diagnosed with dementia whose daughter is concerned because the client is more confused today.
    5. The 37-year-old client who has a Stage 4 pressure sore and the dressing needs to be changed this morning.

69. While ambulating in the hallway with the nurse, the client diagnosed with myocardial infarction complains of chest pain. Which interventions should the nurse implement? **Select all that apply.**
    1. Administer nitroglycerin 0.4 mg sublingual STAT.
    2. Have the client walk back to the room.
    3. Take the client's vital signs.
    4. Place the client on supplemental oxygen.
    5. Ask the ward secretary to call the healthcare provider for orders.

70. The nurse received an aPTT report on a client receiving heparin via continuous drip infusion. According to the report, the client's drip rate should be decreased by 100 units per hour. The heparin comes prepared as 25,000 units in 500 mL of fluid. The current rate of infusion is 26 mL per hour. At what rate should the nurse set the pump? _____

CARDIAC CLINICAL SCENARIO

Ms. Teresa is the 7a–7p charge nurse on 24-bed telemetry unit. There are four RNs, two LPNs, two UAPs, two telemetry technicians, and one unit secretary working on the unit along with Ms. Teresa. There are 20 clients in the unit.

1. Which client should Ms. Teresa assign to the most experienced RN on the unit?
   1. The client diagnosed with atrial fibrillation who is receiving the first dose of praxada (dabigatran).
   2. The client diagnosed with congestive heart failure who is coughing up pink, frothy sputum.
   3. The client diagnosed with a myocardial infarction who is exhibiting occasional premature ventricular contractions.
   4. The client diagnosed with mitral valve prolapse who is complaining of shortness of breath when sitting in the chair.

2. The telemetry technician tells the primary nurse the client in room 420 has a straight line. Which intervention should the primary nurse implement first?
   1. Instruct the UAP to take the crash cart to room 420.
   2. Tell the telemetry technician to call the Rapid Response Team.
   3. Determine if the client has an apical pulse and blood pressure.
   4. Check to see if the client has the telemetry leads on the chest.

3. The primary nurse has instructed the unlicensed assistive personnel (UAP) to assist the client in 410 to the bathroom for a shower. Which action by the UAP warrants intervention by the primary nurse?
   1. The UAP did not notify the desk the telemetry was being removed.
   2. The UAP did not remove the electrodes from the client's chest.
   3. The UAP placed a bath chair in the shower for the client.
   4. The UAP stayed in the client's bathroom while the client showered.

4. Ms. Teresa is looking over the morning laboratory results. Which client warrants Ms. Teresa notifying the healthcare provider (HCP)?
   1. The client receiving IVP digoxin who has a digoxin level of 2.4 mg/dL.
   2. The client receiving Coumadin (warfarin) who has an INR of 1.2.
   3. The client receiving furosemide who has a potassium level of 3.5 mEq/L.
   4. The client receiving nystatin who has a cholesterol level of 205.

5. Which client should Ms. Teresa assign to the LPN?
   1. The client who was just admitted from the emergency department to the unit.
   2. The client who is exhibiting supraventricular tachycardia on the telemetery.
   3. The client who had a left femoral cardiac catheterization this morning.
   4. The client who needs teaching concerning coronary artery disease.

6. Ms. Teresa is transcribing the healthcare provider's admissions orders for a client being admitted for R/O myocardial infarction. Which HCP's order should Ms. Teresa question?
   1. Draw cardiac isoenzymes every 6 hours.
   2. Provide low-fat, low-cholesterol diet.
   3. Administer morphine IVP 2 mg every 5 minutes for chest pain.
   4. Schedule client for endoscopy in a.m.

7. Which nursing task is most appropriate for Ms. Teresa to delegate to the UAP?
   1. Request the UAP to obtain the newly admitted client's weight.
   2. Ask the UAP to clean the room for the client who has been discharged.
   3. Tell the UAP to take the vital signs on the client who is hypovolemic.
   4. Instruct the UAP to discuss the low-fat, low-cholesterol diet with the client.

8. The client in room 420 is complaining of severe chest pain of 10 on a 1-to-10 pain scale. Which intervention should the nurse implement first?
   1. Check the client's MAR for the last time medication was administered.
   2. Assess the client's apical pulse, blood pressure, and lung sounds.
   3. Administer a sublingual nitroglycerin to the client.
   4. Place oxygen via nasal cannula at 6 L/min.

9. The client is in ventricular tachycardia. Which intervention should the nurse implement first?
   1. Defibrillate the client.
   2. Assess the carotid pulse.
   3. Administer epinephrine IVP.
   4. Start cardiopulmonary resuscitation.

10. Ms. Teresa is completing discharge teaching for the client diagnosed with angina. Which statement indicates the client needs more teaching?
    1. "I must keep my nitroglycerin tablets in a dark bottle at all times."
    2. "I should walk at least 30 minutes at least three times a week."
    3. "I will decrease the number of cigarettes I smoke daily."
    4. "I am going to take one baby aspirin every day."

ANSWERS AND RATIONALES

The correct answer number and rationale for why it is the correct answer are given in **boldface type**. Rationales for why the other possible answer options are incorrect also are given, but they are not in boldface type.

1. 1. **This client may or may not be stable. The client may have "no complaints" at this time, but the nurse must assess this client first to determine whatever the complaint was that brought the client to the ED has stabilized. This client should be seen first.**
   2. It is important for the nurse to assess for pain relief in a timely manner, but this client has been medicated and the pain was a 3. The nurse can evaluate the amount of pain relief after making sure that the ED admission is stable.
   3. This client has been back from the procedure and a bilateral pedal pulse indicates the client is stable; therefore, this client does need to be seen first.
   4. Psychological issues are important, but not more so than a physiological issue, and the client admitted from the ED may have a physiological problem.

   Content – Medical/Surgical: **Category of Health Alteration** *– Cardiovascular:* **Integrated Processes** *– Nursing Process: Planning:* **Client Needs** *– Safe and Effective Care Environment: Management of Care:* **Cognitive Level** *– Synthesis*

MAKING NURSING DECISIONS: The test taker should use some tool as a reference to guide in the decision-making process. In this situation, Maslow's Hierarchy of Needs should be applied. Physiological needs have priority over psychosocial ones.

2. 1. The cardiac glycoside, such as digoxin, should not be administered unless the apical pulse is 60 or above.
   2. Because the client's serum K+ level is already low, the nurse should question administering a loop diuretic.
   3. **The client in ventricular fibrillation is in a life-threatening situation; therefore, the antidysrhythmic, such as lidocaine or amiodorone, should be administered first.**
   4. The client's blood pressure is above 90/60, so the calcium-channel blocker can be administered but it is not priority over a client who is in a life-threatening situation.

Content – Medical/Surgical: **Category of Health Alteration–** *Cardiovascular:* **Integrated Processes –** *Nursing Process: Assessment:* **Client Needs** *– Safe and Effective Care Environment: Management of Care:* **Cognitive Level** *– Analysis*

MAKING NURSING DECISIONS: The test taker should know which medications are priority, such as life-threatening medications, insulin, and mucolytics (Carafate). These medications should be administered first by the nurse.

3. 1. The nurse would expect the client with a deep vein thrombosis to have an edematous right calf, so the nurse would not need to assess this client first.
   2. The nurse would expect the client with mitral valve stenosis to have heart palpitations (sensations of rapid, fluttering heartbeat).
   3. The nurse would expect the client with arterial occlusive disease to have intermittent claudication (leg pain), so the nurse would not need to assess this client first.
   4. **The client would not expect the client with congestive heart failure to have pink, frothy sputum because this is a sign of pulmonary edema. This client should be assessed first.**

   Content – Medical/Surgical: **Category of Health Alteration** *– Cardiovascular:* **Integrated Processes –** *Nursing Process: Planning:* **Client Needs** *– Safe and Effective Care Environment: Management of Care:* **Cognitive Level** *– Synthesis*

MAKING NURSING DECISIONS: The test taker must determine which sign/symptom is not expected for the disease process. If the sign/symptom is not expected, then the nurse should assess the client first. This type of question is determining if the nurse is knowledgeable of signs/symptoms of a variety of disease processes.

4. 1. This client is at high risk for complications related to necrotic myocardial tissue and will need extensive teaching; therefore, this client should not be assigned to a new graduate.
   2. Unstable angina means this client is at risk for life-threatening complications and should not be assigned to a new graduate.
   3. **A new graduate should be able to complete a pre-procedural checklist and get this client to the catheterization lab.**

4. Chest pain means this client could be having a myocardial infarction and should not be assigned to a new graduate.
Content – Medical/Surgical: **Category of Health Alteration –** *Cardiovascular:* **Integrated Nursing Process** *– Planning:* **Client Needs** *– Safe and Effective Care Environment: Management of Care:* **Cognitive Level** *– Synthesis*

MAKING NURSING DECISIONS: When the test taker is deciding which client should be assigned to a new graduate, the most stable client should be assigned to the least experienced nurse.

5. 1. An LPN can perform sterile procedures such as inserting indwelling catheters and IV catheters. An RN should perform the functions that require nursing judgment, such as planning and evaluating the care of the clients.
2. Although an LPN could administer most intravenous piggyback (IVPB) medications, only qualified RNs may administer intravenous push (IVP) medications and chemotherapy.
3. **A UAP is capable of performing the morning care. This is an appropriate nursing task to delegate.**
4. Writing a care plan for a client requires nursing judgment; therefore, an RN should be assigned this function.
Content – Medical/Surgical: **Category of Health Alteration –** *Cardiovascular:* **Integrated Processes** *– Nursing Process: Planning:* **Client Needs** *– Safe and Effective Care Environment: Management of Care:* **Cognitive Level** *– Synthesis*

MAKING NURSING DECISIONS: An RN cannot delegate assessment, teaching, evaluation, medications, or an unstable client to a UAP. Tasks that cannot be delegated are nursing interventions that require nursing judgment. Remember that in most instances, options with the word "all" (options 1 and 2) can be eliminated because if the test taker can think of one time when some other level of licensure could safely perform the task, then the option automatically becomes wrong.

6. 1. Unless the information shared is directly connected to healthcare issues, the nurse should not share confidential information with anyone else. The nurse should inform clients that information directly affecting the client's healthcare will be shared on a need-to-know basis only.
2. **The case manager's job is to ensure continuity and adequacy of care for the client. This individual has a "need to know."**
3. The case manager is part of the healthcare team; therefore, information should be shared.

4. The client gave permission when being admitted to the hospital for information to be shared among those providing care. The case manager does not need to obtain further consent.
Content – Medical/Surgical: **Category of Health Alteration –** *Cardiovascular:* **Integrated Processes** *– Nursing Process: Implementation:* **Client Needs** *– Safe and Effective Care Environment: Management of Care:* **Cognitive Level** *– Knowledge*

MAKING NURSING DECISIONS: The test taker must be knowledgeable of the role of each member of the multidisciplinary healthcare team as well as HIPAA rules and regulations. These topics will be tested on the NCLEX-RN® exam.

7. 1. The telemetry strip indicates an artifact, so there is no need for the UAP or any staff member to call a Code Blue, which is used when someone has arrested.
2. **The UAP should be instructed to check the telemetry lead placement; this reading cannot be ventricular fibrillation because the client is talking to the nurse over the intercom system. This telemetry is an artifact; therefore, the leads should be checked and the UAP can do this because the client is stable.**
3. The UAP can take care of this problem; there is no need for the primary nurse to check the client.
4. The strip indicates an artifact, but there is no indication that the client should be removed from telemetry.
Content – Medical/Surgical: **Category of Health Alteration –** *Cardiovascular:* **Integrated Processes** *– Nursing Process: Implementation:* **Client Needs** *– Safe and Effective Care Environment, Management of Care:* **Cognitive Level** *– Application*

MAKING NURSING DECISIONS: An RN cannot delegate assessment, teaching, evaluation, medications, or an unstable client to a UAP. Tasks that cannot be delegated are nursing interventions requiring nursing judgment.

8. 1. The nurse who just has surgical nursing experience would not be the choice to float to the emergency department.
2. **The nurse with critical care experience would be the best choice to float to the emergency department.**
3. The nurse just returning from sick leave would not be a good choice to send to the emergency department, which may be very busy at times.
4. This nurse has not had experience in critical care; therefore, this nurse would not be the best choice to float to the emergency department.

Content – Medical/Surgical: **Category of Health Alteration** *– Cardiovascular:* **Integrated Processes** *– Nursing: Process: Planning:* **Client Needs** *– Safe and Effective Care Environment: Management of Care:* **Cognitive Level** *– Synthesis*

MAKING NURSING DECISIONS: The nurse needs to know management issues for the RN-NCLEX®. The nurse with experience in certain areas of nursing would be most appropriate to float to the areas with related types of clients, such as critical care and the emergency department.

9.   Correct Answer: 5, 4, 3, 2, 1

   5. The nurse must first obtain informed consent prior to administering the blood product.
   4. The nurse needs to complete the pre-transfusion assessment including assessing for any signs of allergic reaction prior to administering the unit of blood.
   3. The blood must be hung with Y-tubing and normal saline, and an 18-gauge angiocatheter is preferred.
   2. The nurse must check the unit of blood from the laboratory with another nurse and with the client's blood band.
   1. During the first 15 minutes, the blood transfusion must be administered slowly to determine if the client is going to have an allergic reaction.

   Content – Adult Health, Cardiac: **Category of Health Alteration** *– Cardiovascular:* **Integrated Processes** *– Nursing Process: Implementation:* **Client Needs** *– Physiological Integrity: Reduction of Risk Potential:* **Cognitive Level** *– Analysis*

MAKING NURSING DECISIONS: This is an alternate type of question included in the NCLEX-RN® blueprint. The nurse must be able to perform skills in the correct order. Obtaining informed consent and assessment should always be the first interventions.

10. 1. The charge nurse is responsible for all clients. At times it is necessary to see clients with a psychosocial need before other clients who have situations that are expected and are not life threatening.
   2. An elevated CPK-MB, cardiac isoenzyme, level is expected in a client with an acute myocardial infarction; therefore, the charge nurse would not see this client first.
   3. The INR is within the normal limits of 2 to 3; therefore, this client does not need to be assessed first.
   4. This client is being transferred to the cardiac unit; therefore, the client is stable and does

not require the charge nurse to see this client first.

   Content – Medical/Surgical: **Category of Health Alteration** *– Cardiovascular:* **Integrated Processes** *– Nursing Process: Assessment:* **Client Needs** *– Psychosocial Integrity:* **Cognitive Level** *– Analysis*

MAKING NURSING DECISIONS: The test taker must determine if any of the assessment data is normal or abnormal for the client's diagnosis. If the data is abnormal, then this client should be seen first. If the data is normal then a client with a psychosocial problem is the client the nurse should assess first.

11. Correct Answer: 3, 2, 4, 5, 1

   3. Because this is less than 1 mL, the nurse should draw this medication up in a 1-mL tuberculin syringe to ensure accuracy of dosage.
   2. The nurse should dilute the medication with normal saline to a 5- to 10-mL bolus to help decrease pain during administration and maintain the IV site longer. Administering 0.25 mg of digoxin in 0.5 mL is very difficult, if not impossible, to push over 5 full minutes, which is the manufacturer's recommended administration rate. If the medication is diluted to a 5- to 10-mL bolus, it is easier for the nurse to administer the medication over 5 minutes.
   4. The nurse must check two identifiers according to the Joint Commission safety guidelines.
   5. The nurse should clamp the tubing between the port and the primary IV line so that the medication will enter the vein, not ascend up the IV tubing.
   1. Cardiovascular and narcotic medications are administered over 5 minutes.

   Content – Medical/Surgical: **Category of Health Alteration** *– Cardiovascular:* **Integrated Processes** *– Nursing Process: Implementation:* **Client Needs** *– Physiological Integrity: Reduction of Risk Potential:* **Cognitive Level** *– Application*

MAKING NURSING DECISIONS: This is an alternate type of question that is included in the NCLEX-RN® blueprint. The nurse must be able to perform skills in the correct order.

12. 1. The nurse should first discontinue the medication that is causing the increase in the client's blood pressure prior to doing anything else.
   2. The nurse should notify the HCP but not prior to taking care of the client's elevated blood pressure.

3. The client may need a medication to decrease the blood pressure but the nurse should first discontinue the medication causing the elevated blood pressure.
4. The nurse must first decrease the client's blood pressure prior to assessing the client.
Content – Medical/Surgical: Category of Health Alteration – Cardiovascular: Integrated Processes – Nursing Process: Assessment: Client Needs – Physiological Integrity: Reduction of Risk Potential: Cognitive Level – Analysis

MAKING NURSING DECISIONS: The test taker should remember that when the client is in distress, do not assess. The nurse must intervene and take care of the client. If any of the options is assessment data the HCP will need or an intervention that will help the client, then the test taker should not select the option to notify the HCP.

13. 1. The client with rheumatic heart fever is expected to have carditis and should be on bed rest. The nurse needs to talk to the client about the importance of being on bed rest but this client is not in a life-threatening situation and does not need the most experienced nurse.
2. These ABG values are within normal limits; therefore, a less experienced nurse could care for this client.
3. **Multifocal PVCs are an emergency and are possibly life threatening. An experienced nurse should care for this client.**
4. A cardiac catheterization is a routine procedure and would not require the most experienced nurse.
Content – Medical/Surgical: Category of Health Alteration – Cardiovascular: Integrated Processes – Nursing Process: Planning: Client Needs – Safe and Effective Care Environment: Management of Care: Cognitive Level – Synthesis

MAKING NURSING DECISIONS: The test taker must determine which client is the most unstable and would require the most experienced nurse, thus making this type of question an "except" question. Three clients are either stable or have non–life-threatening conditions.

14. 1. All clients in the ICU are on telemetry, and the UAP could bathe the client. This would not warrant intervention by the charge nurse.
2. The UAP can perform glucometer checks at the bedside, and there is nothing that indicates the client is unstable. This would not warrant intervention by the charge nurse.

3. The UAP can assist with helping the client sit up for a portable chest x-ray as long as the UAP is not pregnant and wears a shield.
4. **This client is at risk for choking and is not stable; therefore, the charge nurse should intervene and not allow the UAP to feed this client.**
Content – Medical/Surgical: Category of Health Alteration – Cardiovascular: Integrated Processes – Nursing Process: Implementation: Client Needs – Safe and Effective Care Environment, Management of Care: Cognitive Level – Application

MAKING NURSING DECISIONS: This is an "except" question. The test taker could ask which task is appropriate to delegate to the UAP; three options would be appropriate to delegate and one would not be. Remember the RN cannot delegate assessment, teaching, evaluation, medications, or an unstable client to the UAP.

15. 1. **The client receiving a CCB should avoid grapefruit juice because it can cause the CCB to rise to toxic levels. Grapefruit juice inhibits cytochrome P450-3A4 found in the liver and the intestinal wall. This inhibition affects the metabolism of some drugs and can, as is the case with CCBs, lead to toxic levels of the drug. For this reason, the nurse should investigate any medications the client is taking if the client drinks grapefruit juice.**
2. The apical heart rate should be greater than 60 beats/minute before administering the medication; therefore, the nurse would not question administering this medication.
3. Nonsteroidal anti-inflammatory drugs (NSAIDs) should be taken with foods to prevent gastric upset; therefore, the nurse would not question administering this medication.
4. The INR therapeutic level for warfarin (Coumadin), an anticoagulant, is 2 to 3; therefore, the nurse would not question administering this medication.
Content – Medical/Surgical: Category of Health Alteration – Cardiovascular: Integrated Processes – Nursing Process: Planning: Client Needs – Physiological Integrity: Pharmacological and Parenteral Therapies: Cognitive Level – Knowledge

MAKING NURSING DECISIONS: The test taker must be knowledgeable of medications. In most scenarios, there is no test-taking hint to help the test taker when answering medication questions except common nursing interventions, such as do not administer cardiac medications if client has AP <60 or B/P <90/60, do not administer medications with grapefruit juice or antacids, or

most medications are administered with food to prevent GI distress.

16. 1. This is a win-lose strategy wherein, during the conflict, one party (charge nurse) exerts dominance and the other (staff nurse) submits.
2. **This is a win-win strategy that focuses on goals and attempts to meet the needs of both parties. The charge nurse keeps an experienced nurse and the staff nurse keeps her position. Both parties win.**
3. This is negotiation in which the conflicting parties give and take on the issue. The staff nurse gets one more chance and the charge nurse's authority is still intact.
4. This is not an example of a win-win strategy and is not an appropriate action for the staff nurse to take. The opinion of the staff should not influence the charge nurse's action.
*Content – Medical/Surgical: **Category of Health Alteration** – Cardiovascular: **Integrated Processes –** Nursing Process: Implementation: **Client Needs** – Safe and Effective Care Environment: Management of Care: **Cognitive Level** – Application*

MAKING NURSING DECISIONS: There will be management questions on the NCLEX-RN®. In many instances, there is no test-taking strategy; the nurse must be knowledgeable of management issues.

17. 1. The client with pericarditis is expected to have chest pain with inspiration; therefore, this client does not warrant immediate intervention.
2. The client with mitral valve regurgitation is expected to have thready peripheral pulses and cool, clammy extremities. Therefore, this client does not warrant immediate intervention.
3. The client with Marfan syndrome is expected to have a chest that sinks in or sticks out, known as funnel chest or pectus excavatum; therefore, this client does not warrant immediate intervention.
4. **Slurred speech and drooling are signs of a cerebrovascular accident (stroke or brain attack) and is not normal for a client with atherosclerosis; therefore, this client should be assessed first.**
*Content – Medical/Surgical: **Category of Health Alteration** – Cardiovascular: **Integrated Processes –** Nursing Process: Assessment: **Client Needs** – Physiological Integrity: Reduction of Risk Potential: **Cognitive Level –** Analysis*

MAKING NURSING DECISIONS: The test taker should ask "is the assessment data normal for" the disease process. If it is normal for the disease process, the nurse would not need to intervene; if it is not normal for the disease process, then this warrants intervention by the nurse.

18. 1. The family may be allowed to bring in food occasionally from home, but what they bring may not adhere to a low-sodium diet, and the family should not be required to provide three meals per day for the client. This is the facility's responsibility.
2. **Assessing the client's intake will help the nurse to determine the extent of the client's complaints. This is the first intervention.**
3. This may be true but does not help the client adjust to a lack of sodium in the diet.
4. A referral to the dietician should be made after the nurse fully assesses the situation.
*Content – Medical/Surgical: **Category of Health Alteration** – Cardiovascular: **Integrated Processes –** Nursing Process: Implementation: **Client Needs –** Physiological Integrity: Physiological Adaptation: **Cognitive Level** – Knowledge*

MAKING NURSING DECISIONS: Assessment is the first step of the nursing process, and the test taker should use the nursing process or some other systematic process to assist in determining priorities.

19. 1. The client with mitral valve stenosis can live with this diagnosis and it is not a life-threatening condition.
2. The client with asymptomatic sinus bradycardia is stable and because the client is not exhibiting any signs/symptoms, this client does not need to be assigned to the most experienced nurse.
3. **A client with fulminant pulmonary edema is experiencing an acute, life-threatening problem. The most experienced nurse should be assigned to this client.**
4. A client with acute atrial fibrillation is not in a life-threatening situation; therefore, this client would not be assigned to the most experienced nurse.
*Content – Medical/Surgical: **Category of Health Alteration** – Cardiovascular: **Integrated Processes –** Nursing Process: Planning: **Client Needs** – Safe and Effective Care Environment: Management of Care: **Cognitive Level** – Synthesis*

MAKING NURSING DECISIONS: The test taker must determine which client is the most unstable and would require the most experienced nurse, thus making this type of question an "except" question. Three clients are either stable or have non–life-threatening conditions.

20. 1. **The client's International Normalized Ratio (INR) is 3.4. The therapeutic range is 2 to 3 for a client diagnosed with atrial fibrillation. This client is at risk for bleeding. The nurse should hold the medication and discuss the warfarin with the HCP.**
   2. Metoclopramide is used to stimulate gastric emptying. Nothing in the stem or the MAR indicates a problem with administering this medication. The nurse would administer this medication.
   3. Docusate is a stool softener. Nothing in the stem or the MAR indicates a problem with administering this medication. The nurse would administer this medication.
   4. Atorvastatin is a lipid-lowering medication. Nothing in the stem or the MAR indicates a problem with administering this medication. The nurse would administer this medication.

   Content – Medical/Surgical: ***Category of Health Alteration*** *– Cardiovascular:* ***Integrated Process:*** *Nursing Process: Assessment:* ***Client Needs** – Physiological Integrity: Reduction of Risk Potential:* ***Cognitive Level** – Analysis*

MAKING NURSING DECISIONS: This is an alternate type question included in the NCLEX-RN® blueprint. The test taker must be able to read a medication administration record (MAR), be knowledgeable of medications, and be able to make an appropriate decisions as to the nurse's most appropriate intervention.

21. 1. The first step in cardiopulmonary resuscitation according to the AHA guidelines is to establish unresponsiveness by "shaking and shouting." If the client does not respond to being shaken, then the nurse can proceed to the next step, which is to "look, listen, and feel" for breaths. This is assessment and, according to AHA guidelines, the UAP could perform this function if alone. However, the nurse should assess the client before a UAP.
   2. Administering chest compressions is performed after establishing unresponsiveness and lack of respiration.
   3. **The nurse can tell the UAP to get the crash cart while the nurse assesses the client. This is the best task to assign the UAP at this time because this client may be unstable and until that is determined, the nurse should not delegate any client care.**
   4. The nurse should place the client in the recumbent position before attempting to perform chest compressions; the nurse

should send the UAP for help and the crash cart.

Content – Medical/Surgical: ***Category of Health Alteration*** *– Cardiovascular:* ***Integrated Processes*** *– Nursing Process: Implementation:* ***Client Needs*** *– Safe and Effective Care Environment: Management of Care:* ***Cognitive Level** – Application*

MAKING NURSING DECISIONS: This is an "except" question. The test taker could ask which task is appropriate to delegate to the UAP; three options would be appropriate to delegate and one would not be. Remember the RN cannot delegate assessment, teaching, evaluation, medications, or an unstable client to the UAP.

22. 1. **The nurse should care for the client as if the DNR order was not on the chart. A DNR order does not mean the client no longer wishes treatment. It means the client does not want CPR or to be placed on a ventilator if the client's heart stops beating.**
   2. The information about the DNR status is already inside the chart. It may need to be placed on the outside of the chart and a special armband or other notification made to other healthcare personnel.
   3. The client has a DNR order, but this does not imply that there may be 6 months or less life expectancy for the client. (Hospice care may be requested for clients with less than a 6-month life expectancy.) An order for hospice must be written by the attending healthcare provider before making this referral.
   4. The client should be allowed as many visitors as the hospital policy allows.

Content – Medical/Surgical: ***Category of Health Alteration*** *– Cardiovascular:* ***Integrated Processes*** *– Nursing Process: Planning:* ***Client Needs** – Physiological Integrity: Basic Care and Comfort:* ***Cognitive Level** – Knowledge*

MAKING NURSING DECISIONS: The NCLEX-RN® blueprint includes nursing care that is ruled by legal requirements. The nurse must be knowledgeable of these issues.

23. 1. **The nurse should be aware that sexual activity is important to most adults and should not decide that the client is not sexually active because of a client's age. The nurse should provide instructions regarding sexual activity before the client is discharged. This is the question that should be asked because many clients may be embarrassed to bring up the subject.**

2. The client should not drive a motor vehicle until released to do so by the healthcare provider (HCP). This is not an appropriate question at this time.

3. The client should be discharged with a prescription for oral pain medications to be taken as directed by the surgeon. The nurse should not encourage the client to use old medications the client may have at home. This is not an appropriate question.

4. The nurse is providing discharge instructions and should tell the client when to call the healthcare provider (HCP). This is not an appropriate question.

Content – Medical/Surgical: **Category of Health Alteration** *– Cardiovascular:* **Integrated Processes** *– Nursing Process: Assessment:* **Client Needs** *– Physiological Integrity: Physiological Adaptation:* **Cognitive Level** *– Analysis*

24. 1. **The LPN can contact the HCP and give pertinent information. The INR is high (therapeutic is 2 to 3), and the HCP should be informed.**

2. The RN cannot assign assessment to an LPN.

3. The INR is elevated, but this will not affect the client's atrial fibrillation. The client is at risk for abnormal bleeding, not a life-threatening dysrhythmia.

4. The normal INR is 2 to 3; therefore, some action should be implemented.

Content – Medical/Surgical: **Category of Health Alteration** *– Cardiovascular:* **Integrated Processes** *– Nursing Process: Implementation:* **Client Needs** *– Physiological Integrity: Reduction of Risk Potential:* **Cognitive Level** *– Application*

MAKING NURSING DECISIONS: The nurse cannot assign assessment, teaching, evaluation, or an unstable client to an LPN. The LPN can transcribe HCP orders and can call them on the phone to obtain orders for a client.

25. 1. In a disaster, the nurse should utilize as many individuals as possible to help control the situation; therefore, this is an inappropriate intervention.

2. The unlicensed assistive personnel (UAP) cannot assess clients; therefore, this is not an appropriate action.

3. **Unlicensed assistive personnel (UAP) have the ability to keep the victims calm; therefore, this is an appropriate action. This action is not critical to the safety of the victims.**

4. The paramedics do not need civilians assisting them as they stabilize and transport the victims. This is not an appropriate action.

Content – Medical/Surgical: **Category of Health Alteration** *– Cardiovascular:* **Integrated Processes** *– Nursing Process: Planning:* **Client Needs** *– Safe and Effective Care Environment: Management of Care:* **Cognitive Level** *– Synthesis*

MAKING NURSING DECISIONS: The test taker must be knowledgeable of the role of each member of the multidisciplinary healthcare team as well as HIPAA rules and regulations. These topics will be tested on the NCLEX-RN® exam.

26. 1. The clinic nurse should not correct the UAP in front of the client. This is embarrassing to the UAP and makes the client uncomfortable.

2. The clinic nurse must correct the UAP's behavior. The client's weight gain should not be announced in the office area so that all staff, clients, and visitors can hear. This is a violation of confidentiality.

3. **The clinic nurse should correct the UAP's behavior, but it should be done in private and with an explanation as to why the action is inappropriate. This is a violation of confidentiality because the scale is located in the office area and any client or visitor passing by, as well as other staff members, can hear the comment.**

4. The clinic nurse should handle this situation. If the UAP's behavior shows a pattern of behavior, then it should be reported to the director of nurses.

Content – Medical/Surgical: **Category of Health Alteration** *– Cardiovascular:* **Integrated Processes** *– Nursing Process: Implementation:* **Client Needs** *– Safe and Effective Care Environment: Management of Care:* **Cognitive Level** *– Application*

MAKING NURSING DECISIONS: In any business, including a healthcare facility, arguments or discussions of confidential information should not occur among staff of any level where the customers—in this case, the clinic clients—can hear it or see it.

27. 1, 2, 3, and 5 are correct.

1. **Case managers help coordinate healthcare between multiple sources of healthcare attempting to contain healthcare cost.**

2. **The case manager is a client advocate and helps with communication between the client and healthcare providers, which, it is hoped, enhances the client's quality of life.**

3. **The case manager coordinates outpatient care and in-patient care, and helps with referrals for the client.**

4. Case management is not a form of health insurance.

5. **The case manager is involved in assessing, planning, facilitating, and advocating for health services for a client, which, it is hoped, provide quality care. Trying to coordinate this is often exhausting and frustrating for the client and family.**
   Content – Medical/Surgical: *Category of Health Alteration* – Cardiovascular: *Integrated Processes* – Nursing Process: Implementation: *Client Needs* – Safe and Effective Care Environment: Safety and Infection Control: *Cognitive Level* – Application

MAKING NURSING DECISIONS: The test taker must be knowledgeable of the role of each member of the multidisciplinary healthcare team as well as HIPAA rules and regulations. These topics will be tested on the NCLEX-RN® exam. This is an alternate type question wherein the test taker must select more than one option as correct and must select all appropriate options to receive credit for a correct answer.

28. 1. If the client takes the loop diuretic in the morning, then going to the bathroom frequently in the morning would not warrant intervention.

2. Rising from a sitting position slowly helps prevent orthostatic hypotension, which is a potential side effect of all the medications. This statement would not warrant intervention.

3. This statement indicates the client is adhering to a low-sodium diet, as he should be. No intervention is warranted.

4. **Grapefruit juice can cause calcium channel blockers to rise to toxic levels. Grapefruit juice inhibits cytochrome P450-3A4 found in the liver and intestinal wall. This statement warrants intervention by the nurse.**
   Content – Medical/Surgical: *Category of Health Alteration* – Cardiovascular: *Integrated Processes* – Nursing Process:Assessment: *Client Needs* – Physiological Integrity: Physiological Adaptation: *Cognitive Level* – Analysis

MAKING NURSING DECISIONS: The test taker must be knowledgeable of medications. In most scenarios, there is no test-taking hint to help the test taker when answering medication questions except common nursing interventions, such as do not administer cardiac medications if client has AP <60 or B/P <90/60, do not administer medications with grapefruit juice or antacids, or most medications are administered with food to prevent GI distress.

29. 1. This is a win-win strategy that focuses on goals (to have adequate staff) and attempts to meet the needs of both parties. The director of nurses keeps an experienced nurse, and the UAP keeps her position. Both parties win.

2. This is a possible win-win strategy in which both parties win. The UAP keeps her job, and the director of nurses can hire a UAP who will be able to work the assigned hours.

3. **This is a win-lose strategy during which the conflict shows one party (the director of nurses) exerts dominance and the other party (UAP) must submit and loses.**

4. This is a negotiation in which the conflicting parties give and take on the issues. The UAP gets one more chance, and the director of nurse's authority is still intact.
   Content – Medical/Surgical: *Category of Health Alteration* – Cardiovascular: *Integrated Processes* – Nursing Process: Implementation: *Client Needs* – Safe and Effective Care Environment: Management of Care: *Cognitive Level* – Application

MAKING NURSING DECISIONS: There will be management questions on the NCLEX-RN®. In many instances, there is no test-taking strategy; the nurse must be knowledgeable of management issues.

30. 1. A full sharps container is a violation of Occupational Health and Safety Administration (OSHA) regulations, and because the UAP has not done it after being asked twice, a third request is not necessary.

2. The nurse should discuss why the sharps container has not been changed, but it is not the first intervention.

3. **A full sharps container is a violation of Occupational Health and Safety Administration (OSHA) regulations and may result in a $25,000 fine. The nurse should first take care of this situation immediately and then discuss it with the UAP. This is modeling appropriate behaviour.**

4. The situation should be documented because the UAP was told twice, but documentation is not the first intervention.
   Content – Medical/Surgical: *Category of Health Alteration* – Cardiovascular: *Integrated Process*: Nursing Process: Implementation: *Client Needs* – Safe and Effective Care Environment: Management of Care: *Cognitive Level* – Application

MAKING NURSING DECISIONS: The NCLEX-RN® blueprint includes nursing care that is ruled by legal requirements. The nurse must be knowledgeable of these issues. The nurse may have to

take action first and then take further action if necessary.

31. 1. The wife should call 911, but the American Heart Association recommends chewing a baby aspirin at the onset of chest pain.
    2. **The AHA recommends the client having chest pain chew an aspirin to help decrease platelet aggregation. This is the first intervention the clinic nurse should tell the wife to do. The client is in distress; therefore, the nurse should have the wife do something.**
    3. This question could be asked to determine whether the pain is secondary to a gallbladder attack or gastric irritation, but this is not the first intervention.
    4. The clinic nurse could possibly talk to the client while the wife is getting an aspirin, but this is not the first intervention.

    Content – Medical/Surgical: ***Category of Health Alteration** – Cardiovascular:* ***Integrated Processes** – Nursing Process: Implementation:* ***Client Needs** – Physiological Integrity: Reduction of Risk Potential:* ***Cognitive Level** – Analysis*

MAKING NURSING DECISIONS: The test taker should apply the nursing process when the question asks the nurse, "Which intervention should be implemented first?" If the client is in distress, do not assess; if the client is in distress, do something.

32. 1. This blood pressure—148/92—is elevated, but it would not be life threatening for someone diagnosed with hypertension; therefore, the nurse would not contact this client first.
    2. A pulse oximeter reading of 93% is low but still within normal limits, and a client with cystic fibrosis, a chronic respiratory condition, would be expected to have a chronically low oxygen level. This client would not need to be contacted first.
    3. The client with CHF would be expected to have edematous feet; this client would not need to be contacted first.
    4. **The client with chronic atrial fibrillation is at risk for pulmonary emboli, a potentially life-threatening complication. Chest pain is a common symptom of pulmonary embolism. The nurse should contact this client first.**

    Content – Medical/Surgical: ***Category of Health Alteration** – Cardiovascular:* ***Integrated Processes** – Nursing Process: Assessment:* ***Client Needs** – Physiological Integrity: Reduction of Risk Potential:* ***Cognitive Level** – Analysis*

MAKING NURSING DECISIONS: When deciding which client to assess first, the test taker should determine whether the signs/symptoms the client is exhibiting are normal or expected for the client situation. After eliminating the expected option, the test taker should determine which situation is more life threatening.

33. 1. **The nurse's first intervention is to assist the client to a sitting position to decrease the workload of the heart by decreasing venous return and maximizing lung expansion. This will, it is hoped, help relieve the client's respiratory distress.**
    2. The nurse should assess the client's vital signs, but the first intervention is to help the client breathe.
    3. The nurse should contact the paramedics if the client does not improve after being placed in a sitting position, but this is not the nurse's first intervention.
    4. The nurse should auscultate the client's lungs, but the first intervention is to help the client breathe more easily.

    Content – Medical/Surgical: ***Category of Health Alteration** – Cardiovascular:* ***Integrated Processes** – Nursing Process: Implementation:* ***Client Needs** – Physiological Integrity: Physiological Adaptation:* ***Cognitive Level** – Application*

MAKING NURSING DECISIONS: The nurse should remember that if a client is in distress and the nurse can do something to relieve the distress, that action should be done first, before assessment. The test taker should select an option that directly helps the client's condition.

34. 1. The HH nurse can contact the agency's chaplain to provide spiritual support for the client's family, but the first intervention is to pronounce the client's death.
    2. **Nurses in home health have been given the authority to pronounce death for clients who are on service and death is imminent. This intervention should be implemented first.**
    3. The family should be able to stay at the bedside, but if for some reason they need to leave, the nurse's asking them to leave is not the first intervention. The nurse can assess the apical pulse with the family at the bedside.
    4. The client's funeral home needs to be contacted, but it is not the nurse's first action, and often the family will call the funeral home.

    Content – Medical/Surgical: ***Category of Health Alteration** – Cardiovascular:* ***Integrated Processes** – Nursing Process: Implementation:* ***Client Needs** – Safe*

and Effective Care Environment: Management of Care:
***Cognitive Level** – Application*

**MAKING NURSING DECISIONS: The NCLEX-RN®
blueprint includes nursing care that is ruled by
legal requirements. The nurse must be knowledgeable of these issues. The nurse must be
aware of the rules and regulations of the various
areas of nursing.**

35. 1. The therapeutic range for INR is 2 to 3;
    therefore, this client would not need to be
    contacted first.
   2. The client's serum potassium level is within
    the normal range—3.5 to 5.5 mEq/L.
    Therefore, this client would not need to
    be contacted first.
   3. **The client's digoxin level is higher than
    the therapeutic level for digoxin, which
    is 0.8 to 2 mg/dL. This client should
    be contacted first to assess for signs/
    symptoms of digoxin toxicity.**
   4. The glycosylated hemoglobin, which is the
    average of blood glucose levels over 3 months,
    should not be more than 8%. This client, with
    a level of 6%, does not need to be contacted.
   *Content – Medical/Surgical: **Category of Health
   Alteration** – Cardiovascular: **Integrated Processes** –
   Nursing Process: Assessment: **Client Needs** –
   Physiological Integrity: Reduction of Risk Potential:
   Cognitive Level – Analysis*

**MAKING NURSING DECISIONS: The test taker
must know normal laboratory data.**

36. 1. The client should be encouraged to exercise,
    but it should be in a supervised setting
    such as a cardiac rehabilitation unit because
    the client has diabetes and hypertension.
   2. The client should adhere to a low-fat,
    low-cholesterol, carbohydrate-counting
    diet, but this is not the priority intervention.
    The client needs to be in a supervised
    setting, and diet teaching is included in
    cardiac rehabilitation.
   3. **Cardiac rehabilitation includes progres-
    sive exercise, diet teaching, and classes
    on modifying risk factors. This supervised
    setting would be the priority intervention
    for this client when the client is discharged
    from HH.**
   4. The client should lose weight slowly, but the
    priority intervention for this client would be
    a referral to a supervised setting where the
    client can lose weight slowly and safely.
   *Content – Medical/Surgical: **Category of Health
   Alteration** – Cardiovascular: **Integrated Processes** –
   Nursing Process: Planning: **Client Needs** – Physiological*

*Integrity: Physiological Adaptation: **Cognitive Level** –
Synthesis*

**MAKING NURSING DECISIONS: The test taker
must be knowledgeable of the role of each
member of the multidisciplinary healthcare team
as well as HIPAA rules and regulations. These
topics will be tested on the NCLEX-RN® exam.**

37. 1. The nurse should prepare the needed
    equipment, but it is not the nurse's first
    intervention.
   2. The nurse should call and arrange a time
    convenient for the visit, but the nurse should
    first review the client referral so the nurse is
    aware of the need for the visit.
   3. **The nurse should review the client's
    referral form and other pertinent data
    concerning the client's condition first
    before taking any further steps. The
    nurse may need to contact the referring
    agency if the information is unclear or if
    important information is missing. This is
    assessment.**
   4. The nurse will not know which referrals will
    be needed until after the first visit.
   *Content – Medical/Surgical: **Category of Health
   Alteration** – Cardiovascular: **Integrated Processes** –
   Nursing Process: Assessment: **Client Needs** – Safe and
   Effective Care Environment: Management of Care:
   Cognitive Level – Analysis*

**MAKING NURSING DECISIONS: Assessment is the
first step of the nursing process, and the test
taker should use the nursing process or some
other systematic process to assist in determining
priorities. The client is not in distress because
he/she is at home.**

38. 1. If the client or family is intoxicated, hostile,
    or obnoxious, the nurse should leave and
    reschedule the visit. There is no need to call
    the police unless the nurse thinks he or she
    will be hurt.
   2. The HH nurse should wear the agency iden-
    tification on the shirt or blouse; it should be
    visible to anyone talking to the nurse.
   3. To be eligible for HH visits, the client must
    be homebound, and all visits should be done
    in the daylight hours as a safety precaution.
   4. **The agency should be informed of the
    schedule so the nurse can be located if
    the nurse does not return when expected.**
   *Content – Medical/Surgical: **Category of Health
   Alteration** – Cardiovascular: **Integrated Processes** –
   Nursing Process: Implementation: **Client Needs** – Safe
   and Effective Care Environment: Safety and Infection
   Control: **Cognitive Level** – Application*

MAKING NURSING DECISIONS: The test taker must be knowledgeable of all the various areas of nursing and the role of each member of the multidisciplinary healthcare team, as well as HIPAA rules and regulations. These topics will be tested on the NCLEX-RN® exam.

39. 1. This is professional boundary crossing. Even though the grandson is not the client, he is related to the client. The HH aide should not go out with him.
  2. **This statement protects the HH aide. This is professional boundary crossing. The employee should not date any relatives of the client because this may pose a conflict of interest. The HH aide should wait until the client is no longer on service.**
  3. The nurse's best response is to tell the HH aide the facts about dating relatives of clients. The director would tell the HH aide the same information.
  4. The HH aide could date the grandson when the client is no longer on service. So this statement is not the nurse's best response.

  Content – Medical/Surgical: ***Category of Health Alteration*** *– Cardiovascular:* ***Integrated Processes*** *– Nursing Process: Implementation:* ***Client Needs*** *– Safe and Effective Care Environment: Management of Care:* ***Cognitive Level*** *– Application*

MAKING NURSING DECISIONS: There will be management questions on the NCLEX-RN®. In many instances, there is no test-taking strategy; the nurse must be knowledgeable of management issues. Boundary crossings is a very important area every nurse must be aware.

40. **1, 2, 4, and 5 are correct.**
  1. **A 2-lb weight gain indicates the client is retaining fluid and should contact the HCP. This is an appropriate teaching intervention.**
  2. **Keeping the head of the bed elevated will help the client breathe easier; therefore, this is an appropriate teaching intervention.**
  3. The loop diuretic should be taken in the morning to prevent nocturia. This is not an appropriate teaching intervention.
  4. **Sodium retains water. Telling the client to avoid eating foods high in sodium is an appropriate teaching intervention.**
  5. **Isotonic exercise, such as walking or swimming, helps tone the muscles, and discussing this with the client is an appropriate teaching intervention.**

Content – Medical/Surgical: ***Category of Health Alteration*** *– Cardiovascular:* ***Integrated Processes*** *– Nursing Process: Planning:* ***Client Needs*** *– Physiological Integrity: Physiological Adaptation:* ***Cognitive Level*** *– Synthesis*

MAKING NURSING DECISIONS: This is an alternate type of question included in the NCLEX-RN®. The nurse must be able to select all the options that answer the question correctly. There are no partially correct answers.

41. 1. The INR is not at a therapeutic level yet; the nurse should administer this medication.
  2. **This potassium level is very low. Hypokalemia potentiates dysrhythmias in clients receiving digoxin. This nurse should discuss potassium replacement with the HCP before administering this medication.**
  3. An aspartate aminotransferase (AST) test measures the amount of this enzyme in the blood. The enzyme is part of the liver function panel. The normal is 14–20 U/L for males and 10–36 U/L for females.
  4. Creatinine level is reflective of renal status. Normal is 0.6–1.2 mg d/L.

  Content – Medical/Surgical: ***Category of Health Alteration*** *– Cardiovascular:* ***Integrated Processes*** *– Nursing Process: Assessment:* ***Client Needs*** *– Physiological Integrity: Pharmacological and Parenteral Therapies:* ***Cognitive Level*** *– Analysis*

MAKING NURSING DECISIONS: The test taker must know normal laboratory data.

42. 1. Assessment of the client's spiritual needs in end-of-life issues is a key consideration but is the chaplain's responsibility, when he/she is a member of the hospice team.
  2. The client's financial situation can be assessed, but it is not priority over the client's spiritual needs when death is near.
  3. **The client's support system is the priority assessment for the hospice nurse. The client will be cared for in the home and the nurse must know who is available to help the client.**
  4. The client's medical diagnosis is important when addressing the grieving process but there is nothing the nurse can do about the medical diagnosis, which is why assessing, supporting, and addressing the client's spiritual needs will be carried out prior to the medical diagnosis.

  Content – Medical/Surgical: ***Category of Health Alteration*** *– Cardiovascular:* ***Integrated Processes*** *– Nursing Process: Assessment:* ***Client Needs*** *– Physiological Integrity: Physiological Adaptation:* ***Cognitive Level*** *– Synthesis*

MAKING NURSING DECISIONS: The test taker must be knowledgeable of all the various areas of nursing and the role of each member of the multidisciplinary healthcare team, as well as HIPAA rules and regulations. These topics will be tested on the NCLEX-RN® exam.

43. 1. The client's HCP will need to determine time of death but it is not the nurse's first intervention.
2. The Rapid Response Team would not be notified because the client has a DNR.
3. **The nurse should stay with the client and her husband and not make any life-rescuing interventions while the client is dying. The husband should not be left alone.**
4. The UAP can perform post-mortem care but it is not the first intervention when the client's husband tells the nurse his wife has quit breathing.

*Content – Medical/Surgical: **Category of Health Alteration** – Cardiovascular **Integrated Processes** – Nursing Process: Implementation: **Client Needs** – Safe and Effective Care Environment: Safety and Infection Control: **Cognitive Level** – Application*

MAKING NURSING DECISIONS: A do not resuscitate (DNR) is a written physician's order instructing healthcare providers not to attempt CPR. A new term recently introduced is "allow natural death" (AND). The nurse cannot legally perform CPR on a client who has a DNR.

44. 1. This client should be seen, but a client who is terminally ill and is refusing to eat is not an emergency situation.
2. The client has a right to rescind the out-of-hospital DNR but paperwork is not priority over a client who is in pain.
3. **One of the main goals of hospice is pain and symptom control. This client should be seen first so that appropriate pain control can be obtained immediately.**
4. A Stage 1 pressure ulcer must be assessed and treatment started but this is not priority over pain control.

*Content – Medical/Surgical: **Category of Health Alteration** – Cardiovascular: **Integrated Processes** – Nursing Process: Assessment: **Client Needs** – Physiological Integrity: Physiological Adaptation: **Cognitive Level** – Synthesis*

MAKING NURSING DECISIONS: The nurse can use Maslow's Hierarchy of Needs to determine which client to assess first. Pain is a physiological need.

45. 1. Encouraging the client to review his or her life experiences assists the client to

come to a closure of his or her life. This is an important intervention the volunteer can perform.
2. This is the job of the UAP, not the volunteer.
3. This is the job of the chaplain, not the volunteer.
4. This is the job of the nurse or occupational therapist, not the volunteer.

*Content – Medical/Surgical: **Category of Health Alteration** – Cardiovascular: **Integrated Processes** – Nursing Process: Planning: **Client Needs** – Safe and Effective Care Environment: Management of Care: **Cognitive Level** – Synthesis*

MAKING NURSING DECISIONS: When the test taker is deciding which option is the most appropriate task to delegate/assign, the test taker should choose the task that allows each staff member to function within his or her full scope of practice. Do not assign a task to a staff member that falls outside the staff member's or volunteer's expertise.

46. 1. **The nurse should provide instruction and support to the UAP. This is the best response.**
2. This is a callous statement and does not help the UAP learn to provide post-mortem care.
3. This is not hearing the UAP's concern.
4. The nurse should assist the UAP to learn to perform the duties of a UAP, not circumvent the workload.

*Content – Medical/Surgical: **Category of Health Alteration** – Cardiovascular: **Integrated Processes** – Nursing Process: Planning: **Client Needs** – Safe and Effective Care Environment: Management of Care: **Cognitive Level** – Synthesis*

47. 1. If the HCP is called, the nurse should perform this task, not the UAP. A UAP cannot take a telephone order; only a licensed nurse can take telephone orders.
2. The UAP cannot administer a medication, not even Tylenol.
3. **The nurse should immediately go to the client's room and assess the client. Sometimes the nurse may need the client's chart and medical administration record (MAR) to assist in the assessment of findings. The UAP can bring these documents to the room.**
4. The UAP should not be asked to relay such information. This is the nurse's or HCP's responsibility.

*Content – Medical/Surgical: **Category of Health Alteration** – Cardiovascular: **Integrated Processes** – Nursing Process: Planning: **Client Needs** – Safe and Effective Care Environment: Management of Care: **Cognitive Level** – Synthesis*

MAKING NURSING DECISIONS: When the test taker is deciding which option is the most appropriate task to delegate/assign, the test taker should choose the task that allows each staff member to function within his or her full scope of practice. Do not assign a task to a staff member that requires a higher level of expertise than that staff member has. Conversely, do not assign a task to a staff member when that task could be performed by a staff member with a lower level of expertise.

48. 1. The LPN can feed a client who is stable but unable to feed him or herself because of medical equipment. This is an appropriate task to assign.
   2. **The nurse cannot assign assessment. This is the inappropriate task to assign to the LPN.**
   3. The LPN can discharge a client who had a procedure and who does not require extensive teaching.
   4. The LPN can administer a routine IVPB medication.
   *Content – Medical/Surgical: **Category of Health Alteration** – Cardiovascular: **Integrated Processes** – Nursing Process: Planning: **Client Needs** – Safe and Effective Care Environment: Management of Care: **Cognitive Level** – Synthesis*

MAKING NURSING DECISIONS: The nurse cannot assign assessment, teaching, evaluation, or an unstable client to an LPN. The LPN can transcribe HCP orders and can call HCPs on the phone to obtain orders for a client.

49. 1. The UAP should encourage the client to remain independent as long as possible. If the client is unable to perform activities of daily living (ADLs), then the UAP should perform the tasks.
   2. This may be true, but the UAP cannot and should not distance himself or herself from the clients. The UAP should maintain a professional relationship with the clients.
   3. **This is an important statement for the UAP to understand. If information revealed to the UAP is necessary to provide appropriate care to the client, then the information must be shared on a need-to-know basis with the healthcare team.**
   4. Clients should be encouraged to discuss their life because life review may help clients accept their death.
   *Content – Medical/Surgical: **Category of Health Alteration** – Cardiovascular: **Integrated Processes** – Nursing Process: Diagnosis: **Client Needs** – Safe and Effective Care Environment: Safety and Infection Control: **Cognitive Level** – Analysis*

MAKING NURSING DECISIONS: The test taker must be knowledgeable of the role of each member of the multidisciplinary healthcare team as well as HIPAA rules and regulations. These topics will be tested on the NCLEX-RN® exam.

50. 1. The nurse in the client's room notifies the hospital operator of a code situation.
   2. **Answering the call lights of the other clients on the unit can be delegated to the UAP.**
   3. In a hospital, the respiratory therapist assumes the responsibility for ventilations.
   4. The nursing supervisor is responsible for requesting the family to leave the room. The UAP does not have the authority to make this request.
   *Content – Medical/Surgical: **Category of Health Alteration** – Cardiovascular: **Integrated Processes** – Nursing Process: Planning: **Client Needs** – Safe and Effective Care Environment: Management of Care: **Cognitive Level** – Synthesis*

MAKING NURSING DECISIONS: When the test taker is deciding which option is the most appropriate task to delegate/assign, the test taker should choose the task that allows each member of the staff to function within his or her full scope of practice. Do not assign a task to a staff member that requires a higher level of expertise or that a staff member with a lower level of expertise could perform.

51. 1. **If the family is not causing a disruption in the code, the family member should be allowed to stay in the room with the supervisor remaining near the family member and explaining why the interventions are being implemented will help the client to survive. The supervisor should be ready to escort the family member out of the code if the family member becomes disruptive.**
   2. This will cause ill will on the part of the family and could result in the filing of a needless lawsuit.
   3. The HCP is busy with the care of the client. This is not the time to ask an HCP a question the supervisor can handle.
   4. Ignoring the family member could cause a problem; the supervisor should be proactive in managing the situation.
   *Content – Medical/Surgical: **Category of Health Alteration** – Cardiovascular: **Integrated Processes** – Nursing Process: Implementation: **Client Needs** – Safe and Effective Care Environment: Safety and Infection Control: **Cognitive Level** – Application*

MAKING NURSING DECISIONS: The nurse should always try and support the client or the family's request if it does not violate any local, state, or federal rules and regulations. This is the test taker's best decision if unsure of the correct answer.

52. 1. **Federal law requires that clients presenting to an emergency department must be assessed and treated without regard to payment. The nurse should initiate steps to assess the client.**
2. The nurse must assess the client. If a transfer is made, it will be after the client has been stabilized and the receiving hospital has accepted the transfer.
3. Federal law requires that clients presenting to an emergency department must be assessed and treated without regard to payment. The hospital will attempt to recover the costs after the client has been treated,
4. This is irrelevant information.

Content – *Medical/Surgical:* **Category of Health Alteration** – *Cardiovascular:* **Integrated Processes** – *Nursing Process: Implementation:* **Client Needs** – *Safe and Effective Care Environment: Management of Care:* **Cognitive Level** – *Application*

MAKING NURSING DECISIONS: The NCLEX-RN® blueprint includes nursing care that is ruled by legal requirements. The nurse must be knowledgeable of these issues.

53. 1. **The client with angina should be asymptomatic; when the client is complaining of chest pain, this is abnormal data. Therefore, this client should be assessed first. Remember Maslow's Hierarchy of Needs identifies physiological needs as priority and pain is priority.**
2. In a client diagnosed with CHF, 4+ edema is expected. The nurse would not need to assess this client first.
3. The client diagnosed with endocarditis is expected to have a fever. The nurse would not need to assess this client first.
4. The client diagnosed with aortic valve stenosis has the classic triad of syncope, angina, and exertional dyspnea; therefore, this client would not be assessed first.

Content – *Medical/Surgical:* **Category of Health Alteration** – *Cardiovascular:* **Integrated Processes** – *Nursing Process: Assessment:* **Client Needs** – *Physiological Integrity: Reduction of Risk Potential:* **Cognitive Level** – *Analysis*

MAKING NURSING DECISIONS: The test taker must determine which sign/symptom is not expected for the disease process. If the sign/symptom is not expected then the nurse should assess the client first. This type of question is

posed to determine whether the nurse is knowledgeable of the signs/symptoms of a variety of disease processes.

54. 1. **First-dose intravenous antibiotic medications are priority medications and should be administered within 1 to 2 hours of when the order was written. This should be the first medication administered.**
2. Antiplatelet medication, aspirin, is not a priority medication.
3. A coronary vasodilator patch, nitroglycerin, is not a priority medication.
4. A statin medication that decreases cholesterol level should be administered in the evening when the enzyme for cholesterol metabolism is at its highest peak.

Content – *Medical/Surgical:* **Category of Health Alteration** – *Drug Administration:* **Integrated Processes** – *Nursing Process: Planning:* **Client Needs** – *Physiological Integrity: Pharmacological and Parenteral Therapies:* **Cognitive Level** – *Synthesis*

MAKING NURSING DECISIONS: The test taker should know which are priority medications, such as life-threatening medications, insulin, and mucolytics (Carafate). As the rationale explains, antibiotic therapy should be initiated as soon as possible; a delay could cause death of the client.

55. 1. The nurse checks an apical pulse, not a radial pulse, prior to administering digoxin.
2. There is no serum amiodorone level; therefore, the nurse cannot implement this intervention.
3. **Intravenous heparin increases the client's partial thromboplastin time and causes an anticoagulant effect. The nurse should always be aware of the client's most current PTT levels when therapeutic heparin is being administered.**
4. The nurse should monitor the client's renal function, creatinine level, not the liver function.

Content – *Medical/Surgical:* **Category of Health Alteration** – *Drug Administration:* **Integrated Processes** – *Nursing Process: Implementation:* **Client Needs** – *Safe and Effective Care Environment: Management of Care:* **Cognitive Level** – *Application*

MAKING NURSING DECISIONS: The nurse must be aware of interventions that must be implemented prior to administering medications. The nurse must know what to monitor prior to administering medications because untoward reactions and possibly death can occur.

56. 1. The client would be expected to be drowsy after a narcotic preoperative medication. The

nurse would not need to call a time-out for this client.

2. **Whenever there is a discrepancy on the chart or with what the client says, the nurse should call an immediate time-out until the situation has been resolved.**

3. The client's allergy must be documented on the client's chart and identification band; therefore, this would not warrant a time-out.

4. Because this is what is supposed to happen, the nurse would not need to call a time-out.

*Content – Medical/Surgical: **Category of Health Alteration** – Cardiovascular: **Integrated Processes** – Nursing Process: Implementation **Client Needs** – Physiological Integrity: Reduction of Risk Potential: **Cognitive Level** – Knowledge*

MAKING NURSING DECISIONS: The NCLEX-RN® blueprint includes nursing care that is ruled by the current National Patient Safety Goals. The nurse must be knowledgeable of these goals.

57. 1. The day shift nurse should check the client's potassium and digoxin levels prior to administering the digoxin. The digoxin has been administered for the day.

2. A partial thromboplastin time is monitored for IV heparin, not Coumadin.

3. **The nurse should monitor the INR prior to administering warfarin (Coumadin). The therapeutic level for warfarin is 2 to 3.**

4. This should be done immediately prior to administering the medication at the bedside.

*Content – Medical/Surgical: **Category of Health Alteration** – Cardiovascular: **Integrated Processes** – Nursing Process: Implementation: **Client Needs** – Physiological Integrity: Reduction of Risk Potential: **Cognitive Level** – Synthesis*

MAKING NURSING DECISIONS: This is an alternate type question included in the NCLEX-RN® blueprint. The test taker must be able to read a medication administration record (MAR), be knowledgeable of medications, and be able to make an appropriate decision as to the nurse's most appropriate intervention.

58. 1. Lasix should be administered to the client who has an adequate urinary output.

2. Lovenox is prescribed to prevent deep vein thromboses (DVT) in clients who are immobile, such as a postsurgical client.

3. **The nurse should not administer an antiplatelet medication to a client going to surgery because this will increase postoperative bleeding. The nurse should hold this medication and discuss this with the surgeon.**

4. The client's blood pressure is within an acceptable range. The nurse should administer this medication.

*Content – Medical/Surgical: **Category of Health Alteration** – Drug Administration: **Integrated Processes** – Nursing Process: Assessment: **Client Needs** – Physiological Integrity: Pharmacological and Parenteral Therapies: **Cognitive Level** – Analysis*

MAKING NURSING DECISIONS: The nurse must be knowledgeable of interventions when administering medications to clients undergoing surgery, such as the client should not receive any PO medications or should not receive any medications that could increase bleeding.

59. 1. The nurse and respiratory therapist, not the UAP, are responsible for monitoring the ABGs.

2. Infusion of blood and blood products, even the client's own, cannot be delegated to a UAP.

3. **The UAP can assist with hygiene needs; this is one of the main tasks that may be delegated to UAPs.**

4. The nurse must assess the surgical site for bleeding, infection, and healing. The UAP cannot perform assessments.

*Content – Medical/Surgical: **Category of Health Alteration** – Cardiovascular: **Integrated Processes** – Nursing Process: Planning: **Client Needs** – Safe and Effective Care Environment: Management of Care: **Cognitive Level** – Synthesis*

MAKING NURSING DECISIONS: An RN cannot delegate assessment, teaching, evaluation, medications, or an unstable client to a UAP. Tasks that cannot be delegated are nursing interventions requiring nursing judgment.

60. 1. **The nurse should administer a unit of blood over the greatest length of time possible (4 hours) to a client diagnosed with congestive heart failure to prevent fluid volume overload. The nurse should question this order.**

2. Administering a diuretic to a client diagnosed with CHF who is receiving blood is an appropriate order. The nurse would not question this HCP order.

3. Restricting fluids to a client diagnosed with CHF is an appropriate order depending on the severity of the client's condition. The nurse would not question this order, especially when administering IV fluids to the client.

4. The HCP should evaluate the effects of the two units of blood. The nurse would not question this HCP order.

*Content – Medical/Surgical; **Category of Health Alteration** – Cardiovascular: **Integrated Processes** – Nursing Process: Assessment: **Client Needs** – Safe and Effective Care Environment: Safety and Infection Control: **Cognitive Level** – Synthesis*

MAKING NURSING DECISIONS: When the stem asks the nurse to determine which healthcare provider's order to question, the test taker needs to realize this is an "except" question. Three of the options are appropriate for the HCP to prescribe and one is not appropriate for the client's disease process or procedure.

61. 1. The nurse should not document that the client fell unless the nurse observed the client fall. The nurse should never write "incident report" in a chart. This becomes a red flag to a lawyer.
    2. **The nurse should document exactly what was observed. This statement is the correct documentation.**
    3. This statement is not substantiated and should not be placed in the chart.
    4. This statement is documenting something the nurse did not observe, a fall.

    *Content – Medical/Surgical: **Category of Health Alteration** – Cardiovascular: **Integrated Processes** – Nursing Process: Implementation: **Client Needs** – Safe and Effective Care Environment, Management of Care: **Cognitive Level** – Application*

MAKING NURSING DECISIONS: The nurse must be able to document nursing care safely; it includes accurate, timely documentation; it meets professional, legislative, and agency standards; it facilitates communication between nurses and other healthcare providers; and it is comprehensive.

62. 1. Cooking and cleaning are jobs that can be arranged through some home health agencies, but these jobs would be done by a housekeeper, not by the UAP.
    2. **The home health aide is responsible for assisting the client with activities of daily living and transferring from the bed to the chair. Sitting outside is good for the client and is a task that can be delegated to the home health aide.**
    3. This is boundary crossing by the UAP and could create legal difficulties if the UAP had an accident.
    4. This is assessment and cannot be delegated to a UAP.

    *Content – Medical/Surgical: **Category of Health Alteration** – Cardiovascular: **Integrated Processes** – Nursing Process: Planning: **Client Needs** – Safe and Effective Care Environment: Management of Care: **Cognitive Level** – Synthesis*

MAKING NURSING DECISIONS: When the test taker is deciding which option is the most appropriate task to delegate/assign, the test taker should choose the task that allows each staff member to function within his or her full scope of practice. Do not assign a task to a staff member that falls outside the staff member's or volunteer's expertise. Remember the RN cannot delegate assessment, teaching, evaluation, medications, or an unstable client to the UAP.

63. 1. If the client is in distress, assessment is not the first intervention if there is an action the nurse can take to relieve the distress. The nurse should administer the nitroglycerin first.
    2. Calling for an electrocardiogram and troponin level should be implemented but not before administering the nitroglycerin.
    3. **Placing nitroglycerin under the client's tongue may relieve the client's chest pain and provide oxygen to the heart muscle. This is the nurse's first intervention.**
    4. Notification of the HCP can be done after the nurse has stabilized the client.

    *Content – Medical/Surgical: **Category of Health Alteration** – Cardiovascular: **Integrated Processes** – Nursing Process: Implementation: **Client Needs** – Physiological Integrity: Reduction of Risk Potential: **Cognitive Level** – Application*

MAKING NURSING DECISIONS: The nurse should remember that if a client is in distress and the nurse can do something to relieve the distress, that action should be done first, before assessment. The test taker should select an option that directly helps the client's condition.

64. 1. The supervisor can take notes documenting the code until relieved, but the supervisor needs to be free to supervise the code and coordinate room assignments and staffing.
    2. **The first intervention for the supervisor is to ensure that all the jobs in the code are being filled.**
    3. This is the responsibility of the supervisor, but it is not the first intervention.
    4. The supervisor can administer medications, but the supervisor needs to be flexible to complete the duties of the supervisor.

    *Content – Medical/Surgical: **Category of Health Alteration** – Cardiovascular: **Integrated Processes** – Nursing Process: Implementation: **Client Needs** – Safe and Effective Care Environment: Safety and Infection Control: **Cognitive Level** – Synthesis*

MAKING NURSING DECISIONS: The test taker must be knowledgeable of the role of each member of the multidisciplinary healthcare team as

well as HIPAA rules and regulations. These topics will be tested on the NCLEX-RN® exam. The administrative manager is responsible for the other members of the healthcare team.

65. 1. This client is being treated, and if the blood is almost finished, then it can be assumed that the client is tolerating the blood without incident.
2. **The client has been given devastating news. When all the information in the options is expected and not life threatening, then psychological issues have priority. This client should be seen first.**
3. The client has eaten. The nurse could arrange for the dietician to consult with the client about food preferences, but this client does not need to be assessed first.
4. Dyspnea on exertion is not priority if the client is exerting himself or herself.

Content – Medical/Surgical: *Category of Health Alteration* – Cardiovascular: *Integrated Processes* – Nursing Process: Assessment: *Client Needs* – Psychosocial Integrity: *Cognitive Level* – Analysis

MAKING NURSING DECISIONS: The test taker must determine if the assessment data is normal or abnormal for the client's diagnosis or situation. If the data is abnormal then this client should be seen first. If the data is normal then a client with a psychosocial problem is the client the nurse should assess first.

66. 1. This medication could be administered but it will not have as rapid an impact as the SL dose.
2. Nitroglycerin is administered first because it will dilate the vessels and resolve the cause of the chest pain. If the chest pain still is present after three (3) NTG then the morphine should be administered.
3. Oxycodone and acetaminophen will not address the chest pain specifically.
4. **The nurse should administer the medication that will have the most rapid onset and directly resolve the problem. Nitroglycerin is a potent vasodilator and will dissolve rapidly under the tongue (sublingually).**

Content – Medical/Surgical: *Category of Health Alteration* – Cardiovascular: *Integrated Processes* – Nursing Process: Assessment: *Client Needs* – Physiological Integrity: Pharmacological and Parenteral Therapies: *Cognitive Level* – Analysis

MAKING NURSING DECISIONS: This is an alternate type question included in the NCLEX-RN® blueprint. The test taker must be able to read a medication administration record (MAR), be

knowledgeable of medications, and be able to make an appropriate decision as to the nurse's most appropriate intervention.

67. 1. A client with a DVT on a heparin drip should have an aPTT in this range. The charge nurse should make sure that the drip is maintaining the client in the therapeutic range, but the safety of the client going to surgery is first priority.
2. **This client is scheduled for surgery this morning; therefore, the charge nurse must make sure that he is stable for the procedure and notify the surgeon if there is any reason to question the safety of the client having the procedure this morning.**
3. This client is postprocedure and unless there is a situation that arises from the nurse's assessment then this client is not priority.
4. Gall bladder disease is not life threatening, although it can be very uncomfortable. This client is not priority.

Content – Medical/Surgical: *Category of Health Alteration* – Cardiovascular: *Integrated Processes* – Nursing Process: Assessment: *Client Needs* – Physiological Integrity: Reduction of Risk Potential: *Cognitive Level* – Analysis

MAKING NURSING DECISIONS: This is an alternate type of question included in the NCLEX-RN® blueprint. The test taker must be able to read a chart, be knowledgeable of laboratory data, and be able to make appropriate decisions as to the nurse's most appropriate action.

68. Correct Answer: 3, 1, 4, 2, 5
3. **This client may be chilling, indicting a potential rise in temperature. The nurse should assess the client and the temperature to see if interventions should be initiated based on a progression of the septicemia.**
1. **This client should be assessed to be sure that the client is stable because there was chest pain during the last shift.**
4. **The nurse should assess the client next because although confusion is expected, the nurse must determine whether any new situation is occurring.**
2. **This client has a psychosocial need but it must be addressed and steps implemented to resolve the problem.**
5. **A dressing change can take some time to complete. This is a physiological situation but not a life-threatening one and the nurse should see this client when he/she has time to perform the dressing change.**

*Content – Medical/Surgical: **Category of Health Alteration** – Cardiovascular: **Integrated Processes** – Nursing Process Planning: **Client Needs** – Safe and Effective Care Environment: Management of Care: **Cognitive Level** – Synthesis*

MAKING NURSING DECISIONS: This is an alternate type of question which requires the nurse to assess clients in order of priority. This requires the nurse to evaluate each client's situation and determine which situations are life threatening, which situations are expected for the client's situation, or which client has a psychosocial problem.

69. 1, 3, and 4 are correct.
    1. **Nitroglycerin tablets are vasodilators that are administered to dilate the coronary vessels and provide oxygen to the heart muscle.**
    2. The client should be made to sit down immediately. Exercise is the probable cause of the chest pain; therefore, the activity should immediately stop.
    3. **The nurse should assess the client's vital signs as part of the assessment of the client's current situation.**
    4. **Supplemental oxygen will assist in getting higher concentrations of oxygen to the heart muscle.**
    5. A ward secretary cannot take orders; only a nurse should discuss the client with the healthcare provider.

*Content – Medical/Surgical: **Category of Health Alteration** – Cardiovascular: **Integrated Processes** – Nursing Process: Implementation: **Client Needs** – Safe and Effective Care Environment: Safety and Infection Control: **Cognitive Level** – Analysis*

MAKING NURSING DECISIONS: This is an alternate type of question included in the NCLEX-RN®. The nurse must be able to select all the options that answer the question correctly. There are no partially correct answers.

70. Answer: 24 mL per hour
    25,000 divided by 500 mL = 50 units of heparin per mL.
    26 (current rate) × 50 = 1300 units of heparin currently infusing.
    1300 − 100 = 1200 units of heparin needed as new infusion rate.
    1200 divided by 50 = 24 mL per hour to infuse

*Content – Medical/Surgical: **Category of Health Alteration** – Drug Administration: **Integrated Processes** – Nursing Process: Implementation: **Client Needs** – Physiological Integrity: Pharmacological and Parenteral Therapies: **Cognitive Level** – Application*

MAKING NURSING DECISIONS: This is an alternate type of question included in the NCLEX-RN®. The nurse must know how to solve math questions.

CARDIAC CLINICAL SCENARIO ANSWERS AND RATIONALES

The correct answer number and rationale for why it is the correct answer are given in boldface type. Rationales for why the other possible answer options are incorrect also are given, but they are not in boldface type.

1. 1. Praxada is a medication specifically prescribed to prevent clotting in clients who have atrial fibrillation. Any nurse could administer the first dose of the medication; it would not have to be the most experienced nurse.
   2. **Pink, frothy sputum indicates pulmonary edema, which is a serious complication of CHF; therefore, the most experienced nurse should be assigned this client.**
   3. Occasional premature ventricular contractions are experienced by most individuals and this client would not require the most experienced nurse.
   4. Clients with mitral valve prolapse exhibit signs of congestive heart failure; therefore, SOB is expected and the most experienced nurse should not be assigned to this client.

2. 1. The crash cart would need to be brought to the room if the client was coding, but first the nurse should determine if the client's leads are on the chest.
   2. The Rapid Response Team is called if the client is in a potentially life-threatening situation and the nurse must first determine if the leads are on the client.
   3. The nurse should assess the client's vital signs but because the telemetry technician reports the client is flat-lined the nurse should first check if the leads are in place on the chest.
   4. **The nurse should first determine if the client's telemetry leads are in place on the chest. If the leads are off then it will show as a flat line at the telemetry station. The telemetry technician cannot leave the station.**

3. 1. **This warrants intervention because the telemetry technician needs to know if the client's telemetry is being removed so the technician won't think the client is in asystole.**
   2. The electrodes attached to the client's chest do not have to be removed when the client showers, so this would not warrant intervention. The telemetry must be removed, not the electrodes.
   3. Placing a bath chair in the shower is an appropriate intervention so the client won't get tired during the shower; this would not warrant intervention.
   4. The UAP should stay near the client in the shower in case the client needs assistance; this would not warrant intervention.

4. 1. **The therapeutic digoxin level is 0.8 to 2.0 mg/dL; therefore, Ms. Teresa should notify the client's HCP because this is above the therapeutic level.**
   2. The therapeutic INR level is 2 to 3; therefore, Ms. Teresa would not notify the HCP.
   3. The normal potassium level is 3.5 to 5.5 mEq/L, so Ms. Teresa would not notify the HCP.
   4. Normal cholesterol level is below 200, but 205 is not life threatening and would not warrant notifying the HCP.

5. 1. This client must have an admission assessment completed and Ms. Teresa cannot assign assessment to an LPN.
   2. The client with SVT will need intravenous adenosine; therefore, this client should not be assessed to an LPN.
   3. **The LPN could care for a client who has had a diagnostic test; this would be an appropriate client assignment.**
   4. Ms. Teresa cannot assign teaching to the LPN.

6. 1. The client would need to have cardiac isoenzymes to determine if a myocardial infarction has occurred; therefore, this HCP would not be questioned.
   2. The client probably has coronary artery disease and a low-fat, low-cholesterol diet would be expected.
   3. Intravenous morphine is the drug of choice for chest pain; therefore, this order would not be questioned.
   4. **An endoscopy is not an usual diagnostic test for a client diagnosed with R/O myocardial infarction; therefore, Ms. Teresa should question this order.**

7. 1. **The UAP can obtain the client's weight. The nurse cannot delegate assessment, teaching, evaluation, medications, or an unstable client.**
   2. The custodial or housekeeping department is responsible for cleaning the room, not the UAP.
   3. The nurse cannot delegate assessment, teaching, evaluation, medications, or an unstable

client. A client who is hypovolemic is not stable; therefore, this task cannot be delegated.

4. The nurse cannot delegate assessment, teaching, evaluation, medications, or an unstable client. Discussing the diet is teaching, which cannot be delegated to a UAP.

8. 1. The nurse can check the MAR but it is not the first intervention when the client is having acute chest pain. Remember, the nurse does not treat paperwork.

2. When the client is in distress the nurse should not assess. The nurse should treat the client's pain immediately; therefore, this is not the first intervention.

3. **The nurse should treat the pain, so administering sublingual nitroglycerin, a coronary vasodilator, is the nurse's first intervention.**

4. The nurse should administer oxygen but not prior to addressing the client's chest pain first.

9. 1. The nurse must first determine if the client has a pulse. If the client does not have a pulse then the nurse must defibrillate the client. If the client has a pulse then the nurse should not defibrillate the client.

2. **The nurse must determine if the client has a pulse or not prior to taking any further action; therefore, this is the nurse's first intervention.**

3. This is the first medication administered during a code but the nurse first determines if the client has a pulse.

4. This is appropriate intervention if the client has no pulse but the nurse first determines if the client has a pulse.

10. 1. Nitroglycerin tablets lose efficacy when exposed to sunlight; therefore, keeping the tablets in a dark bottle indicates the client understands the teaching.

2. A sedentary lifestyle is a modifiable risk factor for atherosclerosis, which causes angina, so walking three times a week is an appropriate intervention.

3. **This is a modifiable risk factor; the client must stop smoking altogether. Decreasing the number of cigarettes a day indicates the client needs more teaching.**

4. A daily aspirin will help prevent platelet aggregation; therefore, this indicates the client understands the discharge teaching.

Peripheral Vascular Management

Not everything that can be counted counts, and not everything that counts can be counted.

—Albert Einstein

QUESTIONS

1. The nurse has finished receiving the morning change-of-shift report. Which client should the nurse assess first?
   1. The client diagnosed with arterial occlusive disease who has intermittent claudication.
   2. The client on strict bed rest who is complaining of calf pain and has a reddened calf.
   3. The client who complains of low back pain when lying supine in the bed.
   4. The client who is upset because the food doesn't taste good and is cold all the time.

2. The nurse is caring for clients on a vascular disorder unit. Which laboratory data warrant immediate intervention by the nurse?
   1. The PTT of 98 seconds for a client diagnosed with deep vein thrombosis (DVT).
   2. The hemoglobin 11.4 for a client diagnosed with Raynaud's phenomenon.
   3. The white blood cell (WBC) count of 11,000 for a client with a stasis venous ulcer.
   4. The triglyceride level of 312 mmol/L in a client diagnosed with hypertension (HTN).

3. The unlicensed assistive personnel (UAP) tells the nurse the client has a blood pressure of 78/46 and a pulse of 116 using a vital signs machine. Which intervention should the nurse implement first?
   1. Notify the healthcare provider immediately.
   2. Have the UAP recheck the client's vital signs manually.
   3. Place the client in Trendelenburg position.
   4. Assess the client's cardiovascular status.

4. The charge nurse on a vascular unit is working with a new unit secretary. Which statement concerning laboratory data is most important for the charge nurse to tell the unit secretary?
   1. "Be sure to show me any lab information that is called in to the unit."
   2. "Make sure to file the reports on the correct client's chart."
   3. "Do not take any laboratory reports over the telephone."
   4. "Verify all telephone reports by calling back to the lab."

5. The nurse on the vascular unit is preparing to administer medications to clients on a medical unit. Which medication should the nurse question administering?
   1. Vitamin K (AquaMephyton), a vitamin, to a client with an International Normal Ratio (INR) of 2.8.
   2. Propranolol (Inderal), a beta-adrenergic, to a client with arterial hypertension.
   3. Nifedipine (Procardia), a calcium channel blocker, to a client with Raynaud's disease.
   4. Enalapril (Vasotec), an angiotensin-converting enzyme (ACE) inhibitor, to a client with a sodium level of 138 mEq/L.

6. The nurse has received the shift report. Which client should the nurse assess first?
   1. The client with a deep vein thrombosis who is complaining of dyspnea and coughing.
   2. The client diagnosed with Buerger's disease who has intermittent claudication.
   3. The client diagnosed with an aortic aneurysm who has an audible bruit.
   4. The client with acute arterial ischemia who has bilateral palpable pedal pulses.

7. The female client diagnosed with atherosclerosis tells the clinic nurse her stomach hurts after she takes her morning medications. The client is taking a calcium channel blocker, a daily aspirin, and a statin. Which intervention should the nurse implement first?
   1. Assess the client for abnormal bleeding.
   2. Instruct the client to stop taking the aspirin.
   3. Recommend the client take an enteric-coated aspirin.
   4. Instruct the client to notify the HCP.

8. The nurse educator on a vascular unit is discussing delegation guidelines to a group of new graduates. Which statement from the group indicates the need for more teaching?
   1. "The UAP will be practicing on my brand-new nursing license."
   2. "I will still retain accountability for what I delegate to the UAP."
   3. "I must make sure the UAP to whom I delegate is competent to perform the task."
   4. "When I delegate, I must follow up with the UAP and evaluate the task."

9. The nurse is reviewing the literature to identify evidence-based practice research that supports a new procedure using a new product when changing the central line catheter dressing. Which research article would best support the nurse's proposal for a change in the procedure?
   1. The article in which the study was conducted by the manufacturer of the product used.
   2. The research article that included 10 subjects participating in the study.
   3. The review-of-literature article that cited ambiguous statistics about the product.
   4. The review-of-literature article that cited numerous studies supporting the product.

10. The nurse and the unlicensed assistive personnel are caring for clients on a vascular unit. Which task is most appropriate for the nurse to delegate?
    1. Provide indwelling catheter care to a client on bed rest.
    2. Evaluate the client's 8-hour intake and output.
    3. Give a bath to the client who is third-spacing.
    4. Administer a cation-exchange resin enema to a client.

11. The nurse asks the female UAP to apply the sequential compression devices (SCDs) to a client who is on strict bed rest. The UAP tells the nurse that she has never done this procedure. Which action would be priority for the nurse to take?
    1. Tell another UAP to put the SCDs on the client.
    2. Demonstrate the procedure for applying the SCDs.
    3. Perform the task and apply the SCDs to the client.
    4. Request the UAP watch the video demonstrating this task.

12. The nurse in the vascular critical care unit is working with an LPN who was pulled to the unit as a result of high census. Which task is most appropriate for the nurse to assign to the LPN?
    1. Assess the client who will be transferred to the medical unit in the morning.
    2. Administer a unit of blood to the client who is 1 day postoperative.
    3. Hang the bag of heparin for a client diagnosed with a pulmonary embolus.
    4. Assist the HCP with the insertion of a client's Swan-Ganz line.

13. The nurse is administering one unit of packed red blood cells to a client. Fifteen minutes after initiation of the blood transfusion, the client becomes restless and complains of itching on the trunk and arms. Which intervention should the nurse implement first?
    1. Assess the client's vital signs.
    2. Notify the HCP.
    3. Maintain a patent IV line.
    4. Stop the transfusion at the hub.

14. The staff nurse on a vascular disorder unit asks the charge nurse, "What should I be looking for when I read a research article?" Which response indicates the charge nurse does not understand how to read a nursing research article?
   1. "You should be able to determine why the research was done."
   2. "You should look to find out how much money was used for the study."
   3. "You should evaluate which research method was used for the study."
   4. "You should read the method section to find out what setting was used."

15. The nurse calls the HCP for an order for pain medication for a client who is 2 days postoperative aortic aneurysm repair. The HCP gives the nurse an order for "Demerol 50 mg IVP now and then every 4 hours as needed." Which action should the nurse implement first?
   1. Write the order in the chart with the words "per telephone order (TO)."
   2. Request another nurse to verify the HCP's order on the phone.
   3. Read back the order to the HCP before hanging up the phone.
   4. Transcribe the order to the medication administration record.

16. The charge nurse on the vascular unit is reviewing laboratory blood work. Which result warrants intervention by the charge nurse?
   1. The client whose INR is 2.3.
   2. The client whose H&H is 11 g/dL and 36%.
   3. The client whose platelet count is 65,000 per milliliter of blood.
   4. The client whose red blood cell count is 4.8×10 mm^6.

17. A client on the vascular unit tells the day shift primary nurse that the night nurse did not answer the call light for almost 1 hour. Which statement would be most appropriate by the day shift primary nurse?
   1. "The night shift often has trouble answering the lights promptly."
   2. "I am sorry that happened and I will answer your lights promptly today."
   3. "I will notify my charge nurse to come and talk to you about the situation."
   4. "There might have been an emergency situation so your light was not answered."

18. The nurse is preparing to administer a unit of packed red blood cells to an elderly client who is 1 day postoperative abdominal aortic aneurysm. Which interventions should the nurse implement? List in order of performance.
   1. Obtain the unit of blood from the blood bank.
   2. Start an IV access with normal saline at a keep-open rate.
   3. Have the client sign the permit to receive blood products.
   4. Check the unit of blood with another nurse at the bedside.
   5. Initiate the transfusion at a slow rate for 15 minutes.

19. The elderly client diagnosed with deep vein thrombosis is complaining of chest pain during inhalation. Which intervention should the nurse implement first?
   1. Ask the HCP to order a stat lung scan.
   2. Place oxygen on the client via nasal cannula.
   3. Prepare to administer intravenous heparin.
   4. Tell the client not to ambulate and remain in bed.

20. Which laboratory data should the nurse in the long-term care unit notify the healthcare provider about?
   1. The client receiving digoxon who has a digoxin level of 2.6.
   2. The client receiving enoxaparin (Levonox) who has a PT of 12.9 seconds.
   3. The client receiving ticlopidine (Ticlid) who has a platelet count of 160,000.
   4. The client receiving furosemide (Lasix) who has a potassium level of 4.2 mEq/L.

21. The occupational nurse is caring for the client who just severed two fingers from the right hand. Which intervention should the occupational nurse implement first?
   1. Place the severed fingers in a sterile cloth and then in an ice chest.
   2. Instruct the client to elevate the right arm over the heart.
   3. Don non-sterile gloves on both hands.
   4. Apply direct pressure to the right radial pulse.

22. The clinic nurse is making assignments to the staff. Which assignment/delegation is most appropriate?
    1. Request the LPN to escort the client to the examination room.
    2. Ask the unlicensed assistive personnel (UAP) to prepare the room for the next client.
    3. Instruct the RN to administer the tetanus shot to the client.
    4. Tell the clinic secretary to call in a new prescription for a client.

23. The female client tells the charge nurse the unlicensed assistive personnel (UAP) did not know how to take her blood pressure. Which action should the charge nurse implement first?
    1. Discuss the client's comment with the UAP.
    2. Retake the BP and inform the client of her BP reading.
    3. Explain that the UAP knows how to take a BP reading.
    4. Ask the UAP to demonstrate taking a BP reading.

24. Which medication is most appropriate for the nurse to assign to the LPN to administer?
    1. The intravenous push antiemetic to the client who is nauseated and vomiting.
    2. The subcutaneous low-molecular-weight heparin to the client with a pulmonary embolus.
    3. The PO pentoxifylline (Trental) to the client who has intermittent claudication.
    4. The sublingual nitroglycerin to the client who is complaining of chest pain.

25. The clinic nurse is assessing a client who is complaining of right leg calf pain. The right calf is edematous and warm to the touch. Which intervention should the nurse implement first?
    1. Notify the clinic HCP immediately.
    2. Ask the client how long the leg has been hurting.
    3. Complete a neurovascular assessment on the leg.
    4. Place the client's right leg on two pillows.

26. The fire alarm starts going off in the family practice clinic. Which action should the nurse take first?
    1. Determine whether there is a fire in the clinic.
    2. Evacuate all the people from the clinic.
    3. Immediately call 911 and report the fire.
    4. Instruct clients to stay in their rooms and close the doors.

27. The female unlicensed assistive personnel (UAP) tells the clinic nurse, "One of the medical interns asked me out on a date. I told him no but he keeps asking." Which statement is the nurse's best response?
    1. "I will talk to the intern and tell him to stop."
    2. "Did anyone hear the intern asking you out?"
    3. "He asks everyone out; that is just his way."
    4. "You should inform the clinic's director of nurses."

28. The clinic nurse overhears another staff nurse telling the pharmaceutical representative, "If you bring us lunch from the best place in town, I will make sure you get to see the HCP." Which action should the clinic nurse take?
    1. Tell the pharmaceutical representative the staff nurse's statement was inappropriate.
    2. Report this behavior to the clinic's director of nurses immediately.
    3. Do not take any action and wait for the food to be delivered.
    4. Inform the HCP of the staff nurse's and pharmaceutical representative's behaviors.

29. The home health (HH) nurse in the office is notified the female client on warfarin (Coumadin), an oral anticoagulant, has an International Normalized Ratio (INR) of 3.8. Which action should the HH nurse implement first?
    1. Document the result of the INR in the client's chart.
    2. Contact the client and ask whether or not she has any abnormal bleeding.
    3. Notify the client's healthcare provider of the INR results.
    4. Schedule an appointment with the client to draw another INR.

30. The home health (HH) nurse is caring for a client with arterial hypertension who has had a cerebrovascular accident. Which priority intervention should the nurse discuss with the client when teaching about arterial hypertension?
    1. Discuss the importance of the client adhering to a low-salt diet.
    2. Explain the need for the client to take antihypertensive medications as prescribed.
    3. Tell the client to check and record their blood pressure readings daily.
    4. Encourage the client to walk at least 30 minutes three times a week.

31. Which action by the unlicensed assistive personnel (UAP) indicates to the nurse the UAP understands the correct procedure for applying compression stockings to the client recovering from a pulmonary embolus?
    1. The UAP instructs the client to sit in the chair when applying the stockings.
    2. The UAP cannot insert one finger under the proximal end of the stocking.
    3. The UAP ensures the toe opening is placed on the top side of the feet.
    4. The UAP checked to make sure the client's toes were warm after putting the stockings on.

32. The home health (HH) nurse enters the yard of a client and is bitten on the leg by the client's dog. Which intervention should the nurse implement first?
    1. Clean the dog bite with soap and water and apply antibiotic ointment.
    2. Obtain the phone number and contact the client's veterinarian.
    3. Contact the HH care agency and complete an occurrence report.
    4. Ask the client whether the dog has had all the required vaccinations.

33. The nurse on the vascular unit is caring for a client diagnosed with arterial occlusive disease. Which statement by the client warrants immediate intervention by the nurse?
    1. "My legs start to hurt when I walk to check my mail."
    2. "My legs were so cold I had to put a heating pad on them."
    3. "I hang my legs off the side of my bed when I sleep."
    4. "I noticed that the hair on my feet and up my leg is gone."

34. The home health (HH) nurse has completed a home assessment on a client and finds out there are no smoke detectors in the home. The client tells the nurse they just cannot afford them. Which action should the nurse implement first?
    1. Purchase at least one smoke detector for the client's home.
    2. Notify the HH care agency social worker to discuss the situation.
    3. Ask the client whether a family member could buy a smoke detector.
    4. Contact the local fire department to see if they can provide smoke detectors for the client.

35. The nurse is admitting a 72-year-old female client and notes multiple bruises on the face, arms, and legs along with possible cigarette burns on her upper arms. The client states she fell on an ashtray and doesn't want to talk about it. Which nursing intervention is priority?
    1. Document the objective findings in the client's chart.
    2. Tell the client she must talk about the situation with the nurse.
    3. Report the situation to the Adult Protective Services.
    4. Take photographs of the bruises and cigarette burns.

36. The nurse is admitting a client diagnosed with deep vein thrombosis (DVT) in the right leg. Which statement by the client warrants immediate intervention by the nurse?
    1. "I take a baby aspirin every day at breakfast."
    2. "I have ordered myself a medical alert bracelet."
    3. "I eat spinach and greens at least twice a week."
    4. "I got a new recliner so I can elevate my legs."

37. The male client with peripheral vascular disease tells the nurse, "I know my foot is really bad. My doctor told me I don't have any choice and I must have an amputation, but I don't want one." Which action supports the nurse being a client advocate?
    1. Support the medical treatment, and recommend the client have the amputation.
    2. Recommend the client talk to his wife and children about his decision.
    3. Explain to the client that he has a right to a second opinion if he doesn't want an amputation.
    4. Tell the client she will go with him to discuss his decision with the doctor.

38. The charge nurse observes the unlicensed assistive personnel (UAP) crying after the death of a client. Which is the charge nurse's best response to the UAP?
    1. "If you cry every time a client dies, you won't last long on the unit."
    2. "It can be difficult when a client dies. Would you like to take a break?"
    3. "You need to stop crying and go on about your responsibilities."
    4. "Did you not realize that clients die in a healthcare facility?"

39. The nursing staff confronts the hospice nurse overseeing the care of a client in a long-term care facility. The nursing staff wants to send the client who is diagnosed with gangrene of the left leg secondary to peripheral occlusive disease to the hospital for treatment. Which intervention should the nurse implement first?
    1. Check with the client to see whether or not the client wants to go to a hospital.
    2. Explain that the client can be kept comfortable at the long-term care facility.
    3. Discuss the hospice concept of comfort measures only with the staff.
    4. Call a client care conference immediately to discuss the conflict.

40. The client diagnosed with an abdominal aortic aneurysm died unexpectedly, and the nurse must notify the significant other. Which statement made by the nurse is the best over the telephone?
    1. "I am sorry to tell you, but your loved one has died."
    2. "Could you come to the hospital? The client is not doing well."
    3. "The HCP has asked me to tell you of your family member's death."
    4. "Do you know whether the client wished to be an organ donor?"

41. The nurse has been pulled from a medical unit to work on the vascular unit for the shift. Which client should the charge nurse assign to the medical unit nurse?
    1. The client with the femoral-popliteal bypass who has paraesthesia of the foot.
    2. The client with an abdominal aortic aneurysm who is complaining of low back pain.
    3. The client newly diagnosed with chronic venous insufficiency who needs teaching.
    4. The client with varicose veins who is complaining of deep, aching pain of the legs.

42. The charge nurse in the vascular intensive care unit assigns three clients to the staff nurse. The staff nurse thinks this is an unsafe assignment. Which action should the staff nurse implement first?
    1. Refuse to take the assignment and leave the hospital immediately.
    2. Tell the supervisor that he or she is concerned about the unsafe assignment.
    3. Document his or her concerns in writing and give it to the supervisor.
    4. Take the assignment for the shift but turn in his or her resignation.

43. At 2230, the nurse is preparing to administer pain medication to a male client who rates his pain as a 4 on the numeric pain scale. Which medication should the nurse administer?

Client: Mr. C	Admit Number: 432165		Allergies: Ibuprofen
Date: Today	Height: 65 inches Weight: 64.2 kg 141.2 pounds		Diagnosis: Chronic vein insufficiency
Medication	0701–1500	1501–2300	2301–0700
Morphine sulfate mg IVP q 2 hours PRN	0930 DN2		
Promethazine (Phenergan) 12.5 mg IVP q 4 hours PRN		1845 EN	
Prochlorperazine (Compazine) 5 mg PO tid PRN			
Hydrocodone (Vicodin) 5 mg PO q 4–6 hours PRN		1730 EN	
Ibuprofen (Motrin) 600 mg PO q 3–4 hours PRN			
Nurse's Name/Initials	Day Nurse RN/DN	Evening Nurse RN/EN	Night Nurse RN/NN

1. Administer morphine 2 mg IVP.
2. Administer promethazine 12.5 mg IVP.
3. Administer hydrocodone 5 mg PO.
4. Administer ibuprofen 600 mg PO.

44. The matriarch of a family has died on the vascular unit. The family tells the nurse the daughter is coming to the hospital from a nearby city to see the body. Which intervention should the nurse implement?
1. Plan to allow the daughter to see the client in the room.
2. Take the client to the morgue for the daughter to view.
3. Request the family call the daughter and tell her not to come.
4. Explain to the daughter that the unit is too busy for family visitation.

45. The unit manager on the vascular unit is planning a change in the way post-mortem care is provided. Which is the first step in the change process?
1. Collect data.
2. Identify the problem.
3. Select an alternative.
4. Implement a plan.

46. The nurse is preparing to administer the third unit of packed red blood cells (PRBCs) to a client with a ruptured aortic aneurysm. Which interventions should the nurse implement? **Select all that apply.**
1. Hang a bag of D₅NS to keep open (TKO).
2. Change the blood administration set.
3. Check the client's current vital signs.
4. Assess for allergies to blood products.
5. Obtain a blood warmer for the blood.

47. The nurse and the unlicensed assistive personnel (UAP) are caring for clients on a vascular unit. Which task should the nurse delegate to the UAP?
1. Apply bilateral sequential compression devices to the client with deep vein thrombosis.
2. Accompany the client with thromboangiitis obliterans outside to smoke a cigarette.
3. Elevate the leg of the client who is one day postoperative femoral-popliteal bypass.
4. Perform Doppler studies on the client with right upper extremity lymphedema.

48. The charge nurse on a vascular postsurgical unit observes a new graduate telling an elderly client's spouse not to push the client's patient-controlled analgesia (PCA) pump button. Which action should the charge nurse implement?
1. Encourage the visitor to push the button for the client.
2. Ask the nurse to step into the hallway to discuss the situation.
3. Discuss the hospital protocol for the use of PCA pumps.
4. Continue to perform the charge nurse's other duties.

49. Which client should the nurse assess first after receiving the shift report?
1. The client with a right above-the-knee amputation who is complaining of right foot pain.
2. The client with arterial hypertension who is complaining of a severe headache.
3. The client with lymphedema who has 4+ pitting edema of the left lower leg.
4. The client with gangrene of the right foot who has a foul-smelling discharge.

50. The nurse observes an LPN crushing nifedipine (Procardia XL) before administering the medication to a client with arterial hypertension who has difficulty swallowing pills. Which intervention should the nurse implement first?
1. Tell the LPN to take the client's blood pressure.
2. Take no action since this is appropriate behaviour.
3. Show the LPN where to find pudding for the client.
4. Tell the LPN this medication cannot be crushed.

51. A 90-year-old male client was recently widowed after more than 60 years of marriage. The client was admitted to a long-term care facility and is refusing to eat. Which intervention is an example of the ethical principle of autonomy?
1. Place a nasogastric feeding tube and feed the client.
2. Discuss why the client does not want to eat anymore.
3. Arrange for the family to bring food for the client.
4. Allow the client to refuse to eat if he wants to.

52. The nurse is admitting a client with an abdominal aortic aneurysm who is a member of the Church of Jesus Christ of Latter-Day Saints (Mormon). Which action by the nurse indicates cultural sensitivity to the client?
1. The nurse does not insist on administering a blood transfusion.
2. The nurse pins the client's amulet to the client's pillow.
3. The nurse keeps the client's undershirt on during the bath.
4. The nurse notifies the client's curandero of the admission.

53. Which client should the nurse on the vascular unit assess first after receiving the shift report?
1. The client with lymphedema whose ABG results are pH 7.33, PaO_2 89, $PaCO_2$ 47, HCO_3 25.
2. The client with Raynaud's phenomenon who has bluish cold upper extremities.
3. The client with chronic venous insufficiency who has an ulcerated area on the right foot.
4. The client receiving intravenous heparin infusion who has a PTT on 78.

54. The charge nurse of a long-term care facility is making assignments. Which client should be assigned to the most experienced unlicensed assistive personnel (UAP)?
    1. The client with arterial occlusive disease who must dangle the legs off the side of the bed.
    2. The client with congestive heart failure who is angry about the family not visiting.
    3. The client with an above the knee amputation who needs a full body lift to get in the wheelchair.
    4. The client with Buerger's disease who is particular about the way things are done.

55. The client complains of chest pain on deep inspiration. Which intervention should the nurse implement first?
    1. Place the client on oxygen.
    2. Assess the client's lungs.
    3. Notify the respiratory therapist.
    4. Assess the client's pulse oximeter reading.

56. Which of the staff nurse's personal attributes is an important consideration for the unit manager when discussing making an experienced nurse a preceptor for new graduates? **Select all that apply.**
    1. The nurse's need for the monetary stipend.
    2. The nurse's ability to organize the work.
    3. The ability of the nurse to interact with others.
    4. The quality of care the nurse provides.
    5. The nurse's willingness to be a preceptor.

57. The nurse just received the a.m. shift report. Which client should the nurse assess first?
    1. The client who is 6 hours post-op vein ligation who has absent pedal pulses.
    2. The client diagnosed with deep vein thrombosis who is complaining of calf pain.
    3. The client with Raynaud's disease who has throbbing and tingling in the extremities.
    4. The client with Buerger's disease who has intermittent claudication of the feet and arms.

58. The intensive care department nurse is calculating the total intake for a client diagnosed with hypertensive crisis. The client has received 950 mL of D_5W, 2 IVPB of 100 mL of 0.9% NS, 16 ounces of water, 8 ounces of milk, and 6 ounces of chicken broth. The client has had a urinary output of 2,200 mL. What is the total intake for this client? _____

59. The nurse is teaching the client diagnosed with arterial occlusive disease. Which statement indicates the client needs more teaching?
    1. "I will wash my legs and feet daily in warm water."
    2. "I should buy my shoes in the afternoon."
    3. "I must wear knee-high stockings."
    4. "I should not elevate my legs."

60. The nurse is caring for clients on a vascular unit. Which nursing task is most appropriate to delegate to an unlicensed assistive personnel (UAP)?
    1. Tell the UAP to obtain the glucometer reading of the client who is dizzy and lightheaded.
    2. Request the UAP to elevate the feet of the client with chronic venous insufficiency.
    3. Ask the UAP to take the vital signs of the client who has numbness of the right arm.
    4. Instruct the UAP to administer a tap water enema to the client with an aorta aneurysm.

61. A client is 2 days postoperative abdominal aortic aneurysm repair. Which data require immediate intervention from the nurse?
    1. The client refuses to take deep breaths and cough.
    2. The client's urinary output is 300 mL in 8 hours.
    3. The client has hypoactive bowel sounds.
    4. The client's vital signs are T 98, P 68, R 16, and BP 110/70.

62. The nurse is caring for clients on a vascular surgical floor. Which client should be assessed first?
    1. The client who is 2 days postoperative right below-the-knee amputation who has phantom pain in the right foot.
    2. The client who is 1 day postoperative abdominal aortic aneurysm who is complaining of numbness and tingling of both feet.
    3. The client with superficial thrombophlebitis of the left arm who is complaining of tenderness to the touch.
    4. The client with arterial occlusive disease who is complaining of calf pain when ambulating down the hall.

63. The nurse is caring for a client receiving heparin sodium via constant infusion. The heparin protocol reads to increase the IV rate by 100 units/hour if the PTT is less than 50 seconds. The current PTT level is 46 seconds. The heparin comes in 500 mL of D_5W with 25,000 units of heparin added. The current rate on the IV pump is 20 mL per hour. At what rate should the nurse set the pump? _____

64. The unlicensed assistive personnel (UAP) is caring for a client diagnosed with chronic venous insufficiency. Which action would warrant immediate intervention from the nurse?
    1. The UAP assists the client to apply compression stockings.
    2. The UAP elevates the client's leg while sitting in the recliner.
    3. The UAP assists the client to the bathroom for a.m. care.
    4. The UAP is cutting the client's toenails after soaking the client's feet in tepid water.

65. The nurse has just received the a.m. shift report. Which client would the nurse assess first?
    1. The client with a venous stasis ulcer who is refusing to eat the high protein meal.
    2. The client with varicose veins who is refusing to wear thromboembolic hose.
    3. The client with arterial occlusive disease who is refusing to elevate their legs.
    4. The client with deep vein thrombosis who is refusing to stay in the bed.

66. At 1000 a client who has had femoral popliteal surgery on the right leg is complaining of severe right upper quadrant pain of 10 out of 10 on the pain scale. Based on the information in the chart below, what should the nurse do for the client?

Client Name: Mr. B.A.	Account Number: 0101223		Allergies: Codeine	
Height: 72 inches	Weight in pounds: 220 Weight in kg: 100		Date of Birth: 02/05/1982	
Date: Today	Medication Morphine Sulfate 2 mg IVP every 4 hour PRN pain	2301–0700 0445 NN	0701–1500 0845DN	1501–2300
	Oxycodone 7.5/ acetaminophen 325 mg PO every 3 hours PRN pain	0030 NN 0545 NN		
	Maalox 30 mL PO PRN indigestion			
	Nitroglycerin 0.4 mg SL every 5 minutes up to 3 tablets PRN Chest pain			
Signature/Initials		Night Nurse RN/NN	Day Nurse RN/DN	

    1. Administer the oxycodone and acetaminophen PO.
    2. Help the client to practice guided imagery for the pain.
    3. Call the surgeon for an increase in pain medication.
    4. Administer a dose of morphine to the client.

67. The client on a surgical unit is scheduled to receive an antibiotic piggyback over 1 hour. The piggyback is prepared in 150 mL of solution. At what rate should the nurse set the piggyback if the administration set delivers 20 drops per mL? _____

68. The client in the day surgical unit is scheduled to have vein ligation on the right leg. The client states, "I am having surgery on my left leg." Which intervention should the nurse implement first?
1. Have the client sign the surgical operative permit.
2. Assess the client's neurological status.
3. Ask when the client last took a drink of water or ate anything.
4. Call a time out until clarifying which leg is having the vein ligation.

69. The 63-year-old client is diagnosed with an abdominal aortic aneurysm. Which area on the figure should the nurse place a stethoscope to assess for a bruit?

1. A
2. B
3. C
4. D

70. The male post-op femoral popliteal client notifies the desk via the intercom system he has fallen and is now bleeding. Which interventions should the nurse implement? Rank in order of performance.
1. Apply pressure directly to the bleeding site.
2. Notify the surgeon of the fall and the bleeding.
3. Redress the site with a sterile dressing.
4. Assist the client to a recumbent position in the bed.
5. Make out an occurrence report and document the fall.

PERIPHERAL VASCULAR DISEASE CLINICAL SCENARIO

DH is the charge nurse on a medical unit. She has three primary nurses, JC, who has been a nurse on the unit for 12 years; BN, who has been on the unit for 1 year; and PN, who is a new graduate. There are 3 UAPs, BA, BE, and AM.

1. JC just received the a.m. shift report. Which client should JC assess first?
   1. The client diagnosed with coronary artery disease who has a BP of 170/100.
   2. The client diagnosed with deep vein thrombosis who is complaining of calf pain.
   3. The client diagnosed with arterial occlusive disease who has intermittent claudication.
   4. The client diagnosed with aortic abdominal aneurysm who has low back pain.

2. Which assessment data would warrant immediate intervention by DH, charge nurse for the client diagnosed with arterial occlusive disease?
   1. The client has decreased hair on his or her calf.
   2. The client has no palpable dorsal pedal pulse.
   3. The client has paralysis and parasthesia.
   4. The client hangs his or her legs off the side of bed.

3. The nurse and the unlicensed assistive personnel (UAP) are caring for a client who is 4 hours postoperative right femoral–popliteal bypass surgery. Which nursing task should JC delegate to the UAP?
   1. Check the client's pedal pulse with the Doppler.
   2. Assist the client to ambulate down the hall.
   3. Review the client's neurovascular assessment.
   4. Elevate the client's leg on two pillows.

4. Which interventions should DH discuss with the client diagnosed with atherosclerosis? **Select all that apply.**
   1. Take a baby aspirin daily.
   2. Eat a low-fat, low-cholesterol diet.
   3. Maintain a sedentary lifestyle as much as possible.
   4. Decrease all foods high in fiber.
   5. Walk 30 minutes a day at least 3 days a week.

5. The client is 2 days postoperative abdominal aortic aneurysm. Which intervention should BN implement first when making initial rounds?
   1. Auscultate the client's bowel sounds.
   2. Assess the client's surgical dressing.
   3. Encourage the client to splint the incision.
   4. Monitor the client's intravenous therapy.

6. The client is diagnosed with a small abdominal aortic aneurysm. Which statement by the client indicates to BN the client needs more discharge teaching?
   1. "I should not lift more than 5 pounds for at least 4 to 6 weeks."
   2. "I attend a support group to help me quit smoking."
   3. "I will need to wear a truss at all times after the surgery."
   4. "If I get a temperature of 101 or higher I will call my doctor."

7. PN is assigned the following clients. Which client should PN assess first?
   1. The client who is 4 days postoperative abdominal surgery and is complaining of abdominal pain when ambulating.
   2. The client who 1 day postoperative femoral-popliteal repair has a 3+ posterior tibial pulse.
   3. The client who had an abdominal aortic repair who had a urine output of 150 mL in the last 8 hours.
   4. The client with deep vein thrombosis who is complaining about being unable to get out of the bed.

8. PN is caring for a client receiving heparin sodium via constant infusion. The heparin protocol reads to decrease the IV rate by 100 units/hour if the PTT is between 78 to 90 seconds. The current PTT level is 85 seconds. The heparin comes in 500 mL of D_5W with 25,000 units of heparin added. The current rate on the IV pump is 18 mL per hour. At what rate should the nurse set the pump? _____

9. The unlicensed assistive personnel (UAP) is caring for the client diagnosed with chronic venous insufficiency. Which action would warrant immediate intervention by PN?
   1. The UAP is elevating the client's legs on two pillows.
   2. The UAP is massaging the client's calf muscles.
   3. The UAP is instructing the client to stay in the bed.
   4. The UAP is calculating the client's shift intake and output.

10. An 80-year-old client is being discharged home after having surgery to débride a chronic venous ulcer on the right ankle. Which referral is most appropriate for DH, the charge nurse, to make?
    1. Hospice.
    2. Home health.
    3. Physical therapist.
    4. Cardiac rehabilitation.

ANSWERS AND RATIONALES

The correct answer number and rationale for why it is the correct answer are given in **boldface type.** Rationales for why the other possible answer options are incorrect also are given, but they are not in boldface type.

1. 1. Intermittent claudication is a symptom of arterial occlusive disease; therefore, this client does not need to be assessed first.

   2. The client with calf pain could be experiencing deep vein thrombosis (DVT), a complication of immobility, which may be fatal if a pulmonary embolus occurs; therefore, this client should be assessed first.

   3. The client experiencing low back pain when sitting in a chair should be assessed but not prior to the client with suspected DVT.

   4. The nurse should address the client's concern about the food, but it is not priority over a physiological problem.

   Content – Medical/Surgical: **Category of Health Alteration** *– Peripheral Vascular:* **Integrated Processes** *– Nursing Process: Assessment:* **Client Needs** *– Physiological Integrity: Reduction of Risk Potential:* **Cognitive Level** *– Analysis*

MAKING NURSING DECISIONS: When deciding which client to assess first, the test taker should determine whether the signs/symptoms the client is exhibiting are normal or expected for the client situation. After eliminating the expected options, the test taker should determine which situation is more life threatening.

2. 1. **Therapeutic levels for PTT should be 1½ to 2 times the normal value, which is 39 seconds; therefore, this client is at risk for bleeding. The prolonged PTT indicates the client is receiving heparin (drug of choice to treat DVT). The nurse should stop the infusion and follow the facility protocol.**

   2. The hemoglobin is within normal range and the client with Raynaud's disease does not have a problem with bleeding.

   3. The WBC count is elevated (normal is 5,000 to 10,000), but it would be elevated in a client who has an infection such as venous stasis ulcer.

   4. The nurse should notify the HCP on rounds of any laboratory data that are abnormal but not immediately life threatening. The triglyceride level is high, but it will take weeks to

months of a heart healthy diet, exercise, and possibly medications to lower this level.

Content – Medical/Surgical: **Category of Health Alteration** *– Peripheral Vascular:* **Integrated Processes** *– Nursing: Implementation:* **Client Needs** *– Safe and Effective Care Environment: Safety and Infection Control:* **Cognitive Level** *– Synthesis*

MAKING NURSING DECISIONS: When a question asks for immediate intervention, the test taker must decide whether there is an intervention the nurse can implement immediately or whether the HCP must be notified. If the data are abnormal—but not life threatening—then the option can be eliminated as a possible correct answer.

3. 1. The nurse should first assess the client to determine the status prior to notifying the HCP.

   2. The unlisted assistive personnel (UAP) has notified the nurse of a potentially serious situation. The nurse must first assess the client prior to taking any action.

   3 The nurse might place the client in Trendelenburg position once cardiovascular shock is determined.

   4. The nurse should immediately go to the client's room to assess the client.

   Content – Medical/Surgical: **Category of Health Alteration** *– Peripheral Vascular:* **Integrated Processes** *– Nursing Process: Assessment:* **Client Needs** *– Physiological Integrity: Reduction of Risk Potential:* **Cognitive Level** *– Analysis*

MAKING NURSING DECISIONS: Any time the nurse receives information about a client (who may be experiencing a complication) from another staff member, the nurse must assess the client. The nurse should not make decisions about the client's needs based on another staff member's information.

4. 1. **Because laboratory values called into a unit usually include critical values, the charge nurse should tell the unit secretary "to show me any lab information that is called in immediately." The charge nurse must evaluate this information immediately.**

   2. Posting laboratory results is the responsibility of the laboratory staff, not the nursing staff.

   3. This is unrealistic because laboratory data are important information that must be called in to a unit when there is a critical value so that immediate action can be taken for the client's

welfare. The secretary must know how to process the information.

4. The unit secretary should verify the information by repeating back the information at the time of the call, not by making a second telephone call to the lab.

Content – Medical/Surgical: ***Category of Health Alteration*** *– Peripheral Vascular:* ***Integrated Processes** – Nursing Process: Planning:* ***Client Needs*** *– Safe and Effective Care Environment: Management of Care:* ***Cognitive Level*** *– Synthesis*

MAKING NURSING DECISIONS: The test taker must be knowledgeable of the roles of all members of the multidisciplinary healthcare team, as well as HIPAA rules and regulations. The nurse must ensure the healthcare team member knows appropriate actions to take in specific situations. These will be tested on the NCLEX-RN®.

5. 1. **Vitamin K is the antidote for warfarin (Coumadin) overdose and is administered to a client when his or her INR level is above the therapeutic 2–3; therefore, the nurse should question administering this medication.**
2. Inderal is administered to clients diagnosed with hypertension; therefore, the nurse would not question administering this medication.
3. Procardia reduces the number of vasospastic attacks in clients with Raynaud's disease; therefore, the nurse should question administering this medication to a client with hypotension.
4. Vasotec, an ACE inhibitor, is administered to clients with diabetes to help prevent diabetic nephropathy. The nurse would not question administering this medication.

Content – Medical/Surgical: ***Category of Health Alteration*** *– Peripheral Vascular:* ***Integrated Processes** – Nursing Process: Assessment:* ***Client Needs*** *– Safe and Effective Care Environment: Safety and Infection Control:* ***Cognitive Level*** *– Analysis*

MAKING NURSING DECISIONS: The nurse must be aware of interventions that must be implemented prior to administering medications. The nurse must know what to monitor prior to administering medications because untoward reactions and possibly death can occur.

6. 1. **This client is exhibiting signs/symptoms of a potentially fatal complication of DVT—pulmonary embolism. The nurse should assess this client first.**
2. Intermittent claudication of the feet, hands, and arms is a symptom of Buerger's disease; therefore, this client should not be assessed first.

3. The client with an aortic aneurysm is expected to have an audible bruit and does not indicate any life-threatening condition; therefore, this client does not need to be assessed first.
4. The client with acute arterial ischemia should have unpalpable pedal pulses to be considered a medical emergency; therefore, this client does not need to be assessed first.

Content – Medical/Surgical: ***Category of Health Alteration*** *– Peripheral Vascular:* ***Integrated Processes** – Nursing Process: Assessment:* ***Client Needs*** *– Physiological Integrity: Reduction of Risk Potential:* ***Cognitive Level*** *– Analysis*

MAKING NURSING DECISIONS: The test taker must determine which sign/symptom is not expected for the disease process. If the sign/symptom is not expected, then the nurse should assess the client first. This type of question is determining if the nurse is knowledgeable of the signs/symptoms of a variety of disease processes.

7. 1. **Because the client has been on the daily aspirin for more than a year, the nurse should assess for bleeding by asking questions such as, "Do your gums bleed after brushing teeth?" or "Do you notice blood when you blow your nose?"**
2. Because aspirin can cause gastric distress, the nurse could instruct the client to stop taking it; however, because this is a daily medication being used as an antiplatelet agent, the nurse should provide information that would allow the client to continue the medication.
3. The nurse should realize the stomach discomfort is probably secondary to daily aspirin, and enteric-coated aspirin would be helpful to decrease the stomach discomfort and allow the client to stay on the medication, but the nurse should first assess the client for bleeding.
4. Because aspirin is not a prescription medication, the nurse can recommend a different form of aspirin, such as one that is enteric coated. However, if the enteric-coated aspirin does not relieve the pain, the HCP should then be notified.

Content – Medical/Surgical: ***Category of Health Alteration*** *– Peripheral Vascular:* ***Integrated Processes** – Nursing Process: Assessment:* ***Client Needs*** *– Physiological Integrity: Reduction of Risk Potential:* ***Cognitive Level*** *– Analysis*

MAKING NURSING DECISIONS: Assessment is the first step of the nursing process, and the test taker should use the nursing process or some other systematic process to assist in determining priorities.

8. 1. This statement indicates the new graduate needs more teaching because the nurse is responsible for delegating the right task to the right individual. Absolutely no one works on the nurse's license but the nurse holding the license.

2. The nurse does retain accountability for the task delegated; therefore, the new graduate does not need more teaching.

3. The nurse must make sure the unlicensed assistive personnel (UAP) is able to perform the task safely and competently; therefore, the new graduate does not need more teaching.

4. The nurse must make sure the delegated task was completed correctly; therefore, the new graduate does not need more teaching.

Content – Medical/Surgical: ***Category of Health Alteration*** *– Peripheral Vascular:* ***Integrated Processes*** *– Nursing Process: Planning:* ***Client Needs*** *– Safe and Effective Care Environment: Management of Care:* ***Cognitive Level*** *– Synthesis*

MAKING NURSING DECISIONS: An RN cannot delegate assessment, teaching, evaluation, medications, or an unstable client to a UAP. Tasks that cannot be delegated are nursing interventions requiring nursing judgment. The nurse must be aware of delegation rules and regulations.

9. 1. The manufacturer of a product would provide biased information and would not provide the best data to support a change proposal.

2. Research studies with a limited number of participants indicate the need for further research and would not be the best research to support a change proposal.

3. Research should provide clear statistical data that support the research problem or hypothesis.

4. **The more research articles there are that support a change proposal, the more valid is the information, which increases the possibility for change to be considered by the healthcare facility.**

Content – Medical/Surgical: ***Category of Health Alteration*** *– Peripheral Vascular:* ***Integrated Processes*** *– Nursing Process: Evaluation:* ***Client Needs*** *– Physiological Integrity: Reduction of Risk Potential:* ***Cognitive Level*** *– Knowledge*

MAKING NURSING DECISIONS: The NCLEX-RN® blueprint includes nursing care based on evidence-based practice. The nurse must be knowledgeable of nursing research.

10. 1. The unlicensed assistive personnel (UAP) can clean the perineal area of a client who is on bed rest and who has an indwelling catheter. Because the client is stable, this nursing task could be delegated to the UAP.

2. The UAP can obtain the client's intake and output, but the nurse must evaluate the data to determine whether interventions are needed or whether interventions are effective.

3. A client who is third-spacing is unstable and in a life-threatening situation; therefore, the nurse cannot delegate the UAP to give this client a bath.

4. This is a medication enema, and the UAP cannot administer medications. In addition, if a cation-exchange resin enema is ordered, the client is unstable and has excessively high serum potassium (K^+) level.

Content – Medical/Surgical: ***Category of Health Alteration*** *– Peripheral Vascular:* ***Integrated Processes*** *– Nursing Process: Planning:* ***Client Needs*** *– Safe and Effective Care Environment: Management of Care:* ***Cognitive Level*** *– Synthesis*

MAKING NURSING DECISIONS: An RN cannot delegate assessment, teaching, evaluation, medications, or an unstable client to a UAP. Tasks that cannot be delegated are nursing interventions requiring nursing judgment.

11. 1. Although the nurse could request another unlicensed assistive personnel (UAP) to perform the task, this is not the best action because the nurse should demonstrate applying SCDs so that the UAP can learn how to complete the task.

2. **This is the priority action because the nurse will ensure the UAP knows how to apply SCDs correctly, thereby enabling the nurse to delegate the task to the UAP successfully in the future.**

3. The nurse could do the task, but if the UAP is not shown how to do it, then the UAP will not be able to perform the task the next time it is delegated.

4. The UAP could watch a video demonstrating this task, but the priority action is that the nurse should demonstrate SCD application to the UAP.

Content – Medical/Surgical: ***Category of Health Alteration*** *– Peripheral Vascular:* ***Integrated Processes*** *– Nursing Process: Implementation:* ***Client Needs*** *– Safe and Effective Care Environment: Safety and Infection Control:* ***Cognitive Level*** *– Application*

MAKING NURSING DECISIONS: The nurse cannot delegate any task in which the UAP admits to not being able to perform. It is the nurse's responsibility to know what can be delegated and

when. **The nurse may have to complete the task if the UAP is not competent to do so.**

12. 1. The nurse should not assign assessment of a client to an LPN even if the client is stable.

2. The LPN cannot initiate administration of blood; therefore, this task must be completed by the nurse.

3. **The LPN can administer medications; therefore, the LPN could hang a bag of heparin on an IV pump to this client.**

4. The nurse must assess for dysrhythmias during the insertion, and the nurse assisting the HCP should be experienced in inserting the line. An LPN pulled from another unit should not be assigned this task.

Content – *Medical/Surgical:* **Category of Health Alteration** – *Peripheral Vascular:* **Integrated Processes** – *Nursing Process: Planning:* **Client Needs** – *Safe and Effective Care Environment: Management of Care:* **Cognitive Level** – *Synthesis*

MAKING NURSING DECISIONS: The nurse cannot assign assessment, teaching, evaluation, or an unstable client to a LPN. The LPN can transcribe HCP orders and can call HCPs on the phone to obtain orders for a client.

13. 1. The client is having signs/symptoms of a blood transfusion reaction. The nurse must stop the transfusion immediately and then assess the client's vital signs.

2. The HCP needs to be notified, but not before the nurse stops the blood transfusion.

3. The nurse should maintain a patent IV so that medications can be administered, but this is not the first intervention.

4. **Any time the nurse suspects the client is having a reaction to blood or blood products, the nurse should stop the infusion at the spot closest to the client and not allow any more of the blood to enter the client's body. This is the nurse's first intervention.**

Content – *Medical/Surgical:* **Category of Health Alteration** – *Peripheral Vascular:* **Integrated Processes** – *Nursing Process: Implementation:* **Client Needs** – *Physiological Integrity: Reduction of Risk Potential:* **Cognitive Level** – *Application*

MAKING NURSING DECISIONS: The nurse should remember: If a client is in distress and the nurse can do something to relieve the distress, it should be done first, before assessment. The test taker should select an option that directly helps the client's condition.

14. 1. A research article should answer the question "why": Why was the research done? This

statement indicates the charge nurse understands how to read a research article.

2. **The cost of the research is not pertinent when reading a research article and determining whether the research supports evidence-based practice. This statement indicates the charge nurse does not understand how to read a research article.**

3. A research article should answer the question "what": What research method was used? This statement indicates the charge nurse understands how to read a research article.

4. A research article should answer the question "where": In what setting was the research conducted? This statement indicates the charge nurse understands how to read a research article.

Content – *Medical/Surgical:* **Category of Health Alteration** – *Peripheral Vascular:* **Integrated Processes** – *Nursing Process: Evaluation:* **Client Needs** – *Safe and Effective Care Environment: Management of Care:* **Cognitive Level** – *Application*

MAKING NURSING DECISIONS: The NCLEX-RN® blueprint includes nursing care based on evidence-based practice. The nurse must be knowledgeable of nursing research.

15. 1. The nurse should write the order on the HCP's order and write "per telephone order (TO)," but this is not the nurse's first intervention.

2. The nurse does not need to have another nurse verify the HCP's telephone order.

3. **The Joint Commission has implemented this requirement for all telephone orders. The nurse should document on the HCP's order "repeat order verified."**

4. The nurse should transcribe the order to the MAR, but it is not the first intervention.

Content – *Medical/Surgical:* **Category of Health Alteration** – *Peripheral Vascular:* **Integrated Processes** – *Nursing Process: Implementation:* **Client Needs** – *Safe and Effective Care Environment: Management of Care:* **Cognitive Level** – *Knowledge*

MAKING NURSING DECISIONS: The NCLEX-RN® blueprint includes nursing care that is ruled by legal requirements as well as rules and regulations of the Joint Commission, Centers for Medicare & Medicaid Services, Centers for Disease Control and Prevention, and the Occupational Safety and Health Administration. The nurse must be knowledgeable of these standards.

16. 1. The therapeutic level for a client on warfarin (Coumadin) is an INR of 2 to 3; therefore, this client does not warrant intervention.

2. These hemoglobin/hematocrit levels are a little low but not so critical that this would warrant intervention by the charge nurse.

3. **A platelet count of less than 100,000 per milliliter of blood indicates thrombocytopenia; therefore, this client warrants intervention by the charge nurse.**

4. This is a normal red blood cell count; therefore, the charge nurse would not need to intervene.

Content – Medical/Surgical: ***Category of Health Alteration*** *– Peripheral Vascular:* ***Integrated Processes –*** *Nursing Process: Assessment:* ***Client Needs*** *– Physiological Integrity, Reduction of Risk Potential:* ***Cognitive Level*** *– Synthesis*

MAKING NURSING DECISIONS: The nurse must be knowledgeable of normal laboratory values. These values must be memorized and the nurse must be able to determine if the laboratory value is normal for the client's disease process or medications the client is taking.

17. 1. This statement is not supporting the night shift and makes the unit look bad. The nurse should not "bad-mouth" the night shift.

2. The nurse has no idea what happened that delayed answering the call light; it could have been a code or other type of life-threatening situation. The day shift primary nurse may not be able to answer the light in some certain situations and should not falsely reassure the client.

3. **The nurse should have someone come talk to the client who is in a position to then investigate what happened on the night shift and determine why this happened. The day shift primary nurse does not have this authority.**

4. This is negating the client's feeling, and the client does not need to know what was going on in the critical care unit.

Content – Medical/Surgical: ***Category of Health Alteration*** *– Peripheral Vascular:* ***Integrated Processes –*** *Nursing Process: Implementation:* ***Client Needs*** *– Physiological Integrity: Basic Care and Comfort:* ***Cognitive Level*** *– Application*

MAKING NURSING DECISIONS: There will be management questions on the NCLEX-RN®. In many instances, there is no test-taking strategy for these questions; the nurse must be knowledgeable of management issues.

18. **Correct Answer: 3, 2, 1, 4, 5**

3. **The client must agree to the risks and benefits of a blood transfusion before the nurse can administer the blood product. This is the first intervention.**

2. **The nurse has only 30 minutes from the time the blood is retrieved from the blood bank until the transfusion is initiated. The nurse should make sure the client has a patent IV access before obtaining the blood from the blood bank.**

1. **The nurse can obtain the unit of packed cells when the client has signed the permit and has a patent IV access.**

4. **The nurse should always check the blood product with another nurse at the client's bedside against the client's hospital identification band and blood bank crossmatch band.**

5. **After the nurse has followed the procedure to ensure the correct blood product is being administered, with a second nurse then the transfusion of packed cells can be initiated. The blood is initiated at a slow rate—10 mL per hour for the first 15 minutes—so that the nurse can observe the client for potential complications.**

Content – Medical/Surgical: ***Category of Health Alteration*** *– Peripheral Vascular:* ***Integrated Processes –*** *Nursing Process: Implementation:* ***Client Needs*** *– Safe and Effective Care Environment: Management of Care:* ***Cognitive Level*** *– Application*

MAKING NURSING DECISIONS: This is an alternate type of question included in the NCLEX-RN® blueprint. The nurse must be able to perform skills in the correct order. Obtaining informed consent and performing an assessment should always be the first interventions.

19. 1. This should be an anticipated order if the nurse suspects a pulmonary embolus, but it is not the first intervention.

2. **The nurse should suspect the client has a pulmonary embolus, a complication of the thrombophlebitis. Pulmonary emboli decrease the oxygen supply to the body, and the nurse should immediately administer oxygen to the client.**

3. An anticoagulant infusion will be ordered for the client once it is determined that the client is experiencing a pulmonary embolus.

4. Getting oxygen to the body is a priority; telling the client not to ambulate can be done after initiating the oxygen.

Content – Medical/Surgical: ***Category of Health Alteration*** *– Peripheral Vascular:* ***Integrated Processes –*** *Nursing Process: Implementation:* ***Client Needs*** *– Physiological Integrity: Reduction of Risk Potential:* ***Cognitive Level*** *– Application*

MAKING NURSING DECISIONS: Physiological problems have the highest priority when deciding on a course of action. If the client is in distress, then the nurse must intervene with a nursing action that attempts to alleviate or control the problem. The test taker should not choose a diagnostic test if there is an option that directly treats the client.

20. 1. The therapeutic level for digoxin is 0.8 to 2.0 so this warrants notifying the HCP.
2. There is no serum blood level to monitor Levonox, which is a low-molecular-weight heparin administered to prevent deep vein thrombosis.
3. The platelet level is within normal level of 150,000 to 400,000, so this would not warrant notifying the HCP.
4. The normal potassium level is 3.5 to 5.5 mEq/L, so this result would not warrant notifying the HCP.
   Content – Medical/Surgical: **Category of Health Alteration** *– Peripheral Vascular:* **Integrated Processes** *– Nursing Process: Assessment:* **Client Needs** *– Physiological Integrity: Reduction of Risk Potential:* **Cognitive Level** *– Analysis*

MAKING NURSING DECISIONS: The nurse must be knowledgeable of normal laboratory values. These values must be memorized and the nurse must be able to determine if the laboratory value is normal for the client's disease process or for medications the client is taking.

21. 1. This is the correct procedure to help preserve the fingers so the surgeon can reattach the fingers, but is not the first intervention.
2. Elevating the right arm will help decrease bleeding, but it is not the first intervention.
3. **The nurse should first put on non-sterile gloves to protect from getting any blood-borne diseases.**
4. Applying direct pressure is an appropriate intervention, but the first intervention is to apply gloves to protect the nurse.
   Content – Medical/Surgical: **Category of Health Alteration** *– Peripheral Vascular:* **Integrated Processes** *– Nursing Process: Implementation:* **Client Needs** *– Safe and Effective Care Environment: Safety and Infection Control:* **Cognitive Level** *– Application*

MAKING NURSING DECISIONS: The test taker must remember: If the client is in distress, do not assess, but Standard Precautions take priority. The nurse must always put Standard Precautions as a priority when caring for all clients, especially when blood and body fluids are present.

22. 1. The unlicensed assistive personnel (UAP) could escort the client to the room so that the LPN could be assigned tasks that are within the LPN's scope of practice.
2. **The UAP can make sure the room is clear of the previous client's gown and equipment used with the previous client. The UAP can also make sure there are gowns, tongue blades, and additional equipment in the examination room.**
3. The LPN can administer medication; therefore, it would be more appropriate to assign this task to the LPN, so that the RN could be assigned tasks that are beyond the scope of practice of an LPN and within the RN scope of practice.
4. The clinic secretary is unlicensed personnel and does not have the authority to call in a new prescription for a client.
   Content – Medical/Surgical: **Category of Health Alteration** *– Peripheral Vascular:* **Integrated Processes** *– Nursing Process: Planning:* **Client Needs** *– Safe and Effective Care Environment: Management of Care:* **Cognitive Level** *– Synthesis*

MAKING NURSING DECISIONS: When the test taker is deciding which option is the most appropriate task to delegate/assign, the test taker should choose the task that requires each member of the staff to function within his or her full scope of practice. Do not assign a task to a staff member that requires a higher level of expertise than the staff member has, and do not assign a task to a staff member when the task could be delegated/assigned to a staff member with a lower level of expertise.

23. 1. The nurse should discuss the client's comment, but it is not the nurse's first intervention.
2. **The nurse should first take the client's BP correctly and address the client's concern.**
3. If the nurse's BP reading and the UAP's BP reading are close to the same, the nurse could reassure the client that the UAP does know how to take BP readings. However, this is not the nurse's first intervention.
4. This is an appropriate action, but it is not the first intervention. The nurse is responsible for making sure the UAP has the ability to perform any delegated tasks correctly.
   Content – Medical/Surgical: **Category of Health Alteration** *– Peripheral Vascular:* **Integrated Processes** *– Nursing Process: Implementation:* **Client Needs** *– Safe and Effective Care Environment: Management of Care:* **Cognitive Level** *– Application*

MAKING NURSING DECISIONS: The nurse should address client needs first, including answering the client's questions, verifying the client's vital signs, or assessing the client if the client is not in distress.

24. 1. Intravenous push medications cannot be assigned to an LPN. It is the most dangerous route for administering medication, and only an RN (or HCP) can perform this task.
    2. The client who is diagnosed with a pulmonary embolus is not stable; therefore, this medication is not the best medication to be assigned to the LPN.
    3. **Trental is a PO medication prescribed specifically to treat intermittent claudication. It increases erythrocyte flexibility and reduces blood viscosity.**
    4. The client may be having a myocardial infarction; therefore, this client is unstable and should not be assigned to an LPN.

    *Content – Medical/Surgical: **Category of Health Alteration** – Peripheral Vascular: **Integrated Processes** – Nursing Process: Planning: **Client Needs** – Safe and Effective Care Environment: Management of Care: **Cognitive Level** – Synthesis*

MAKING NURSING DECISIONS: The test taker must determine which option absolutely is included within the LPN's scope of practice. LPNs are not routinely taught how to administer intravenous push medications. The test taker must also determine which client is the most stable, which makes this an "except" question. Three clients are either unstable or have potentially life-threatening conditions and should not be assigned to an LPN.

25. 1. **The nurse should realize the client probably has deep vein thrombosis, which is a medical emergency. The HCP should be notified immediately so the client can be started on IV heparin and admitted to the hospital.**
    2. This information may be needed, but the nurse should notify the HCP based on the signs/symptoms alone.
    3. A neurovascular assessment should be completed, but not before notifying the HCP. The signs/symptoms alone indicate a potentially life-threatening condition.
    4. The client's leg should be elevated, but this is a potentially life threatening emergency and the nurse should first call the HCP.

    *Content – Medical/Surgical: **Category of Health Alteration** – Peripheral Vascular: **Integrated Processes** – Nursing Process: Assessment: **Client Needs** – Physiological Integrity: Reduction of Risk Potential: **Cognitive Level** – Analysis*

MAKING NURSING DECISIONS: The test taker needs to read all of the options carefully before choosing the option that says, "Notify the HCP." If any of the options will provide information the HCP needs to know in order to make a decision, the test taker should choose that option. If, however, the HCP does not need any additional information to make a decision and the nurse suspects the condition is serious or life threatening, the priority intervention is to call the HCP.

26. 1. **The nurse should first determine whether there is a fire or whether someone accidentally or purposefully pulled the fire alarm. Because this is a clinic, not a hospital, the nurse should keep calm and determine the situation before taking action.**
    2. The nurse should not evacuate clients, visitors, and staff unless there is a real fire.
    3. The nurse should assess the situation before contacting the fire department.
    4. This is an appropriate intervention, but this is not the first intervention. The nurse should first assess to determine whether there is a fire.

    *Content – Medical/Surgical: **Category of Health Alteration** – Peripheral Vascular: **Integrated Processes** – Nursing Process: Implementation: **Client Needs** – Safe and Effective Care Environment: Safety and Infection Control: **Cognitive Level** – Knowledge*

MAKING NURSING DECISIONS: The nurse must be knowledgeable of emergency preparedness. Employees receive this information in employee orientation and are responsible for implementing procedures correctly. The NCLEX-RN® blueprint includes questions on safe and effective care environment.

27. 1. The clinic nurse should allow the director to address sexual harassment allegations. This is a matter that should be handled legally.
    2. This is an appropriate question to ask when investigating sexual harassment allegations, but the clinic nurse should allow the director of nurses to pursue this situation.
    3. The clinic nurse is responsible for taking the appropriate action when sexual allegations are reported. This statement shows that the clinic nurse is not taking the allegations seriously and could result in disciplinary action against the nurse.
    4. **This is the most appropriate response because sexual harassment allegations are a legal matter. The clinic nurse implemented the correct action by making sure the unlicensed assistive personnel (UAP)**

reported the allegation to the director of nurses.

*Content – Medical/Surgical: **Category of Health Alteration** – Peripheral Vascular: **Integrated Processes** – Nursing Process: Implementation: **Client Needs** – Safe and Effective Care Environment: Management of Care: **Cognitive Level** – Application*

MAKING NURSING DECISIONS: There will be management questions on the NCLEX-RN®. In many instances, there is no test-taking strategy for these questions. The nurse must be knowledgeable of which management issues must comply with local, state, and federal requirements.

28. 1. The clinic nurse should not discuss the staff nurses' statement with the pharmaceutical representative because the staff member's behavior is unethical and could have repercussions. The clinic nurse should notify the director of nurses.
    2. **This behavior is unethical and is making promises that the staff nurse may or may not be able to keep. Because this situation includes the HCP, an outside representative, and the staff nurse, this situation should be reported to the director of nurses for further action.**
    3. This behavior must be reported. This is bribing the pharmaceutical representative and using a meeting with the HCP as the reward.
    4. The clinic nurse should maintain the chain of command and report this to the nursing supervisor, not to the HCP.

*Content – Medical/Surgical: **Category of Health Alteration** – Peripheral Vascular: **Integrated Processes** – Nursing Process: Implementation: **Client Needs** – Safe and Effective Care Environment: Management of Care: **Cognitive Level** – Application*

MAKING NURSING DECISIONS: There will be management questions on the NCLEX-RN®. In many instances, there is no test-taking strategy for these questions. The nurse must be knowledgeable of management issues.

29. 1. The nurse should document the results in the client's chart, but this is not the nurse's first intervention.
    2. **The therapeutic value for INR is 2 to 3; levels higher than that increase the risk of bleeding. The nurse should first contact the client and determine whether she has any abnormal bleeding and then instruct the client to not take any more Coumadin.**
    3. The nurse should notify the client's HCP, but the nurse should first determine whether

the client has any abnormal bleeding so that can be reported to the HCP.

4. The client will need to have another INR drawn, but it is not the nurse's first intervention.

*Content – Medical/Surgical: **Category of Health Alteration** – Peripheral Vascular: **Integrated Processes** – Nursing Process: Assessment: **Client Needs** – Physiological Integrity: Pharmacological and Parenteral Therapies: **Cognitive Level** – Analysis*

MAKING NURSING DECISIONS: Any time the nurse receives information from another source about a client who may be experiencing a complication, the nurse must assess the client. In this scenario, the nurse assesses the client by talking to him or her on the phone. The nurse should not make decisions about client needs unless the nurse talks to the client.

30. 1. A low-salt diet is used to treat arterial hypertension, but it is not the priority intervention.
    2. **The priority intervention for the client with arterial hypertension is to take antihypertensive medications.**
    3. Taking and documenting blood pressure readings is important, but it does not treat the arterial hypertension; therefore, it is not the priority intervention.
    4. Walking will help decrease the client's high blood pressure in some situations, but it is not priority.

*Content – Medical/Surgical: **Category of Health Alteration** – Peripheral Vascular: **Integrated Processes** – Nursing Process: Planning: **Client Needs** – Physiological Integrity: Physiological Adaptation: **Cognitive Level** – Synthesis*

MAKING NURSING DECISIONS: All options are plausible in questions that ask the test taker to identify a priority intervention. The test taker must identify the most important intervention.

31. 1. Stockings should be applied after the legs have been elevated for a period of time—when the amount of blood in the leg vein is at its lowest. Applying the stockings when the client is sitting in a chair indicates the home health (HH) aide does not understand the correct procedure for applying compression stockings.
    2. If a finger cannot be inserted under the proximal end of the stocking, the compression hose is too tight, and the HH worker does not understand the correct procedure for applying the stockings.
    3. The toe opening should be placed on the plantar side of the foot. Placing the toe opening on

the top side of the foot indicates the HH aide does not understand the correct procedure for applying compression stockings.

4. **Warm toes mean the stockings are not too tight and there is good circulation. Checking that the toes are warm indicates the HH aide understands the correct procedure for applying the compression stockings.**

Content – Medical/Surgical: ***Category of Health Alteration*** *– Peripheral Vascular:* ***Integrated Processes*** *– Nursing Process: Evaluation:* ***Client Needs*** *– Safe and Effective Care Environment: Management of Care:* ***Cognitive Level*** *– Synthesis*

MAKING NURSING DECISIONS: The nurse must ensure the UAP can perform any tasks that are delegated. It is the nurse's responsibility to evaluate the task, demonstrate, and/or teach the UAP how to perform the task.

32. 1. **The nurse should first take care of the bite and then determine whether the dog is up to date on the required vaccinations. The nurse should be concerned about the possibility of rabies.**
    2. If the dog is not up to date on the required vaccinations, then the veterinarian should be notified to quarantine the dog to check for rabies.
    3. The nurse should complete an occurrence report and document the dog bite. If the nurse must pay for anything concerning the dog bite, it should be covered by workers' compensation.
    4. Besides an infection of the dog bite, the worst complication would be the nurse contracting rabies. If the dog is up to date on the required vaccinations, then this should not be a concern.

Content – Medical/Surgical: ***Category of Health Alteration*** *– Peripheral Vascular:* ***Integrated Processes*** *– Nursing Process: Implementation:* ***Client Needs*** *– Safe and Effective Care Environment: Safety and Infection Control:* ***Cognitive Level*** *– Application*

MAKING NURSING DECISIONS: The test taker should apply the nursing process when the question asks, "Which intervention should be implemented first?" If the client is in distress, do not assess; if the client is in distress, take action.

33. 1. This would not warrant immediate intervention because intermittent claudication, pain when walking, is the hallmark sign of arterial occlusive disease.
    2. **This comment warrants immediate intervention because the client's legs have decreased sensation secondary to the arterial**

occlusive disease, and a heating pad could burn the client's legs without the client's realizing it. The client should not use a heating pad to keep the legs warm.

3. Hanging his or her legs off the bed helps increase the arterial blood supply to the legs, which, in turn, helps decrease the leg pain. This comment would not warrant immediate intervention by the nurse.
4. Hair growth requires oxygen, and the client has decreased oxygen to the legs; therefore, decreased hair growth would be expected and not require immediate intervention.

Content – Medical/Surgical: ***Category of Health Alteration*** *– Peripheral Vascular:* ***Integrated Processes*** *– Nursing Process: Evaluation:* ***Client Needs*** *– Physiological Integrity: Physiological Adaptation:* ***Cognitive Level*** *– Analysis*

MAKING NURISNG DECISIONS: When the question asks, "Which warrants immediate intervention?" it is an "except" question. Three of the comments indicate the client understands the teaching and one indicates the client does not understand the teaching.

34. 1. The nurse cannot purchase supplies for the client. This is crossing a professional boundary.
    2. The social worker does assist with financial concerns and referrals for the client, but purchasing smoke detectors is not within the social worker's scope of practice.
    3. The nurse should not encourage the client to be dependent on family members for purchasing supplies for the client's home. This may be a possibility when all other avenues have been pursued.
    4. **The nurse should contact the fire department. Many fire departments will supply and install smoke detectors for people who cannot afford them. The nurse should investigate this option first because it is the most immediate response to the safety need.**

Content – Medical/Surgical: ***Category of Health Alteration*** *– Peripheral Vascular:* ***Integrated Processes*** *– Nursing Process: Implementation:* ***Client Needs*** *– Safe and Effective Care Environment; Safety and Infection Control:* ***Cognitive Level*** *– Application*

MAKING NURSING DECISIONS: The nurse must be knowledgeable of emergency preparedness in the hospital as well as in the community. Employees receive this information in employee orientation and are responsible for implementing procedures correctly. The NCLEX-RN® blueprint includes questions on safe and effective care environment.

35. 1. The nurse should document the objective findings in the chart, but this is not the priority intervention.
2. The nurse cannot force the client to talk about the situation.
3. **The bruises and burns should make the nurse suspect elder abuse, and the nurse is mandated by law to report this to Adult Protective Services.**
4. The nurse should let Adult Protective Services take pictures of the suspected abuse because there is a legal chain of custody that must be followed if the case goes to court.

Content – Medical/Surgical: **Category of Health Alteration** *– Peripheral Vascular:* **Integrated Processes** *– Nursing Process: Implementation:* **Client Needs** *– Safe and Effective Care Environment: Safety and Infection Control:* **Cognitive Level** *– Application*

MAKING NURSING DECISIONS: The NCLEX-RN® blueprint includes nursing care that is ruled by legal requirements. The nurse is legally obligated to report possible child abuse or adult abuse. The nurse must be knowledgeable of these issues.

36. 1. **Aspirin, an antiplatelet agent, puts the client at risk for bleeding. The client diagnosed with deep vein thrombosis will be on warfarin (Coumadin), an anticoagulant, which puts the client at risk for bleeding; therefore, this comment requires immediate intervention by the nurse.**
2. The client should wear a medical alert bracelet to notify any emergency HCP of the client's condition and medication. This statement would not warrant immediate intervention.
3. Most books recommend not eating green, leafy vegetables that are high in vitamin K, because doing so is the antidote to Coumadin toxicity. The client would have to eat green, leafy vegetables more than twice a week to counteract the Coumadin; therefore, this comment would not warrant immediate intervention as much as the client's taking of daily aspirin.
4. Elevating the client's legs would not warrant intervention by the nurse.

Content – Medical/Surgical: **Category of Health Alteration** *– Peripheral Vascular:* **Integrated Processes** *– Nursing Process: Evaluation:* **Client Needs** *– Physiological Integrity: Pharmacological and Parenteral Therapies:* **Cognitive Level** *– Synthesis*

MAKING NURSING DECISIONS: This question asks the nurse to identify which statement warrants immediate intervention, which indicates

three of the options are appropriate for the disease process or disorder and one is inappropriate. This is an "except" question, but it does not say all the options are correct "except."

37. 1. The nurse should be a client advocate and support the client's wishes, not support the HCP's recommendation even if it is best for the client.
2. Recommending the client talk to his family may be an appropriate action, but it does not support the nurse being a client advocate.
3. The client does have a right to a second opinion, but this action is not supporting the client's decision not to have an amputation, and thus is not client advocacy.
4. **This action shows the nurse being the client's advocate. Offering to go talk to the HCP about the amputation and making sure the HCP hears the client's opinion is being a client advocate. Another discussion may change the client's decision, but either way, client advocacy is supporting the client's decision.**

Content – Medical/Surgical: **Category of Health Alteration** *– Peripheral Vascular:* **Integrated Processes** *– Nursing Process: Planning:* **Client Needs** *– Physiological Integrity: Physiological Adaptation:* **Cognitive Level** *– Synthesis*

MAKING NURSING DECISIONS: There will be management questions on the NCLEX-RN® addressing client advocacy. A client advocate acts as a liaison between clients and healthcare providers to help improve or maintain a high quality of healthcare.

38. 1. Crying at a death is a universal human response. Although the statement may be true, the nurse should recognize the UAP's need for a short time to compose him- or herself.
2. **Hospital personnel are not immune to human emotions. The UAP needs a short time to compose him- or herself. The nurse should offer the UAP compassion. If this occurred with every death, the UAP could be counselled to transfer to a different area of the hospital.**
3. This is not accepting the UAP's feelings.
4. This is not accepting the UAP's feelings.

Content – Medical/Surgical: **Category of Health Alteration** *– Peripheral Vascular:* **Integrated Processes** *– Nursing Process: Implementation:* **Client Needs** *– Safe and Effective Care Environment: Management of Care:* **Cognitive Level** *– Application*

MAKING NURSING DECISIONS: There will be management questions on the NCLEX-RN®. In many instances, there is no test-taking strategy for these questions. The nurse must be knowledgeable of management issues.

39. 1. Clients receiving hospice can decide to discontinue the service and resume standard healthcare practices and treatments whenever they wish. The nurse should assess the client's wishes before continuing.
   2. This is true, but if the client wants to be treated, it is the client's decision. If the client does not want treatment, then the nurse should discuss the client's wishes with the long-term care facility staff.
   3. If the client does not want treatment, then the nurse should discuss the client's wishes with the long-term care facility staff.
   4. If the staff continues to try to get the client to accept futile treatment, a client conference should be called. This is not the first action for the hospice nurse because a client conference is a scheduled event and would not take place immediately.

   *Content – Medical/Surgical: **Category of Health Alteration** – Peripheral Vascular: **Integrated Processes** – Nursing Process: Assessment: **Client Needs** – Safe and Effective Care Environment: Management of Care: **Cognitive Level** – Analysis*

MAKING NURSING DECISIONS: This question requires the test taker to have a basic knowledge of hospice and hospice goals. The nurse must also be aware of basic referrals.

40. 1. Telling the family over the telephone could cause the client's significant other to have an accident while driving to the hospital. The nurse should avoid disclosing this type of information over the telephone.
   2. **This response allows the family/ significant other to know there has been some incident, but it does not disclose the death. This is the best statement for the nurse at this time. The family will be able to arrive safely at the hospital before hearing the news their loved one has died.**
   3. Telling the family over the telephone could cause the client to have an accident while driving to the hospital. The nurse should avoid disclosing this type of information over the telephone.
   4. This is a backward way of telling the family that the client died and should be avoided.

   *Content – Medical/Surgical: **Category of Health Alteration** – Peripheral Vascular: **Integrated Processes** – Nursing Process: Implementation: **Client Needs** – Physiological Integrity: Basic Care and Comfort: **Cognitive Level** – Application*

MAKING NURSING DECISIONS: There will be management questions on the NCLEX-RN®. In many instances, there is no test-taking strategy for these questions. The nurse must be knowledgeable of management issues.

41. 1. The client is experiencing a complication of the surgical procedure and should be assigned to a nurse who is more experienced in caring for clients with vascular complications.
   2. Low back pain could indicate a leaking abdominal aortic aneurysm and should not be assigned to a floating nurse. A more experienced vascular nurse should care for this client.
   3. Since this client needs extensive teaching, this client should not be assigned to a floating nursing but a more experienced vascular nurse.
   4. **The client with varicose veins would be expected to have deep aching pain in the legs; therefore, the nurse who is being floated to the vascular unit could be assigned to this client.**

   *Content – Medical/Surgical: **Category of Health Alteration** – Peripheral Vascular: **Integrated Processes** – Nursing Process: Planning: **Client Needs** – Safe and Effective Care Environment: Management of Care: **Cognitive Level** – Synthesis*

MAKING NURSING DECISIONS: The nurse should assign the most stable client to the least experienced nurse.

42. 1. Leaving the facility will make client care even more strained.
   2. **The nurse should notify the supervisor that the nurse is concerned that the assignment will not allow the nurse to provide adequate care to any of the three clients. This is the first step the nurse should implement.**
   3. This is the second step. The nurse should put his or her concerns in writing and present the documentation to the supervisor. In states that have a "safe harbor" clause in the Nursing Practice Act, this will prevent the nurse from losing his or her license should a poor outcome result from the assignment.
   4. If the staffing continues to be unsafe, the nurse may choose to resign, but the resignation should follow accepted business practices.

   *Content – Medical/Surgical: **Category of Health Alteration** – Peripheral Vascular: **Integrated Processes** – Nursing Process: Implementation: **Client Needs** – Safe and Effective Care Environment: Management of Care: **Cognitive Level** – Application*

MAKING NURSING DECISIONS: There will be management questions on the NCLEX-RN®. In

many instances, there is no test-taking strategy for these questions; the nurse must be knowledgeable of management issues. If the nurse thinks the assignment is a violation of the state's Nursing Practice Act, then the nurse must notify the supervisor immediately.

43. 1. Morphine is a potent narcotic analgesic. A 4 on the 1-to-10 pain scale is considered moderate pain and should be treated with a less potent pain medication.
    2. Promethazine is administered for nausea.
    3. **Hydrocodone is a narcotic analgesic that is less potent than morphine. It has been 5 hours since the hydrocodone was last administered, and no other pain medication has been required by the client. This is the best medication for moderate pain.**
    4. Ibuprofen may be effective for moderate pain, but the client is allergic to ibuprofen. The nurse should tag the medical administration record (MAR) and chart to notify the HCP to discontinue this medication.

    Content – Medical/Surgical: ***Category of Health Alteration*** *– Drug Administration:* ***Integrated Processes*** *– Nursing Process: Assessment:* ***Client Needs*** *– Physiological Integrity: Pharmacological and Parenteral Therapies:* ***Cognitive Level*** *– Analysis*

MAKING NURSING DECISIONS: This is an alternate type question included in the NCLEX-RN® blueprint. The test taker must be able to read a medication administration record (MAR), must be knowledgeable of medications, and be able to make an appropriate decision as to the nurse's most appropriate intervention.

44. 1. **The daughter lives in a "nearby" city. The client should not be moved anywhere until the daughter arrives.**
    2. A morgue is a difficult place to view a body. This could be appropriate if the daughter was going to take hours to days to get to the hospital.
    3. Many people feel it is necessary to view the body. Not allowing the daughter time to view the body before transfer to a funeral home or the morgue could cause hurt feelings and impede the grieving process.
    4. Many people feel it is necessary to view the body. Not allowing the daughter time to view the body before transfer to a funeral home or the morgue could cause hurt feelings and impede the grieving process.

    Content – Medical/Surgical: ***Category of Health Alteration*** *– Peripheral Vascular:* ***Integrated Processes*** *– Nursing Process: Implementation:* ***Client Needs*** *– Psychosocial Integrity:* ***Cognitive Level*** *– Application*

MAKING NURSING DECISIONS: The nurse should always try and support the client's or family's request, if it does not violate any local, state, or federal rules and regulations. This is the test taker's best decision if unsure of the correct answer.

45. 1. **The change process can be compared to the nursing process. The first step of each process is to assess the problem. Assessment involves collecting the pertinent data that support the need for a change.**
    2. The second step is to identify the problem or, in the nursing process, identify possible nursing diagnoses.
    3. The third step is to select an alternative to implement to fix the problem. This is similar to choosing a specific nursing diagnosis.
    4. The fourth step is to implement a plan of action. This is similar to implementing the nursing care plan.

    Content – Medical/Surgical: ***Category of Health Alteration*** *– Peripheral Vascular:* ***Integrated Processes*** *– Nursing Process: Assessment:* ***Client Needs*** *– Safe and Effective Care Environment: Management of Care:* ***Cognitive Level*** *– Analysis*

MAKING NURSING DECISIONS: Assessment is the first step of the nursing process, and the test taker should use the nursing process or some other systematic process to assist in determining priorities.

46. **2 and 3 are correct.**
    1. The only solution compatible with blood is normal saline. Dextrose causes the blood to coagulate.
    2. **The blood administration set is changed after every two units.**
    3. **The nurse must assess the client's vital signs before every unit of blood is administered.**
    4. The nurse should assess for allergies prior to administering medications. Before administering blood products, the nurse should assess to determine compatibility with the client's blood type. The client may have an incompatible blood type, but this is not an allergy.
    5. A blood warmer is used when the client has identified cold agglutinins. This is not in the stem of the question.

    Content – Medical/Surgical: ***Category of Health Alteration*** *– Peripheral Vascular:* ***Integrated Processes*** *– Nursing Process: Implementation:* ***Client Needs*** *– Physiological Integrity: Safety and Infection Control:* ***Cognitive Level*** *– Application*

MAKING NURSING DECISIONS: This is an alternate type of question included in the NCLEX-RN®. The nurse must be able to select all the options that answer the question correctly. There are no partially correct answers.

47. 1. The client with a deep vein thrombosis is placed on strict bed rest and should not have any type of pressure on his or her calf, which may cause the clot to dislodge and cause a pulmonary embolus. This task should not be delegated to an unlicensed assistive personnel (UAP).
    2. The number one intervention for a client with thromboangiitis obliterans is to stop smoking; therefore, this task should not be elevated. The UAP should be on the unit caring for clients, not outside to allow a client to smoke.
    3. **The leg should be elevated to prevent postoperative edema; therefore, this task could be delegated to the UAP.**
    4. The UAP cannot perform Doppler studies; a trained technician must perform this test.

    Content – Medical/Surgical: **Category of Health Alteration** *– Peripheral Vascular:* **Integrated Processes** *– Nursing Process: Planning:* **Client Needs** *– Safe and Effective Care Environment: Management of Care:* **Cognitive Level** *– Synthesis*

MAKING NURSING DECISIONS: An RN cannot delegate assessment, teaching, evaluation, medications, or an unstable client to a UAP. Tasks that cannot be delegated are nursing interventions requiring nursing judgment.

48. 1. Only the client should activate the PCA pump. Allowing family or significant others to push the button places the client at risk for an overdose.
    2. The nurse is acting appropriately; there is no reason to discuss the instructions further.
    3. The nurse is acting appropriately; there is no reason to discuss the instructions further.
    4. **The nurse is acting appropriately, and there is no reason to discuss the instructions further. The charge nurse should continue with other duties.**

    Content – Medical/Surgical: **Category of Health Alteration** *– Peripheral Vascular:* **Integrated Processes** *– Nursing Process: Implementation:* **Client Needs** *– Safe and Effective Care Environment: Management of Care:* **Cognitive Level** *– Application*

MAKING NURSING DECISIONS: There will be management questions on the NCLEX-RN®. In many instances, there is no test-taking strategy for these questions; the nurse must be knowledgeable of management issues concerning personnel. The nurse is responsible for evaluating the behaviour of subordinates when caring for clients.

49. 1. **This client may be having phantom pain, but it must be assessed and the client must be medicated. The nurse should assess this client first.**
    2. The client's blood pressure must be taken to determine if the headache is due to hypertensive crisis, but it is not priority for postoperative surgical pain.
    3. The client with lymphedema would be expected to have edema of the lower leg; therefore, the nurse would not assess this client first.
    4. The client with gangrene would be expected to have a foul-smelling discharge; therefore, this client would not be assessed first.

    Content – Medical/Surgical: **Category of Health Alteration** *– Peripheral Vascular:* **Integrated Processes** *– Nursing Process: Assessment:* **Client Needs** *– Physiological Integrity: Reduction of Risk Potential:* **Cognitive Level** *– Analysis*

MAKING NURSING DECISIONS: When deciding which client to assess first, the test taker should determine whether the signs/symptoms the client is exhibiting are normal or expected for the client situation. After eliminating the expected option, the test taker should determine which situation is more life threatening.

50. 1. The LPN should not administer the medication if the client's BP is less than 90/50, but this is not the first action the nurse should take.
    2. This medication cannot be crushed and the nurse needs to intervene and correct the LPN's behaviour.
    3. The LPN should be shown where to find pudding or applesauce to mix in crushed medications, but this medication should not be crushed.
    4. **The XL in the name of the medication indicates that this medication is a sustained-released formulation and should not be crushed. The nurse should speak directly with the LPN to correct the behaviour.**

    Content – Medical/Surgical: **Category of Health Alteration** *– Drug Administration:* **Integrated Processes** *– Nursing Process: Implementation:* **Client Needs** *– Safe and Effective Care Environment, Management of Care:* **Cognitive Level** *– Application*

MAKING NURSING DECISIONS: The nurse must be aware of interventions that must be implemented prior to administering medications. The nurse must know which medications cannot be crushed. The nurse is responsible for evaluating the behavior and actions of their subordinates.

51. 1. This is an example of paternalism or beneficence.
2. This is an example of beneficence.
3. This is an example of nonmalfeasance or beneficence.
4. **This is an example of autonomy.**
*Content – Medical/Surgical: **Category of Health Alteration** – Peripheral Vascular: **Integrated Processes** – Nursing Process: Implementation: **Client Needs** – Physiological Integrity: Basic Care and Comfort: **Cognitive Level** – Application*

MAKING NURSING DECISIONS: The NCLEX-RN® blueprint includes nursing care that addresses ethical principles, including autonomy, beneficence, justice, and veracity, to name a few.

52. 1. This would be culturally sensitive to a client who is a Jehovah's Witness.
2. Mormons do not wear amulets.
3. **The devout Mormon client wears a religious undershirt that should not be removed; this action indicates cultural sensitivity on the part of the nurse.**
4. Mormons do not consult curanderos. Some Hispanic cultures consult curanderos.
*Content – Medical/Surgical: **Category of Health Alteration** – Peripheral Vascular: **Integrated Processes** – Nursing Process: Implementation: **Client Needs** – Physiological Integrity: Basic Care and Comfort: **Cognitive Level** – Application*

MAKING NURSING DECISIONS: The NCLEX-RN® blueprint includes nursing care that addresses cultural diversity. The nurse needs to be aware of cultural differences.

53. 1. **These ABGs show respiratory acidosis, which needs immediate intervention; therefore, this client should be assessed first.**
2. The client with Reynaud's phenomenon would be expected to have bluish, cold upper extremities; therefore, the nurse would not need to assess the client first.
3. The client with chronic venous insufficiency has ulceration on the feet; therefore, this nurse would not need to assess the client first.
4. The PTT is 1.5 to 2 times the normal; therefore, the nurse would not need to assess this client first. Normal PTT is 39 seconds; therefore, therapeutic PTT is 58 to 78.
*Content – Medical/Surgical: **Category of Health Alteration** – Peripheral Vascular: **Integrated Processes** – Nursing Process: Assessment: **Client Needs** – Physiological Integrity: Reduction of Risk Potential: **Cognitive Level** – Analysis*

MAKING NURSING DECISIONS: The test taker must determine which sign/symptom is not

expected for the disease process. If the sign/symptom is not expected, then the nurse should assess the client first. This type of question is determining if the nurse is knowledgeable of signs/symptoms of a variety of disease processes.

54. 1. The client with arterial occlusive disease dangles the feet off the side of the bed to increase the blood supply to the legs; therefore, a less experienced unlicensed assistive personnel (UAP) could care for this client.
2. The nurse should be assigned to care for this client, who is angry about the family's not visiting, because the client requires assessment, nursing judgment, and therapeutic communication and intervention, which are not within the UAP's scope of practice.
3. **This client requires an experienced UAP who is skilled in client lifts, so the client is lifted safely and the UAP is not injured in the process. The most experienced UAP should be assigned this client.**
4. The experienced UAP could care for this client, but then other UAPs would not learn to care for the client. This client should be rotated through the UAPs so that all the UAPs can learn to care for the client who is particular about the way things are done.
*Content – Medical/Surgical: **Category of Health Alteration** – Peripheral Vascular: **Integrated Processes** – Nursing Process: Planning: **Client Needs** – Safe and Effective Care Environment: Management of Care: **Cognitive Level** – Synthesis*

MAKING NURSING DECISIONS: When the test taker is deciding which option is the most appropriate task to delegate/assign, the test taker should choose the task that allows each staff member to function within his or her full scope of practice. Remember: The RN cannot delegate assessment, teaching, evaluation, medications, or an unstable client to the UAP.

55. 1. **Chest pain on deep inspiration is a symptom of pulmonary embolism. The nurse should first place the client on oxygen.**
2. The first intervention is to provide the client with oxygen. The test taker should not assess when the client is in distress.
3. The respiratory therapist can be notified, but it is not the nurse's first intervention. The nurse should first address the client's needs.
4. The nurse should not select equipment over addressing the client's needs.
*Content – Medical/Surgical: **Category of Health Alteration** – Cardiovascular: **Integrated Processes** – Nursing Process: Implementation: **Client Needs** – Physiological Integrity: Reduction of Risk Potential: **Cognitive Level** – Synthesis*

MAKING NURSING DECISIONS: The nurse should remember: If a client is in distress and the nurse can do something to relieve the distress, that should be done first, before assessment. The test taker should select an option that directly helps the client's condition.

56. **2, 3, 4, and 5 are correct.**
    1. Monetary need is not a good reason to select a nurse to become a preceptor.
    2. **The nurse should be able to organize his or her own workload before becoming a role model for a new nurse. If the nurse is not organized, taking on new responsibilities will be very frustrating for the preceptor and for the preceptee.**
    3. **The nurse who acts as a preceptor should have good people skills and be approachable.**
    4. **The nurse should consistently provide quality care that others should emulate.**
    5. **The nurse should be willing to take on this responsibility or the preceptor will resent the new nurse.**

    Content – Medical/Surgical: **Category of Health Alteration** *– Peripheral Vascular:* **Integrated Processes** *– Nursing Process: Planning:* **Client Needs** *– Safe and Effective Care Environment: Management of Care:* **Cognitive Level** *– Synthesis*

MAKING NURSING DECISIONS: This is an alternate type of question included in the NCLEX-RN®. The nurse must be able to select all the options that answer the question correctly. There are no partially correct answers.

57. 1. **This client is experiencing neurovascular compromise and requires immediate attention. The client with venous problems should have palpable pedal pulses. This procedure is for clients with varicose veins.**
    2. The calf pain is expected with a client diagnosed with deep vein thrombosis; therefore, the nurse would not assess this client first.
    3. The client with Raynaud's phenomenon has coldness and numbness in the vasoconstriction phase followed by throbbing, aching pain, tingling, and swelling in the hyperemic phase. The nurse would not see this client first since these are expected signs/symptoms.
    4. Buerger's disease (thromboangiitits obliterans) is often confused with peripheral arterial disease (PAD). As the disease progresses, rest pain develops along with color and temperature changes in the affected limb or limbs.

    Content – Medical/Surgical: **Category of Health Alteration** *– Peripheral Vascular:* **Integrated Processes** *Nursing Process: Assessment:* **Client Needs** *– Safe and*

Effective Care Environment: Management of Care: **Cognitive Level** *– Synthesis*

MAKING NURSING DECISIONS: The test taker must determine which sign/symptom is not expected for the disease process. If the sign/symptom is not expected, then the nurse should assess the client first. This type of question is determining if the nurse is knowledgeable of signs/symptoms of a variety of disease processes.

58. **Answer: 2,050 mL total intake.** The urinary output is not used in this calculation. The nurse must add up both intravenous fluids and oral fluids to obtain the total intake for this client: 950 + 200 = 1,150 IV fluids; (1 ounce = 30 mL) 16 ounces × 30 mL = 480 mL, 8 ounces × 30 mL = 240 mL, 6 ounces × 30 mL = 180 mL; 480 + 240 + 180 = 900 oral fluids. Total intake is 1,150 + 900 = 2,050.

    Content – Medical/Surgical: **Category of Health Alteration** *– Cardiovascular:* **Integrated Processes** *– Nursing Process: Implementation:* **Client Needs** *– Physiological Integrity: Pharmacological and Parenteral Therapies:* **Cognitive Level** *– Analysis*

MAKING NURSING DECISIONS: This is an alternate type question included in the NCLEX-RN®. The nurse must be knowledgeable on how to perform math questions.

59. 1. Cold water causes vasoconstriction and hot water may burn the client's feet; therefore, warm water should be used and the feet should be cleaned daily. This indicates the client understands the teaching.
    2. Shoes should be purchased in the afternoon when the feet are the largest. This indicates the client understands the teaching.
    3. **This statement indicates the client needs more teaching because knee-high stockings will further decrease circulation to the legs.**
    4. The client should not elevate legs because it further decreases arterial blood flow to the legs. The client should dangle his or her legs off the side of the bed, which increases arterial blood flow to the lower extremities. This indicates that the client understand the teaching.

    Content – Medical/Surgical: **Category of Health Alteration** *– Peripheral Vascular:* **Integrated Processes** *– Nursing Process: Evaluation:* **Client Needs** *– Physiological Integrity: Physiological Adaptation:* **Cognitive Level** *– Analysis*

MAKING NURSING DECISIONS: When the question says "needs more teaching," it is an "except" question. Three of the comments indicate the client understands the teaching and one indicates the client does not understand the teaching.

60. 1. The nurse cannot delegate a client who is unstable to the unlicensed assistive personnel (UAP). The client is experiencing hypoglycemia and is not stable.
2. **The client is stable and elevating the feet is an appropriate intervention for a client with venous problems; therefore, the UAP could feed this client.**
3. The nurse cannot delegate a client who is unstable to the UAP. The client has numbness of the right arm and should be assessed by the nurse.
4. The client with an abdominal aortic aneurysm should not have any increased pressure in the abdomen because it may cause the aneurysm to rupture; therefore, this should not be implemented by anyone.

Content – Medical/Surgical: *Category of Health Alteration* – Peripheral Vascular: *Integrated Processes* – Nursing Process: Planning: *Client Needs* – Safe and Effective Care Environment: Management of Care: *Cognitive Level* – Synthesis

MAKING NURSING DECISIONS: This is an "except" question. The test taker could ask which task is appropriate to delegate to the UAP; three options would be appropriate to delegate and one would not be. Remember: The RN cannot delegate assessment, teaching, evaluation, medications, or an unstable client to the UAP.

61. 1. **The nurse needs to intervene because the client is at high risk for developing pneumonia, especially due to the abdominal incision.**
2. The client must have 30 mL urinary output every hour, and 300 mL in 8 hours is adequate urinary output. Clients who are postoperative AAA are at high risk for renal failure because of the anatomical location of the AAA near the renal arteries.
3. The client should have hypoactive bowel sounds on the second day postoperative. The client was NPO prior to surgery and NPO until bowel sounds returned, so hypoactive bowel sounds would be expected.
4. These vital signs are within normal limits and would not warrant immediate intervention by the nurse.

Content – Medical/Surgical: *Category of Health Alteration* – Peripheral Vascular: *Integrated Processes* – Nursing Process: Assessment: *Client Needs* – Physiological Integrity: Reduction of Risk Potential: *Cognitive Level* – Analysis

MAKING NURSING DECISIONS: The test taker should ask "are the assessment data normal for" the disease process. If they are normal for the disease process, then the nurse would not need to intervene; if they are not normal for the disease process, then this warrants intervention by the nurse.

62. 1. The nurse should assess the client's right foot pain, but not prior to a potentially life-threatening situation.
2. **Parasthesia (numbness and tingling) indicates a graft occlusion from the surgical procedure, which is a potentially life-threatening complication; therefore, this client should be assessed first.**
3. The most common cause of superficial thrombophlebitis is IV therapy, and tenderness to the touch, redness, and warmth are expected. This is not a medical emergency; therefore, the nurse would not assess this client first.
4. The client with arterial occlusive disease would be expected to have pain in the calf when ambulating, which is called intermittent claudication.

Content – Medical/Surgical: *Category of Health Alteration* – Peripheral Vascular: *Integrated Processes* – Nursing Process: Assessment: *Client Needs* – Physiological Integrity: Reduction of Risk Potential: *Cognitive Level* – Analysis

MAKING NURSING DECISIONS: When deciding which client to assess first, the test taker should determine whether the signs/symptoms the client is exhibiting are normal or expected for the client's situation. After eliminating the expected option, the test taker should determine which situation is more life threatening.

63. **Answer: 20 mL/hour.** To determine the rate, the test taker must first determine how many units are in each mL of fluid: 25,000 divided by 500 = 50 units of heparin in each mL of fluid, and 50 divided into 100 = 2, and 2 + 20 = 22.

Content – Medical/Surgical: *Category of Health Alteration* – Drug Administration: *Integrated Processes* – Nursing Process: Implementation: *Client Needs* – Physiological Integrity: Pharmacological and Parenteral Therapies: *Cognitive Level* – Application

MAKING NURSING DECISIONS: This is an alternate type of question included in the NCLEX-RN®. The nurse must be knowledgeable on how to solve math questions.

64. 1. Compression stockings are used to treat chronic venous insufficiency; therefore, this action does not warrant intervention by the nurse.

2. The client's legs should be elevated; therefore, this action would not warrant immediate intervention.

3. The client can ambulate with assistance; therefore, this action does not warrant intervention.

4. **The client should have a podiatrist cut his or her toenails. The unlicensed assistive personnel (UAP) should not do this because if the UAP accidently cuts the skin, it could cause a sore that may not heal, and then result in amputation of the extremity.**

*Content – Medical/Surgical: **Category of Health Alteration** – Peripheral Vascular: **Integrated Processes** – Nursing Process: Evaluation: **Client Needs** – Safe and Effective Care Environment: Management of Care: **Cognitive Level** – Analysis*

MAKING NURSING DECISIONS: The nurse cannot delegate any task in which the UAP admits to not being able to perform. Delegation means the nurse is responsible for the UAP's actions; therefore, the nurse must intervene if the UAP is performing unsafely.

65. 1. The client with a venous stasis ulcer should eat a diet high in protein (meat, beans, cheese, tofu), vitamin A (green, leafy vegetables), vitamin C (citrus fruits, tomatoes, cantaloupe), and zinc (meat, seafood). The nurse needs to talk to this client, but it is not a life-threatening condition or a complication; therefore, the client is not assessed first.

2. The client should wear thromboembolic hose, but this is not a life-threatening condition or a complication; therefore, the client does not have to be assessed first.

3. The client with arterial occlusive disease should not elevate the feet because it further decreases oxygen to the extremity; therefore, this action is not required to be assessed by the nurse.

4. **The nurse should assess this client first because if the client does not stay in the bed, the clot in the calf muscle may dislodge and result in a pulmonary embolus. The client with a DVT must be on bed rest.**

*Content – Medical/Surgical: **Category of Health Alteration** – Peripheral Vascular: **Integrated Processes** – Nursing Process: Assessment: **Client Needs** – Physiological Integrity: Reduction of Risk Potential: **Cognitive Level** – Analysis*

MAKING NURSING DECISIONS: The nurse must determine if the client's behavior is potentially unsafe for the client's disease process. If the

client is putting him- or herself at risk, then the nurse must assess this client first.

66. 1. Oral pain medications provide relief for mild to moderate pain. A 10 is considered to be severe pain.

2. Guided imagery will not alleviate severe pain.

3. **If the current pain regimen is not working for this client, the nurse should notify the surgeon for an adjustment in the pain medication.**

4. It has only been 1 hour and 15 minutes since the pain medication was administered. It is too soon for the nurse to administer the morphine.

*Content – Medical/Surgical: **Category of Health Alteration** – Peripheral Vascular: **Integrated Processes** – Nursing Process: Implementation: **Client Needs** – Physiological Integrity: Basic Care and Comfort: **Cognitive Level** – Application*

MAKING NURSING DECISIONS: This is an alternate type of question included in the NCLEX-RN® blueprint. The test taker must be able to read a medication administration record (MAR), must be knowledgeable of medications, and must be able to make an appropriate decisions as to the nurse's most appropriate intervention.

67. Answer: 50 drops per minute
150 mL divided by 60 = 2.5 mL per minute to infuse
2.5 times 20 = 50

*Content – Medical/Surgical: **Category of Health Alteration** – Drug Administration: **Integrated Processes** – Nursing Process: Implementation: **Client Needs** – Physiological Integrity: Pharmacological and Parenteral Therapies: **Cognitive Level** – Application*

MAKING NURSING DECISIONS: This is an alternate type question included in the NCLEX-RN®. The nurse must be knowledgeable on how to perform math questions.

68. 1. The nurse needs to have the surgical operative permit signed by the client, but not until the discrepancy between what operative permit says and what the client said is resolved.

2. The nurse can assess the client's neurological status, but not prior to calling a time out. Calling a time out is the priority intervention.

3. Determining if the client had anything by mouth is an appropriate intervention, but not priority to clarifying which leg will the surgical procedure be performed.

4. **The nurse must stop everything and clarify which leg will have the surgical procedure. This is the first and priority intervention the nurse must implement.**

*Content – Medical/Surgical: **Category of Health
Alteration** – Peripheral Vascular: **Integrated Processes** –
Nursing Process: Implementation: **Client Needs** – Safe
and Effective Care Environment: Safety and Infection
Control: **Cognitive Level** – Application*

MAKING NURSING DECISIONS: The NCLEX-RN®
blueprint includes nursing care administered
by the current National Patient Safety Goals.
The nurse must be knowledgeable of these
goals.

69. 1. The abdominal bruit is located at the mid-
abdominal area above the umbilicus.
   2. The mid-scapula area is not an appropriate
area to auscultate an abdominal aortic
aneurysm.
   3. An abdominal aortic aneurysm is diagnosed when the client has an abdominal
bruit. An abdominal bruit is a murmur that
corresponds to the cardiac cycle. It is heard
best with the diaphragm of the stethoscope, usually over the abdominal aorta.
   4. The nurse cannot auscultate a bruit on the
feet.

*Content – Medical/Surgical: **Category of Health
Alteration** – Peripheral Vascular: **Integrated Processes** –
Nursing Process: Assessment: **Client Needs** – Physiological
Integrity: Basic Care and Comfort: **Cognitive Level** –
Analysis*

MAKING NURSING DECISIONS: This is an alternate type question included in the NCLEX-RN®.
It is a picture and the nurse must be able to point
the curser at the appropriate area. It is called a
hot spot.

70. **Correct Answer: 1, 4, 3, 2, 5**
   1. The bleeding must be stopped. The
nurse should don unsterile gloves and
apply pressure to the bleeding site for a
minimum of 5 minutes.
   4. When the bleeding has stopped, the
client can be assisted back to bed so a
thorough assessment of the injuries can
be performed.
   3. The site should be redressed when possible to protect the wound from infectious
organisms.
   2. Once the nurse has been able to assess
the client and has the client in a safe environment, then the nurse should notify
the surgeon.
   5. The occurrence should be noted on a report form and the appropriate hospital
personnel notified, but this can be done
after caring for the client.

*Content – Medical/Surgical: **Category of Health
Alteration** – Peripheral Vascular: **Integrated Processes** –
Nursing Process: Implementation: **Client Needs** – Safe
and Effective Care Environment: Management of Care:
Cognitive Level – Analysis*

MAKING NURSING DECISIONS: This is an alternate
type of question included in the NCLEX-RN®.
The nurse must be able to place the interventions in order of priority. The nurse can use
Maslow's Hierarchy of Needs to prioritize the
interventions. Written documentation is the last
action taken in an emergency or life-threatening
situation.

CLINICAL SCENARIO ANSWERS AND RATIONALES

The correct answer number and rationale for why it is the correct answer are given in boldface type. Rationales for why the other possible answer options are incorrect also are given, but they are not in boldface type.

1. 1. The client has an elevated blood pressure, but it is not life threatening; therefore, the client does not need to be seen first.
   2. The client with a DVT would be expected to be complaining of calf pain; therefore, this client would not be seen first.
   3. The client with peripheral vascular disease would be expected to have intermittent claudication; therefore, this client would not be seen first.
   4. **The client with a triple AAA who has a low back pain could have a leak, which could be life threatening; therefore, this client should be assessed first.**

2. 1. Increased hair loss occurs due to decreased oxygen to the lower extremities, but this is not life threatening; therefore, this information would not warrant immediate intervention.
   2. The client with arterial occlusive disease would be expected to have an absent dorsal pedal pulse; therefore, this would not warrant immediate intervention.
   3. **Numbness, tingling, and inability to move his or her toes would warrant intervention by the nurse. This indicates no arterial blood flow to the extremities.**
   4. The client hangs his or her legs off the bed to help increase arterial oxygen blood flow to the lower extremities. This would not warrant immediate intervention.

3. 1. JC cannot delegate assessment, teaching, evaluation, medications, or an unstable client to the UAP. Checking the pedal pulse is assessment.
   2. The client who is 4 hours postoperative leg surgery would not be able to ambulate down the hall. The client will be on bed rest for at least 24 hours.
   3. JC cannot delegate assessment, teaching, evaluation, medications, or an unstable client to the UAP.
   4. **The leg should be elevated to help decrease edema secondary to surgery and this can be delegated to a UAP.**

4. **3 and 4 are correct.**
   1. A daily aspirin is recommended as an anticoagulant to clients with atherosclerosis.

2. A low-fat, low-cholesterol diet is recommended to help decrease plaque formation in the vessels.
   3. **Sedentary life style is a "couch potato" lifestyle, which is not recommended for clients with atherosclerosis.**
   4. **The client should eat foods high in fiber to help decrease his or her cholesterol level.**
   5. Walking is an excellent isotonic exercise, which is recommended to help lose weight, develop collateral circulation, and decrease stress.

5. 1. BN should auscultate the bowel sounds, but BN should first assess the client's surgical incision, since the client is 2 days postoperative.
   2. **BN should first assess the surgical dressing to assess for bleeding or any type of drainage, then continue with the rest of the assessment, including bowel sounds, vital signs, and IV therapy.**
   3. The nurse should assess first, since it is the first part of the nursing process when the client is not in distress.
   4. Monitoring the intravenous therapy should be done by BN, but assessment is the first intervention.

6. 1. The client should not lift more than 5 pounds; doing so might cause the surgical incision to have dishensence. This statement indicates the client understands the teaching.
   2. The number one factor for developing atherosclerosis and increased blood pressure is smoking cigarettes; therefore, the client must quit. This statement indicates the client understands the teaching.
   3. **A truss is a kind of surgical appliance used for clients with a hernia. It provides support for the herniated area using a pad and belt arrangement to hold it in the correct position. This client would not be prescribed a truss; therefore, the client needs more discharge teaching.**
   4. The client should notify the healthcare provider if there is an elevated temperature because this indicates that the client has a postoperative infection. This statement indicates the client understands the teaching.

7. 1. PN would expect the client to have pain in the surgical area and, though this client's pain needs to be assessed, it would not be prior to a client in renal failure.

2. The 3+ posterior tibial pulse indicates the blood supply to the foot is adequate and would not require the client to be seen first by PN.

3. **The client is going into renal failure (should be 30 mL/hr), which is a potentially life-threatening complication of triple AAA surgery; therefore, this client must be assessed first.**

4. The client complaint needs to be addressed, but not prior to a physiological potentially life-threatening complication.

8. **Answer: 16 mL/hour.** To determine the rate, the test taker must first determine how many units are in each mL of fluid; 25,000 divided by 500 = 50 units of heparin in each mL of fluid, and 50 divided into 100 = 2, 18-2 = 16.

9. 1. The client should elevate the lower extremities to help decrease the edema and help the unoxgenated blood go up the inferior cava.

2. Massaging the legs would not warrant intervention for this client; it would be inappropriate for a client with deep vein thrombosis. Varicose veins will not dislodge a clot.

3. **The client with varicose veins should not be on bed rest. The client should have bathroom privileges and up ad lib.**

4. The UAP can calculate the client's I&O, not evaluate the I&O.

10. 1. Hospice is for a client whose healthcare provider determines the client has less than 6 months to live. This client does not have this diagnosis.

2. **The home health nurse is an appropriate referral for this client. The client's home should be assessed to determine if the client needs assistance in the home.**

3. The physical therapist addresses gait training and transferring.

4. Cardiac rehabilitation helps clients who have had myocardial infarctions, cardiac bypass surgery, or congestive heart failure recover.

Respiratory Management

If a man does his best, what else is there?

—General George S. Patton

QUESTIONS

1. The nurse on a medical unit has a client with adventitious breath sounds, but the nurse is unable to determine the exact nature of the situation. Which multidisciplinary team member should the nurse consult first?
   1. The healthcare provider.
   2. The unit manager.
   3. The respiratory therapist.
   4. The case manager.

2. The nurse is working with a licensed practical nurse (LPN) and an unlicensed assistive personnel (UAP) to care for a group of clients. Which nursing task should not be delegated or assigned?
   1. The routine oral medications for the clients.
   2. The bed baths and oral care.
   3. Evaluating the client's progress.
   4. Transporting a client to dialysis.

3. Which client should the charge nurse assign to the new graduate on the respiratory unit?
   1. The client diagnosed with lung cancer who has rust-colored sputum and chest pain of 10 on a scale of 1 to 10.
   2. The client diagnosed with atelectasis who is having shortness of breath and difficulty breathing.
   3. The client diagnosed with tuberculosis who has a non-productive cough and orange colored urine.
   4. The client diagnosed with pneumonia who has a pulse oximeter reading of 91% and has a CRT >3 seconds.

4. Which tasks are appropriate to assign to the unlicensed assistive personnel (UAP)?
   Select all that apply.
   1. Perform mouth care on the client with pneumonia.
   2. Apply oxygen via nasal cannula to the client.
   3. Empty the trashcans in the clients' rooms.
   4. Take the empty blood bag back to the laboratory.
   5. Show the client how to ambulate on the walker.

5. Which client should the medical unit nurse assess first after receiving the shift report?
    1. The 84-year-old client diagnosed with pneumonia who is afebrile but getting restless.
    2. The 25-year-old client diagnosed with influenza who is febrile and has a headache.
    3. The 56-year-old client diagnosed with a left-sided hemothorax with tidaling in the water-seal compartment of the Pleurvac.
    4. The 38-year-old client diagnosed with a sinus infection who has green drainage from the nose.

6. The client who is 2 days postoperative following a left pneumonectomy has an apical pulse (AP) rate of 128 beats per minute and a blood pressure (BP) of 80/50 mm Hg. Which intervention should the nurse implement first?
    1. Notify the healthcare provider (HCP) immediately.
    2. Assess the client's incisional wound.
    3. Prepare to administer dopamine, a vasopressor.
    4. Increase the client's intravenous (IV) rate.

7. The client who is 1 day postoperative following chest surgery is having difficulty breathing, has bilateral rales, and is confused and restless. Which intervention should the nurse implement first?
    1. Assess the client's pulse oximeter reading.
    2. Notify the Rapid Response Team.
    3. Place the client in the Trendelenburg position.
    4. Check the client's surgical dressing.

8. The client in the post-anesthesia care unit (PACU) has noisy and irregular respirations (Rs) with a pulse oximeter reading of 89%. Which intervention should the PACU nurse implement first?
    1. Increase the client's oxygen rate via nasal cannula.
    2. Notify the respiratory therapist to draw arterial blood gases.
    3. Tilt the head back and push forward on the angle of the lower jaw.
    4. Obtain an intubation tray and prepare for emergency intubation.

9. The day surgery admission nurse is obtaining operative permits for clients having surgery. Which client should the nurse question signing the consent form?
    1. The 16-year-old married client who is diagnosed with an ectopic pregnancy.
    2. The 39-year-old client diagnosed with paranoid schizophrenia.
    3. The 50-year-old client who admits to being a recovering alcoholic.
    4. The 84-year-old client diagnosed with chronic obstructive pulmonary disease (COPD).

10. The intensive care unit (ICU) nurse is caring for a client on a ventilator who is exhibiting respiratory distress. The ventilator alarms are going off. Which intervention should the nurse implement first?
    1. Notify the respiratory therapist immediately.
    2. Ventilate with a manual resuscitation bag.
    3. Check the ventilator to resolve the problem.
    4. Auscultate the client's lung sounds.

11. The charge nurse on the critical care respiratory unit is evaluating arterial blood gas (ABG) values of several clients. Which client would require an immediate intervention by the charge nurse?
    1. The client with chronic obstructive pulmonary disease who has a pH 7.34, PaO_2 70, $PaCO_2$ 55, HCO_3 24.
    2. The client with Adult Respiratory Distress Syndrome who has a pH 7.35, PaO_2 75, $PaCO_2$ 50, HCO_3 26.
    3. The client with reactive airway disease with a pH 7.48, PaO_2 80, $PaCO_2$ 30, HCO_3 23.
    4. The client with a pneumothorax with a pH 7.41, PaO_2 98, $PaCO_2$ 43, HCO_3 25.

12. The primary nurse in the critical care respiratory unit is very busy. Which nursing task should be the nurse's priority?
   1. Assist the HCP with a sterile dressing change for a client with a left pneumonectomy.
   2. Obtain a tracheostomy tray for a client who is exhibiting air hunger.
   3. Transcribe orders for a client with cystic fibrosis who was transferred from the ED.
   4. Assess the client diagnosed with mesothelioma who is upset, angry, and crying.

13. The nurse is caring for a client diagnosed with flail chest who has had a chest tube for 3 days. The nurse notes there is no tidaling in the water-seal compartment. Which initial action should be taken by the nurse?
   1. Check the tubing for any dependent loops.
   2. Auscultate the client's posterior breath sounds.
   3. Prepare to remove the client's chest tubes.
   4. Notify the HCP that the lungs have re-expanded.

14. The client with a right-sided pneumothorax had chest tubes inserted 2 hours ago. There is no fluctuation in the water-seal chamber of the Pleurovac. Which intervention should the nurse implement first?
   1. Assess the client's lung sounds.
   2. Check for any kinks in the tubing.
   3. Ask the client to take deep breaths.
   4. Turn the client from side to side.

15. Which client requires the immediate attention of the intensive care unit nurse?
   1. The client with histoplasmosis who is having excessive diaphoresis and neck stiffness.
   2. The client with acute respiratory distress syndrome (ARDS) who has difficulty breathing.
   3. The client with pulmonary sarcoidosis who has a dry cough and mild chest pain.
   4. The client with asbestosis who has a productive cough and chest tightness.

16. The client in the intensive care unit is on a ventilator. Which interventions should the nurse implement? **Select all that apply.**
   1. Ensure there is a manual resuscitation bag at the bedside.
   2. Monitor the client's pulse oximeter reading every shift.
   3. Assess the client's respiratory status every 2 hours.
   4. Check the ventilator settings every 4 hours.
   5. Collaborate with the respiratory therapist.

17. The unlicensed assistive personnel (UAP) is bathing the client diagnosed with adult acute respiratory distress syndrome (ARDS) who is on a ventilator. The bed is in the high position with the opposite side rail elevated. Which action should the ICU nurse take?
   1. Demonstrate the correct technique when giving a bed bath.
   2. Encourage the UAP to put the bed in the lowest position.
   3. Explain that the client on a ventilator should not be bathed.
   4. Give the UAP praise for performing the bath safely.

18. The female charge nurse on the respiratory unit tells the male nurse, "You are really cute and have a great body. Do you work out?" Which action should be taken by the male nurse if he thinks he is being sexually harassed?
   1. Document the comment in writing and tell another staff nurse.
   2. Ask the charge nurse to stop making comments like this.
   3. Notify the clinical manager of the sexual harassment.
   4. Report this to the corporate headquarters office.

19. The client diagnosed with abdominal pain of unknown etiology has a nasogastric tube draining green bile and reports abdominal pain of 8 on a scale of 1 to 10. The client's arterial blood gas values are pH 7.48, PaO_2 98, $PaCO_2$ 36, HCO_3 28. Which intervention should the nurse implement based on the client's ABGs?
1. Assess the client to rule out any complications secondary to the client's pain.
2. Determine the last time the client was medicated for abdominal pain.
3. Check the amount of suction on the client's nasogastric tube.
4. Administer intravenous sodium bicarbonate to the client.

20. The charge nurse in the intensive care unit asks a nurse to float from the medical/surgical unit to the ICU. Which client should the charge nurse assign to the float nurse?
1. The client who is 3 hours postoperative lung transplant.
2. The client who has a central venous pressure of 13 cm H_2O.
3. The client who is diagnosed with bacterial pneumonia.
4. The client who is diagnosed with Hantavirus pulmonary syndrome.

21. The client has arterial blood gas values of pH 7.38, PaO_2 77, $PaCO_2$ 40, HCO_3 24. Which intervention should the critical care nurse implement?
1. Administer oxygen 6 L/min via nasal cannula.
2. Encourage the client to take deep breaths.
3. Administer intravenous sodium bicarbonate.
4. Assess the client's respiratory status.

22. The husband of a client diagnosed with a terminal lung cancer asks the nurse, "How am I going to take care of my wife when we go home?" Which action by the nurse is most appropriate?
1. Notify the social worker about the husband's concerns.
2. Contact the hospital chaplain to talk to the husband.
3. Leave a note on the chart for the HCP to talk to the husband.
4. Reassure the husband that everything will be all right.

23. The clinic nurse is scheduling a chest x-ray for a female client who may have pneumonia. Which question is most important for the nurse to ask the client?
1. "Have you ever had a chest x-ray before?"
2. "Can you hold your breath for a minute?"
3. "Do you smoke or have you ever smoked cigarettes?"
4. "Is there any chance you may be pregnant?"

24. The clinic nurse is returning phone messages from clients. Which phone message should the nurse return first?
1. The elderly client with pneumonia who reports being dizzy when getting up.
2. The client with cystic fibrosis who needs a prescription for pancreatic enzymes.
3. The client with lung cancer on chemotherapy who reports nausea.
4. The client with pertussis who reports coughing spells so severe that they cause vomiting.

25. The client diagnosed with active tuberculosis tells the public health nurse, "I am not going to take any more medications. I am tired of them." Which statement is the nurse's best response?
1. "You are tired of taking your tuberculosis medications."
2. "You must take your TB medications. It is not an option."
3. "You must discuss this with your healthcare provider."
4. "As long as you wear a mask, you do not have to take the meds."

26. The nurse is working in an outpatient clinic along with a licensed practical nurse (LPN). Which client should the nurse assign to the LPN?
   1. The client whose purified protein derivative (PPD) induration of the left arm is 14 mm.
   2. The client diagnosed with pneumonia whose pulse oximeter reading is 90%.
   3. The client with acute bronchitis who has a chronic clear mucous cough and low fever.
   4. The client with reactive airway disease who has bilateral wheezing.

27. The unlicensed assistive personnel (UAP) tells the clinic nurse that the male client in Room 1 is "really breathing hard and can't seem to catch his breath." Which instruction should the nurse give to the UAP?
   1. Put 4 mL oxygen on the client.
   2. Sit the client upright in a chair.
   3. Go with the nurse to the client's room.
   4. Take the client's vital signs.

28. The clinic nurse is scheduling a 14-year-old client for a tonsillectomy. Which intervention should the clinic nurse implement?
   1. Obtain informed consent from the client.
   2. Send a throat culture to the laboratory.
   3. Discuss the need to cough and deep breathe.
   4. Request the laboratory to draw a PT and a PTT.

29. The client calls the clinic nurse and asks, "What is the best way to prevent getting influenza?" Which statement is the nurse's best response?
   1. "Take prophylactic antibiotics for 10 days after being exposed to influenza."
   2. "Stay away for large crowds and wear a scarf over your mouth during cold weather."
   3. "The best way to prevent getting influenza is to get a yearly flu vaccine."
   4. "You must eat three well-balanced meals a day and exercise daily to prevent influenza."

30. The clinic nurse is evaluating vital signs for clients being seen in the outpatient clinic. Which client would require nursing intervention?
   1. The 10-month-old infant who has a pulse rate of 140 beats per minute.
   2. The 3-year-old toddler who has a respiratory rate of 28 breaths per minute.
   3. The 24-week gestational woman who has a BP of 142/96 mm Hg.
   4. The 42-year-old client who has a temperature of 100.2°F (37.8°C).

31. The nurse is accidentally stuck with a needle used to administer an intradermal injection for a PPD. Which intervention should the nurse implement first?
   1. Complete the accident/occurrence report.
   2. Immediately wash the area with soap and water.
   3. Ask the client whether he or she has AIDS or hepatitis.
   4. Place an antibiotic ointment and bandage on the site.

32. The clinic nurse is reviewing laboratory results for clients seen in the clinic. Which client requires additional assessment by the nurse?
   1. The client who has a hemoglobin of 9 g/dL and a hematocrit of 29%.
   2. The client who has a WBC count of 9.0 mm^3.
   3. The client who has a serum potassium level of 4.8 mEq/L.
   4. The client who has a serum sodium level of 137 mEq/L.

33. The Hispanic female client diagnosed with bacterial pneumonia is being admitted to the medical unit. The Hispanic husband answers questions even though the nurse directly asks the client. Which action should the nurse take?
    1. Ask the husband to allow his wife to answer the questions.
    2. Request the husband to leave the examination room.
    3. Continue to allow the husband to answer the wife's questions.
    4. Do not ask any further questions until the client starts answering.

34. The clinic nurse encounters a client who does not respond to verbal stimuli and initiates cardiopulmonary resuscitation (CPR). What should the nurse do? Prioritize the nurse's actions from first (1) to last (5).
    1. Open the client's airway.
    2. Check the client's carotid pulse.
    3. Assess the client for unresponsiveness.
    4. Perform compressions at a 30:2 rate.
    5. Pinch the nose and give two breaths.

35. The home health nurse is visiting the client diagnosed with end-stage chronic obstructive pulmonary disease (COPD) while the unlicensed assistive personnel (UAP) is providing care. Which action by the UAP would warrant intervention by the nurse?
    1. Keeping the bedroom at a warm temperature.
    2. Maintaining the client's oxygen rate at 2 L/min.
    3. Helping the client sit in the orthopneic position.
    4. Allowing the client to sleep in the recliner.

36. Which task is most appropriate for the home health nurse to delegate to unlicensed assistive personnel (UAP)?
    1. Changing the client's subclavian dressing.
    2. Reinserting the client's Foley catheter.
    3. Demonstrating ambulation with a walker.
    4. Getting the client up in a chair three times a day.

37. In the local restaurant, the nurse overhears another hospital staff member talking to a friend about a client. The staff member discloses that the client was just diagnosed with lung cancer. What is the most appropriate action by the nurse?
    1. Do not approach the staff member in the restaurant.
    2. Ask the staff member not to discuss anything about the client.
    3. Contact the staff member's clinical manager and report the behavior.
    4. Tell the client that the staff member was discussing confidential information.

38. The 92-year-old client has a hospital bed in the home and is on strict bed rest. The unlicensed assistive personnel (UAP) cares for the client in the morning 5 days a week. Which statement indicates that the UAP needs additional education by the nurse?
    1. "I do not give her a lot of fluids so she won't wet the bed."
    2. "I perform passive range-of-motion exercises every morning."
    3. "I put her on her side so that there will be no pressure on her butt."
    4. "I do not pull her across the sheets when I am moving her in bed."

39. The home health client is diagnosed with chronic obstructive disease. The unlicensed assistive personnel (UAP) tells the home health nurse that the client has trouble breathing when the client lies in a supine position. Which priority instruction should the nurse provide to the UAP?
    1. To ensure the client's oxygen is in place correctly.
    2. To allow the client to sleep in a recliner.
    3. To allow a fan to blow on the client when lying in bed.
    4. To have the client take slow, deep breaths.

40. The wife of a client diagnosed as terminal is concerned that the client is not eating or drinking. Which is the home health nurse's best response?
1. "I will start an IV if your husband continues to refuse to eat or drink."
2. "You should discuss placing a PEG feeding tube in your husband with the HCP."
3. "This is normal at the end of life; the dehydration produces a type of euphoria."
4. "You are right to be concerned. Would you like to talk about your worry?"

41. The client has just been told a medical condition cannot be treated successfully and the client has a life expectancy of about 6 months. To whom should the nurse refer the client at this time?
1. A home health nurse.
2. The client's pastor.
3. A hospice agency.
4. The social worker.

42. The hospice client asks the nurse, "What should I do about my house? My son and daughter are fighting over it." Which statement is the nurse's best response?
1. "I think you should tell your children that you will leave the house to a charity."
2. "I would sell the house and go on an extended vacation and spend the money."
3. "What do you want to happen to your house? It is your decision."
4. "Wait and let your children fight over the house after you are gone."

43. The female nurse manager is discussing the yearly performance evaluation with a male nurse. Which information regarding communication styles should the nurse manager employ when talking with the employee?
1. Men tend to see the work from a global perspective centering on feelings.
2. Men often see the work environment from a logical, focused perspective.
3. Men ask many more questions than women and require specific answers.
4. Men and women communicate similarly in a nursing environment.

44. The newly hired nurse manager has identified that whenever a specific staff member is unhappy with an assignment, the entire unit has a bad day. Which action should the unit manager take to correct this problem?
1. Determine why the staff member is unhappy.
2. Discuss the staff member's attitude and the way it affects the unit.
3. Place the staff member on a counseling record for the behavior.
4. Suspend the staff member until the behavior improves.

45. The healthcare facility where the nurse works uses e-mail to notify the staff of in-services and mandatory requirements. Which is important information for the nurse manager to remember when using e-mail to disseminate information?
1. Give as much information as possible in each e-mail.
2. Use e-mail for all communications with the staff.
3. Use capital letters to get a point across with emphasis.
4. Make the e-mail notices quick and easy to read.

46. At 1700, the HCP is yelling at the nursing staff because the early morning lab work is not available for a client's chart. Which is the most appropriate response by the charge nurse?
1. Call the lab and have the lab supervisor talk with the HCP.
2. Discuss the HCP's complaints with the nursing supervisor.
3. Form a committee of lab and nursing personnel to fix the problem.
4. Tell the HCP to stop yelling and calm down.

47. The nurse is caring for a client who has a chest tube. What should the nurse do? Prioritize the nurse's actions from first (1) to last (5).
  1. Assess the client's lung sounds.
  2. Note the amount of suction being used.
  3. Check the chest tube dressing for drainage.
  4. Make sure that the chest tube is securely taped.
  5. Place a bottle of sterile saline at the bedside.

48. The nurse is assessing clients on a respiratory unit. Which client should be the nurse's first priority?
  1. The client diagnosed with bronchiectasis who has clubbing of the fingernails.
  2. The client diagnosed with byssinosis who reports chest tightness.
  3. The client diagnosed with cystic fibrosis who has a pulse oximeter reading of 91%.
  4. The client diagnosed with pneumoconiosis who has shortness of breath.

49. The nurse is developing a nursing care plan for a client diagnosed with chronic obstructive pulmonary disease (COPD). What should be the client's priority nursing diagnosis?
  1. Activity intolerance.
  2. Altered coping.
  3. Impaired gas exchange.
  4. Self-care deficit.

50. The nurse assists with the insertion of a chest tube in a client diagnosed with a spontaneous pneumothorax. Which data indicates that the treatment has been effective?
  1. The chest x-ray indicates consolidation.
  2. The client has bilateral breath sounds.
  3. The suction chamber has vigorous bubbling.
  4. The client has crepitus around the insertion site.

51. The healthcare provider ordered the loop diuretic, bumetanide (Bumex), to be administered STAT to a client diagnosed with pulmonary edema. After 4 hours, which of the following assessment data indicates the client may be experiencing a complication of the medication?
  1. The client develops jugular vein distention.
  2. The client has bilateral rales and rhonchi.
  3. The client complains of painful leg cramps.
  4. The client's output is greater than the intake.

52. The client involved in a motor vehicle accident is being prepped for surgery when the client asks the emergency department nurse, "What happened to my child?" The nurse knows the child is dead. Which statement is an example of the ethical principle of nonmalfeasance?
  1. "I will find out for you and let you know after surgery."
  2. "I am sorry but your child died at the scene of the accident."
  3. "You should concentrate on your surgery right now."
  4. "You are concerned about your child. Would you like to talk?"

53. The new graduate has accepted a position at a facility that is accredited by the Joint Commission. Which statement describes the purpose of this organization?
  1. The Commission reviews facilities for compliance with standards of care.
  2. Accreditation by the Commission guarantees the facility will be reimbursed for care provided.
  3. Accreditation by the Commission reduces liability in a legal action against the facility.
  4. The Commission eliminates the need for Medicare to survey a hospital.

54. The client in a critical care unit died. What action should the nurse implement first?
1. Stay with the significant other.
2. Gather the client's belongings.
3. Perform post-mortem care.
4. Ask about organ donation.

55. The nurse caring for client BC is preparing to administer medications. Based on the laboratory data given in this table, which intervention should the nurse implement?

Client's Name: BC	Account Number: 55678-78	Allergies: Sulfa
Diagnosis: Deep Vein Thrombosis	Height: 70 inches	Weight: 150 pounds

Laboratory Report		
Lab Test	Client Value	Normal Value
PT	19.3	10–13 seconds
INR	1.7	2.0–3.0 (therapeutic)
PTT	53	34 seconds

1. Administer warfarin (Coumadin) IVP.
2. Continue the heparin drip.
3. Hold the next dose of warfarin.
4. Administer the daily aspirin.

56. In the intensive care unit (ICU), the critical care nurse assesses a client diagnosed with an asthma attack who has a respiration rate of 10 and an oxygen saturation of 88%. Which intervention should the nurse implement first?
1. Call a Rapid Response Team (RRT).
2. Increase the oxygen to 10 LPM.
3. Check the client's ABG results.
4. Administer the fast-acting inhaler.

57. The client in the intensive care unit (ICU) has been on a ventilator for 2 weeks with an endotracheal tube in place. Which intervention should the nurse prepare the client for next?
1. Transfer to a long-term care facility.
2. Daily arterial blood gases.
3. Removal of life support.
4. Placement of a tracheostomy.

58. The nurse is teaching the parents of a child diagnosed with cystic fibrosis. Which information is priority to teach the parents?
1. Explain that the child's skin tastes salty.
2. Observe the consistency of the stools daily.
3. Give pancreatic enzymes with every meal.
4. Increase the intake of salt in the child's diet.

59. The UAP enters the elderly female client's room to give the bath, but the client is watching her favorite soap opera. Which instructions should the nurse give to the UAP?
1. Tell the UAP to complete the bath at this time.
2. Have the UAP skip the client's bath for the day.
3. Instruct the UAP to give the bath after the program.
4. Document the attempt to give the bath as refused.

60. The nurse has been made the chairperson of a quality improvement committee. Which statement is an example of effective group process?
    1. The nurse involves all committee members in the discussion.
    2. The nurse makes sure all members of the group agree with the decisions.
    3. The nurse asks two of the committee members to do the work.
    4. The nurse does not allow deviation from the agenda to occur.

61. While the nurse is caring for a client on a ventilator the ventilator alarm sounds. What is the first action taken by the nurse?
    1. Silence the ventilator alarm.
    2. Notify the respiratory therapist.
    3. Assess the client's respiratory status.
    4. Ventilate the client using a manual resuscitation bag.

62. The client diagnosed with acute respiratory distress syndrome (ARDS) is having increased difficulty breathing. The arterial blood gas indicates an arterial oxygen level of 54% on O_2 at 10 LPM. Which intervention should the intensive care unit nurse implement first?
    1. Prepare the client for intubation.
    2. Bag the client with a bag/mask device.
    3. Call a Code Blue and initiate cardiopulmonary resuscitation (CPR).
    4. Start an IV with an 18-gauge catheter.

63. The client's arterial blood gas (ABG) results are pH 7.34, $PaCO_2$ 50, HCO_3 24, PaO_2 87. Which intervention should the nurse implement first?
    1. Have the client turn, cough, and deep breathe.
    2. Place the client on oxygen via nasal cannula.
    3. Check the client's pulse oximeter reading.
    4. Notify the HCP of the ABG results.

64. The client is admitted to the emergency department with an apical pulse rate of 134, respiration rate of 28, and BP of 92/56, and the skin is pale and clammy. What action should the nurse perform first?
    1. Type and crossmatch the client for PRBCs.
    2. Start two IVs with large-bore catheters.
    3. Obtain the client's history and physical.
    4. Check the client's allergies to medications.

65. The charge nurse of the respiratory care unit is making assignments. Which clients should be assigned to the intensive care nurse who is working on the respiratory care unit for the day? **Select the patient/patients that apply.**
    1. The client who had four coronary artery bypass grafts 3 days ago.
    2. The client who has anterior and posterior chest tubes after a motor vehicle accident.
    3. The client who will be moved to the intensive care unit when a bed is available.
    4. The client who has a do not resuscitate order and is requesting to see a chaplain.
    5. The client who is on multiple intravenous drip medications needed to be titrated.

66. The emergency department nurse is preparing to assist the surgeon to insert chest tubes in a client with a right hemothorax. Which position is appropriate for the procedure?
    1. Have the client sit upright and bend over the over bed table.
    2. Place the client in the left lateral recumbent position.
    3. Have the client sit on the side of the bed with the back arched like a Halloween cat.
    4. Place the client lying on the back with the head of the bed up 45 degrees.

67. The nurse is admitting a patient diagnosed with pneumonia. Which healthcare provider's order should be implemented first?
    1. 1,000 mL normal saline at 125 mL/hour.
    2. Obtain sputum for Gram stain and culture.
    3. Ceftriaxone (Rocephin) 1,000 mg IVPB every 12 hours.
    4. Ultrasonic nebulization treatment every 6 hours.

68. The nurse is preparing to make rounds after receiving shift report. Which client should the nurse assess first?
   1. The patient diagnosed with end-stage COPD complaining of shortness of breath after ambulating to the bathroom.
   2. The patient diagnosed with a deep vein thrombosis who is requesting an anti-anxiety medication.
   3. The patient diagnosed with cystic fibrosis who has a sputum specimen to be taken to the laboratory.
   4. The patient diagnosed with an empyema who has a temperature of 100.8°F, pulse of 118, respiration rate of 26, and BP of 148/64.

69. The respiratory unit nurse is calculating the shift intake and output for a client diagnosed with right-sided chest tube. The client has received 1,500 mL of D5W, IVPB of 100 mL of 0.9% NS, 12 ounces of water, 6 ounces of milk, and 4 ounces of chicken broth. The client has had a urinary output of 800 mL and chest drainage of 125 mL. What is the total intake and output for this client? _____

70. Which client should the charge nurse on the respiratory unit assign to the graduate nurse who just completed orientation?
   1. The client diagnosed with bronchiolitis who has a wheezy cough and rapid breathing.
   2. The client diagnosed with pneumonia who has dull percussion and vocal fremitus.
   3. The client diagnosed with a flail chest who has paradoxical movement of the chest wall.
   4. The client diagnosed with reactive airway disease who has bilateral wheezing.

RESPIRATORY CLINICAL SCENARIO

Ms. Gail is the charge nurse for the 7a-7p shift. The staff includes three RNs, one LPN, and two UAPs for a 16-bed unit.

1. Ms. Gail is making shift assignments. Which client should be assigned to the most experienced RN?
   1. The client diagnosed with pneumonia who has bilateral crackles and a pulse oximeter reading of 96%.
   2. The client whose pulse oximeter reading keeps decreasing after receiving high levels oxygen via nasal cannula.
   3. The client who had a Caldwell Luc procedure 1 day ago and has purulent drainage on the drip pad.
   4. The client who had a tonsillectomy this morning who is complaining of throat pain rated 8 on a pain scale of 1 to 10.

2. The client diagnosed with a community-acquired pneumonia is being admitted to the unit. Which healthcare provider's order should be implemented first?
   1. Administer Rocephin 50 mg IVPB every 24 hours.
   2. Apply oxygen 2 L via nasal cannula.
   3. Obtain a sputum specimen for culture and sensitivity.
   4. Place client in respiratory isolation.

3. The client diagnosed with an exacerbation of COPD is in respiratory distress. Which intervention should the nurse implement first?
   1. Place the client in the orthopnic position.
   2. Administer 6 L oxygen via nasal cannula.
   3. Assess the client's pulse oximeter reading.
   4. Notify the respiratory therapist.

4. Which client should Ms. Gail assign to the licensed practical nurse (LPN)?
   1. The client who had a laryngectomy 2 days ago and has crepitus.
   2. The client with respiratory difficulty who is confused and keeps climbing out of bed.
   3. The client newly diagnosed with active tuberculosis who needs medication teaching.
   4. The client diagnosed with asthma who has a pulse oximetry reading of 90%.

5. Ms. Gail and the UAP are caring for the following clients. Which information provided by the UAP requires immediate intervention by Ms. Gail?
   1. The client diagnosed with active tuberculosis who is in respiratory isolation and has orange urine in the urinary catheter.
   2. The client who has a right upper lobectomy on the patient controlled analgesia (PCA) pump has level 4 pain on a scale of 1 to 10.
   3. The client with a left-sided pneumothorax has 200 mL of blood in the collection chamber of the Pleuravac.
   4. The client diagnosed with bacterial pneumonia who has an elevated temperature and chills.

6. One of Ms. Gail's staff nurses is preparing to administer a.m. medications to clients. Which medication should the nurse question administering to the client?
   1. Carafate for the client who has not had breakfast.
   2. Digoxin to the client with a digoxin level of 1.9 mg/dL.
   3. Hanging the heparin bag to a client with a PT/PTT of 12.9/78.
   4. The aminoglycoside antibiotic to the client with an elevated trough level.

7. The client is getting out of bed, becomes very anxious, and has a feeling of impending doom. The nurse reports these findings to Ms. Gail. Which intervention should Ms. Gail tell the nurse to implement first after placing the client in the high-Fowler's position?
   1. Administer oxygen via nasal cannula.
   2. Prepare the client for a ventilation/perfusion scan.
   3. Notify the client's healthcare provider.
   4. Auscultate the client's lung sounds.

8. The client with a right-sided chest tube is complaining of pain rated 6 on a pain scale of 1 to 10. Which intervention should the nurse implement first?
   1. Document the client's pain complaint in the nurse's notes.
   2. Instruct the client to take slow, deep breaths and exhale slowly.
   3. Assess the client's respiratory status and chest tube insertion site.
   4. Check the client's MAR to determine when the last pain medication was administered.

9. Ms. Gail is discussing the care of a client with a right-sided chest tube secondary to a pneumothorax with a graduate nurse. Which interventions should Ms. Gail discuss with the graduate nurse? **Select all that apply.**
   1. Place the client in the high-Fowler's position.
   2. Assess the chest tube drainage system every shift.
   3. Maintain strict bed rest for the client.
   4. Ensure the tubing has no dependent loops.
   5. Mark the collection chamber for drainage every shift.

10. Ms. Gail is making client assignments. Which client should Ms. Gail assign to the LPN?
    1. The client who is suspected of having acute respiratory distress syndrome.
    2. The client with a hemothorax who needs two units of blood.
    3. The client with chest tubes who has jugular vein distention and BP of 96/60.
    4. The client who is scheduled for a bronchoscopy to R/O lung cancer.

ANSWERS AND RATIONALES

The correct answer number and rationale for why it is the correct answer are given in **boldface type**. Rationales for why the other possible answer options are incorrect also are given, but they are not in boldface type.

1. 1. The client's HCP should be consulted if the nurse determines a need, but at this time, the nurse should discuss the client with the respiratory therapist.
   2. The unit manager may or may not be capable of helping the nurse assess a client with adventitious breath sounds; therefore, this is not the first person the nurse should consult.
   3. **Respiratory therapists assess and treat clients with lung problems multiple times every day. Therefore, this is the best person to consult when the nurse needs help identifying a respiratory problem.**
   4. The case manager is usually capable of maneuvering through the maze of healthcare referrals, but is not necessarily an expert in lung sounds.
   Content – Medical/Surgical: **Category of Health Alteration** *– Respiratory:* **Integrated Processes** *– Nursing Process: Planning:* **Client Needs** *– Safe and Effective Care Environment: Management of Care:* **Cognitive Level** *– Analysis*

MAKING NURSING DECISIONS: The test taker must be knowledgeable of the role of all members of the multidisciplinary healthcare team as well as HIPAA rules and regulations. These will be tested on the NCLEX-RN® exam.

2. 1. The LPN may be assigned to administer the routine oral medications to the clients.
   2. Bed baths and oral care can be performed by the UAP.
   3. **The nurse cannot delegate or assign tasks that require nursing judgment, such as evaluating a client's progress.**
   4. The UAP can transport a client to dialysis.
   Content – Medical/Surgical: **Category of Health Alteration** *– Respiratory:* **Integrated Processes** *– Nursing Process: Planning:* **Client Needs** *– Safe and Effective Care Environment: Management of Care:* **Cognitive Level** *– Synthesis*

MAKING NURSING DECISIONS: The nurse cannot delegate assessment, evaluation, teaching, or administration of medications to any client or the care of an unstable client to a UAP. Also, the nurse cannot assign assessment, evaluation,

teaching, or tasks that require nursing judgment to an LPN.

3. 1. The client with lung cancer is expected to have rust-colored sputum; however, complaining of pain rated as a 10 warrants a more experienced nurse to assess the cause of the pain and medicate as needed.
   2. The client with atelectasis (collapsed lung) who is having difficulty breathing needs a more experienced nurse to assess the client. This client is not stable.
   3. **The orange-colored urine is secondary to rifampin, an antitubercular medication, and a non-productive cough is expected. Therefore, this client is stable and should be assigned to a new graduate nurse.**
   4. The client is exhibiting respiratory compromise and is not stable. The pulse oximeter reading should be greater than 93% and the CRT should be less than 3 seconds.
   Content – Medical/Surgical: **Category of Health Alteration** *– Respiratory:* **Integrated Processes** *– Nursing Process: Planning:* **Client Needs** *– Safe and Effective Care Environment: Management of Care:* **Cognitive Level** *– Synthesis*

MAKING NURSING DECISIONS: The charge nurse should assign the most stable client to the new graduate nurse. The test taker must determine which client is exhibiting expected signs/symptoms and this client should be assigned to the new graduate nurse. Client's exhibiting signs/symptoms not expected for the client should be assigned to a more experienced nurse.

4. 1 and 4 are correct.
   1. **The UAP can perform mouth care on a client who is stable.**
   2. Oxygen is a medication and the nurse cannot delegate medication administration to the UAP.
   3. The housekeeping staff empty trashcans, not the UAP. Remember not to assign tasks that should be done by another hospital department.
   4. **The UAP can take the empty blood bag to the laboratory.**
   5. The nurse cannot delegate teaching to the UAP.
   Content – Medical/Surgical: **Category of Health Alteration** *– Respiratory:* **Integrated Processes** *– Nursing Process: Planning:* **Client Needs** *– Safe and Effective Care Environment: Management of Care:* **Cognitive Level** *– Synthesis*

MAKING NURSING DECISIONS: The nurse should not delegate assessment, teaching, evaluation, medications, or an unstable client to the UAP.

5. 1. Elderly clients diagnosed with pneumonia may not present with the "normal" symptoms, such as fever. The client's increased restlessness may indicate a decrease in oxygen to the brain. This client should be seen first.

2. The client with influenza would be expected to have an elevated temperature and a headache; therefore, this client would not need to be assessed first.

3. Tidaling in the water-seal compartment is expected; therefore, the nurse would not need to assess this client first.

4. Sinus drainage is to be expected in a client diagnosed with a sinus infection.

Content – Medical/Surgical: **Category of Health Alteration** *– Respiratory:* **Integrated Processes** *– Nursing Process: Assessment:* **Client Needs** *– Physiological Integrity: Reduction of Risk Potential* **Cognitive Level** *– Synthesis*

MAKING NURSING DECISIONS: The test taker must determine which sign/symptom is not expected for the disease process. If the sign/symptom is not expected then the nurse should assess the client first. This type of question is determining if the nurse is knowledgeable of signs/symptoms of a variety of disease processes.

6. 1. The HCP should be notified, but this is not the first intervention. The HCP will require other information, such as what the incision looks like and whether there is any bleeding that can be seen, before making any decisions. The nurse, therefore, should first provide emergency care to the client—in this case, support the client's circulatory system by increasing the IV rate—and then assess the patient before reporting to the HCP.

2. The incisional wound should be assessed, but the priority is maintaining circulatory status because the client's vital signs indicate shock.

3. The client may require medication, such as dopamine, to increase the blood pressure, but the client's circulatory system needs immediate support, which increasing the IV rate will provide. That, then, is the priority.

4. **Increasing the IV rate will provide the client with circulatory volume immediately. Therefore, this is the first intervention.**

Content – Medical/Surgical: **Category of Health Alteration** *– Respiratory:* **Integrated Processes** *– Nursing Process: Implementation:* **Client Needs** *– Physiological Integrity: Reduction of Risk Potential:* **Cognitive Level** *– Synthesis*

MAKING NURSING DECISIONS: Remember: "If the client is in distress, do not assess." Situations such as those in this question require the nurse to intervene to prevent the client's status from deteriorating. Before selecting "notify the HCP" as the correct answer, the test taker must examine the other three options. If any of the other options contain data that will relieve the client's distress, prevent a life-threatening situation, or provide information the HCP will need to make an informed decision, then the test taker should eliminate the "notify the HCP" option.

7. 1. The client is in distress; therefore, the nurse should do something to help the client.

2. **The Rapid Response Team was mandated by The Joint Commission. It is a team of healthcare professionals who respond to clients who are breathing but who the nurse thinks are in an emergency situation. A code is called if the client is not breathing.**

3. The Trendelenburg position is used for a client who is in hypovolemic shock, so this would not be appropriate for a client in respiratory distress.

4. The stem of the question provides enough information to indicate the client is in distress, and assessing the surgical dressing will not help the client.

Content – Medical/Surgical: **Category of Health Alteration** *– Respiratory:* **Integrated Processes** *– Nursing Process: Implementation:* **Client Needs** *– Physiological Integrity: Reduction of Risk Potential:* **Cognitive Level** *– Synthesis*

MAKING NURSING DECISIONS: The nurse must determine if the client is in distress; remember: if in distress do not assess. The nurse must intervene to help the client. Do not select equipment over the client's body. The **NCLEX-RN®** blueprint includes nursing care that is ruled by the current National Patient Safety Goals. The nurse must be knowledgeable of these goals.

8. 1. Increasing the oxygen rate will not help open the client's airway, which is the first intervention. Oxygen can be increased after the airway is patent.

2. The respiratory therapist could be notified and arterial blood gases (ABGs) drawn if positioning does not increase the pulse oximeter reading, but this is not the first intervention.

3. **The client is exhibiting signs/symptoms of hypopharyngeal obstruction, and this maneuver pulls the tongue forward and opens the air passage.**

4. The client may need to be intubated if positioning does not open the airway, but this is not the first intervention.

Content – Medical/Surgical: **Category of Health Alteration** – *Respiratory:* **Integrated Processes** – *Nursing Process: Assessment:* **Client Needs** – *Physiological Integrity: Reduction of Risk Potential:* **Cognitive Level** – *Analysis*

MAKING NURSING DECISIONS: Physiological problems have the highest priority when deciding on a course of action. If the client is in distress, then the nurse must intervene with a nursing action that attempts to alleviate or control the problem. The test taker should not choose a diagnostic test if there is an option that directly treats the client.

9. 1. An emancipated minor under the age of 18 but married or independently earning his or her own living would not warrant the nurse's questioning whether she should sign the permit. "Married" indicates an independently functioning individual.
    2. **An incompetent client cannot sign the consent form. An incompetent client is an individual who is not autonomous and cannot give or withhold consent, for example, individuals who are cognitively impaired, mentally ill, neurologically incapacitated, or under the influence of mind-altering drugs. The client may be able to sign the permit, but the nurse should question the client's ability to sign the permit because paranoid schizophrenia is a mental illness.**
    3. A recovering alcoholic is not considered incapacitated. If the client is currently under the influence of alcohol, then the permit could not legally be signed by the client.
    4. The elderly client is considered competent until deemed incompetent in a court of law or meets the criteria to be considered incompetent.
    Content – Management of Care: **Category of Health Alteration** – *Preoperative:* **Integrated Processes** – *Nursing Process: Implementation:* **Client Needs** – *Safe and Effective Care Environment: Management of Care:* **Cognitive Level** – *Knowledge*

MAKING NURSING DECISIONS: The NCLEX-RN® blueprint includes nursing care that is ruled by legal requirements. The nurse must be knowledgeable of these issues.

10. 1. The nurse must first address the client's acute respiratory distress and then notify other members of the multidisciplinary team.
    2. If the ventilator system malfunctions, the nurse must ventilate the client with a manual resuscitation bag (Ambu) until the problem is resolved. The nurse should determine

whether the nurse can remedy the situation by assessing the ventilator before beginning manual ventilations.
    3. **The client is having respiratory distress and the ventilator is sounding an alarm; therefore, the nurse should first assess the ventilator to determine the cause of the problem and correct it because the client is totally dependent on the ventilator for breathing. This is one of the few situations wherein the nurse would assess the equipment before assessing the client.**
    4. In most situations, assessing the client is the first intervention, but because the client is totally dependent on the ventilator for breathing, the nurse should first assess the ventilator to determine the cause of the alarms.
    Content – Medical/Surgical: **Category of Health Alteration** – *Respiratory:* **Integrated Processes** – *Nursing Process: Implementation:* **Client Needs** – *Safe and Effective Care Environment: Management of Care:* **Cognitive Level** – *Application*

MAKING NURSING DECISIONS: The nurse must determine if the client is in distress; remember: if in distress do not assess. The nurse must intervene to help the client. In most situations the nurse should not select equipment over the client's body but because the ventilator is breathing for the client, the ventilator should be assessed first.

11. 1. Although these are abnormal ABG values, respiratory acidosis, they are expected in a client with COPD; therefore, the nurse would not need to see this client first.
    2. The client with ARDS would be expected to have a low arterial oxygen level; therefore, the nurse would not assess this client first.
    3. **The ABG shows respiratory alkalosis; therefore, the nurse should assess this client first to determine if the client is hyperventilating, in pain, or has an elevated temperature.**
    4. These are normal ABGs; therefore, the nurse would not need to assess this client first.
    Content – Medical/Surgical: **Category of Health Alteration** – *Respiratory:* **Integrated Processes** – *Nursing Process: Assessment:* **Client Needs** – *Physiological Integrity: Reduction of Risk Potential:* **Cognitive Level** – *Analysis*

MAKING NURSING DECISIONS: The nurse must be knowledgeable of normal laboratory values. These values must be memorized and the nurse must be able to determine if the laboratory value is normal for the client's disease process or medications the client is taking.

12. 1. Changing the dressing is not priority over a client who is in respiratory distress.
2. **The client who is exhibiting air hunger indicates respiratory distress; therefore, a tracheostomy tray should be obtained first.**
3. The transcribing of orders is important, but not more important than a client in respiratory distress.
4. The client who is angry and upset needs to be assessed but not priority over the client who is in respiratory distress.
   Content – Medical/Surgical: **Category of Health Alteration** – Respiratory: **Integrated Processes** – Nursing Process: Assessment: **Client Needs** – Physiological Integrity: Reduction of Risk Potential: **Cognitive Level** – Analysis

MAKING NURSING DECISIONS: The nurse should use some tool as a reference to guide in the decision-making process. In this situation, apply Maslow's Hierarchy of Needs. Physiological needs have priority over psychosocial ones.

13. 1. After 3 days, the nurse should suspect that the lung has re-expanded. The nurse should not expect dependent loops to have caused this situation.
2. **After 3 days, the nurse should assess the lung sounds to determine whether the lungs have re-expanded. This would be the nurse's first intervention.**
3. This will be done if it is determined the lungs have re-expanded, but it is not the first intervention.
4. The nurse should notify the HCP if it is determined the lungs have re-expanded; a chest x-ray can be taken prior to removing the chest tubes.
   Content – Medical/Surgical: **Category of Health Alteration** – Respiratory: **Integrated Processes** – Nursing Process: Implementation: **Client Needs** – Physiological Integrity: Reduction of Risk Potential: **Cognitive Level** – Analysis

MAKING NURSING DECISIONS: The nurse must determine if the client is in distress; remember: if in distress, do not assess. If the client is not in distress then the nurse should assess, the first part of the nursing process.

14. 1. The nurse should assess the client's breath sounds but not prior to determining why there is no tidaling in the water-seal chamber.
2. **The nurse should first determine why there is no tidaling in the water-seal chamber. Since the client just had the** chest tubes inserted, it is probably a kink or a dependent loop, or the client is lying on the tubing. The nurse should first check for this prior to taking any other action.
3. The nurse should encourage the client to take deep breaths and cough, which may push a clot through the tubing, but should not do so before checking for a kink.
4. Turning the client side to side will not help determine why there is no tidaling in the water-seal compartment of the Pleurovac.
   Content – Medical/Surgical: **Category of Health Alteration** – Respiratory: **Integrated Processes** – Nursing Process: Implementation: **Client Needs** – Physiological Integrity: Reduction of Risk Potential: **Cognitive Level** – Synthesis

MAKING NURSING DECISIONS: When the test question asks the test taker to determine which intervention should be implemented first it means that all the options could be possible. This is one of the few times the nurse should check equipment before assessing the client.

15. 1. The client with histoplasmosis would be expected to have excessive sweating and neck stiffness; therefore, this client would not be seen first. Histoplasmosis is an infection in the lungs caused by inhaling the spores of a fungus.
2. **The client with ARDS is expected to have difficulty breathing but of these four clients, the client with breathing difficulty has priority. Apply Maslow's Hierarchy of Needs. ARDS is the sudden failure of the respiratory system. A person with ARDS has rapid breathing, difficulty getting enough air into the lungs and low blood oxygen levels.**
3. The client with pulmonary sarcoidosis would be expected to have a dry cough and mild chest pain; therefore, this client would not be seen first. In pulmonary sarcoidosis, small patches of inflamed cells can appear on the lungs' small alveoli, bronchioles, or lymph nodes. The lungs can become stiff and may not be able to hold as much air as healthy lungs.
4. The client with asbestosis would be expected to have a productive cough and chest tightness; therefore, this client would not be seen first. Asbestosis is a disease that involves scarring of lung tissue as a result of breathing in asbestos fibers.
   Content – Medical/Surgical: **Category of Health Alteration** – Respiratory: **Integrated Processes** – Nursing Process: Assessment: **Client Needs** – Physiological

Integrity: Reduction of Risk Potential: **Cognitive Level** *– Analysis*

MAKING NURSING DECISIONS: The nurse should determine if the signs/symptoms the client is experiencing is expected or normal; if they are then the client would not warrant immediate intervention. If all the clients have expected signs/symptoms, then apply Maslow's Hierarchy of Needs and oxygenation is priority.

16. 1, 3, 4, and 5 are correct.
    1. There must be a manual resuscitation bag at the bedside in case the ventilator does not work appropriately. The nurse must use this to bag the client.
    2. The pulse oximeter reading should be done more often than every shift.
    3. The client's respiratory status should be assessed frequently—every 2 hours.
    4. The ventilator's settings should be monitored throughout the shift.
    5. The respiratory therapist is the member of the multidisciplinary team who is responsible for ventilators.
    Content – Medical/Surgical: **Category of Health Alteration** *– Respiratory:* **Integrated Processes** *– Nursing Process: Implementation:* **Client Needs** *– Physiological Integrity: Basic Care and Comfort:* **Cognitive Level** *– Application*

MAKING NURSING DECISIONS: In questions that request the test taker to "select all that apply," the test taker must select from one to all five options as the correct answer. The RN-NCLEX® does not give partial credit for these types of questions.

17. 1. This is the correct technique when bathing a client; therefore, the nurse does not need to demonstrate the correct technique to give a bath.
    2. The bed should be at a comfortable height for the UAP to bathe the client, not in the lowest position.
    3. All clients should receive a bath; therefore, this would not be an appropriate action for the nurse to take.
    4. Part of the delegation process is to evaluate the UAP's performance and the nurse should praise any action on the part of the UAP that ensures the client's safety.
    Content – Management of Care: **Category of Health Alteration** *– Respiratory:* **Integrated Processes** *– Nursing Process: Implementation:* **Client Needs** *– Safe and Effective Care Environment: Safety and Infection Control:* **Cognitive Level** *– Application*

MAKING NURSING DECISIONS: The nurse must ensure the unlicensed assistive personnel (UAP) can perform any tasks that are delegated. It is the nurse's responsibility to evaluate the task, demonstrate, and/or teach the UAP how to perform the task.

18. 1. The male nurse should document the comment and tell other people, such as family, friends, and staff, but this is not the nurse's first intervention.
    2. **The first action is to ask the person directly to stop. The harasser needs to be told in clear terms that the behavior makes the nurse uncomfortable and that he wants it to stop immediately.**
    3. The male nurse could take this action, but it is not the first action.
    4. This male nurse could take this action, but only if direct contact and the chain of command at the hospital do not stop the charge nurse's behavior.
    Content – Medical/Surgical: **Category of Health Alteration** *– Respiratory:* **Integrated Processes** *– Nursing Process: Implementation:* **Client Needs** *– Safe and Effective Care Environment: Management of Care:* **Cognitive Level** *– Application*

MAKING NURSING DECISIONS: There will be management questions on the NCLEX-RN®. In many instances, there is no test-taking strategy; the nurse must be knowledgeable of management issues that must comply with local, state, and federal requirements.

19. 1. The client is in metabolic alkalosis, so this intervention is not appropriate for the client's ABGs.
    2. The client is in metabolic alkalosis, so this intervention is not appropriate for the client's ABGs.
    3. **The ABG indicates metabolic alkalosis, which could be caused by too much hydrochloric acid being removed via the N/G tube. Therefore, the nurse should check the N/G wall suction.**
    4. Sodium bicarbonate is administered for metabolic acidosis not metabolic alkalosis.
    Content – Medical/Surgical: **Category of Health Alteration** *– Respiratory:* **Integrated Processes** *– Nursing Process: Assessment:* **Client Needs** *– Physiological Integrity: Reduction of Risk Potential:* **Cognitive Level** *– Analysis*

MAKING NURSING DECISIONS: The nurse must be knowledgeable of normal laboratory values. These values must be memorized and the nurse must be able to determine if the laboratory value is normal for the client's disease process or medications the client is taking.

20. 1. This client is critical and there is a possibility of organ rejection; therefore, this client should not be assigned to a float nurse.
 2. The normal CVP is 4–10 cm H_2O and an elevated CVP indicates right ventricular failure or volume overload; therefore, this client should not be assigned to a float nurse.
 3. The float nurse from the medical unit is able to administer antibiotic therapy and complete respiratory assessments; therefore, this client would be the most appropriate client to assign to the float nurse.
 4. Hantavirus pulmonary syndrome is a disease that results from contact with infected rodents or their urine, droppings, or saliva. HPS is potentially deadly. There is no specific treatment for HPS, and there is no cure. This client should be assigned to a more experienced nurse.
 Content – Management of Care: ***Category of Health Alteration** – Respiratory:* ***Integrated Processes** – Nursing Process: Planning :**Client Needs** – Safe and Effective Care Environment: Management of Care:* ***Cognitive Level** – Synthesis*

MAKING NURSING DECISIONS: The test taker must determine which client is most stable and assign that client to a float nurse. The clients who are more critical should be assigned to more experienced intensive care nurses.

21. 1. **The client's PaO_2 is below the normal level of 80–100; therefore, the nurse should administer oxygen.**
 2. The client should take deep breaths if the client's $PaCO_2$ is greater than 45.
 3. The nurse should administer sodium bicarbonate if the client's HCO_3 is less than 22.
 4. The client needs oxygen due to the low arterial oxygen level; the client does not need a respiratory assessment.
 Content – Medical/Surgical: ***Category of Health Alteration** – Respiratory:* ***Integrated Processes** – Nursing Process: Implementation: **Client Needs** – Physiological Integrity: Reduction of Risk Potential:* ***Cognitive Level** – Application*

MAKING NURSING DECISIONS: The nurse must be knowledgeable of normal laboratory values. These values must be memorized and the nurse must be able to determine if the laboratory value is normal for the client's disease process or medications the client is taking.

22. 1. **A social worker is qualified to assist the client with referrals to any agency or personnel that may be needed after the client is discharged home.**
 2. The chaplain should be contacted if spiritual guidance is required, but the stem did not specify this need.
 3. The HCP can talk to the husband but will not be able to address his concerns of taking care of his wife when she is discharged home.
 4. This is false reassurance and does not address the husband's concern after his wife is discharged home. The nurse does not know whether everything is going to be all right.
 Content – Medical/Surgical: ***Category of Health Alteration** – Respiratory:* ***Integrated Processes** – Nursing Process: Implementation :**Client Needs** – Physiological Integrity: Basic Care and Comfort:* ***Cognitive Level** – Application*

MAKING NURSING DECISIONS: The test taker must be knowledgeable of the role of all members of the multidisciplinary healthcare team as well as HIPAA rules and regulations. These will be tested on the NCLEX-RN® exam.

23. 1. The nurse could ask this question because the radiologist may need to compare the previous chest x-ray with the current one, but this is not the most important question.
 2. The client will have to hold her breath when the chest x-ray is taken, but this is not the most important question.
 3. Smoking or a history of smoking is pertinent to the diagnosis of pneumonia, but it is not the most important question.
 4. This is the most important question because if the client is pregnant, the x-rays can harm the fetus.
 Content – Management of Care: ***Category of Health Alteration** – Respiratory:* ***Integrated Processes** – Nursing Process: Assessment: **Client Needs** – Safe and Effective Care Environment: Safety and Infection Control:* ***Cognitive Level** – Analysis*

MAKING NURSING DECISIONS: The test taker should realize that for any female client of childbearing age, the most important questions or concerns will probably address the chance of pregnancy. Most medications and many diagnostic tests and treatments can harm the fetus.

24. 1. **The elderly client should be called first so that the nurse can determine whether the dizziness when getting up is the result of medication or some other reason. Orthostatic hypotension can be life threatening; therefore, this client may need to be assessed immediately.**
 2. Ordering a prescription is not priority over a client with a physiological problem.
 3. Nausea is often expected with chemotherapy; therefore, this client's phone call would not

be returned prior to calling a client with a potentially life-threatening problem.

4. Pertussis—known as whooping cough—is a serious, very contagious disease that causes severe, uncontrollable coughing fits. The coughing makes it difficult to breathe and often ends with a "whoop" noise. Because coughing spells are expected, the nurse would not call this client first.

Content – Medical/Surgical: **Category of Health Alteration** *– Respiratory:* **Integrated Processes** *– Nursing Process: Implementation:* **Client Needs** *– Physiological Integrity: Reduction of Risk Potential:* **Cognitive Level** *– Application*

MAKING NURSING DECISIONS: The test taker should apply some systematic approach when answering priority questions. All of the clients are experiencing physiological problems, the first priority according to Maslow's Hierarch of Needs. Once that is established, then the test taker should determine which physiological problem is most life threatening—in this case, dizziness when standing because of its possible cause, hypotension, which can be life threatening.

25. 1. This is a therapeutic response with the goal of having the client ventilate feelings. This is not appropriate for the client's comment the nurse must give factual information.
2. **The client with active TB must take the medication as prescribed for 9–12 months. If the client refuses to take the medication, a court order will be obtained to make the client take the medication because tuberculosis is a community threat.**
3. The nurse should provide factual information when possible and not "pass the buck" to the HCP.
4. This is not a true statement. The client must be on the prescribed medications.

Content – Medical/Surgical: **Category of Health Alteration** *– Respiratory:* **Integrated Processes** *– Nursing Process: Implementation:* **Client Needs** *– Physiological Integrity: Physiological Adaptation:* **Cognitive Level** *– Application*

MAKING NURSING DECISIONS: The nurse must be knowledgeable of diseases that pose a threat to the community. The nurse should provide factual information to the client.

26. 1. An induration greater than 10 mm is positive for tuberculosis. This client needs to be assessed and followed up to rule out tuberculosis. This client should not be assigned to an LPN.
2. A pulse oximeter reading less than 93% is life threatening; therefore, this client should not be assigned to an LPN.

3. **Acute bronchitis is an inflammation of the bronchial tubes, the major airways into the lungs. The client is exhibiting expected signs/symptoms; therefore, the LPN could care for this client.**
4. The client is exhibiting wheezing, an acute exacerbation of reactive airway disease. This client should be assigned to a nurse.

Content – Medical/Surgical: **Category of Health Alteration** *– Respiratory:* **Integrated Processes** *– Nursing Process: Planning:* **Client Needs** *– Safe and Effective Care Environment: Management of Care:* **Cognitive Level** *– Synthesis*

MAKING NURSING DECISIONS: The nurse should assign the LPN the client who has the lowest level of need but for whom the task still remains in the LPN's scope of practice. The nurse cannot assign assessing, teaching, evaluating, or an unstable client to an LPN.

27. 1. The UAP cannot administer oxygen to a client. Oxygen is considered a medication.
2. The nurse should not depend on the UAP to care for the client who is experiencing a potentially life-threatening condition.
3. **This is the first intervention because the nurse must assess the client. Asking the UAP to accompany the nurse will allow the nurse to stay with the client while the UAP obtains any needed equipment.**
4. The nurse should immediately assess the client. The UAP does not have the knowledge or skills to care for the client experiencing shortness of breath.

Content – Management of Care: **Category of Health Alteration** *– Respiratory:* **Integrated Processes** *– Nursing Process: Implementation:* **Client Needs** *– Physiological Integrity: Reduction of Risk Potential:* **Cognitive Level** *– Analysis*

MAKING NURSING DECISIONS: Any time the nurse receives information from another staff member about a client who may be experiencing a new problem, complication, or life-threatening problem, the nurse must assess the client. The nurse should not make decisions about client needs based on another staff member's information.

28. 1. The parent/guardian must sign the consent for surgery because the client is under the age of 18.
2. The client has already been diagnosed with tonsillitis; therefore, a throat culture is not needed prior to surgery.
3. The client should not cough after this surgery because it could cause bleeding from the incision site.

4. **A PT/PTT will assess the client for any bleeding tendencies. This is priority before this surgery because bleeding is a life-threatening complication.**
   Content – Medical/Surgical: **Category of Health Alteration –** *Respiratory:* **Integrated Processes –** *Nursing Process: Implementation:* **Client Needs –** *Safe and Effective Care Environment: Management of Care:* **Cognitive Level –** *Application*

MAKING NURSING DECISIONS: The NCLEX-RN®️ blueprint includes perioperative nursing care. The nurse must be knowledgeable of preoperative and postoperative care that is generic for all clients undergoing surgery.

29. 1. Influenza, or the flu, is a serious respiratory illness caused by a virus. Antibiotics are not prescribed to treat influenza.
    2. Staying away from large crowds and a scarf over the mouth is not the best way to prevent getting influenza.
    3. **Influenza, or flu, is a serious respiratory illness. It is easily spread from person to person and can lead to severe complications, even death. The best way to prevent the influenza is to get a flu vaccine every year. The influenza virus is constantly changing. Each year, scientists work together to identify the virus strains that they believe will cause the most illness, and a new vaccine is made based on their recommendations.**
    4. Three meals a day and daily exercise will help the client stay healthy in general but it is not the best way to prevent getting influenza.
    Content – Medical/Surgical: **Category of Health Alteration –** *Respiratory:* **Integrated Processes –** *Nursing Process: Evaluation:* **Client Needs –** *Health Promotion and Maintenance:* **Cognitive Level –** *Analysis*

MAKING NURSING DECISIONS: The nurse must be knowledgeable of immunizations for both children and adults. This is a knowledge-based question that is included on the NCLEX-RN®️ exam.

30. 1. The normal pulse rate for a 1- to 11-month-old is 100 to 150. This client would not warrant immediate intervention.
    2. The normal respiratory rate for a toddler is 20 to 30. This client would not warrant immediate intervention.
    3. **A 24-week gestational woman with a BP of 142/96 would warrant intervention because the average systolic BP should be between 90 and 140 mm Hg and the diastolic BP should be between 60 and**

85 mm Hg. This BP could indicate pregnancy-induced hypertension.
    4. This is an elevated temperature, but it would not warrant intervention from the nurse. This is not a potentially life-threatening temperature.
    Content – Medical/Surgical: **Category of Health Alteration –** *Respiratory:* **Integrated Processes –** *Nursing Process: Assessment:* **Client Needs –** *Physiological Integrity: Reduction of Risk Potential:* **Cognitive Level –** *Analysis*

MAKING NURSING DECISIONS: The nurse must be knowledgeable of vital signs. This is basic nursing care that is tested on the NCLEX-RN®️.

31. 1. The documentation of the accident must be completed but it is not priority over caring for the wound first.
    2. **The nurse should wash the area with soap and water and attempt to squeeze the area to make it bleed.**
    3. The nurse should not ask this question directly to the client. The nurse could ask whether the client would agree to have blood drawn for testing, but not directly ask whether the client has AIDS or hepatitis.
    4. The puncture site would not require antibiotic ointment unless it is infected, which it wouldn't be immediately after the incident.
    Content – Medical/Surgical: **Category of Health Alteration –** *Respiratory:* **Integrated Processes –** *Nursing Process: Implementation:* **Client Needs –** *Safe and Effective Care Environment: Safety and Infection Control:* **Cognitive Level –** *Application*

MAKING NURSING DECISIONS: The NCLEX-RN®️ blueprint includes adhering to Standard Precautions when providing nursing care to clients. Remember: The nurse should always address the problem directly prior to completing documentation.

32. 1. **The normal hemoglobin level is 12 to 15 g/dL, and normal hematocrit is 39% to 45%. This client's H&H is low. The nurse should contact the client and make an immediate appointment.**
    2. The normal WBC count is 4.0 to 10.0 mm³. This client's WBC count is within normal range and does not warrant intervention from the clinic nurse.
    3. The normal serum potassium level is 3.5 to 5.5 mEq/L. This client's level is within normal range and does not warrant intervention from the clinic nurse.
    4. The normal serum sodium level is 135 to 145 mEq/L. This client's level is within the normal range, and the client does not warrant intervention from the clinic nurse.

Content – Medical/Surgical: ***Category of Health Alteration*** *– Respiratory:* ***Integrated Processes –*** *Nursing Process: Assessment:* ***Client Needs*** *– Safe and Effective Care Environment: Safety and Infection Control:* ***Cognitive Level*** *– Analysis*

MAKING NURSING DECISIONS: The nurse must be knowledgeable of normal laboratory values. These values must be memorized and the nurse must be able to determine if the laboratory value is normal for the client's disease process or medications the client is taking.

33. 1. In the Hispanic culture, the husband often speaks for the wife and family, and requesting the husband not to speak may be insulting. This action may cause the wife to leave as well.
    2. In the Hispanic culture, the husband often is the spokesperson and makes decisions for the wife and family. Asking the husband to leave the room may cause the client to leave as well.
    3. **This behavior may be cultural, and the nurse should continue to allow the husband to answer the questions, while the nurse looks at the client. The nurse must be respectful of the client's culture. The nurse can, however, ask whether the client agrees with the husband's answers.**
    4. This is disrespectful to the client's culture. Many times the nurse must honor the client's culture while caring for the client.
    Content – Management of Care: ***Category of Health Alteration*** *– Respiratory:* ***Integrated Processes –*** *Nursing Process: Evaluation:* ***Client Needs*** *– Physiological Integrity: Basic Care and Comfort:* ***Cognitive Level*** *– Analysis*

MAKING NURSING DECISIONS: The NCLEX-RN® blueprint includes nursing care addressing cultural diversity. The nurse needs to be aware of cultural differences.

34. Correct Answer: 3, 4, 1, 5, 2
    3. **The nurse needs to determine if the client is unresponsive prior to taking any action. If the client is unresponsive, then perform compressions.**
    4. **The American Heart Association recommends 30 compressions followed by two breaths.**
    1. **After completing compressions, open the client's airway to ensure a patent airway.**
    5. **The nurse should then administer two breaths while the client's nose is pinched.**
    2. **The nurse then must determine whether the client's heart is pumping by checking the carotid pulse.**
    Content – Medical/Surgical: ***Category of Health Alteration*** *– Respiratory:* ***Integrated Processes –*** *Nursing Process: Implementation:* ***Client Needs*** *– Safe*

and Effective Care Environment: Management of Care: ***Cognitive Level*** *– Analysis*

MAKING NURSING DECISIONS: This is an alternate type of question included in the NCLEX-RN® blueprint. The nurse must be able to perform skills in the correct order.

35. 1. **The client with end-stage COPD usually prefers a cool climate, with fans to help ease breathing. A warm area would increase the effort the client would require to breathe. This action would warrant intervention by the nurse.**
    2. The client with end-stage COPD should be maintained on a low oxygen rate, such as 2 L/min to prevent depression of the hypoxic drive. High levels of oxygen will depress the client's ability to breathe. This action would not warrant intervention by the nurse.
    3. The client will usually sit in the orthopneic position, usually slumped over a bedside table, to help ease breathing. This is called the three-point stance. This action would not warrant intervention by the nurse.
    4. The client in end-stage COPD has great difficulty breathing; therefore, sleeping in a recliner is sometimes the only way the client can sleep. This action would not warrant intervention by the nurse.
    Content – Medical/Surgical: ***Category of Health Alteration*** *– Respiratory:* ***Integrated Processes –*** *Nursing Process: Implementation:* ***Client Needs*** *– Safe and Effective Care Environment: Management of Care:* ***Cognitive Level*** *– Analysis*

MAKING NURSING DECISIONS: The nurse only delegates tasks in which the UAP has been trained to perform. Delegation means the nurse is responsible for the UAPs actions; therefore, the nurse must evaluate the UAPs understanding of the procedure the UAP is asked to perform.

36. 1. The UAP cannot perform sterile dressing changes.
    2. The UAP cannot perform sterile procedures.
    3. The UAP cannot teach the client.
    4. **The UAP can transfer the client from the bed to the chair three times a day.**
    Content – Management of Care: ***Category of Health Alteration*** *– Respiratory:* ***Integrated Processes –*** *Nursing Process: Planning :* ***Client Needs*** *– Safe and Effective Care Environment, Management of Care:* ***Cognitive Level*** *– Synthesis*

MAKING NURSING DECISIONS: The nurse cannot delegate assessment, evaluation, teaching, medications, or an unstable client to a UAP.

37. 1. The staff member is violating HIPAA, and the nurse should take action immediately.

2. The nurse should first ask the staff member not to discuss the client with a friend. Discussing any information about a client is a violation of HIPAA.

3. The nurse should address the staff member in the restaurant. The nurse could tell the clinical manager, but the nurse must stop the conversation in the restaurant immediately.

4. The nurse should not tell the client about the breach of confidentiality.

   Content – *Management of Care: **Category of Health Alteration** – Respiratory: **Integrated Processes** – Nursing Process: Implementation: **Client Needs** – Safe and Effective Care Environment: Management of Care: **Cognitive Level** – Application*

MAKING NURSING DECISIONS: There will be management questions on the NCLEX-RN®. In many instances, there is no test-taking strategy; the nurse must be knowledgeable of management issues. The Health Insurance Portability and Accountability Act (HIPAA) passed into law in 1996 to standardize exchange of information between healthcare providers and to ensure patient record confidentiality.

38. 1. **This statement warrants intervention because fluids will help prevent dehydration and renal calculi. The nurse should explain the client needs to increase fluids.**

    2. ROM exercises help prevent deep vein thrombosis (DVT). This statement does not require intervention by the nurse. The UAP can perform skills if taught and performance is evaluated by the nurse.

    3. Keeping the client off the buttocks is an appropriate intervention for a client on strict bed rest. This comment does not require intervention by the nurse.

    4. Pulling the client across the sheets will cause skin breakdown. Because the UAP is not doing this, no intervention by the nurse is needed.

       Content – *Medical/Surgical: **Category of Health Alteration** – Respiratory: **Integrated Processes** – Nursing Process: Planning: **Client Needs** – Safe and Effective Care Environment: Management of Care: **Cognitive Level** – Analysis*

MAKING NURSING DECISIONS: Delegation means the nurse is responsible for the UAP's actions and performance. The nurse must correct the UAP's performance to ensure the client is cared for safely in the hospital or the home.

39. 1. The client's oxygen should always be placed correctly but it is not the priority intervention for difficulty breathing.

    2. **Because the client has difficulty breathing while lying in bed, allowing the client to**

sit in a recliner will help the client; therefore, this is the priority intervention.

3. Often clients report a fan blowing on the face helps with difficulty breathing but this is not a priority intervention.

4. Slow, deep breaths will not help the client with difficulty breathing as much as will sitting in a recliner.

   Content – *Medical/Surgical: **Category of Health Alteration** – Respiratory: **Integrated Processes** – Nursing Process: Planning: **Client Needs** – Physiological Integrity: Basic Care and Comfort: **Cognitive Level** – Synthesis*

MAKING NURSING DECISIONS: In questions that ask the test taker to identify a priority intervention all the options are something a nurse can implement. The test taker must identify the most important intervention.

40. 1. The body naturally begins to slow down, and clients may not wish to take in liquids or nourishment. This can produce a natural euphoria and make the dying process easier on the client. IV fluids would interfere with this process and would increase secretions the client cannot handle, thus making the client more uncomfortable.

    2. A PEG feeding tube would increase the intake of the client and would increase secretions the client cannot handle. This can require suctioning the client and further augmenting the client's discomfort.

    3. **Refusal to take in food and liquids produces a natural euphoria and makes the dying process easier on the client. This is an appropriate teaching statement.**

    4. This is a therapeutic response, but factual information is needed by the wife to accept the process.

       Content – *Medical/Surgical: **Category of Health Alteration** – Respiratory: **Integrated Processes** – Nursing Process: Implementation: **Client Needs** – Psychosocial Integrity: **Cognitive Level** – Application*

MAKING NURSING DECISIONS: The NCLEX-RN® addresses questions concerned with end of life care. This is included in the Psychosocial Integrity section of the test blueprint.

41. 1. The home health nurse may be a possibility if a hospice organization is not available, but hospice is the best referral.

    2. The nurse would not refer the client to his or her own pastor. The nurse could place a call to notify the pastor at the client's request, but this would not be considered a referral.

    3. **One of the guidelines for admission to a hospice agency is a terminal process with a life expectancy of 6 months or less.**

These organizations work to assist the client and family to live life to its fullest while providing for comfort measures and a peaceful, dignified death.

4. The hospital social worker is not an appropriate referral at this time.

Content – Medical/Surgical: **Category of Health Alteration** – Respiratory: **Integrated Processes** – Nursing Process: Planning: **Client Needs** – Physiological Integrity: Physiological Adaptation: **Cognitive Level** – Synthesis

MAKING NURSING DECISIONS: The nurse must be knowledgeable about appropriate referrals and implement the referral to the most appropriate person/agency.

42. 1. This is advising and crossing professional boundaries. The nurse should not try to influence the client in these types of concerns.
    2. This is advising and crossing professional boundaries. The nurse should not try to influence the client in these types of concerns.
    3. **This response allows the client to make his or her own decision. It validates that the nurse heard the concern but does not advise the client.**
    4. This is advising and crossing professional boundaries. The nurse should not try to influence the client in these types of concerns.

Content – Management of Care: **Category of Health Alteration** – Respiratory: **Integrated Processes** – Nursing Process: Implementation :**Client Needs** – Psychosocial Integrity: **Cognitive Level** – Application

MAKING NURSING DECISIONS: The nurse must always remember that nurses have positions of authority in a healthcare environment. Nurses must maintain professional boundaries at all times and refuse to cross professional boundaries.

43. 1. Women tend to see the big picture and seek solutions based on what makes people feel comfortable rather than on logic.
    2. **Men often see the world from a logical perspective and focus on a specific intervention.**
    3. Men tend to ask fewer questions than women, especially if the man perceives that asking the question will make him look foolish or ignorant.
    4. Men and women communicate very differently. The female manager of a male employee should recognize the difference when attempting to arrive at a common goal.

Content – Medical/Surgical: **Category of Health Alteration** – Respiratory: **Integrated Processes** – Nursing Process: Communication: **Client Needs** – Safe and Effective Care Environment: Management of Care: **Cognitive Level** – Application

MAKING NURSING DECISIONS: There will be management questions on the NCLEX-RN®. In many instances, there is no test-taking strategy; the nurse must be knowledgeable of management issues.

44. 1. The attitude of the staff member changes from one day to the next. The "why" is not important for the manager to know. The important thing for the manager to know is whether the staff member can control the attitude.
    2. **The first step is an informal meeting with the staff member to discuss the inappropriate attitude and how it affects the staff. The manager should document the conversation informally with the date and time (the staff member does not need to see this documentation) for future reference. If the situation is not resolved, a formal counseling must take place.**
    3. This step would follow the informal discussion if the attitude did not improve.
    4. This is a step sometimes used to get the attention of the staff member when formal counseling has not been effective. This step occurs just before termination.

Content – Management of Care: **Category of Health Alteration** – Respiratory: **Integrated Processes** – Nursing Process: Implementation: **Client Needs** – Safe and Effective Care Environment: Management of Care: **Cognitive Level** – Application

MAKING NURSING DECISIONS: There will be management questions on the NCLEX-RN®. In many instances, there is no test-taking strategy; the nurse must be knowledgeable of management issues.

45. 1. E-mails should be easy to read and concise. Individuals may not take the time to read and understand poorly worded, lengthy e-mails.
    2. Some communication is appropriate by e-mail, but when discussing a problem with an individual, it is best to use face-to-face communication in which both parties can give and receive feedback.
    3. Capital letters in e-mails may be interpreted as shouting or yelling at the receiver.
    4. **E-mail communication should be concise and easy to read. If the e-mail requires a lot of information, then the writer should use bullets to separate information.**

Content – Medical/Surgical: **Category of Health Alteration** – Communication: **Integrated Processes** – Nursing Process: Implementation: **Client Needs** – Safe and Effective Care Environment: Management of Care: **Cognitive Level** – Application

MAKING NURSING DECISIONS: There will be management questions on the NCLEX-RN®. In many instances, there is no test-taking strategy; the nurse must be knowledgeable of management issues.

46. 1. **The problem is not a nursing problem. The HCP should be discussing the problem with an individual from the department that "owns" the problem.**
    2. This is not a nursing problem.
    3. This is not a nursing problem.
    4. This will only make the HCP angrier. The HCP should be directed to discuss the problem with the department that can "fix" the problem.
    *Content – Management of Care: **Category of Health Alteration** – Respiratory: **Integrated Processes** – Nursing Process: Implementation: **Client Needs** – Safe and Effective Care Environment: Management of Care: **Cognitive Level** – Application*

MAKING NURSING DECISIONS: There will be management questions on the NCLEX-RN®. In many instances, there is no test-taking strategy; the nurse must be knowledgeable of management issues.

47. **Correct Answer: 1, 4, 3, 2, 5**
    1. **The nurse should begin the care by assessing the client. Remember the nursing process.**
    4. **The nurse should have the client's chest and dressing exposed and should check to make sure the chest tube is securely taped at this time.**
    3. **The nurse then follows the chest tube to the drainage system and assesses the system.**
    2. **The last part of the chest tube drainage system to assess is the suction system.**
    5. **The nurse should make sure that emergency supplies are at the bedside last.**
    *Content – Medical/Surgical: **Category of Health Alteration** – Respiratory :**Integrated Processes** – Nursing Process: Assessment: **Client Needs** – Safe and Effective Care Environment: Management of Care: **Cognitive Level** – Analysis*

MAKING NURSING DECISIONS: This is an alternate type of question included in the NCLEX-RN® blueprint. The nurse must be able to perform skills in the correct order. Assessment should always be the first intervention if the client is not in distress.

48. 1. Bronchiectasis is a condition in which the lungs' airways are abnormally stretched and widened. This is caused by mucous blockage, which allows bacteria to grow and leads to

infection. Signs/symptoms include coughing, abnormal breath sounds, and clubbing; therefore, the nurse would not assess this client first.
    2. Byssinosis (brown lung disease) is a lung disease caused by exposure to dust from cotton processing, hemp, and flax. Signs/symptoms include chest tightness, cough, and wheezing; therefore, this client would not be assessed first.
    3. **Cystic fibrosis (CF) is an inherited disease that causes thick, sticky mucus to form in the lungs, pancreas, and other organs. In the lungs, this mucus blocks the airways, causing lung damage and making it hard to breathe. A pulse oximeter reading of 90% equates to approximately a 60% arterial saturation. The nurse should assess this client first.**
    4. Pneumoconiosis, known as black lung disease, is an occupational lung disease caused by inhaling coal dust. The signs/symptoms are shortness of breath and chronic cough; therefore, this client would not be assessed first.
    *Content – Medical/Surgical: **Category of Health Alteration** – Respiratory: **Integrated Processes** – Nursing Process: Assessment: **Client Needs** – Physiological Integrity: Reduction of Risk Potential: **Cognitive Level** – Analysis*

MAKING NURSING DECISIONS: The test taker must determine which sign/symptom is not expected for the disease process. If the sign/symptom is not expected then the nurse should assess the client first. This type of question is determining if the nurse is knowledgeable of signs/symptoms of a variety of disease processes.

49. 1. Activity intolerance is not priority over gas exchange. If gas exchange does not occur, the client will die.
    2. Coping is a psychosocial problem, and physiological problems are priority.
    3. **Impaired gas exchange is the priority problem for this client. If the client does not have adequate gas exchange, the client will die. Remember Maslow's Hierarchy of Needs.**
    4. Self-care deficit is not priority over gas exchange.
    *Content – Medical/Surgical: **Category of Health Alteration** – Respiratory: **Integrated Processes** – Nursing Process: Assessment: **Client Needs** – Physiological Integrity: Physiological Adaptation: **Cognitive Level** – Analysis*

MAKING NURSING DECISIONS: The NCLEX-RN® integrates the nursing process throughout the

Client Needs categories and subcategories. The nursing process is a scientific, clinical reasoning approach to client care that includes assessment, analysis, planning, implementation, and evaluation. The nurse will be responsible for identifying nursing diagnosis for clients.

50. 1. Consolidation indicates fluid or exudates in the lung—pneumonia. This would not indicate the client is improving.
    2. **Bilateral breath sounds indicate the left lung has re-expanded and the treatment is effective.**
    3. Vigorous bubbling in the suction chamber indicates that there is a leak in the system, but this does not indicate the treatment is effective.
    4. Crepitus (subcutaneous emphysema) indicates that oxygen is escaping into the subcutaneous layer of the skin, but this does not indicate the lung has re-expanded, which is the goal of the treatment.

    Content – Medical/Surgical: **Category of Health Alteration** *– Respiratory:* **Integrated Processes** *– Nursing Process: Assessment:* **Client Needs** *– Safe and Effective Care Environment: Safety and Infection Control:* **Cognitive Level** *– Analysis*

MAKING NURSING DECISIONS: The nurse should realize a normal finding indicates the medical treatment is effective. If the nurse is vacillating between two options and one option is equipment the nurse should select the client's body as the correct answer.

51. 1. Jugular vein distention would indicate the client has CHF. This is not a complication of a loop diuretic.
    2. Rales and rhonchi are symptoms of pulmonary edema, not a complication of a loop diuretic.
    3. **Leg cramps may indicate a low serum potassium level, which can occur as a result of the administration of a diuretic.**
    4. This would indicate the medication is effective and is not a complication of the medication.

    Content – Medical/Surgical : **Category of Health Alteration** *– Respiratory:* **Integrated Processes** *– Nursing Process: Assessment:* **Client Needs** *– Physiological Integrity: Pharmacological and Parenteral Therapies:* **Cognitive Level** *– Analysis*

MAKING NURSING DECISIONS: The nurse must be aware of expected actions of medications. The nurse must be aware of assessment data indicating the medication is effective or the medication is causing a side effect or an adverse effect.

52. 1. **Nonmalfeasance means to do no harm. This statement is letting the client know**

that the concern has been heard but does not give the client bad news before surgery. The nurse is aware that someone having surgery should be of sound mind, and finding out your child is dead would be horrific.
    2. This is an example of veracity.
    3. This is an example of paternalism, telling the client what he or she should do.
    4. This is a therapeutic response, not an example of nonmalfeasance.

    Content – Medical/Surgical: **Category of Health Alteration** *– Ethics:* **Integrated Processes** *– Nursing Process: Implementation:* **Client Needs** *– Safe and Effective Care Environment: Management of Care:* **Cognitive Level** *– Application*

MAKING NURSING DECISIONS: The NCLEX-RN® blueprint includes nursing care that addresses ethical principles, including autonomy, beneficence, justice, and veracity, to name a few.

53. 1. **The Joint Commission is an organization that monitors healthcare facilities for compliance with standards of care. Accreditation is voluntary, but most third-party payers will not reimburse a facility that is not accredited by some outside organization.**
    2. Accreditation does not guarantee reimbursement, although most third-party payers require some accreditation by an outside organization.
    3. Accreditation does not reduce the hospital's liability.
    4. Medicare/Medicaid will not review a facility routinely if the Joint Commission has accredited the facility, but a representative will review the facility in cases of reported problems.

    Content – Management of Care: **Category of Health Alteration** *– Respiratory:* **Integrated Processes** *– Nursing Process: Implementation:* **Client Needs** *– Safe and Effective Care Environment: Management of Care:* **Cognitive Level** *– Application*

MAKING NURSING DECISIONS: The NCLEX-RN® blueprint includes nursing care that is ruled by legal requirements as well as Joint Commission, Medicare & Medicaid Services, Centers for Disease Control and Prevention, and Occupational Safety and Health Administration rules and regulations. The nurse must be knowledgeable of these standards.

54. 1. The nurse should "offer self" to the significant other. Ignoring the needs of the significant other at this time makes the significant other feel that the nurse does not care, and if the nurse does not care

for "me," then did the nurse provide adequate care to my loved one? This action is very important to assist in the grieving process.

2. The UAP can gather the deceased client's belongings.
3. The UAP can perform post-mortem care.
4. The representative of the organ donation team will make this request. Organ banks think it is best for specially trained individuals to discuss organ donation with the significant others.

*Content – Medical/Surgical: **Category of Health Alteration** – Respiratory: **Integrated Processes** – Nursing Process: Implementation: **Client Needs** – Psychosocial Integrity: **Cognitive Level** – Application*

MAKING NURSING DECISIONS: The NCLEX-RN® addresses questions concerned with end-of-life care. This is included in the Psychosocial Integrity section of the test blueprint. If unsure of the correct option, selecting an option addressing an individual is a better choice.

55. 1. Coumadin is an oral, not intravenous, medication.
 2. **The therapeutic PTT results should be 1.5 to 2 times the control, or 51 to 68 seconds. The client's value of 53 is within the therapeutic range. The nurse should continue the heparin drip as is.**
 3. The INR is not up to therapeutic range yet, so warfarin (Coumadin) should be administered.
 4. These lab values do not provide any information about aspirin administration, but the nurse should ask the HCP whether aspirin (an antiplatelet) should be discontinued because the client is receiving two anticoagulants—heparin and warfarin.

*Content – Medical/Surgical: **Category of Health Alteration** – Respiratory: **Integrated Processes** – Nursing Process: Implementation: **Client Needs** – Physiological Integrity: Reduction of Risk Potential: **Cognitive Level** – Application*

MAKING NURSING DECISIONS: This is an alternate type of question included in the NCLEX-RN® blueprint. The test taker must be able to read a chart, must be knowledgeable of laboratory data, and must be able to make appropriate decisions as to the nurse's most appropriate action.

56. 1. A Rapid Response Team (RRT) is called when the nurse assesses a client whose condition is deteriorating. The purpose of an RRT is to intervene to prevent a code. In the scenario described, the situation has not progressed to an arrest. The nurse should call an

RRT, but administering oxygen is the first intervention.
 2. **The first action is to increase the client's oxygen to 100%.**
 3. The nurse could check the ABG results, but the client is in distress and the nurse should implement an intervention to relieve the distress.
 4. A fast-acting inhaler should be used, but not until after the oxygen has been increased and an RRT called.

*Content – Medical/Surgical: **Category of Health Alteration** – Respiratory: **Integrated Processes** – Nursing Process: Implementation: **Client Needs** – Physiological Integrity: Reduction of Risk Potential: **Cognitive Level** – Synthesis*

MAKING NURSING DECISIONS: The nurse should remember: If a client is in distress and the nurse can do something to relieve the distress, that should be done first, before assessment. The test taker should select an option that directly helps the client's condition.

57. 1. The client may eventually need to be transferred to a facility that accepts long-term ventilator-dependent clients, but the nurse would not anticipate this at this time.
 2. The client on a ventilator will have blood gases ordered more often than daily.
 3. The stem does not indicate that the client is ready to be removed from the ventilator.
 4. **A client who has been intubated for 10 to 14 days and still requires mechanical ventilation should have a surgically placed tracheostomy to prevent permanent vocal cord damage.**

*Content – Medical/Surgical: **Category of Health Alteration** – Respiratory: **Integrated Processes** – Nursing Process: Analysis: **Client Needs** – Physiological Integrity: Reduction of Risk Potential: **Cognitive Level** – Knowledge*

MAKING NURSING DECISIONS: The nurse must be knowledgeable of expected medical treatment for the client. This is a knowledge-based question.

58. 1. The child's skin will normally taste salty, but this is not the priority intervention to teach.
 2. The parents should be asked about the client's stools during an assessment because the effectiveness of the pancreatic enzymes is evaluated by the consistency of the stool. This is not the priority intervention because the child must take the enzymes before monitoring the consistency of the stool.
 3. **Cystic fibrosis is a genetic condition that results in blockage of the pancreatic ducts. The child needs pancreatic**

enzymes to be administered with every meal and snack so the enzymes will be available when the food gets to the small intestine.

4. Cystic fibrosis is one of the few diseases that requires salt replacement, but salt replacement is not more important than taking the pancreatic enzymes.

Content – Medical/Surgical: ***Category of Health Alteration*** *– Respiratory:* ***Integrated Processes** – Nursing Process: Implementation:* ***Client Needs** – Physiological Integrity: Physiological Adaptation:* ***Cognitive Level** – Knowledge*

MAKING NURSING DECISIONS: The nurse must be knowledgeable of expected medical treatment for the client. This is a knowledge-based question.

59. 1. The UAP should be sensitive to the client's preferences and not insist that the client miss the program.
2. The UAP should arrange an acceptable time for the client, and the UAP can return to complete the task at the agreed-on time.
3. **This is the best instruction for the nurse to give to the UAP.**
4. The bath has not been refused. The client does not want the program interrupted.

Content – Management of Care: ***Category of Health Alteration*** *– Respiratory:* ***Integrated Processes** – Nursing Process: Implementation:* ***Client Needs** – Physiological Integrity: Basic Care and Comfort:* ***Cognitive Level** – Synthesis*

MAKING NURSING DECISIONS: Delegation means the nurse is responsible for the UAP's actions and performance. The nurse must provide guidance to the UAP.

60. 1. **Effective group process involves all members of the group.**
2. Unanimous decisions may indicate group-think, which can be a problem in a group process.
3. Effective group process involves all members of the group, not just two.
4. Not allowing deviation from the agenda is an autocratic style and limits the creativity and involvement of the group.

Content – Management of Care: ***Category of Health Alteration*** *– Respiratory:* ***Integrated Processes** – Nursing Process: Implementation:* ***Client Needs** – Psychosocial Integrity:* ***Cognitive Level** – Application*

MAKING NURSING DECISIONS: There will be management questions on the NCLEX-RN®. In many instances, there is no test-taking strategy; the nurse must be knowledgeable of management issues.

61. 1. **The ventilator should be checked to determine which alarm is sounding. This is the first step in assessing the client's problem.**
2. The nurse should assess the ventilator and the client and then notify the respiratory therapist, if needed.
3. The client should be assessed, but the ventilator may require only a simple adjustment to fix the problem and turn off the alarm. This is one instance in which the nurse should assess the machine prior to assessing the client because the machine is breathing for the client.
4. The client should be manually ventilated if the nurse cannot determine the cause of the ventilator alarm.

Content – Medical/Surgical: ***Category of Health Alteration*** *– Respiratory:* ***Integrated Processes** – Nursing Process: Implementation:* ***Client Needs** – Physiological Integrity: Reduction of Risk Potential:* ***Cognitive Level** – Application*

MAKING NURSING DECISIONS: The nurse must determine if the client is in distress. Remember: If in distress, do not assess. The nurse must intervene to help the client. In most situations, the nurse should not select equipment over the client's body; however, when the equipment is breathing for the client the equipment should be assessed first.

62. 1. **Acute respiratory distress syndrome is diagnosed when the client has an arterial blood gas of less than 50% while receiving oxygen at 10 LPM. The nurse should prepare for the client to be intubated.**
2. The nurse should intervene while the client is breathing by calling the HCP and assisting in the intubation and setup of the mechanical ventilator. If the client has an arrest before this can be arranged, the client would be ventilated with a bag/mask device.
3. If the nurse does not intervene immediately, an arrest situation will occur, at which time a Code Blue would be called and CPR started.
4. If the client does not have a patent IV, the nurse should start one, but not before preparing for intubation.

Content – Medical/Surgical: ***Category of Health Alteration*** *– Respiratory:* ***Integrated Processes** – Nursing Process: Implementation:* ***Client Needs** – Physiological Integrity: Reduction of Risk Potential:* ***Cognitive Level** – Knowledge*

MAKING NURSING DECISIONS: The nurse must be knowledgeable of expected medical treatment for the client. This is a knowledge-based question.

63. **1.** **These blood gases indicate respiratory acidosis that could be caused by ineffective cough, with resulting air trapping. The nurse should encourage the client to turn, cough, and deep breathe.**
2. The PaO_2 level is within normal limits, 80 to 100. Administering oxygen is not the first intervention.
3. The nurse knows the arterial blood gas oxygen level, which is an accurate test. The pulse oximeter only provides an approximate level.
4. This is not the first intervention. The nurse can intervene to treat the client before notifying the HCP.

Content – Medical/Surgical: **Category of Health Alteration** *– Respiratory:* **Integrated Processes** *– Nursing Process: Implementation:* **Client Needs** *– Physiological Integrity: Reduction of Risk Potential:* **Cognitive Level** *– Knowledge*

MAKING NURSING DECISIONS: The nurse must be knowledgeable of expected medical treatment for the client. This is a knowledge-based question.

64. 1. The nurse should first prevent circulatory collapse by starting two IVs and initiating normal saline or Ringer's lactate. The cross-match may be needed if the shock condition is caused by hemorrhage.
2. **The client is exhibiting symptoms of shock. The nurse should start IV lines to prevent the client from progressing to circulatory collapse.**
3. All clients have a history taken and physical examination performed as part of the admission process to the emergency department, but this is not the first intervention.
4. Checking the client's allergies to medications is important, but it is not the first intervention in a client exhibiting signs of shock.

Content – Medical/Surgical: **Category of Health Alteration** *– Respiratory:* **Integrated Processes** *– Nursing Process: Implementation:* **Client Needs** *– Physiological Integrity: Reduction of Risk Potential:* **Cognitive Level** *– Synthesis*

MAKING NURSING DECISIONS: The nurse should remember if a client is in distress and the nurse can do something to relieve the distress, that should be done first, before assessment. The test taker should select an option that directly helps the client's condition.

65. 1. This client is nearing discharge status. Postoperative clients are progressed rapidly. A medical-surgical nurse could take care of this client.

2. Chest tubes are frequently cared for on a medical-surgical unit, the medical-surgical nurse can care for this client.
3. **This client's status is uncertain. The ICU nurse would be an appropriate assignment for this client since the patient will be moved to ICU soon.**
4. A medical-surgical nurse can care for this client.
5. **The intensive care nurse should care for this client requiring titration of multiple medications simultaneously.**

Content – Medical/Surgical: **Category of Health Alteration** *– Respiratory:* **Integrated Processes** *– Nursing Process: Planning :* **Client Needs** *– Safe and Effective Care Environment: Management of Care:* **Cognitive Level** *– Synthesis*

MAKING NURSING DECISIONS: The charge nurse must decide which clients need a higher level of expertise to make this decision. Those clients requiring a higher level of expertise should be assigned to the nurse with the greatest knowledge in certain areas.

66. **1.** **This position allows for access to the client's back area. The chest tube for a hemothorax is positioned low and posterior to allow for gravity to assist in the removal of fluid from the thoracic area.**
2. This is the position for giving an enema.
3. This is the position used to assist with a lumbar puncture.
4. This is a resting position; it is not preparing for a chest tube placement.

Content – Medical/Surgical: **Category of Health Alteration** *– Respiratory:* **Integrated Processes** *– Nursing Process: Implementation:* **Client Needs** *– Physiological Integrity: Physiological Adaptation:* **Cognitive Level** *– Analysis*

MAKING NURSING DECISIONS: The nurse must have knowledge of basic anatomy and physiology to answer this question. "Hemo" means blood and "thorax" refers to the thoracic cavity. Blood is in the area where the lung needs to expand. Blood is heavier than air so the client should be positioned to access the area where dependent drainage will occur.

67. 1. Starting an intravenous line must be done prior to being able to initiate a piggyback medication.
2. **In order to treat the client with the most effective medication and not skew the results of a sputum culture, the specimen must be obtained prior to initiating antibiotics.**
3. New orders for intravenous antibiotics must be considered a priority to prevent the client

from going into gram-negative sepsis, a potentially lethal situation. However, in order to initiate the antibiotic the nurse must make sure a correct diagnosis is able to be made.

4. Respiratory treatments are important, but not before starting the antibiotics.

Content – Medical/Surgical: **Category of Health Alteration** – Respiratory: **Integrated Processes** – Nursing Process: Implementation: **Client Needs** – Physiological Integrity: Reduction of Risk Potential: **Cognitive Level** – Application

MAKING NURSING DECISIONS: To arrive at the correct priority intervention, the test taker must decide if one option must be accomplished prior to initiating other options.

68. 1. Shortness of breath after ambulating is expected for a patient diagnosed with COPD.
2. **Patients diagnosed with deep vein thrombosis are at risk for pulmonary embolism (PE). Anxiety is a symptom of PE. The nurse must determine if interventions are needed for PE, a life-threatening emergency.**
3. Anyone can take a specimen to the laboratory.
4. An empyema is an abscess in the thoracic cavity. These vital signs would be expected for this patient.

Content – Medical/Surgical: **Category of Health Alteration** – Respiratory: **Integrated Processes** – Nursing Process: Assessment: **Client Needs** – Physiological Integrity: Reduction of Risk Potential: **Cognitive Level** – Analysis

MAKING NURSING DECISIONS: When deciding which patient to assess first, there are rules. 1. Is the situation life threatening or life altering? 2. Is the information/data presented abnormal or unexpected? 3. Is the information expected for the disease process? Or is the problem a psychosocial one? 4. Are the data within normal limits? The test taker should choose the correct answer based on 1 first, 2 next, 3 next, and 4 last.

69. Answer: 2160 mL intake and 925 mL output. The urinary output is not used in this calculation. The nurse must add up both intravenous fluids and oral fluids to obtain the total intake for this client; 1500 + 100 = 1500 IV fluids; (1 ounce = 30 mL) 12 ounces ¥ 30 mL = 360 mL, 6 ounces ¥ 30 mL = 180 mL, 4 ounces ¥ 30 mL = 120 mL; 360 + 180 + 120 = 660 oral fluids. Total intake is 1,500 + 660 = 2,160. The urinary output 800 mL plus chest drainage 125 mL equals 925 mLs for shift output.

Content – Medical/Surgical: **Category of Health Alteration** – Respiratory: **Integrated Processes** – Nursing Process: Implementation: **Client Needs** – Physiological Integrity: Pharmacological and Parenteral Therapies: **Cognitive Level** – Application

MAKING NURSING DECISIONS: The **NCLEX-RN®** blueprint includes dosage calculations under Pharmacological and Parenteral Therapies. This category is included under Physiological Integrity, which promotes physical health and wellness by providing care and comfort, reducing client risk potential, and managing health alterations.

70. 1. **Bronchiolitis is an inflammation of the bronchioles, which are the small airways in the lungs. Signs/symptoms include wheezy cough, rapid breathing, cyanosis, nasal flaring, muscle retactions, and fever. Because the client is exhibiting expected signs/symptoms this client should be assigned to the graduate nurse.**
2. Dull percussion and vocal fremitus indicate consolidation. Consolidation is fluid instead of air in the alveolar space. This is a potentially life-threatening situation and should not be assigned to a new graduate.
3. Flail chest describes a situation in which a portion of the rib cage is separated from the rest of the chest wall, usually due to a severe blunt trauma, such as a serious fall or a car accident. This affected portion is unable to contribute to expansion of the lungs. Flail chest is a serious condition that can lead to long-term disability and even death. The charge nurse should assign this client to a more experienced nurse.
4. The client with reactive airway disease, asthma, should be asymptomatic; therefore, when the client is wheezing the client is having an acute exacerbation and should be assigned to a more experienced nurse.

Content – Medical/Surgical: **Category of Health Alteration** – Respiratory: **Integrated Processes** – Nursing Process: Planning: **Client Needs** – Safe and Effective Care Environment: Management of Care: **Cognitive Level** – Synthesis

MAKING NURSING DECISIONS: When the test taker is deciding which client should be assigned to a new graduate, the most stable client should be assigned to the least experienced nurse.

CLINICAL SCENARIO ANSWERS AND RATIONALES

The correct answer number and rationale for why it is the correct answer are given in **boldface type.** Rationales for why the other possible answer options are incorrect also are given, but they are not in boldface type.

1. 1. The client with pneumonia is expected to have bilateral crackles, and an SaO_2 of 96% is stable; therefore, this client would not be assigned to the most experienced nursing.
   2. **This client is exhibiting typical signs of adult respiratory distress syndrome (ARDS); therefore, Ms. Gail should assign the most experienced nurse to this client.**
   3. The postoperative client with purulent drainage could be developing an infection and should be assessed but is not priority over a client who is experiencing respiratory distress.
   4. The client with a tonsillectomy is expected to have pain on the same day of surgery; any nurse should be able to care for this client.

2. 1. The nurse should administer the prescribed antibiotic as soon as possible but not prior to obtaining sputum culture.
   2. The client with pneumonia needs more than 2 L oxygen via nasal cannula, which would be appropriate for a client diagnosed with chronic obstructive pulmonary disease.
   3. **The nurse needs to obtain a sputum culture prior to administering antibiotic because the culture and sensitivity will be skewed if the client receives antibiotics. This should be the first HCP implemented.**
   4. The client with pneumonia is not placed in respiratory isolation. This HCP order should be questioned.

3. 1. **Placing the client in the orthopnic position will help the client breathe easier. The position assumed by clients with orthopnea is one in which they are sitting propped up in bed by several pillows.**
   2. The client with COPD must have low oxygen levels less than 3 L/min. COPD clients breathe because of oxygen hunger and high levels of O2 provide so much oxygen that the client loses the stimulus to breathe.
   3. The client is in distress; therefore, the nurse should not assess but instead do something to help the client. The nurse should not treat a machine.
   4. The nurse should implement an intervention first since the client is in distress, then notify the respiratory therapist.

4. 1. **The LPN would be able to care for a client 2 days postoperative; crepitus is air in the subcutaneous tissue but is not life threatening.**
   2. The client who is confused is not stable; therefore, the nurse cannot assign this client to the LPN. The nurse cannot assign assessment, teaching, evaluation, or an unstable client to the LPN.
   3. The nurse cannot assign teaching; therefore, this client cannot be assigned to an LPN.
   4. The client's pulse oximetery is less than 93%; therefore, this client is unstable and cannot be assigned to an LPN.

5. 1. The client with active tuberculosis is usually administered rifampin, which causes urine and bodily fluids to turn orange.
   2. The client who is post-op would be expected to have pain, so this client would not need immediate intervention. The client who has signs/symptoms not expected for the disease process/condition would require immediate intervention.
   3. **The client with a pneumothorax should not have blood in the collection chamber; the client with a hemothorax would be expected to have bloody drainage. This client requires immediate intervention by Ms. Gail.**
   4. A client with bacterial pneumonia would be expected to have elevated temperature and chills; therefore, this client does not require immediate intervention.

6. 1. Carafate coats the stomach and must be administered on an empty stomach; therefore, the nurse would not question administering this medication.
   2. The therapeutic digoxin level is 0.8 to 2.0 mg/dL; therefore, the nurse would not question administering this medication.
   3. The therapeutic PTT for the client receiving heparin is 58–78; therefore, the nurse would not question administering this medication.
   4. **The client on an aminoglycoside antibiotic with an elevated trough level should not receive the medication. The elevation could lead to ototoxicity or nephrotoxicity; therefore, the nurse should question administering this medication.**

7. 1. **The client needs oxygen to help perfuse the lungs, heart, and body; therefore, this is the first intervention Ms. Gail should tell the nurse to implement.**

2. The client will need a ventilation/perfusion scan to confirm the diagnosis of pulmonary embolus, but it is not the nurse's first intervention.
3. The nurse will need to notify the client's healthcare provider but not prior to taking care of the client's body.
4. Assessing the client is indicated, but it is not the first intervention in this situation. Remember: If the client is in distress, do not assess; take an action to help the client.

8. 1. The nurse should document the client's complaints in the nurse's notes but it is not the first intervention. The nurse should first assess the client.
2. Taking slow deep breaths will not address the client's pain of 6 on the pain scale.
3. **The nurse must first determine whether the pain is expected for the client's condition or whether the client is experiencing a complication requiring nursing or medical intervention. This is the nurse's first intervention.**
4. The nurse must check the MAR when it is determined the pain is expected and requires pain medication, but it is not the first intervention.

9. 1, 4, and 5 are correct.
1. **The client should be in a high-Fowler's position to facilitate lung expansion.**

2. The system must be patent and intact to function properly but it should be assessed more often than every shift. It should be assessed every 2 to 4 hours.
3. The client can have bathroom privileges, and ambulation facilitates lung ventilation and expansion.
4. **The tubing should not have any dependent loops. Looping the tubing prevents direct pressure on the chest tube itself and keeps tubing off the floor, addressing both a safety and an infection control issue.**
5. **The collection chamber of the Pleuravac should be marked at the end of every shift and is part of the total output for the client.**

10. 1. The client suspected of having ARDS is not stable and should not be assigned to an LPN. A more experienced nurse should be assigned this client.
2. The LPN cannot administer blood; therefore, this client should not be assigned to the LPN.
3. Jugular vein distention and hypotension are signs of a tension pneumothorax, which is a medical emergency, and the client should be assigned to an RN.
4. **A client scheduled for a bronchoscopy is stable and should be assigned to the LPN. This client is the most stable and least critical.**

Gastrointestinal Management

Let whoever is in charge keep this simple question in her head—NOT how can I always do the right thing myself but how can I provide for this right thing always to be done.

—Florence Nightingale

QUESTIONS

1. The nurse is caring for clients on a medical unit. Which task should the nurse implement first?
   1. Change the abdominal surgical dressing for a client who has ambulated in the hall.
   2. Discuss the correct method of placing Montgomery straps on the client with the UAP.
   3. Assess the male client who called the desk to say he is nauseated and just vomited.
   4. Place a call to the extended care facility to give the report on a discharged client.

2. The nurse is preparing a client diagnosed with peptic ulcer disease for a barium study of the stomach and esophagus. Which nursing intervention is the priority for this client?
   1. Obtain informed consent from the client for the diagnostic procedure.
   2. Discuss the need to increase oral fluid intake after the procedure.
   3. Explain to the client that he or she will have to drink a white, chalky substance.
   4. Tell the client not to eat or drink anything prior to the procedure.

3. Which client warrants immediate intervention from the nurse on the medical unit?
   1. The client diagnosed with dyspepsia who has eructation and bloating.
   2. The client diagnosed with pancreatitis who has steatorrhea and pyrexia.
   3. The client with diverticulitis who has left lower quadrant pain and fever.
   4. The client with Crohn's disease who has right lower abdominal pain and diarrhea.

4. The nurse and the unlicensed assistive personnel (UAP) are caring for clients on a medical-surgical unit. Which task should not be assigned to the UAP?
   1. Instruct the UAP to feed the 69-year-old client who is experiencing dysphagia.
   2. Request the UAP change the linens for the 89-year-old client with fecal incontinence.
   3. Tell the UAP to assist the 54-year-old client with a bowel management program.
   4. Ask the UAP to obtain vital signs on the 72-year-old client diagnosed with cirrhosis.

5. Which behavior by the unlicensed assistive personnel (UAP) requires immediate intervention by the nurse?
   1. The UAP is refusing to feed the client diagnosed with acute diverticulitis.
   2. The UAP would not place the client on the bedside commode who was on bed rest.
   3. The UAP placed the client with a continuous feeding tube in the supine position.
   4. The UAP placed sequential compression devices on the client who is on strict bed rest.

6. The nurse is concerned about the documentation form for blood administration, and other staff members agree the documentation is cumbersome and needs to be revised. Which action is most appropriate for the nurse to implement first?
   1. Discuss the blood administration flow sheet with the chief nursing officer.
   2. Contact an individual to help design a new blood transfusion flow sheet.
   3. Learn to adapt to the present form and do not take any further action.
   4. Volunteer to be on an ad hoc committee to research alternate flow sheets.

7. The charge nurse is transcribing HCP orders for a client scheduled for a barium enema. In addition to the radiology department, which department of the hospital should be notified of the procedure?
   1. The cardiac catheterization department.
   2. The dietary department.
   3. The nuclear medicine department.
   4. The hospital laboratory department.

8. The charge nurse is making assignments on a medical unit. Which client should the nurse assign to the graduate nurse?
   1. The client who has received three units of packed red blood cells (RBCs).
   2. The client scheduled for an esophagogastroduodenoscopy in the morning.
   3. The client with short bowel syndrome who has diarrhea and a K+ level of 3.3 mEq/L.
   4. The client who has just returned from surgery for a sigmoid colostomy.

9. At 0830, the day shift nurse is preparing to administer medications to the client NPO for an endoscopy. Which medication should the nurse question administering? **Select all that apply.**

Client's Name:		Account Number: 123456	Allergies: Penicillin	
Date:	**Medication**	**2301–0700**	**0701–1500**	**1501–2300**
	Lanoxin (digoxin) 0.125 mg PO every day		0900	
	Lasix (furosemide) 40 mg PO bid		0900	1600
	Zantac (ranitidine) 150 mg in 250 mL NS IV continuous infusion every 24 hours	0300 NN@11 mL/hr		
	Vancomycin 850 mg IVPB every 24 hours		0900	2100
	Mylanta 30 mL PO PRN heart burn.			
Signature/Initials		**Day Nurse RN DN**	**Night Nurse RN NN**	

   1. Lanoxin (digoxin) 0.125 mg PO every day.
   2. Lasix (furosemide) 40 mg PO bid.
   3. Zantac (ranitidine) 150 mg in 250 mL NS IV continuous infusion every 24 hours.
   4. Vancomycin 850 mg IVPB every 24 hours.
   5. Mylanta 30 mL PO PRN heartburn.

10. Which client should the nurse assess first after receiving the p.m. shift assessment?
    1. The client with Barrett's esophagus who has dysphagia and pyrosis.
    2. The client with proctitis who has tenesmus and passage of mucus through the rectum.
    3. The client with liver failure who is jaundiced and has ascites.
    4. The client with abdominal pain who has an 8-hour urinary output of 150 mL/hr.

11. The nurse is planning the care of a client diagnosed with acute gastroenteritis. Which nursing problem is priority?
    1. Altered nutrition.
    2. Self-care deficit.
    3. Impaired body image.
    4. Fluid and electrolyte imbalance.

12. The nurse is preparing to administer morning medications to clients on a medical unit. Which medication should the nurse administer first?
    1. Methylprednisolone (Solu-Medrol), a steroid, to a client diagnosed with Crohn's disease.
    2. Donepezil (Aricept), an acetylcholinesterase inhibitor, to a client with dementia.
    3. Sucralfate (Carafate), a mucosal barrier agent, to a client diagnosed with ulcer disease.
    4. Enoxaparin (Lovenox), an anticoagulant, to a client on bed rest after abdominal surgery.

13. The nurse has received the morning shift report on a surgical unit in a community hospital. Which client should the nurse assess first?
    1. The client who is 6 hours postoperative small bowel resection who has hypoactive bowel sounds in all four quadrants.
    2. The client who is scheduled for an abdominal-peritoneal resection this morning and is crying and upset.
    3. The client who is 1 day postoperative for abdominal surgery and has a rigid, hard abdomen.
    4. The client who is 2 days postoperative for an emergency appendectomy and is complaining of abdominal pain, rating it as an 8 on a pain scale of 1 to 10.

14. The charge nurse is reviewing the morning laboratory results. Which data should the charge nurse report to the HCP via telephone?
    1. The client who is 4 hours postoperative for gastric lap banding with a white blood cell (WBC) count of 15,000 mm.
    2. The client who is 1 day postoperative total colectomy with creation of an ileal conduit who has a hemoglobin and hematocrit level of 12/36.
    3. The client who is 4 days postoperative for gastric bypass surgery whose fasting blood glucose level is 180 mg/dL.
    4. The client who is 8 hours postoperative for exploratory laparotomy who has a serum potassium level of 4.5 mEq/L.

15. The nurse is preparing clients for surgery. Which client has the greatest potential for experiencing complications?
    1. The client scheduled for removal of an abdominal mass who is overweight.
    2. The client scheduled for a gastrectomy who has arterial hypertension.
    3. The client scheduled for an open cholecystectomy who smokes two packs of cigarettes per day.
    4. The client scheduled for an emergency appendectomy who smokes marijuana on a daily basis.

QUESTIONS

16. The nurse is performing ostomy care for a client who had an abdominal-peritoneal resection with a permanent sigmoid colostomy. Rank the following interventions in order of priority.
    1. Cleanse the stomal site with mild soap and water.
    2. Assess the stoma for a pink, moist appearance.
    3. Monitor the drainage in the ostomy drainage bag.
    4. Apply stoma adhesive paste to the skin around the stoma.
    5. Attach the ostomy drainage bag to the abdomen.

17. The nurse is transcribing the HCP's orders for a client who is scheduled for an emergency appendectomy and is being transferred from the emergency department (ED) to the surgical unit. Which order should the nurse implement first?
    1. Obtain the client's informed consent.
    2. Administer 2 mg of IV morphine, every 4 hours, PRN.
    3. Shave the lower right abdominal quadrant.
    4. Administer the on-call IVPB antibiotic.

18. The client 1 day postoperative abdominal surgery has an evisceration of the wound. Which intervention should the nurse implement first?
    1. Place sterile normal saline gauze on the eviscerated area.
    2. Reinforce the abdominal dressing with an ABD pad.
    3. Assess the client's abdominal bowel sounds.
    4. Place the client in the left lateral position.

19. The medical-surgical nurse has just received the a.m. shift report. Which client should the nurse assess first?
    1. The client who has a paralytic ileus and has absent bowel sounds.
    2. The client who is 2 days post-op abdominal surgery and has a soft, tender abdomen.
    3. The client who is 6 hours postoperative and has an abdominal wound dehiscence.
    4. The client who had a liver transplant and is being transferred to the rehabilitation unit.

20. The client is being prepared for a colonoscopy in the day surgery center. The charge nurse observes the primary nurse instructing the unlicensed assistive personnel (UAP) to assist the client to the bathroom. Which action should the charge nurse implement?
    1. Take no action because this is appropriate delegation.
    2. Tell the UAP to obtain a bedside commode for the client.
    3. Discuss the inappropriate delegation of the nursing task.
    4. Document the situation in an adverse occurrence report.

21. The nurse is caring for clients on a surgical unit. Which client should the nurse assess first?
    1. The client who has been vomiting for 2 days and has an ABG of pH 7.47, PaO_2 95, $PaCO_2$ 44, HCO_3 30.
    2. The client who is 8 hours postoperative for splenectomy and who is complaining of abdominal pain, rating it as a 9 on a pain scale of 1 to 10.
    3. The client who is 12 hours postoperative abdominal surgery and has dark green bile draining in the nasogastric tube.
    4. The client who is 2 days postoperative for hiatal hernia repair and is complaining of feeling constipated.

22. The unlicensed assistive personnel (UAP) tells the nurse angrily, "You are the worst nurse I have ever worked with and I really hate working with you." Which action should the nurse implement first?
    1. Don't respond to the comment and appraise the situation.
    2. Tell the UAP to leave the unit immediately.
    3. Report this comment and behavior to the charge nurse.
    4. Explain to the UAP that he or she cannot talk to the primary nurse like this.

23. The client is admitted to the critical care unit after a motor vehicle accident. The client asks the nurse, "Do you know if the person in the other car is all right?" The nurse knows the person died. Which statement supports the ethical principle of veracity?
    1. "I am not sure how the other person is doing."
    2. "I will try to find out how the other person is doing."
    3. "You should rest now and try not worry about it."
    4. "I am sorry to have to tell you, but the person died."

24. The client admitted to the critical care unit tells the nurse, "I have an advance directive (AD) and I do not want to have cardiopulmonary resuscitation (CPR)." Which intervention should the nurse implement first?
    1. Ask the client for a copy of the AD so that it can be placed in the chart.
    2. Inform the healthcare provider of the client's request as soon as possible.
    3. Determine whether the client has a durable power of attorney for healthcare.
    4. Request the hospital chaplain to come and talk to the client about this request.

25. The client is diagnosed with esophageal bleeding. Which of the following assessment data warrants immediate intervention by the nurse?
    1. The client's hemoglobin/hematocrit is 11.4/32.
    2. The client's abdomen is soft to touch and non-tender.
    3. The client's vital signs are T 99, AP 114, RR 18, B/P 88/60.
    4. The client's nasogastric tube has coffee ground drainage.

26. Which task should the nurse in the long-term care facility delegate to the unlicensed assistive personnel (UAP)?
    1. Assist the resident up in a wheelchair for meals.
    2. Assess the incontinent client's perianal area.
    3. Discuss requirements with the client for going out on a pass.
    4. Explain how to care for the client's colostomy to the family.

27. The nurse and the unlicensed assistive personnel (UAP) are caring for a client on a medical unit who has difficulty swallowing and is incontinent of urine and feces. Which task should the nurse delegate to the unlicensed assistive personnel (UAP)?
    1. Check the client's PEG feeding tube for patency.
    2. Place DuoDERM wound care patches on the client's coccyx.
    3. Apply non-medicated ointment to the client's perineum.
    4. Suction the client during feeding to prevent aspiration.

28. Which behavior by the unlicensed assistive personnel (UAP) warrants intervention by the long-term care nurse?
    1. The UAP is giving the client with a gastrostomy tube a glass of water.
    2. The UAP is ambulating the client outside using a safety belt.
    3. The UAP is assisting the client with putting a jigsaw puzzle together.
    4. The UAP is giving a back rub to the client who is on bed rest.

29. The nurse is preparing to teach the male client how to irrigate his sigmoid colostomy. Which intervention should the nurse implement first?
    1. Demonstrate the procedure on a model.
    2. Provide the client with written instructions.
    3. Ask the client whether he has any questions.
    4. Show the client all of the equipment needed.

30. The LPN tells the nurse the client diagnosed with liver failure is getting more confused. Which intervention should the nurse implement first?
    1. Assess the client's neurological status.
    2. Notify the client's healthcare provider.
    3. Request a STAT ammonia serum level.
    4. Tell the LPN to obtain the client's vital signs.

31. The nurse is changing the client's colostomy bag. Which interventions should the nurse implement? Rank in the order of priority.
    1. Remove the client's colostomy bag.
    2. Apply the client's new colostomy bag.
    3. Don non-sterile gloves.
    4. Assess the client's stoma site.
    5. Cleanse the area around the client's stoma.

32. Which task is most appropriate for the home healthcare nurse to delegate to the unlicensed assistive personnel (UAP)?
    1. Instruct the UAP to give the herb ginkgo biloba to the client with Alzheimer's.
    2. Ask the UAP to perform the tube feedings for a client with a gastrostomy tube.
    3. Request the UAP to perform the daily colostomy irrigation for the client.
    4. Tell the UAP to wash and dry the client's hair.

33. Which behavior by the UAP warrants intervention by the home health (HH) nurse? The client tells the HH nurse the UAP:
    1. Would not accept a birthday gift from the client.
    2. Gave the client a vase of flowers from the UAP's garden.
    3. Picked up the client's prescriptions from the pharmacy.
    4. Cleaned the client's bathroom, including scrubbing the commode.

34. The female client, diagnosed with diverticulosis, called the home healthcare agency and told the nurse, "I am having really bad pain in my left lower stomach and I think I have a fever." Which action should the nurse take?
    1. Recommend the client take an antacid and lie flat in the bed.
    2. Instruct one of the nurses to visit the client immediately.
    3. Tell the client to have someone drive them to the emergency room.
    4. Ask the client what she has had to eat in the last 8 hours.

35. The client with a sigmoid colostomy has an excoriated area around the stoma that has not improved for more than 2 weeks. Which intervention is most appropriate for the home health nurse (HH) to implement?
    1. Refer the client to the wound care nurse.
    2. Notify the client's healthcare provider.
    3. Continue to monitor the stoma site.
    4. Place Karaya paste over the excoriated area.

36. The client, who is terminally ill, tells the nurse, "I just want to live to see my grandson graduate in 2 months." Which stage of grief is the client experiencing?
    1. Anger.
    2. Bargaining.
    3. Depression.
    4. Acceptance.

37. The nurse is discussing end-of-life care (EOL) with the client diagnosed with pancreatic cancer. Which statements are the goals for end-of-life care? **Select all that apply.**
    1. To provide comfort and supportive care during the dying process.
    2. To plan and arrange the funeral for the client.
    3. To improve the client's quality of life for the remaining time.
    4. To help ensure a dignified death for the client and family.
    5. To assist with the financial cost of the dying process.

38. The male Mexican American client, who is terminally ill, refuses hospice services because he says it is "giving up" and he is not going to die. Which is the most appropriate action by the nurse?
    1. Discuss the philosophy and services of palliative care with the client.
    2. Take no other action and support the client's decision.
    3. Contact the client's healthcare provider to discuss the prognosis.
    4. Talk to the client's family members about his choice to refuse hospice.

39. The nurse is discussing end-of-life issues with a client. The nurse is explaining about a document used for listing the person the client will allow to make healthcare decisions should he or she become unable to make informed decisions for him- or herself. Which document is the nurse discussing with the client?
1. Advance directive.
2. Directive to physicians.
3. Living will.
4. Durable power of attorney for healthcare.

40. The significant other of a client diagnosed with liver cancer and who is dying asks the nurse, "What is bereavement counseling?" Which statement is the nurse's best response?
1. "Bereavement counseling helps the client accept the terminal illness."
2. "It provides support to you and your family in the transition to a life without your loved one."
3. "We provide counseling to you and your loved one during the dying process."
4. "It is group counseling for family members whose loved ones have died."

41. The nurse is working in a digestive disease disorder clinic. Which nursing action is an example of evidence-based practice (EBP)?
1. Turn on the tap water to help a client urinate.
2. Use two identifiers to identify a client before a procedure.
3. Educate a client based on current published information.
4. Read nursing journals about the latest procedures.

42. The charge nurse notices a nurse recapping a needle in a client's room. Which action should the charge nurse take first?
1. Tell the nurse not to recap the needle.
2. Quietly ask the nurse to step into the hall.
3. Reprimand the nurse for not following procedure.
4. Notify the house supervisor of the nurse's behavior.

43. The administrative supervisor is staffing the hospital's medical-surgical units during an ice storm and has received many calls from staff members who are unable to get to the hospital. Which action should the supervisor implement first?
1. Inform the chief nursing officer.
2. Notify the on-duty staff to stay.
3. Call staff members who live close to the facility.
4. Implement the emergency disaster protocol.

44. The nurse is working in a community health clinic. Which nursing task should the nurse delegate to the unlicensed assistive personnel (UAP)?
1. Instruct the UAP to take the client's history.
2. Request the UAP to document the client's complaints.
3. Ask the UAP to obtain the client's weight and height.
4. Tell the UAP to complete the client's follow-up care.

45. The staff nurse is working with a colleague who begins to act erratically and is loud and argumentative. Which action should be taken by the nurse?
1. Ask the supervisor to come to the unit.
2. Determine what is bothering the nurse.
3. Suggest the nurse go home.
4. Smell the nurse's breath for alcohol.

46. The charge nurse is making assignments on a medical-surgical unit. Which client should be assigned to the most experienced nurse?
    1. The client diagnosed with lower esophageal dysfunction who is experiencing regurgitation.
    2. The client diagnosed with Barrett's esophagitis who is scheduled for an endoscopy.
    3. The client diagnosed with gastroesophageal reflux disease who has bilateral wheezes.
    4. The client diagnosed with 1 day post-op hiatal hernia who has pain rated a 4 on a pain scale of 1 to 10.

47. The client is experiencing severe diarrhea and a serum potassium level of 3.3 mEq/L. Which intervention should the nurse implement first?
    1. Notify the client's healthcare provider.
    2. Assess the client for leg cramps.
    3. Place the client on cardiac telemetry.
    4. Prepare to administer intravenous potassium.

48. The unlicensed assistive personnel (UAP) notifies the charge nurse that the male client is angry with the care he is receiving and is packing to leave the hospital. Which intervention should the charge nurse implement first?
    1. Ask the client's nurse why the client is upset.
    2. Discuss the problem with the client.
    3. Notify the healthcare provider (HCP).
    4. Have the client sign the against medical advice (AMA) form.

49. The nurse is caring for a 14-year-old female client diagnosed with bulimia. Which intervention should the nurse delegate to the unlicensed assistive personnel (UAP)?
    1. Talk with the parents about setting goals for the client.
    2. Stay with the client for 15 to 20 minutes after each meal.
    3. Encourage the client to verbalize low self-esteem.
    4. List for the dietician the amount of food the client consumed.

50. The client tells the nurse in the bariatric clinic, "I have tried to lose weight on just about every diet out there but nothing works." Which statement is the nurse's best response?
    1. "Which diets and modifications have you tried?"
    2. "How much weight are you trying to lose?"
    3. "This must be difficult. Would you like to talk?"
    4. "You may need to get used to being overweight."

51. The client 2 days postoperative from a laparoscopic cholecystectomy tells the office nurse, "My right shoulder hurts so bad I can't stand it." Which statement is the nurse's best response?
    1. "This is a result of the carbon dioxide gas used in surgery."
    2. "Call 911 and go to the emergency department immediately."
    3. "Increase the pain medication the surgeon ordered."
    4. "You need to ambulate in the hall to walk off the gas pains."

52. The nurse is administering medications. At 1400, the client diagnosed with gastroenteritis is complaining of being nauseated and has had a formed brown stool. Which intervention should the nurse implement?

Client Name: T.R.	Account Number: 5948726		Allergies: milk	
Height: 5'8"	Weight in pounds: 202		Date of Birth: 07/22/1948	
Date: Today	Medication	2301–0700	0701–1500	1501–2300
	Lomotil 1 or 2 tablets after each stool up to 8 in 24 hours	0400	0900	
	Ondansetron 4–8 mg IVP every 4 hours PRN for nausea	0030 (4 mg)	0630 (4 mg) 1230 (mg)	
Signature/Initials		Night Nurse RN/NN	Day Nurse RN/DN	

1. Administer ondansetron 4 mg IVP.
2. Administer Lomotil 2 tabs PO.
3. Notify the client's healthcare provider.
4. Tell the client nothing can be administered for the nausea.

53. The nurse is caring for a client who is hemorrhaging from a duodenal ulcer. Which collaborative interventions should the nurse implement? **Select all that apply.**
1. Prepare to administer a Sengstaken-Blakemore tube.
2. Assess the client's vital signs.
3. Administer a proton-pump intravenously.
4. Obtain a type and crossmatch for four units of blood.
5. Monitor the client's intake and output.

54. The nurse is caring for a client diagnosed with peptic ulcer disease. Which assessment data would cause the client to require an immediate intervention by the nurse?
1. The client has hypoactive bowel sounds.
2. The client's output is 480 mL for 12-hour shift.
3. The client has T 98.6, AP 98, RR 22, B/P 102/78.
4. The client has coffee ground emesis.

55. The nurse is caring for a client 1 day postoperative sigmoid resection. There is a large amount of bright red blood on the dressing. Which intervention should the nurse implement first?
1. Assess the client's apical pulse and blood pressure.
2. Auscultate the client's bowel sounds.
3. Notify the healthcare provider immediately.
4. Reinforce the dressing with a sterile gauze pad.

56. The nurse is preparing to hang a new bag of total parental nutrition on a client who has had an abdominal perineal resection. The bag has 2,000 mL of 50% dextrose, 10 mL of trace elements, 20 mL of multivitamins, 20 mL of potassium chloride, and 500 mL of lipids. The bag is to infuse over the next 24 hours. At what rate should the nurse set the pump? _____

57. The unlicensed assistive personnel (UAP) tells the nurse a female client, who had a laparoscopic cholecystectomy, is complaining of abdominal pain. Which intervention should the nurse implement first?
1. Check the medication administration record for the last pain medication the client received.
2. Instruct the UAP to ask the client to rate her pain on a 1 to 10 pain scale.
3. Assess the client to rule out any postoperative surgical complications.
4. Tell the UAP to obtain the client's vital signs and pulse oximeter reading.

58. The male client is 30 minutes post-procedure liver biopsy. Which action by the unlicensed assistive personnel (UAP) requires the nurse to intervene?
1. The UAP offered the client a urinal to void.
2. The UAP gave the client a glass of water.
3. The UAP turned the client on the left side.
4. The UAP took the client's vital signs.

59. The client diagnosed with liver failure is experiencing pruritus secondary to severe jaundice and is scratching the upper extremities. Which intervention should the nurse implement first?
1. Request the UAP to assist the client to take a hot, soapy shower.
2. Apply an emollient to the client's upper extremities.
3. Place mittens on both hands of the client.
4. Administer Benadryl 25mg PO to the client.

60. The client with hepatitis asks the nurse, "Is there any herb I can take to help my liver get better?" Which statement is the nurse's best response?
1. "You should ask your healthcare provider about taking herbs."
2. "Milk thistle is a powerful oxidant and promotes liver cell growth."
3. "You should not take any medication that is not prescribed."
4. "Why would you want to take any herbs?"

61. Which task would be most appropriate for the nurse on the GI unit to delegate to the unlicensed assistive personnel (UAP)?
1. Request the UAP to draw the serum liver function test.
2. Ask the UAP to remove the nasogastric tube.
3. Tell the UAP to empty the client's colostomy bag.
4. Instruct the UAP to assist the unit secretary to transcribe HCP orders.

62. The client is diagnosed with gastroenteritis. Which laboratory data warrants immediate intervention by the nurse?
1. A serum sodium level of 152 mEq/L.
2. An arterial blood gas of pH 7.37, Pao_2 95, $Paco_2$ 43, Hco_3 24.
3. A serum potassium level of 4.8 mEq/L.
4. A stool sample that is positive for fecal leukocytes.

63. Which nursing problem is the highest priority for the client diagnosed with gastroenteritis from staphylococcal food poisoning?
1. Fluid and electrolyte imbalance.
2. Alteration in bowel elimination.
3. Nutrition, altered: less than body requirements.
4. Oral mucous membrane, altered.

64. The nurse has received the a.m. shift report. Which client should the nurse assess first?
1. The client with peptic ulcer disease who is complaining of acute epigastric pain.
2. The client with acute gastroenteritis who is upset and wants to go home.
3. The client with inflammatory bowel disease who is receiving total parental nutrition.
4. The client with hepatitis B who is complaining and who is jaundiced and anorexic.

65. The client who has had abdominal surgery is complaining of pain and tells the nurse, "I felt something pop in my stomach." Which intervention should the nurse implement first?
    1. Check the client's apical pulse and blood pressure.
    2. Determine the client's pain on a 1 to 10 pain scale.
    3. Assess the client's surgical wound site.
    4. Administer pain medication intravenously.

66. The client who is 2 days postoperative abdominal surgery has a hemovac drainage tube. Which assessment data indicates the Jackson-Pratt (JP) is functioning appropriately?
    1. The hemovac is round and has 40 mL of fluid.
    2. The drainage tube is pinned to the dressing.
    3. The hemovac insertion site is pink and has no drainage.
    4. The hemovac has suction and is compressed.

67. The nurse is caring for the following clients on a surgical unit. Which client should the nurse assess first?
    1. The client with an inguinal hernia repair who has a urine output of 160 mL in 4 hours.
    2. The client with an emergency appendectomy who was transferred from PACU.
    3. The client who is 4 hours postoperative abdominal surgery who has flatulence.
    4. The client who is 6 hours post-procedure colonoscopy and is being discharged.

68. The client who is morbidly obese is 8 hours postoperative gastric bypass surgery. Which nursing intervention is of the greatest priority?
    1. Instruct the client to use the incentive spirometer.
    2. Weigh the client daily in the same clothes and at the same time.
    3. Apply sequential compression devices to the client's lower extremities.
    4. Assist the client to sit in the bedside chair.

69. The charge nurse has completed report. Which client should be seen first?
    1. The client diagnosed with ulcerative colitis who had five loose stools the previous shift.
    2. The elderly client admitted from another facility who is refusing to be seen by the nurse.
    3. The client with intractable vomiting who has tented skin turgor and dry mucous membranes.
    4. The client with hemorrhoids who had spotting of bright red blood on the toilet tissue.

70. The nurse, a licensed practical nurse (LPN), and an unlicensed assistive personnel (UAP) are caring for clients on a medical floor. Which nursing task is most appropriate to assign/delegate?
    1. Instruct the UAP to discontinue the client's total parenteral nutrition.
    2. Ask the UAP to give the client 30 mL of Maalox for heartburn.
    3. Tell the LPN to administer a bulk laxative to a client diagnosed with constipation.
    4. Request the LPN to assess the abdomen of a client who has had complaints of pain.

GASTROINTESTINAL CLINICAL SCENARIO

Ms. Kathy is the charge nurse on a 36-bed unit that admits clients with gastrointestinal disorders and gastrointestinal surgery. The unit is staffed with four RNs, two LPNs, and two UAPs as well as a ward secretary.

1. Ms. Kathy is making assignments. Which client should be assigned to the graduate nurse who has been on the unit for 1 month?
   1. The client diagnosed with lower esophageal dysfunction who is complaining of pyrosis.
   2. The client who had an endoscopy this morning and has absent bowel sounds.
   3. The client with gastroesophageal reflux disease who has bilateral wheezing.
   4. The client who is 1 day post-op open cholecystectomy and refuses to deep breathe.

2. The client diagnosed with inflammatory bowel disease has a serum potassium level of 4.4 mEq/L. Which intervention should the nurse implement first?
   1. Notify the healthcare provider.
   2. Continue to monitor the client.
   3. Request telemetry for the client.
   4. Prepare to administer potassium IV.

3. The client has been admitted to the hospital with hemorrhaging from a duodenal ulcer. Which independent interventions should Ms. Kathy instruct the primary nurse to implement? **Select all that apply.**
   1. Complete the admission assessment.
   2. Evaluate BP lying, sitting, and standing
   3. Administer antibiotics intravenously.
   4. Administer blood products.
   5. Obtain a hemoglobin and hematocrit.

4. Ms. Kathy is discharging a client with a new sigmoid colostomy. Which statement made by the client indicates to Ms. Kathy the client needs more teaching?
   1. "If my stoma becomes a purple color I will notify my HCP."
   2. "I can eat the foods I used to eat when I go home."
   3. "I should wear a colostomy pouch over my stoma."
   4. "I will irrigate my colostomy every week with 750 mL of tap water."

5. The nurse is preparing to hang a new bag of total parental nutrition on a client who has had an abdominal perineal resection. The bag has 2,000 mL of 50% dextrose, 15 mL of trace elements, 30 mL of multivitamins, 20 mL of potassium chloride, and 200 mL of lipids. The bag is to infuse over the next 24 hours. At what rate should the nurse set the pump? _____

6. The client is admitted to the medical unit with a diagnosis of acute diverticulitis. Which order should Ms. Kathy clarify with the healthcare provider?
   1. Insert a nasogastric tube.
   2. Start IV D_5W at 125 mL/hr.
   3. Schedule the client for a sigmoidoscopy.
   4. Place the client on bed rest with bathroom privileges.

7. Ms. Kathy observes the unlicensed assistive personnel (UAP) turning the client who has just had a liver biopsy to the supine position. Which action should Ms. Kathy implement first?
   1. Tell the UAP to keep the client on bed rest for 2 hours.
   2. Praise the UAP for placing the client in the supine position.
   3. Instruct the UAP to place the client on the right side.
   4. Complete an incident report on the UAP's behavior.

8. One of the primary nurses tells Ms. Kathy she stuck herself in the finger with a "used" needle and cleaned the site with soap and water. Which intervention should Ms. Kathy implement first?
   1. Notify the infection control nurse.
   2. Complete an adverse occurrence report.
   3. Request post-exposure prophylaxis.
   4. Check the hepatitis status of the client.

9. Which nursing task is most appropriate for Ms. Kathy to delegate to the unlicensed assistive personnel (UAP)?
   1. Bathe the client with liver failure who has a Sengstaken-Blakemore tube inflated.
   2. Teach the client with an open cholesectomy to splint the incision when coughing.
   3. Assist the client with pruritis to the bathroom for a shower and a.m. care.
   4. Tell the UAP to assist the nurse performing a paracentesis on the client with liver failure.

10. Ms. Kathy is making rounds on the unit. Which client should Ms. Kathy assess first?
    1. The client diagnosed with peptic ulcer disease who is receiving blood and has a hemoglobin of 10.1 and hematocrit 35.
    2. The client diagnosed with ulcerative colitis who has had 10 loose stools and has a potassium level of 3.5 mEq/L.
    3. The client who is 1 day post-op abdominal surgery with a hard, rigid abdomen and elevated temperature.
    4. The client diagnosed with acute diverticulitis whose nasogastric tube is draining green bile.

ANSWERS AND RATIONALES

The correct answer number and rationale for why it is the correct answer are given in **boldface type**. Rationales for why the other possible answer options are incorrect also are given, but they are not in boldface type.

1. 1. This client should be seen in a timely manner, but not before the client who is vomiting.
   2. This can take some time and should not be hastily completed because the nurse must know the task is being done correctly before delegating it to a UAP. This should be done at a time arranged between the UAP and the nurse.
   3. **This client has experienced a physiological problem and the nurse must assess the client and the emesis to decide on possible interventions.**
   4. The nurse could call the extended care facility after assessing the client who has vomited and after dressing the client's leg.

   Content – Medical/Surgical: *Category of Health Alteration* – Gastrointestinal: *Integrated Processes* – Nursing Process: Implementation: *Client Needs* – Safe and Effective Care Environment: Management of Care: *Cognitive Level* – Analysis

   MAKING NURSING DECISIONS: The test taker should use some tool as a reference to guide in the decision-making process. In this situation, Maslow's Hierarchy of Needs should be applied. Physiological needs have priority over psychosocial ones.

2. 1. A barium study of the upper GI system is an x-ray procedure and does not require the client to sign an informed consent form.
   2. The barium can cause constipation after the procedure; therefore, the client should increase fluid intake, but this is not the priority intervention.
   3. The client will have to drink a white, chalky substance, but the priority intervention is to make sure the client is NPO.
   4. **The test is a barium study of the upper GI system and requires the client's upper GI system to be empty. This client should be made NPO at least 8 to 10 hours before the test.**

   Content – Medical/Surgical: *Category of Health Alteration* – Gastrointestinal: *Integrated Processes* – Nursing Process: Planning: *Client Needs* – Physiological Integrity: Reduction of Risk Potential: *Cognitive Level* – Synthesis

MAKING NURSING DECISIONS: The nurse must be knowledgeable of diagnostic tests. The nurse must know pre-procedure and post-procedure interventions, as well as which ones require informed consent. Remember, with the gastrointestinal system, being NPO is often the priority intervention.

3. 1. The nurse would expect the client with dyspepsia (upset stomach) to have eructation (belching) and bloating; therefore, this client does not warrant immediate intervention.
   2. The nurse would expect the client with pancreatitis to have steatorrhea (fat, frothy stools) and pyrexia (fever); therefore, this client does not warrant immediate intervention.
   3. The nurse would expect the client with diverticulitis to have left lower quadrant pain and fever; therefore, this client does not warrant immediate intervention.
   4. **The client with Crohn's disease should be asymptomatic, so pain and diarrhea warrant intervention by the nurse. Pain could indicate a complication.**

   Content – Medical/Surgical: *Category of Health Alteration* – Gastrointestinal: *Integrated Processes* – Nursing Process: Assessment: *Client Needs* – Physiological Integrity: Reduction of Risk Potential: *Cognitive Level* – Synthesis

MAKING NURSING DECISIONS: "Warrants immediate intervention" means the nurse must determine which client is priority to assess. The nurse would assess a client in pain if all the other options had clients with expected signs/symptoms.

4. 1. **The nurse should not delegate to the UAP feeding a client who is not stable and at risk for complications during feeding, as a result of dysphagia. This requires judgment that the UAP is not expected to possess.**
   2. UAPs can change linens for clients who are incontinent; therefore, this task could be delegated to a UAP.
   3. The UAP can assist the client to the bathroom and document the results of the attempt.
   4. The UAP can obtain the vital signs on a stable client.

   Content – Medical/Surgical: *Category of Health Alteration* – Gastrointestinal: *Integrated Processes* – Nursing Process: Planning: *Client Needs* – Safe and Effective Care Environment: Management of Care: *Cognitive Level* – Synthesis

MAKING NURSING DECISIONS: An RN cannot delegate assessment, teaching, evaluation, medications, or an unstable client to a UAP. Tasks that cannot be delegated are nursing interventions requiring nursing judgment.

5. 1. The client diagnosed with acute diverticulitis should be NPO; therefore, the UAP should not feed a client. This action does not warrant immediate intervention.
   2. The UAP should not allow the client on bed rest to use the bedside commode; therefore, this does not warrant immediate intervention by the nurse.
   3. **A client with a continuous feeding tube should be in the Fowler's or high-Fowler's position to prevent aspiration pneumonia. This action requires immediate intervention by the nurse.**
   4. The UAP can place sequential compression devices on a client; therefore, this does not warrant immediate intervention.

   Content – Medical/Surgical: *Category of Health Alteration* – Gastrointestinal: *Integrated Processes* – Nursing Process: Implementation: *Client Needs* – Safe and Effective Care Environment: Management of Care: *Cognitive Level* – Synthesis

MAKING NURSING DECISIONS: Delegation means the nurse is responsible for the UAP's actions and performance. The nurse must correct the UAP's performance to ensure the client is cared for safely in the hospital or the home.

6. 1. The nurse should go through the chain of command when attempting to make a change.
   2. This may be an appropriate action at some point, but this would not be implemented until after assessing the old form and identifying areas to be changed.
   3. The nurse should be a change agent.
   4. **The staff nurse should be a part of the solution to a problem; volunteering to be on a committee of peers is the best action to effect a change.**

   Content – Medical/Surgical: *Category of Health Alteration* – Gastrointestinal: *Integrated Processes* – Nursing Process: Implementation: *Client Needs* – Safe and Effective Care Environment: Management of Care: *Cognitive Level* – Knowledge

MAKING NURSING DECISIONS: There will be management questions on the NCLEX-RN®. Concepts of Management is included under the category Safe and Effective Environment and subcategory Management of Care. This is a knowledge-based question.

7. 1. Because this procedure is performed in the radiology department and is testing the gastrointestinal system, the cardiac catheter lab does not need to be informed of the procedure.
   2. **The client must be NPO for 8 to 10 hours before the procedure. Therefore, the dietary department should be notified to hold the meal trays.**
   3. The procedure is performed using barium or Gastrografin, neither of which contains any nuclear material. The nuclear medicine department does not need to be informed of the procedure.
   4. The procedure does not involve the clinical laboratory; therefore, this department does not need to be notified.

   Content – Medical/Surgical: *Category of Health Alteration* – Gastrointestinal: *Integrated Processes* – Nursing Process: Implementation: *Client Needs* – Safe and Effective Care Environment: Management of Care: *Cognitive Level* – Application

MAKING NURSING DECISIONS: The test taker must be knowledgeable of the role of all members of the multidisciplinary healthcare team. Referrals are included under the category Safe and Effective Care Environment and subcategory Management of Care.

8. 1. This client is unstable and should not be assigned to a new graduate nurse.
   2. **This client is being prepared for a test in the morning and is the least acute of the clients listed. The new graduate should be assigned to this client.**
   3. This client is hypokalemic secondary to diarrhea and is at risk for cardiac dysrhythmias. This client should be assigned to a more experienced nurse. Short bowel syndrome is a malabsorption disorder caused by the surgical removal of the small intestine or rarely due to the complete dysfunction of a large segment of bowel.
   4. A client returning from surgery with a sigmoid colostomy is at risk for postoperative complications and should be assigned to a more experienced nurse.

   Content – Medical/Surgical: *Category of Health Alteration* – Gastrointestinal: *Integrated Processes* – Nursing Process: Planning: *Client Needs* – Safe and Effective Care Environment: Management of Care: *Cognitive Level* – Synthesis

MAKING NURSING DECISIONS: The test taker must determine which client is the most stable, which makes this an "except" question. Three clients are either unstable or have potentially life-threatening conditions.

9. 1, 2, and 5 are correct.
   1. **The nurse should not administer any PO medications since the client is NPO.**

2. This medication is PO; therefore, this medication should not be administered until after the endoscopy.
3. This is an intravenous medication, so it can be administered even though the client is NPO.
4. This is an intravenous medication, so it can be administered even though the client is NPO.
5. **This is a PRN medication and it is PO; therefore, it should not be administered until after the procedure.**

*Content – Medical/Surgical: **Category of Health Alteration** – Gastrointestinal: **Integrated Processes** – Nursing Process: Implementation: **Client Needs** – Physiological Integrity: Pharmacological and Parenteral Therapies: **Cognitive Level** – Analysis*

MAKING NURSING DECISIONS: This is an alternate type of question included in the NCLEX-RN® blueprint. The test taker must be able to read a medication administration record (MAR), be knowledgeable of medications, and be able to make an appropriate decision as to the nurse's most appropriate intervention.

10. 1. The client with Barrett's esophagus is expected to have dysphagia (difficulty swallowing) and pyroisis (heartburn); therefore, this client would not be assessed first.
2. Proctitis is an inflammation of the anus and the lining of the rectum, affecting only the last 6 inches of the rectum. Symptoms are ineffectual straining to empty the bowels (tenesmus), diarrhea, rectal bleeding and possible discharge, involuntary spasms and cramping during bowel movements, left-sided abdominal pain, passage of mucus through the rectum, and anorectal pain. Since the signs/symptoms are expected, this client would not be assessed first.
3. Jaundice and ascites are expected in a client with liver failure; therefore, the nurse should not assess this client first.
4. **The client has a urinary output of less than 30 mL/hr; therefore, this client may be going into renal failure and should be assessed first.**

*Content – Medical/Surgical: **Category of Health Alteration** – Gastrointestinal: **Integrated Processes** – Nursing Process: Assessment: **Client Needs** – Safe and Effective Care Environment: Management of Care: **Cognitive Level** – Analysis*

MAKING NURSING DECISIONS: The test taker should ask, "Is it normal or expected for the disease process?" If it is normal or expected, then do not assess this client first. If more than one option is not expected or normal, then the test taker should ask which client is in a more

life-threatening situation, needs more assessment, or may need the nurse to notify the healthcare provider.

11. 1. Altered nutrition is a concern, but a client can live for several weeks on minimal intake.
2. Self-care deficit is a psychosocial problem; physiological problems have priority.
3. Impaired body image is a psychosocial problem; physiological problems have priority.
4. **Fluid and electrolyte imbalance can cause cardiac dysrhythmias. This is the priority problem.**

*Content – Medical/Surgical: **Category of Health Alteration** – Gastrointestinal: **Integrated Processes** – Nursing Process: Planning: **Client Needs** – Safe and Effective Care Environment: Management of Care: **Cognitive Level** – Synthesis*

MAKING NURSING DECISIONS: The NCLEX-RN® integrates the nursing process throughout the Client Needs categories and subcategories. The nursing process is a scientific, clinical reasoning approach to client care that includes assessment, analysis, planning, implementation, and evaluation. The nurse will be responsible for identifying nursing diagnoses for clients.

12. 1. This is a routine medication that has a time frame of 30 minutes before and after the scheduled time to be administered. This medication does not need to be the first medication administered.
2. Aricept can be administered within a 30-minute time frame. This medication does not need to be the first medication administered.
3. **A mucosal barrier agent must be administered before the client eats in order for the medication to coat the gastric mucosa. This medication should be administered first.**
4. Lovenox can be administered within the 30-minute time frame. This medication does not need to be the first medication administered.

*Content – Medical/Surgical: **Category of Health Alteration** – Gastrointestinal :**Integrated Processes** – Nursing Process: Implementation: **Client Needs** – Physiological Integrity: Pharmacological and Parenteral Therapies: **Cognitive Level** – Synthesis*

MAKING NURSING DECISIONS: The test taker should know medications that are priority medications, such as life-threatening medications, insulin, and mucolytics (Carafate). These medications should be administered first by the nurse.

13. 1. A client who is 6 hours postoperative abdominal surgery would be expected to have decreased bowel sounds; therefore, this client would not be assessed first.
   2. Surgery is scary, and the client who is crying and upset should be assessed, but not prior to a potentially life-threatening surgical emergency. Psychosocial problems do not take priority over physiological problems.
   3. **A hard, rigid abdomen indicates peritonitis, which is a life-threatening emergency. This client should be assessed first.**
   4. The client who is 2 days postoperative and who is complaining of and rating pain as an 8 should be assessed, but the pain is not life threatening and, therefore, does not take priority over the patient with probable peritonitis.

   Content – Medical/Surgical: ***Category of Health Alteration*** *– Gastrointestinal:* ***Integrated Processes –*** *Nursing Process: Assessment:* ***Client Needs*** *– Safe and Effective Care Environment: Management of Care:* ***Cognitive Level*** *– Analysis*

MAKING NURSING DECISIONS: When deciding which client to assess first, the nurse should determine whether the signs/symptoms the client is exhibiting are normal or expected for the client's situation. After eliminating the expected options, the test taker should determine which situation is more life threatening.

14. 1. **Because a client undergoing an elective procedure such as a gastric lap banding is usually healthy prior to the surgery, an elevated postoperative WBC count—which this client has—may indicate infection and, therefore, requires notifying the HCP.**
   2. The H&H of 12/36 is within normal limits; therefore, this laboratory result does not warrant intervention.
   3. The glucose level is elevated, but many clients who are overweight have diabetes. This client must be at least 50 pounds overweight to have gastric bypass surgery.
   4. A serum potassium level of 4.5 mEq/L is within normal limits; therefore, this does not warrant notifying the healthcare provider.

   Content – Medical/Surgical: ***Category of Health Alteration*** *– Gastrointestinal:* ***Integrated Processes –*** *Nursing Process: Assessment:* ***Client Needs*** *– Physiological Integrity: Reduction of Risk Potential:* ***Cognitive Level*** *– Analysis*

MAKING NURSING DECISIONS: The nurse must be knowledgeable of normal laboratory values. These values must be memorized and the nurse must be able to determine if a laboratory value is normal for the client's disease process or medications the client is taking, or if the healthcare provider should be notified.

15. 1. A client who is overweight and having abdominal surgery is not at a higher risk for postoperative complications than any other client.
   2. The client's high blood pressure should be monitored closely and medications administered to decrease the hypertension, but this would not cause the client to have a higher risk for postoperative complications.
   3. **The location of the incision for a cholecystectomy, the general anesthesia needed, and a heavy smoking history make this client high risk for pulmonary complications.**
   4. Use of marijuana daily does not increase the risk of pulmonary complications for a client having gastric surgery.

   Content – Medical/Surgical: ***Category of Health Alteration*** *– Gastrointestinal:* ***Integrated Processes –*** *Nursing Process: Assessment:* ***Client Needs*** *– Physiological Integrity: Reduction of Risk Potential:* ***Cognitive Level*** *– Analysis*

MAKING NURSING DECISIONS: This is an "except" question but it does not say all the options are correct "except." Only one option would cause the nurse to suspect high risk of postoperative complications. Remember: Smoking cigarettes puts clients at risk for multiple problems, so it would be a good choice.

16. Correct Answer: 3, 2, 1, 4, 5.
   3. **The nurse must first assess the drainage in the bag for color, consistency, and amount.**
   2. **After removing the bag, the nurse should assess the site to ensure circulation to the stoma. A pink, moist appearance indicates adequate circulation.**
   1. **The nurse should cleanse the area with a mild soap and water to ensure that the skin is prepared for the adhesive paste.**
   4. **The nurse should then apply adhesive paste to the clean, dry skin.**
   5. **The ostomy drainage bag is attached last.**

   Content – Medical/Surgical: ***Category of Health Alteration*** *– Gastrointestinal:* ***Integrated Processes –*** *Nursing Process: Implementation:* ***Client Needs*** *– Safe and Effective Care Environment: Management of Care:* ***Cognitive Level*** *– Analysis*

MAKING NURSING DECISIONS: This is an alternate type of question included in the NCLEX-RN® blueprint. The nurse must be able to perform skills in the correct order. Obtaining informed consent and performing an assessment should always be the first interventions.

17. 1. **The nurse must first obtain the operative permit, or determine whether it has been signed by the client, prior to implementing any other orders.**
    2. The client cannot give informed consent after receiving pain medication; therefore, administration of morphine cannot be implemented first.
    3. The operating room staff usually performs shave preps, but the nurse would not implement this prior to medicating the client.
    4. The on-call IVPB is not administered until the operating room (OR) is prepared for the client. New standards recommend that the prophylactic IVPB antibiotic be administered within 1 hour of opening the skin during a surgical procedure.

    Content – Medical/Surgical: **Category of Health Alteration** *– Gastrointestinal:* **Integrated Processes** *– Nursing Process: Implementation:* **Client Needs** *– Safe and Effective Care Environment: Management of Care:* **Cognitive Level** *– Analysis*

MAKING NURSING DECISIONS: The NCLEX-RN® blueprint includes perioperative nursing care. The nurse must be knowledgeable of preoperative and postoperative care, which is generic for all clients undergoing surgery. Obtaining informed consent is a priority intervention.

18. 1. **Evisceration is the removal of viscera (internal organs, especially those in the abdominal cavity). If the bowels protrude from the abdominal incision, the nurse must apply sterile normal saline gauze and then notify the client's surgeon.**
    2. The nurse can place an ADB pad on the normal sterile saline gauze.
    3. The nurse can assess the bowel sounds, but not prior to applying sterile normal saline gauze.
    4. The client should be placed in the supine position; the left lateral position will not affect the client's abdominal evisceration.

    Content – Medical/Surgical: **Category of Health Alteration** *– Gastrointestinal:* **Integrated Processes** *– Nursing Process: Implementation:* **Client Needs** *– Safe and Effective Care Environment: Safety and Infection Control:* **Cognitive Level** *– Analysis*

MAKING NURSING DECISIONS: The test taker should apply the nursing process in questions that ask, "Which intervention should the nurse implement first?" If the client is in distress, do not assess. The nurse should do something directly to help the client's situation.

19. 1. This client with a paralytic ileus would be expected to have absent bowel sounds; therefore, this client should not be assessed first.

2. The client who is postoperative abdominal surgery should have a soft, tender abdomen; therefore, this client should not be assessed first.
3. **Wound dehiscence is the premature "bursting" open of a wound along surgical suture, and is an emergency that would require the nurse to assess this client first.**
4. This client should be prepared for transfer to the rehabilitation unit, but not prior to assessing a client with a complication of surgery.

Content – Medical/Surgical: **Category of Health Alteration** *– Gastrointestinal:* **Integrated Processes** *– Nursing Process: Assessment:* **Client Needs** *– Physiological Integrity: Reduction of Risk Potential:* **Cognitive Level** *– Analysis*

MAKING NURSING DECISIONS: The nurse must determine which client is experiencing an unexpected or abnormal situation for the surgery or condition. All the clients should be assessed and cared for, but the nurse must determine which one should be assessed first.

20. 1. **The primary nurse's instruction to the UAP to assist the client to the bathroom is an appropriate delegation that ensures the safety of the client. It requires no action by the charge nurse.**
    2. There is no information in the stem that indicates the client needs a bedside commode; therefore, this is not an appropriate action.
    3. The UAP can assist a client who is stable to ambulate; therefore, this is not inappropriate delegation.
    4. An adverse occurrence report is completed whenever potential or actual harm has come to the client. Ambulating the client with assistance is not harmful.

    Content – Medical/Surgical: **Category of Health Alteration** *– Gastrointestinal:* **Integrated Processes** *– Nursing Process: Implementation:* **Client Needs** *– Physiological Integrity: Basic Care and Comfort:* **Cognitive Level** *– Application*

MAKING NURSING DECISIONS: The nurse must ensure the UAP can perform any delegated nursing tasks. It is the nurse's responsibility to evaluate the task, and demonstrate and/or teach the UAP how to perform the task.

21. 1. The ABGs reflect metabolic alkalosis, which is expected in a client who has excessive vomiting; therefore, this client would not be assessed first.
    2. **Pain is priority because the nurse must determine if this is expected postoperative pain or a complication of the surgery. This client should be assessed first.**

3. Dark green bile should be draining from the client's nasogastric tube; therefore, this client should not be assessed first.
4. The client who is complaining of being constipated would not be priority over a client with surgical pain.

Content – Medical/Surgical: *Category of Health Alteration* – Gastrointestinal: *Integrated Processes* – Nursing Process: Assessment: *Client Needs* – Safe and Effective Care Environment: Management of Care: *Cognitive Level* – Analysis

MAKING NURSING DECISIONS: When deciding which client to assess first, the nurse should determine whether the signs/symptoms the client is exhibiting are normal or expected for the client situation. After eliminating the expected option, the test taker should determine which situation is more life threatening.

22. 1. **The nurse should first appraise the situation and not do anything. This is the pivotal point at which the nurse can return the anger or reappraise the situation. The most important action to take is to empathize with the UAP and to try to find out the provocation for the behavior.**
    2. The primary nurse could tell the UAP to leave the unit, but this is responding to the anger and not the reason for the anger.
    3. The comment may need to be reported to the charge nurse, but not until the primary nurse can determine what caused the comment. The UAP may be upset about something else entirely.
    4. This is not the first action when dealing with someone who is angry. This comment may cause further angry behavior by the UAP and will not diffuse the situation. The nurse is the professional person and should control the situation.

Content – Medical/Surgical: *Category of Health Alteration* – Gastrointestinal: *Integrated Processes* – Nursing Process: Implementation: *Client Needs* – Safe and Effective Care Environment: Management of Care: *Cognitive Level* – Application

MAKING NURSING DECISIONS: There will be management questions on the NCLEX-RN®. In many instances, there is no test-taking strategy for these questions. The nurse must be knowledgeable of management issues addressing how to deal with conflict and personnel issues.

23. 1. Beneficence is the ethical principle to do good actively for the client. Because the client is in the ICU, the client is critically ill and does not need any type of news that will further upset the client. This statement supports the ethical principle of beneficence.

2. The statement supports beneficence, which is to do good.
3. This statement avoids directly telling the client the other individual is dead.
4. **This statement supports the ethical principle of veracity, which is the duty to tell the truth. This statement will probably further upset the client and cause psychological distress, which may hinder the recovery period.**

Content – Medical/Surgical: *Category of Health Alteration* – Gastrointestinal: *Integrated Processes* – Nursing Process: Implementation: *Client Needs* – Psychosocial Integrity: *Cognitive Level* – Application

MAKING NURSING DECISIONS: The NCLEX-RN® blueprint includes nursing care that addresses ethical principles including autonomy, beneficence, justice, and veracity, to name a few.

24. 1. A copy of the advance directive should be placed in the client's chart, but it is not the nurse's first intervention.
    2. **The nurse should first inform the HCP so the order can be written in the client's chart. The HCP must write the do not resuscitate (DNR) order before the client's wishes can be honored.**
    3. The person with the durable power of attorney for healthcare can make healthcare choices for the client if the client is unable to verbalize his or her wishes, but the first intervention is to have the HCP write a DNR order.
    4. The client has a right to make this request, and the chaplain does not need to talk to the client about the advance directive.

Content – Medical/Surgical: *Category of Health Alteration* – Gastrointestinal: *Integrated Processes* – Nursing Process: Implementation: *Client Needs* – Safe and Effective Care Environment: Management of Care: *Cognitive Level* – Application

MAKING NURSING DECISIONS: There will be management questions on the NCLEX-RN®. Advance Directives is included under the category Safe and Effective Environment and subcategory Management of Care.

25. 1. The client's H&H is not within normal limits, but remember: "Hemoglobin 9 think about transfusion time." This laboratory information does not warrant immediate intervention.
    2. A soft, non-tender abdomen is expected and does not warrant immediate intervention by the nurse.
    3. **The client's apical pulse (AP) is above normal and the B/P is low, which are**

signs of hypovolemic shock, which warrants immediate intervention by the nurse.

4. Coffee ground drainage indicates "old blood," which would not be unexpected in the client who has esophageal bleeding.

Content – Medical/Surgical: **Category of Health Alteration** *– Gastrointestinal:* **Integrated Processes –** *Nursing Process: Assessment:* **Client Needs** *– Physiological Integrity: Reduction of Risk Potential:* **Cognitive Level** *– Synthesis*

MAKING NURSING DECISIONS: The test taker should ask, "Is the assessment data normal for" the disease process? If it is normal for the disease process, then the nurse would not need to intervene; if it is not normal for the disease process, then this warrants intervention by the nurse.

26. 1. Getting a resident up in a wheelchair for meals is an appropriate delegation to an unlicensed assistive personnel (UAP). This task does not require nursing judgment.
2. Assessing an incontinent client's perianal area requires nursing judgment and cannot be delegated to the UAP.
3. Discussing requirements with a client for going out on a pass should be done by the nurse responsible for completing the required documentation and providing any medication that the resident should take along.
4. Explaining colostomy care is teaching, and the RN cannot ask the UAP to teach.

Content – Medical/Surgical: **Category of Health Alteration** *– Gastrointestinal:* **Integrated Processes –** *Nursing Process: Planning:* **Client Needs** *– Safe and Effective Care Environment: Management of Care:* **Cognitive Level** *– Synthesis:*

MAKING NURSING DECISIONS: The nurse cannot delegate assessment, evaluation, teaching, administering medications, or the care of an unstable client to a UAP.

27. 1. Checking the patency of a PEG feeding tube requires nursing judgment, and feeding the client through the tube is based on this judgment. The unlicensed assistive personnel (UAP) should not be asked to perform this task.
2. The nurse should assess the coccyx and the area where the DuoDERM should be placed. The UAP should not be asked to perform this task.
3. **The UAP can apply non-medicated ointment to protect the client's perineum**

when bathing and changing the client's incontinence pads. This will protect the client from skin breakdown.

4. The nurse should not delegate suctioning during feeding to a UAP. This indicates the client is unstable.

Content – Medical/Surgical: **Category of Health Alteration** *– Gastrointestinal:* **Integrated Processes –** *Nursing Process: Planning:* **Client Needs** *– Safe and Effective Care Environment: Management of Care:* **Cognitive Level** *– Synthesis*

MAKING NURSING DECISIONS: When the test taker is deciding which option is the most appropriate task to delegate/assign, the test taker should choose the task that allows each member of the staff to function within his or her full scope of practice. Do not assign a task to a staff member that requires a higher level of expertise than that staff member has; similarly, do not assign a task to a staff member that could be assigned to a staff member with a lower level of expertise.

28. 1. **The client with a gastrostomy tube cannot eat or drink oral fluids; therefore, this behavior warrants intervention by the nurse.**
2. At the long-term care center the clients are allowed to go outside and the unlicensed assistive personnel (UAP) ambulating the client with a safety belt is appropriate behavior.
3. Assisting the client with an activity is an appropriate behavior by the UAP in a long-term care center.
4. Giving a back rub to a client on bed rest is a wonderful thing for the UAP to do for the client.

Content – Medical/Surgical: **Category of Health Alteration** *– Gastrointestinal:* **Integrated Processes –** *Nursing Process: Implementation:* **Client Needs** *– Safe and Effective Care Environment: Management of Care:* **Cognitive Level** *– Synthesis*

MAKING NURSING DECISIONS: The nurse must ensure the UAP can perform any delegated nursing tasks. It is the nurse's responsibility to evaluate the task and demonstrate and/or teach the UAP how to perform the task. It is also the nurse's responsibility to intervene if the UAP is exhibiting an unsafe behavior.

29. 1. The nurse should demonstrate the procedure on a model, but the first intervention should be to assess, to determine whether the client has any questions.
2. The nurse should provide the client with written instructions, but the first interven-

tion should be to assess, to determine whether the client has any questions.

3. **The client cannot learn if he has any questions or concerns. Therefore, the first intervention is to ask the client whether he has any questions. The nurse must allay any of the client's concerns or fears before beginning to teach the client.**

4. The nurse should show the client all the equipment, but the first intervention should be to assess, to determine whether the client has any questions.

*Content – Medical/Surgical: **Category of Health Alteration** – Gastrointestinal: **Integrated Processes** – Nursing Process: Planning: **Client Needs** – Physiological Integrity: Physiological Adaptation: **Cognitive Level** – Synthesis*

MAKING NURSING DECISIONS: The nurse should always apply the nursing process when answering a question requiring the nurse to "determine which intervention to implement first." The first part of the nursing process is to assess.

30. 1. **The nurse should first assess the client's neurological status to determine the status of the client.**

2. The nurse may need to contact the client's HCP, but the nurse should assess the client first, prior to contacting the HCP.

3. Increasing confusion is a symptom of hepatic encephalopathy and checking the client's ammonia level would be appropriate, but not prior to assessing the client.

4. The nurse should assess the client first, prior to the LPN obtaining further data.

*Content – Medical/Surgical: **Category of Health Alteration** – Gastrointestinal: **Integrated Processes** – Nursing Process: Implementation: **Client Needs** – Safe and Effective Care Environment: Management of Care: **Cognitive Level** – Analysis*

MAKING NURSING DECISIONS: Any time the nurse receives information about a client (who may be experiencing a complication) from another staff member, the nurse must assess the client. The nurse should not make decisions about the client's needs based on another staff member's information.

31. Correct Answer: 3, 1, 4, 5, 2

3. The nurse should first put on non-sterile gloves, due to body fluid contamination.

1. The nurse should remove the bag carefully and ensure no drainage in the bag gets on the client's skin.

4. The nurse should ensure the stoma site is moist and pink.

5. The area around the stoma should be cleansed with soap and water and allowed to dry thoroughly.

2. Lastly, the nurse should apply the new colostomy bag.

*Content – Medical/Surgical: **Category of Health Alteration** – Gastrointestinal: **Integrated Processes** – Nursing Process: Implementation: **Client Needs** – Physiological Integrity: Physiological Adaptation: **Cognitive Level** – Analysis*

MAKING NURSING DECISIONS: The nurse must list the interventions in order of priority. This is an alternate type of question included in the NCLEX-RN® blueprint. Remember, Standard Precautions are always a priority.

32. 1. Even though the client is not prescribed this medication by the healthcare provider, the nurse cannot delegate any type of medication administration to the unlicensed assistive personnel (UAP).

2. In some situations, the UAP may be able to perform tube feedings in the home, but the nurse should assign the least invasive procedure to the UAP.

3. In some situations, the UAP may be able to do colostomy irrigations in the home, but the nurse should assign the least invasive procedure to the UAP.

4. **The UAP can wash and dry the client's hair, as this is the least invasive task, so this would be the most appropriate task for the nurse to delegate to the UAP.**

*Content – Medical/Surgical: **Category of Health Alteration** – Gastrointestinal: **Integrated Processes** – Nursing Process: Planning: **Client Needs** – Safe and Effective Care Environment: Management of Care: **Cognitive Level** – Synthesis*

MAKING NURSING DECISIONS: The nurse cannot delegate assessment, teaching, evaluation, medications, or an unstable client to the UAP. The nurse should always assign the least invasive task or the task that requires the least educated employee.

33. 1. Since the UAP cannot accept gifts or money from the client, this would not warrant an intervention.

2. The UAP can bring flowers to the client. This does not violate any rules.

3. **The UAP should not take money from the client to pick up prescriptions and the UAP is not responsible for doing errands for the client. If money is missing or medications are missing, this could result in a difficult situation. The home health (HH) nurse should tell the UAP not to do this type of activity for the client.**

4. Cleaning the house is not part of the UAP's job description, but this would not warrant intervention by the HH nurse.
   *Content – Medical/Surgical: **Category of Health Alteration** – Gastrointestinal: **Integrated Processes** – Nursing Process: Implementation: **Client Needs** – Safe and Effective Environment: Management of Care: **Cognitive Level** – Application*

MAKING NURSING DECISIONS: The nurse is responsible for knowing the scope of practice for the healthcare team members who are his or her subordinates.

34. 1. The client is having signs/symptoms of diverticulitis, which can be potentially life threatening; therefore, the client should get medical assistance immediately.
    2. The client needs to be seen by a medical doctor to be prescribed antibiotics; therefore, there is no reason for an HH nurse to visit the client.
    3. **The nurse must have knowledge of disease processes. The client is verbalizing signs of acute diverticulitis, which requires the client to be NPO and prescribed antibiotics. The client needs to receive immediate medical attention.**
    4. The client is verbalizing signs/symptoms of acute diverticulitis, which requires medical attention. It does not matter what the client has had to eat.
    *Content – Medical/Surgical: **Category of Health Alteration** – Gastrointestinal: **Integrated Processes** – Nursing Process: Implementation: **Client Needs** – Safe and Effective Care Environment: Management of Care: **Cognitive Level** – Analysis*

MAKING NURSING DECISIONS: The nurse must be knowledgeable in expected medical treatments for the client. This is a knowledge-based question.

35. 1. **According to the NCLEX-RN® test blueprint under management of care, the nurse should be knowledgeable of referrals. The wound care nurse is trained to care for clients with colostomy and is knowledgeable in treating complications.**
    2. The most appropriate intervention is to refer the client to a member of the multidisciplinary team who has expertise in the area in which the client is having the problem. In this case, the wound care nurse has the expertise to care for the stoma site.
    3. After 2 weeks, the nurse should obtain further assistance in treating the stoma site.
    4. Karaya paste will not be effective in treating the excoriated area; therefore, this is not an appropriate intervention.

*Content – Medical/Surgical: **Category of Health Alteration** – Gastrointestinal: **Integrated Processes** – Nursing Process: Implementation: **Client Needs** – Safe and Effective Care Environment: Management of Care: **Cognitive Level** – Analysis*

MAKING NURSING DECISIONS: The test taker must be knowledgeable of the role of all members of the multidisciplinary healthcare team as well as HIPAA rules and regulations. These will be tested on the NCLEX-RN® exam.

36. 1. Denial is the first stage of grief. Anger is the second stage of grief: "Why me? It's not fair!" The individual recognizes that denial cannot continue. Because of anger, the person is very difficult to care for due to misplaced feelings of rage and envy.
    2. **Bargaining: "I'll do anything for a few more years." The third stage involves the hope that the individual can somehow postpone or delay death. The client's comments indicate bargaining.**
    3. Depression: "I am so sad, why bother with anything?" During the fourth stage, the dying person begins to understand the certainty of death. Because of this, the individual may become silent, refuse visitors, and spend much of the time crying and grieving.
    4. Acceptance: "It's going to be okay." In this last stage, the individual begins to come to terms with her/his mortality or the mortality of a loved one.
    *Content – Medical/Surgical: **Category of Health Alteration** – Gastrointestinal: **Integrated Processes** – Nursing Process: Evaluation: **Client Needs** – Psychosocial Integrity: **Cognitive Level** – Analysis*

MAKING NURSING DECISIONS: The nurse caring for clients who are dying needs to know the stages of death. Each stage of death requires the nurse to address the psychosocial needs of the client in a different way.

37. 1, 3, and 4 are correct.
    1. **This is a goal for EOL care.**
    2. This will need to be done during the client's dying process, but it is not a goal for EOL care.
    3. **This is a goal for EOL care.**
    4. **This is a goal for EOL care.**
    5. Addressing the financial cost of the dying process is not a goal for EOL care.
    *Content – Medical/Surgical: **Category of Health Alteration** – Gastrointestinal: **Integrated Processes** – Nursing Process: Planning: **Client Needs** – Psychosocial Integrity: **Cognitive Level** – Synthesis*

MAKING NURSING DECISIONS: The nurse must know the role of the other areas of nursing so that the nurse can refer the client and family to the appropriate resource.

38. 1. **Mexican American families are close-knit communities and often prefer to care for their own family members; therefore, they would not seek hospice or palliative care. The nurse should attempt to help the client understand the philosophy, the benefits, and the help hospice can give the client and family.**
    2. The nurse should attempt to help the client and family understand hospice so the client can make an informed decision.
    3. The healthcare provider does not need to be contacted to reaffirm the client is dying.
    4. The nurse should first talk to the client and then to the family.

    Content – Medical/Surgical: **Category of Health Alteration** *– Gastrointestinal:* **Integrated Processes** *– Nursing Process: Planning:* **Client Needs** *– Psychosocial Integrity:* **Cognitive Level** *– Synthesis*

MAKING NURSING DECISIONS: The client has a right to refuse any healthcare, but the nurse first must ensure the client fully understands the focus of the care, especially with cultural differences. When the client fully understands and then refuses the care, the nurse must respect the client's rights. The NCLEX-RN® blueprint includes nursing care addressing cultural diversity.

39. 1. "Advance directive" is a general term used to describe documents that give instructions about future medical care and treatments and who should make them in the event the client is unable to communicate.
    2. A directive to physicians is a written document specifying the client's wish to be allowed to die without heroic or extraordinary measures.
    3. "Living will" is a lay term used frequently to describe any number of documents giving instructions about future medical care and treatments.
    4. **The nurse is specifically describing the term "durable power of attorney for healthcare." It is a document included in an advance directive.**

    Content – Medical/Surgical: **Category of Health Alteration** *– Gastrointestinal:* **Integrated Processes** *– Nursing Process: Planning:* **Client Needs** *– Physiological Integrity: Physiological Adaptation:* **Cognitive Level** *– Knowledge*

MAKING NURSING DECISIONS: The nurse must be aware of documents clients use when addressing end-of-life issues. This is a knowledge-based question, but nurses must be able to ensure the client's last requests are honored.

40. 1. Bereavement counseling is for the survivors, not the client.
    2. **This is the definition of bereavement counseling.**
    3. Bereavement counseling is for the survivors, not the client.
    4. Bereavement counseling may include group counseling, but it could also be individual counseling. This is not the nurse's best response.

    Content – Medical/Surgical: **Category of Health Alteration** *– Gastrointestinal:* **Integrated Processes** *– Nursing Process: Implementation:* **Client Needs** *– Psychosocial Integrity:* **Cognitive Level** *– Application*

MAKING NURSING DECISIONS: The nurse must be able to explain the support provided by hospice. Losing a loved one is a huge loss to most people, and the nurse's responsibility is to help the survivors work through the stages of grief.

41. 1. Many nurses follow this practice, but no research has been completed to support this practice.
    2. This is part of the Joint Commission's Patient Safety Goals, not evidence-based practice.
    3. **Evidence-based practice is the conscientious use of current best evidence in making decisions about nursing care. Using the "evidence," or research, to teach a client is evidence-based practice.**
    4. Reading the journal is a step in EBP, but EBP requires using the information in practice.

    Content – Medical/Surgical: **Category of Health Alteration** *– Gastrointestinal:* **Integrated Processes** *– Nursing Process: Diagnosis:* **Client Needs** *– Safe and Effective Care Environment: Safety and Infection Control:* **Cognitive Level** *– Analysis*

MAKING NURSING DECISIONS: The NCLEX-RN® blueprint includes nursing care based on evidence-based practice. The nurse must be knowledgeable of nursing research.

42. 1. The charge nurse should stop the nurse from recapping the needle, but not in front of the client.
    2. **The charge nurse should not reprimand the nurse in front of the client or client's family. The charge nurse should ask the nurse to step into the hall, where the client cannot hear.**
    3. Reprimanding the nurse is not the first action.
    4. Notifying the house supervisor is not the first action.

    Content – Medical/Surgical; **Category of Health Alteration** *– Gastrointestinal:* **Integrated Processes** *– Nursing Process: Implementation:* **Client Needs** *– Safe*

and Effective Care Environment: Management of Care:
***Cognitive Level** – Analysis*

MAKING NURSING DECISIONS: In any business, including a healthcare facility, correcting a fellow staff member's behavior should not occur in front of a customer or, in this instance, the client.

43. 1. The chief nursing officer should be informed, but this is not the first action.
    2. **The first action for the administrative supervisor is to make sure the clients receive care. The supervisor cannot allow the on-duty staff to leave until replacement staff members have been arranged.**
    3. The supervisor should call any staff that can get to the hospital in an attempt to staff the hospital, but this is not the first action to implement.
    4. An emergency disaster protocol may be implemented, but the first intervention is to ensure the clients have a nurse on duty.

    *Content – Medical/Surgical: **Category of Health Alteration** – Gastrointestinal: **Integrated Processes** – Nursing Process: Implementation: **Client Needs** – Safe and Effective Care Environment: Management of Care: **Cognitive Level** – Application*

MAKING NURSING DECISIONS: The nurse must be knowledgeable of emergency preparedness. Employees receive this information in employee orientation and are responsible for implementing procedures correctly. The NCSBN NCLEX-RN® blueprint includes questions on safe and effective care environment.

44. 1. The nurse cannot delegate any task requiring nursing judgment. Taking a client's history requires knowing which questions need to be asked to assess the client's problems.
    2. Documenting the client's complaints is a nursing responsibility that the nurse must perform. It cannot be delegated to unlicensed assistive personnel (UAP).
    3. **The UAP can obtain the client's height and weight. This is the task the nurse should delegate.**
    4. The client's follow-up care may require teaching, judgment, or further assessment; therefore, the nurse should not delegate this action to a UAP. When delegating to a UAP, the nurse must provide clear, concise, and specific instructions. The nurse cannot delegate teaching.

    *Content – Medical/Surgical: **Category of Health Alteration** – Gastrointestinal: **Integrated Processes** – Nursing Process: Planning: **Client Needs** – Safe and Effective Care Environment, Management of Care: **Cognitive Level** – Synthesis*

MAKING NURSING DECISIONS: An RN cannot delegate assessment, teaching, evaluation, medications, or an unstable client to a UAP. Tasks that cannot be delegated are nursing interventions requiring nursing judgment.

45. 1. **The actions of the colleague indicate possible drug or alcohol impairment. The staff nurse is not in a position of authority to require the potentially impaired nurse to submit to a drug test. The administrative supervisor should assess the situation and initiate the appropriate follow-up. The nurse must make sure an impaired nurse is not allowed to care for clients.**
    2. The nurse is not a counselor, and a staff nurse should not attempt to confront an impaired colleague.
    3. The administrative supervisor and the charge nurse are the only staff members who have the authority to send a nurse home.
    4. The nurse should not attempt to determine the cause of the behavior. This is outside the nurse's authority.

    *Content – Medical/Surgical: **Category of Health Alteration** – Gastrointestinal: **Integrated Processes** – Nursing Process: Implementation: **Client Needs** – Safe and Effective Care Environment: Management of Care: **Cognitive Level** – Application*

MAKING NURSING DECISIONS: There will be management questions on the NCLEX-RN®. Concepts of Management is included under the category Safe and Effective Environment and subcategory Management of Care.

46. 1. Regurgitation (effortless return of food or gastric contents from the stomach into esophagus or mouth) is a common manifestation of GERD; therefore, this client would not be assigned to the most experienced nurse.
    2. Barrett's esophagitis is a complication of GERD; new graduates can prepare a client for a diagnostic procedure.
    3. **This client is exhibiting symptoms of asthma, a complication of GERD; therefore, the client should be assigned to the most experienced nurse.**
    4. Pain is expected with a surgical procedure and a less experienced nurse could administer pain medication.

    *Content – Medical/Surgical: **Category of Health Alteration** – Gastrointestinal: **Integrated Processes** – Nursing Process: Planning: **Client Needs** – Safe and Effective Care Environment: Management of Care: **Cognitive Level** – Synthesis*

MAKING NURSING DECISIONS: The test taker must determine which client is the most unstable and would require the most experienced

nurse, thus making this an "except" type of question. Three clients are either stable or have non–life-threatening conditions.

47. 1. The nurse should notify the HCP, but it is not the first intervention.
  2. The nurse should assess the client for leg cramps, indicating hypokalemia, but the nurse should first ensure the client's cardiac status is stable.
  3. **The client is at high risk for cardiac dysrhythmias, due to hypokalemia. The nurse should first assess the cardiac status, then implement other interventions. Remember Maslow's Hierarchy of Needs.**
  4. The client will need IV potassium, but this requires an HCP order; therefore, this intervention is not implanted first.
  Content – *Medical/Surgical:* **Category of Health Alteration** – *Gastrointestinal:* **Integrated Processes** – *Nursing Process: Implementation:* **Client Needs** – *Physiological Integrity: Reduction of Risk Potential:* **Cognitive Level** – *Analysis*

MAKING NURSING DECISIONS: Before selecting "notify the HCP" as the correct answer, the test taker must examine the other three options. If information in any of the other options contains data that will relieve the client's distress, prevent a life-threatening situation, or provide information the HCP will need to make an informed decision, then the test taker should eliminate the "notify the HCP" option.

48. 1. The charge nurse should discuss the client's anger with the client immediately because the client is preparing to leave the hospital. The charge nurse can talk with the primary nurse after talking with the client.
  2. **This is the first action for the charge nurse. The client is preparing to leave, and a delay in going to the client's room could result in the client leaving before the situation can be resolved.**
  3. The HCP should be notified, but the charge nurse should assess the situation first.
  4. The client will be asked to sign the against medical advice form if he insists on leaving, but the charge nurse should attempt to resolve the situation successfully first.
  Content – *Medical/Surgical:* **Category of Health Alteration** – *Gastrointestinal:* **Integrated Processes** – *Nursing Process: Implementation:* **Client Needs** – *Safe and Effective Care Environment: Safety and Infection Control:* **Cognitive Level** – *Analysis*

MAKING NURSING DECISIONS: The nurse should always apply the nursing process when answering a question requiring the nurse to "determine

which intervention to implement first." The first part of the nursing process is to assess.

49. 1. Planning the care of the client cannot be delegated to an unlicensed assistive personnel (UAP), and the client, not the parents, should set the goals.
  2. The UAP should stay with the client for an hour after a meal. Leaving the client after 20 minutes would allow the client time to induce vomiting.
  3. This requires the nurse to utilize therapeutic conversation and nursing judgment. The nurse cannot delegate this intervention to a UAP.
  4. **The UAP can document the amount of food consumed on a calorie-count form for the dietician to evaluate.**
  Content – *Medical/Surgical:* **Category of Health Alteration** – *Gastrointestinal:* **Integrated Processes** – *Nursing Process: Planning:* **Client Needs** – *Safe and Effective Care Environment: Management of Care:* **Cognitive Level** – *Synthesis*

MAKING NURSING DECISIONS: An RN cannot delegate assessment, teaching, evaluation, medications, or an unstable client to a UAP. Tasks that cannot be delegated are nursing interventions requiring nursing judgment.

50. 1. **This is an assessment question and should be asked to determine what the client has attempted has been unsuccessful.**
  2. The amount of weight loss desired is not as important as assessment of previous unsuccessful strategies.
  3. This is a therapeutic statement, but the nurse should assess the client.
  4. This statement is not helpful, and the nurse working in a bariatric clinic should know that there are many options for weight loss, including surgery.
  Content – *Medical/Surgical:* **Category of Health Alteration** – *Gastrointestinal:* **Integrated Processes** – *Nursing Process: Assessment:* **Client Needs** – *Health Promotion and Maintenance:* **Cognitive Level** – *Analysis*

MAKING NURSING DECISIONS: Assessment is the first step of the nursing process, and the test taker should use the nursing process or some other systematic process to assist in determining priorities.

51. 1. **During a laparoscopic cholecystectomy, carbon dioxide is instilled into the client's abdomen. Postoperatively, the gas migrates to the shoulder by gravity and causes shoulder pain.**
  2. This is not an emergency situation, and the nurse should explain this to the client.
  3. The nurse should not tell the client to increase the pain medication. This is prescribing.

4. These pains are "gas" pains, but they are not intestinal gas pains that can be relieved by ambulation.

*Content – Medical/Surgical: **Category of Health Alteration** – Gastrointestinal: **Integrated Processes** – Nursing Process: Implementation: **Client Needs** – Physiological Integrity: Physiological Adaptation: **Cognitive Level** – Analysis*

MAKING NURSING DECISIONS: The nurse must be knowledgeable of expected medical treatment for the client. This is a knowledge-based question.

52. 1. The medication is ordered every 4 hours and it has been less than 4 hours since the last medication was administered. The nurse cannot administer the PRN medication.
    2. Lomotil is for diarrhea and the client has a soft, brown, formed stool; therefore, the nurse would not administer this medication.
    3. **The nurse should call the healthcare provider to discuss the situation. The client is nauseated and needs something, but there is nothing ordered.**
    4. The nurse should not tell the client there is nothing that can be done. The nurse needs to call the healthcare provider.

*Content – Medical/Surgical: **Category of Health Alteration** – Gastrointestinal: **Integrated Processes** – Nursing Process: Implementation: **Client Needs** – Safe and Effective Care Environment: Management of Care: **Cognitive Level** – Application*

MAKING NURSING DECISIONS: Before selecting "notify the HCP" as the correct answer, the test taker must examine the other three options. If information in any of the other options contains data that will relieve the client's distress, prevent a life-threatening situation, or provide information the HCP will need to make an informed decision, then the test taker should eliminate the "notify the HCP" option.

53. 1, 3, and 4 are correct.
    1. **The HCP must order the insertion of a Sengstaken-Blakemore tube, so this is a collaborative nursing intervention.**
    2. Assessing the client's vital signs does not require an HCP's order, so this is an independent nursing intervention, not a collaborative intervention.
    3. **This is a collaborative intervention that the nurse should implement. It requires an order from the HCP.**
    4. **Obtaining laboratory data requires an HCP's order, so this is a collaborative intervention.**
    5. Monitoring the client's intake and output does not require an HCP's order, so this is

an independent nursing intervention not a collaborative intervention.

*Content – Medical/Surgical: **Category of Health Alteration** – Gastrointestinal: **Integrated Processes** – Nursing Process: Implementation: **Client Needs** – Safe and Effective Care Environment: Management of Care: **Cognitive Level** – Application*

MAKING NURSING DECISIONS: This is an alternate type of question included in the NCLEX-RN®. The nurse must be able to select all the options that answer the question correctly. There are no partially correct answers.

54. 1. Hypoactive bowel sounds are not normal, but it would not warrant immediate intervention. As long as the bowels are moving, it is not an emergency.
    2. The client should have 30 mL of urine output an hour; therefore, this information is normal and does not warrant immediate intervention.
    3. These vital signs are normal; therefore, they do not warrant immediate intervention.
    4. **Coffee ground emesis indicates bleeding and old blood, and warrants intervention by the nurse. Further assessment is needed to determine if the client is hypovolemic and the HCP should be notified.**

*Content – Medical/Surgical: **Category of Health Alteration** – Gastrointestinal: **Integrated Processes** – Nursing Process: Assessment: **Client Needs** – Safe and Effective Care Environment: Management of Care: **Cognitive Level** – Synthesis*

MAKING NURSING DECISIONS: The test taker should ask, "Is the assessment data normal for" the disease process? If it is normal for the disease process, then the nurse would not need to intervene; if it is not normal for the disease process, then this warrants intervention by the nurse.

55. 1. **The nurse should first determine if the client is hypovolemic prior to taking any other action. This will determine the nurse's next action.**
    2. The nurse should auscultate the client's bowel sounds to determine if they are present, but not prior to taking the client's pulse and blood pressure.
    3. The nurse should assess the situation before notifying the HCP.
    4. The nurse may need to reinforce the dressing if the dressing becomes too saturated, but this would occur only after a thorough assessment is completed.

*Content – Medical/Surgical: **Category of Health Alteration** – Gastrointestinal: **Integrated***

Processes – *Nursing Process: Implementation:* **Client Needs** – *Physiological Integrity: Reduction of Risk Potential:* **Cognitive Level** – *Synthesis*

MAKING NURSING DECISIONS: Before selecting "notify the HCP" as the correct answer, the test taker must examine the other three options. If information in any of the other options contains data that will relieve the client's distress, prevent a life-threatening situation, or provide information the HCP will need to make an informed decision, then the test taker should eliminate the "notify the HCP" option.

56. **106 gtts per minute.** The nurse must divide the total amount to be infused by 24 hours to determine the IV rate. 2,550 mL divided by 24 = 106.25

    Content – *Medical/Surgical:* **Category of Health Alteration** – *Gastrointestinal:* **Integrated Processes** – *Nursing Process: Implementation:* **Client Needs** – *Physiological Integrity: Pharmacological and Parenteral Therapies:* **Cognitive Level** – *Application*

MAKING NURSING DECISIONS: The NCLEX-RN® blueprint includes dosage calculations under Pharmacological and Parenteral Therapies. This category is included under Physiological Integrity, which promotes physical health and wellness by providing care and comfort, reducing client risk potential, and managing health alterations.

57. 1. The nurse must check the medication administration record (MAR) to determine the last time the client received any pain medication, but not prior to assessing the client first. Remember: Assessment is the first step of the nursing process.
    2. The nurse must assess the client's pain, not the unlicensed assistive personnel (UAP). The nurse cannot delegate assessment.
    3. **The first part of the nursing process is assessment. The nurse must first assess the client's pain to determine if the pain indicates a complication requiring medical intervention, or if this is routine postoperative pain, which is expected.**
    4. The nurse should not delegate the obtaining of vital signs to a client who may be unstable. The nurse must assess the client.

    Content – *Medical/Surgical:* **Category of Health Alteration** – *Gastrointestinal:* **Integrated Processes** – *Nursing Process: Assessment:* **Client Needs** – *Safe and Effective Care Environment: Management of Care:* **Cognitive Level** – *Analysis*

MAKING NURSING DECISIONS: Any time the nurse receives information about a client (who may be experiencing a complication) from another staff member, the nurse must assess the client. The nurse should not make decisions about the client's needs based on another staff member's information.

58. 1. The client should stay on his or her right side for at least 2 hours post-procedure, so giving the client a urinal to void is an appropriate action and does not warrant intervention.
    2. The client is not NPO after the procedure, so giving the client water is an appropriate action and does not warrant intervention.
    3. **Direct pressure is applied to the site and then the client is placed on the right side to maintain site pressure for at least 2 hours. Turning the client to the left side warrants intervention by the nurse so the client will not hemorrhage.**
    4. The unlicensed assistive personnel (UAP) can take the vital signs for the client who is stable; therefore, this action would not warrant intervention.

    Content – *Medical/Surgical:* **Category of Health Alteration** – *Gastrointestinal:* **Integrated Processes** – *Nursing Process: Evaluation:* **Client Needs** – *Safe and Effective Care Environment: Management of Care:* **Cognitive Level** – *Analysis*

MAKING NURSING DECISIONS: Delegation means the nurse is responsible for the UAP's actions and performance. The nurse must correct the UAP's performance to ensure the client is cared for safely in the hospital or the home.

59. 1. Hot water increases pruritus, and soap will cause dry skin, which increases pruritus; therefore, the nurse should discuss this with the UAP.
    2. This will help prevent dry skin, which will help decrease pruritus, but this is not the client's first intervention. The nurse should first directly protect the client's skin.
    3. **Mittens will help prevent the client from scratching the skin and causing skin breakdown, which is priority for the client with liver failure. The client has decreased Vitamin K, which will lead to bleeding. The client is also immunosuppressed, which will lead to infection.**
    4. Benadryl will help decrease the pruritis, but it will take at least 30 minutes to work. Protecting the client's skin integrity is priority.

    Content – *Medical/Surgical:* **Category of Health Alteration** – *Gastrointestinal:* **Integrated Processes** – *Nursing Process: Implementation:* **Client Needs** – *Physiological Integrity: Basic Care and Comfort:* **Cognitive Level** – *Analysis*

MAKING NURSING DECISIONS: The nurse should remember: If a client is in distress, and the nurse can do something to relieve the distress, that should be done first, before assessment. The test taker should select an option that directly helps the client's condition.

60. 1. This is "passing the buck," and this is not the best option to select. The nurse should answer the client's question.
    2. **Milk thistle has an active ingredient, silymarin, which has been used to treat liver disease for more than 2,000 years. It is a powerful oxidant and promotes liver cell growth. This response gives the client factual information.**
    3. The nurse should not discourage complementary therapies.
    4. This is a judgmental statement and the nurse should encourage the client to ask questions.
    Content – Medical/Surgical: **Category of Health Alteration** *– Complementary Alternative Medicine:* **Integrated Processes** *– Nursing Process: Implementation:* **Client Needs** *– Physiological Integrity: Pharmacological and Parenteral Therapies:* **Cognitive Level** *– Application*

MAKING NURSING DECISIONS: The nurse must be knowledgeable of complementary alternative medicine, which includes herbs used to treat medical conditions.

61. 1. The laboratory technician draws serum blood studies, not the unlicensed assistive personnel (UAP).
    2. The nurse should not request the UAP remove the N/G tube. This is an invasive tube and judgment is required to remove it.
    3. **The UAP can empty feces from a colostomy bag; this is not changing the colostomy bag, just emptying the feces.**
    4. The UAP cannot transcribe HCP orders. The UAP assists the nurse with direct client care.
    Content – Medical/Surgical: **Category of Health Alteration** *– Gastrointestinal:* **Integrated Processes** *– Nursing Process: Planning:* **Client Needs** *– Safe and Effective Care Environment: Management of Care:* **Cognitive Level** *– Synthesis*

MAKING NURSING DECISIONS: An RN cannot delegate assessment, teaching, evaluation, medications, or an unstable client to a UAP. Tasks that cannot be delegated are nursing interventions requiring nursing judgment. The test taker must be knowledgeable of the role of all members of the multidisciplinary healthcare team.

62. 1. **The normal serum sodium level is 135–145 mEq/L; this sodium level is elevated, indicating the client is dehydrated, which warrants intervention by the nurse.**

2. These are normal arterial blood gas results; therefore, the nurse would not need to intervene.
3. The normal serum potassium level is 3.5–5.5 mEq/L; therefore, this laboratory information does not warrant intervention by the nurse.
4. A stool specimen showing fecal leukocytes would support the diagnosis of gastroenteritis and not warrant immediate intervention by the nurse.
Content – Medical/Surgical: **Category of Health Alteration** *– Gastrointestinal:* **Integrated Processes – Nursing Process: Assessment:* **Client Needs** *– Physiological Integrity: Reduction of Risk Potential:* **Cognitive Level** *– Analysis*

MAKING NURSING DECISIONS: The nurse must be knowledgeable of normal laboratory values. These values must be memorized and the nurse must be able to determine if a laboratory value is normal for the client's disease process or medications the client is taking.

63. 1. **Fluid and electrolyte imbalance is priority because of the potential for metabolic acidosis and hypokalemia, which are both life threatening, especially in the elderly.**
    2. The client will have diarrhea, but it is not priority over fluid and electrolyte imbalance.
    3. The client will probably be NPO and will not want to eat, but this diagnosis is not priority over fluid and electrolyte imbalance.
    4. The client's oral mucous membranes may be dry due to vomiting and diarrhea, but it is not priority over fluid and electrolyte imbalance.
    Content – Medical/Surgical: **Category of Health Alteration** *– Gastrointestinal:* **Integrated Processes – Nursing Process: Planning:* **Client Needs** *– Safe and Effective Care Environment: Management of Care:* **Cognitive Level** *– Synthesis*

MAKING NURSING DECISIONS: The NCLEX-RN® integrates the nursing process throughout the Client Needs categories and subcategories. The nursing process is a scientific, clinical reasoning approach to client care that includes assessment, analysis, planning, implementation, and evaluation. The nurse will be responsible for identifying nursing diagnosis for clients.

64. 1. **Pain should be assessed, even if it is expected for the client's diagnosis, if the other clients are stable.**
    2. The nurse needs to talk to this client, but should assess the client with pain first.
    3. The client with IBD who is receiving total parental nutrition is stable and would not be assessed first.

4. The client with hepatitis B would be expected to be jaundiced and anorexic, so this client would not be assessed first.
Content – Medical/Surgical: **Category of Health Alteration** *– Gastrointestinal:* **Integrated Processes** *– Nursing Process: Assessment:* **Client Needs** *– Safe and Effective Care Environment: Management of Care:* **Cognitive Level** *– Analysis*

MAKING NURSING DECISIONS: The test taker should use some tool as a reference to guide in the decision-making process. In this situation, Maslow's Hierarchy of Needs should be applied. Physiological needs have priority over psychosocial ones.

65. 1. The nurse should assess the client for hypovolemia, but the first intervention is to assess the client's surgical wound to determine if wound dehiscence has occurred.
2. The nurse should determine the client's pain, but not prior to determining the cause of the pain.
3. **Assessing the surgical incision is the first intervention because this may indicate the client has wound dehiscence.**
4. The nurse should not administer pain medication without assessing for potential complications first.
Content – Medical/Surgical: **Category of Health Alteration** *– Gastrointestinal:* **Integrated Processes** *– Nursing Process: Assessment:* **Client Needs** *– Physiological Integrity: Reduction of Risk Potential:* **Cognitive Level** *– Analysis*

MAKING NURSING DECISIONS: Assessment is the first step of the nursing process, and the test taker should use the nursing process or some other systematic process to assist in determining priorities.

66. 1. The hemovac should be depressed, which indicates suction is being applied. The hemovac needs to be emptied and suction reapplied, which indicates the hemovac is not functioning appropriately.
2. The tube should be pinned to the dressing to prevent the client drain from accidentally being pulled out of the insertion site, but this does not indicate the hemovac is functioning appropriately.
3. The insertion site should be pink and without any signs of infection, which include drainage, warmth, and redness, but it does not indicate the hemovac is functioning appropriately.
4. **The hemovac should be sunken in or depressed, indicating that suction is being applied, which indicates the hemovac is functioning appropriately.**

Content – Medical/Surgical: **Category of Health Alteration** *– Gastrointestinal:* **Integrated Processes** *– Nursing Process: Assessment:* **Client Needs** *– Physiological Integrity: Reduction of Risk Potential:* **Cognitive Level** *– Analysis*

MAKING NURSING DECISIONS: The NCLEX-RN® includes Safe Use of Equipment as a subcategory under Safety and Infection Control, which addresses content on protecting clients, family/significant others, and healthcare personnel from health and environmental hazards.

67. 1. The client should urinate 30 mL/hour, so 160 mL in 4 hours is appropriate and the nurse should not assess this client first.
2. **This client was just transferred from the Post Anesthesia Care Unit (PACU); therefore, the nurse should assess this client first to perform a baseline assessment and ensure the client is stable.**
3. Flatulence, "gas," indicates the bowels are working, which is normal for a client with abdominal surgery, so this client should not be seen first.
4. The client being discharged would be stable and not a priority for the nurse.
Content – Medical/Surgical: **Category of Health Alteration** *– Gastrointestinal:* **Integrated Processes** *– Nursing Process: Assessment:* **Client Needs** *– Safe and Effective Care Environment: Management of Care:* **Cognitive Level** *– Analysis*

MAKING NURSING DECISIONS: The test taker must determine which sign/symptom is expected for the surgical procedure. Clients being transferred from more intensive nursing area to less intensive areas should be assessed upon arrival to the unit.

68. 1. **The client that is morbidly obese will have a large abdomen that prevents the lungs from expanding, and predisposes the client to respiratory complications. Having the client use an incentive spirometer will help prevent respiratory complications.**
2. The client may be weighed daily, but this is not priority over respiratory complications.
3. Preventing deep vein thrombosis is an important intervention, but oxygenation is priority.
4. The nurse should get the client out of the bed as soon as possible to help prevent deep vein thrombosis, but not priority over oxygenation.
Content – Medical/Surgical: **Category of Health Alteration** *– Gastrointestinal:* **Integrated Processes** *– Nursing Process: Implementation:* **Client Needs** *– Safe and Effective Care Environment: Management of Care:* **Cognitive Level** *– Synthesis*

MAKING NURSING DECISIONS: The test taker should use some tool as a reference to guide in the decision-making process. In this situation, Maslow's Hierarchy of Needs should be applied. Oxygenation is priority.

69. 1. The client with ulcerative colitis can have 10 to 12 loose stools a day; therefore, this client should not be seen first.
    2. This client should be assessed, but not priority over a client with a physiological problem.
    3. **This client has signs of dehydration, which is not expected when a client is vomiting. The client should remain hydrated even when the client is vomiting.**
    4. This is not normal, but it is expected for a client with hemorrhoids.
    *Content – Medical/Surgical: **Category of Health Alteration** – Gastrointestinal: **Integrated Processes** – Nursing Process: Assessment: **Client Needs** – Physiological Integrity: Reduction of Risk Potential: **Cognitive Level** – Analysis*

MAKING NURSING DECISIONS: The test taker must determine which sign/symptom is not

expected for the disease process. If the sign/symptom is not expected, then the nurse should assess that client first. This type of question is determining if the nurse is knowledgeable of signs/symptoms of a variety of disease processes.

70. 1. Total parenteral nutrition is an intravenous medication; the nurse cannot delegate medication administration to the UAP.
    2. The nurse cannot delegate medication administration to the UAP.
    3. **The LPN can administer medications to a client.**
    4. The RN cannot assign assessment to the LPN.
    *Content – Medical/Surgical: **Category of Health Alteration** – Gastrointestinal: **Integrated Processes** – Nursing Process: Planning: **Client Needs** – Safe and Effective Care Environment: Management of Care: **Cognitive Level** – Synthesis*

MAKING NURSING DECISIONS: The nurse cannot assign assessment, teaching, evaluation, or an unstable client to an LPN. The nurse cannot delegate assessment, teaching, evaluation, medications, or an unstable client to the UAP.

CLINICAL SCENARIO ANSWERS AND RATIONALES

The correct answer number and rationale for why it is the correct answer are given in **boldface type.** Rationales for why the other possible answer options are incorrect also are given, but they are not in boldface type.

1. 1. **Pyrosis is heartburn and is expected in a client diagnosed with GERD. The new graduate can care for this client and administer an antacid.**
   2. An endoscopy is a diagnostic test and the client should have bowel sounds; therefore, if the client has no bowel sounds, then this is an unexpected complication and requires a more experienced nurse.
   3. This client is exhibiting symptoms of asthma, a complication of GERD; therefore, the client should be assigned to the more experienced nurse.
   4. An open cholecysectomy incision is just below the diaphragm and the client is at great risk to develop pneumonia, because of the pain and refusal to deep breathe. This client should have a more experienced nurse to ensure the client takes deep breaths.

2. 1. The HCP would not need to be notified since the potassium level is within the normal limits of 3.5–5.5 mEq/L.
   2. **The client's potassium level is within normal limits, so the nurse should continue to monitor the client. The normal level is 3.5 to 5.5 mEq/L.**
   3. Hypokalemia can lead to cardiac dysrhythmias, but the client's potassium level is within normal limits.
   4. The client will need potassium to correct the hypokalemia, but the client's potassium level is within normal limits.

3. **1 and 2 are correct.**
   1. **An admission assessment is an independent intervention that the nurse should implement.**
   2. **Evaluating blood pressure is an independent intervention that the nurse should implement. If the client is able, B/Ps should be taken lying down, sitting, and standing to assess for orthostatic hypotension.**
   3. This is a collaborative intervention that the nurse should implement. It requires an order from the HCP.
   4. Administering blood products is collaborative, requiring an order from the HCP.

5. The HCP must order any laboratory work, so this is not an independent nursing intervention.

4. 1. A purple stoma indicates necrosis and requires immediate intervention, so the client should notify the HCP; therefore, the client understands the teaching.
   2. The client should be on a regular diet, and the colostomy will have been working for several days prior to discharge. The client's statement indicates an understanding of the teaching.
   3. The client should wear a colostomy pouch over the stoma, so it will collect the feces coming from the stoma.
   4. **A sigmoid colostomy must be irrigated daily, so the client will have a bowel movement daily. This statement indicates the client needs more teaching.**

5. **Answer: 94 mL/hour. First determine the total amount to be infused over 24 hours.**

6. 1. The client will have a nasogastric tube because the client will be NPO, which will decompress the bowel and help remove hydrochloric acid.
   2. Preventing dehydration is a priority with the client who is NPO.
   3. **Ms. Kathy should question a sigmoid-oscopy. Invasive tests are not completed during an acute exacerbation of diverticulosis.**
   4. The client is in severe pain and should be on bed rest, which will help rest the bowel.

7. 1. The client should be on bed rest for 2 hours, but must be on the right side to prevent hemorrhaging.
   2. The client must be on the right side for 2 hours to prevent hemorrhaging.
   3. **The client should be placed on the right side, same side as liver, to prevent hemorrhaging after the liver biopsy.**
   4. An incident report may need to be completed, but not prior to taking care of the client by placing the client on the right side.

8. 1. The nurse must notify the infection control nurse as soon as possible so that treatment can start if needed, but this is not the first intervention.
   2. **Ms. Kathy must first have the nurse complete the adverse occurrence report, so there is written documentation concerning the situation. Then Ms. Kathy**

should notify the infection control nurse, who will arrange for post-exposure prophylaxis and then determine if the client has hepatitis.

3. Post-exposure prophylaxis may be needed, but this is not the first action.

4. The infection control nurse will check the status of the client whom the needle was used on before the nurse stuck herself.

9. 1. The client with an inflated Sengstaken-Blakemore tube has acute esophageal varices bleeding and is not stable; therefore, this nursing task cannot be delegated.

2. The nurse cannot delegate assessment, teaching, evaluation, medications, or an unstable client.

3. **The client with pruritis (itching) is stable and the unlicensed assistive personnel (UAP) can assist with showering and a.m. care; therefore, this task can be delegated by Ms. Kathy.**

4. The nurse cannot perform a paracentesis; only an HCP can perform this procedure. Therefore, the UAP cannot assist the nurse.

10. 1. This client's hemoglobin and hematocrit is low, but the client is receiving blood; therefore, this client is stable and does not need to be assessed first.

2. The client with ulcerative colitis would be expected to have 10 loose stools and the potassium level is within normal limits; therefore, this client does not need to be assessed first.

3. **A hard, rigid abdomen and elevated temperature is indicative of peritonitis, which is an acute postoperative complication of abdominal surgery and requires immediate intervention. Ms. Kathy should assess this client first.**

4. Green bile draining from the N/G tube is expected and does not require assessment by Ms. Kathy.

Renal and Genitourinary Management

6

You are the people who are shaping a better world. One of the secrets of inner peace is the practice of compassion.

—Dalai Lama

QUESTIONS

1. The nurse is caring for the following clients on a medical unit. Which client should the nurse assess first?
   1. The client with acute glomerulonephritis who has oliguria and periorbital edema.
   2. The client with benign prostatic hypertrophy who has blood oozing from the intravenous site.
   3. The client with renal calculi who is complaining of flank pain rated as a 5 on a scale of 1 to 10.
   4. The client with nephrotic syndrome who has proteinuria and hypoalbuminemia.

2. The nurse is inserting an indwelling catheter into a male elderly client. Which intervention should the nurse implement first?
   1. Ask the client if he has any prostate problems.
   2. Determine if the client has any betadine allergies.
   3. Lubricate the end of the indwelling catheter.
   4. Ensure urine is obtained in the indwelling catheter.

3. The nurse is preparing to administer intravenous narcotic medication to the client who has renal calculi and is complaining of pain rated as 8 on 1 to 10 pain scale. The client's vital signs are stable. Which intervention should the nurse implement first?
   1. Clamp the IV tubing proximal to the port of medication administration.
   2. Administer the narcotic medication slowly over 2 minutes.
   3. Check the medication administration record (MAR) against the hospital identification band.
   4. Determine if the client's intravenous site is patent.

4. The nurse is administering medications to clients on a surgical unit. Which medication should the nurse administer first?
   1. The narcotic analgesic morphine IV infusion to the client who is 8 hours postoperative and is complaining of pain, rating it as a 7 on a 1 to 10 pain scale.
   2. The aminoglycoside antibiotic vancomycin intravenous piggyback (IVPB) to the client with an infected abdominal wound.
   3. The proton-pump inhibitor pantoprazole (Protonix) IVPB to the client who is at risk for developing a stress ulcer.
   4. The loop-diuretic furosemide (Lasix) intravenous push (IVP) to the client who has undergone surgical debridement of the right lower limb.

5. The nurse and unlicensed assistive personnel (UAP) are caring for clients on a surgical unit. Which action by the UAP warrants immediate intervention?
   1. The UAP empties the indwelling catheter bag for the client with transurethral resection of the prostate (TURP).
   2. The UAP assists a client who received an IV narcotic analgesic 30 minutes ago to ambulate in the hall.
   3. The UAP provides apple juice to the client with a nephrectomy who has just been advanced to a clear liquid diet.
   4. The UAP applies moisture barrier cream to the elderly client with urinary incontinence who has an excoriated perianal area.

6. The charge nurse is making shift assignments to the surgical staff, which consists of two nurses, two licensed practical nurses (LPNs), and two unlicensed assistive personnel (UAP). Which assignment would be most appropriate for the charge nurse to make?
   1. Instruct the nurse to administer all PRN medications.
   2. Instruct the UAP to clean the recently vacated room.
   3. Assign the LPN to change the client's ileal conduit bag.
   4. Request the LPN to complete the admission for a new client.

7. The charge nurse is making assignments in the day surgery center. Which client should be assigned to the most experienced nurse?
   1. The 24-year-old client who had a circumcision and is being prepared for discharge.
   2. The client scheduled for a cystectomy who is crying and upset about the surgery.
   3. The client diagnosed with kidney cancer who is receiving two units of blood.
   4. The client who has end-stage renal disease and had an arteriovenous fistula created.

8. The nurse is completing the admission assessment on the client scheduled for cystectomy with creation of an ileal conduit. The client tells the nurse, "I am taking saw palmetto for my enlarged prostate." Which intervention should the nurse implement first?
   1. Notify the client's HCP to write an order for the herbal supplement.
   2. Ask the client why he is taking an herb for his enlarged prostate.
   3. Consult with the pharmacist to determine any potential drug interactions.
   4. Look up saw palmetto in the *Physicians' Desk Reference* (PDR).

9. The client scheduled for a D&C is upset because the HCP told her she has syphilis. The client asks the nurse, "This is so embarrassing. Do you have to tell anyone about this?" Which statement is the nurse's best response?
   1. "This must be reported to the Public Health Department and your sexual partners."
   2. "According to the Health Insurance Portability and Accountability Act (HIPAA), I cannot report this to anyone without your permission."
   3. "You really should tell your sexual partners, so they can be treated for syphilis."
   4. "I realize you are embarrassed. Would you like to talk about the situation?"

10. The nurse is caring for clients on the renal unit. Which task is most appropriate for the nurse to delegate to the unlicensed assistive personnel (UAP)?
    1. Instruct the UAP to calculate the clients' urinary intake and output.
    2. Request the UAP to double-check a unit of blood that is being administered.
    3. Tell the UAP to change the surgical dressing on the client with a kidney transplant.
    4. Ask the UAP to transfer the client from the renal unit to the intensive care unit.

11. The nurse is caring for clients on a renal unit and making assignments for the day shift. Which client should the nurse assess first?
 1. The client diagnosed with interstitial cystitis who has urinary urgency and pain in the bladder.
 2. The client with acute post–streptococcal glomerulonephritis who has hematuria with a smoky appearance.
 3. The client diagnosed with Goodpasture syndrome who has pallor, anemia, and renal failure.
 4. The client diagnosed with nephrolithiasis who has hematuria and is complaining of pain, rating it as a 9 on 1 to a 10 pain scale.

12. Which action by the licensed practical nurse (LPN) requires intervention by the critical care charge nurse?
 1. The LPN has the trough drawn after hanging the aminoglycoside.
 2. The LPN changes out a "sharps" container that is over the fill line.
 3. The LPN asks another nurse to observe wastage of a narcotic.
 4. The LPN inserts an indwelling urinary catheter into the client.

13. The unlicensed assistive personnel (UAP) reports to the nurse the client's urine output has bright red blood. Which intervention should the nurse implement first?
 1. Instruct the UAP to take a urine specimen to the laboratory.
 2. Document the findings in the client's nursing notes.
 3. Assess the client's urine specimen and complete a renal assessment.
 4. Ask the UAP to take the client's vital signs.

14. The charge nurse is making client assignments. Which client should the nurse assign to the graduate nurse who has just finished orientation?
 1. The client with a cystectomy who had a creation of an ileal conduit.
 2. The client on continuous hemodialysis who is awaiting a kidney transplant.
 3. The client with renal trauma secondary to a motor vehicle accident.
 4. The client who has had abdominal surgery and whose wound has eviscerated.

15. The charge nurse on the renal unit is notified of a bus accident with multiple injuries and clients are being brought to the emergency department (ED). The hospital is implementing the disaster policy. Which action should the nurse take first?
 1. Determine which clients could be discharged home immediately.
 2. Call any off-duty nurses to notify them to come in to work.
 3. Assess the staffing to determine which staff could be sent to ED.
 4. Request all visitors to leave the hospital as soon as possible.

16. The 18-year-old client diagnosed with renal trauma is admitted to the critical care unit after a serious motor vehicle accident resulting from driving under the influence. The mother comes to the unit and starts yelling at her son about "driving drunk." Which action should the nurse implement?
 1. Allow the mother to continue talking to her son.
 2. Notify the hospital security to remove the mother.
 3. Escort the mother to a private area and talk to her.
 4. Tell the mother if she wants to stay, she must be quiet.

17. The nurse is caring for an 84-year-old male client diagnosed with benign prostatic hypertrophy. The client has undergone a transurethral resection of the prostate (TURP) and is complaining of bladder spasms. Which intervention should the nurse implement first?
 1. Administer an antispasmodic medication for bladder spasms.
 2. Calculate the client's urinary output.
 3. Palpate the client's abdomen for bladder distention.
 4. Assess the client's three-way urinary catheter for patency.

18. The nurse is caring for clients on a surgical unit. Which client should the nurse assess first after shift report?
    1. The client diagnosed with polycystic kidney disease who has a B/P 170/100.
    2. The client diagnosed with bladder cancer who has gross painless hematuria.
    3. The client diagnosed with renal calculi who thinks he passed a stone.
    4. The client with acute pyelonephritis who has nausea/vomiting and is dehydrated.

19. The 78-year-old client with Alport syndrome asks the clinic nurse, "What should I do so I won't get sick this winter?" Which priority statement is the nurse's best response?
    1. "You should not be around any crowds during the winter months."
    2. "It is recommended you get a flu vaccine yearly."
    3. "You need to eat three well-balanced meals a day."
    4. "Dress warmly when it is less than 40 degrees Fahrenheit outside."

20. The elderly female client tells the nurse, "I have vaginal dryness and it hurts when my husband and I make love." Which priority intervention should the nurse discuss with the client?
    1. Tell the client to discuss hormone replacement therapy with her HCP.
    2. Encourage the client to refrain from having sexual intercourse.
    3. Recommend the client use a vaginal lubricant prior to intercourse.
    4. Explain to the client that vaginal dryness is not uncommon in the elderly.

21. The elderly female client diagnosed with osteoporosis is prescribed the bisphosphonate medication alendronate (Fosamax). Which intervention is priority when administering this medication?
    1. Administer the medication first thing in the morning.
    2. Ask the client whether she has a history of peptic ulcer disease.
    3. Encourage the client to walk for at least 30 minutes.
    4. Have the client remain upright for 30 minutes after administering the medication.

22. Which nursing task should the nurse on the renal unit assign to the licensed practical nurse (LPN)?
    1. Insert an indwelling urinary catheter before surgery.
    2. Turn and reposition the client every 2 hours.
    3. Measure and record the urine in the bedside commode.
    4. Feed the client who choked on food during the last meal.

23. The nurse on a medical unit has just received the evening shift report. Which client should the nurse assess first?
    1. The client with renal vein thrombosis who has a heparin drip infusion and a PTT of 92.
    2. The client on peritoneal dialysis who has a clear dialysate draining from the abdomen.
    3. The client on hemodialysis whose right upper arm fistula has an audible bruit.
    4. The client diagnosed with cystitis who is complaining of burning on urination.

24. The nurse is preparing to administer medications. Which medication should the nurse administer first?
    1. Digoxin (Lanoxin), a cardiac glycoside, due at 0900.
    2. Furosemide (Lasix), a loop diuretic, due at 0800.
    3. Propoxyphene (Darvon), an analgesic, due in 2 hours.
    4. Acetaminophen (Tylenol), an analgesic, due in 5 minutes.

25. Which intervention should the nurse implement first when assisting a client with a flaccid bladder to urinate?
    1. Perform the Credé's maneuver on the client.
    2. Perform intermittent catheterization on the client.
    3. Place the client on the bedside commode.
    4. Request the client to drink a full glass of water.

26. The nurse is caring for clients in a family practice clinic. Which client should the nurse assess first?
    1. The male client with chronic pyelonephritis who has costrovertebral tenderness.
    2. The female client who is having burning and pain on urination.
    3. The female client with urethritis who reports dysuria, urgency, and frequent urination.
    4. The male client who has hesitancy, terminal dribbling, and intermittency.

27. The nurse and unlicensed assistive personnel (UAP) are working in a family practice clinic. Which task should the nurse delegate to the UAP?
    1. Give the client sample medications for a urinary tract infection (UTI).
    2. Show the client how to use a self-monitoring blood glucometer.
    3. Answer the telephone triage line and take messages from clients.
    4. Take the vital signs of a client scheduled for a physical examination.

28. Which task is most appropriate for the nurse on the renal unit to delegate to the unlicensed assistive personnel (UAP)?
    1. Escort the client with acute polynephritis to the radiology department for a CT scan.
    2. Obtain a sterile urine specimen for the client to rule out (R/O) a urinary tract infection.
    3. Hang the bag of D5W for the client diagnosed with post–streptococcal glomerulonephritis.
    4. Provide discharge instructions for the client diagnosed for nephrotic syndrome.

29. Which task should the employee health nurse delegate to the unlicensed assistive personnel (UAP)?
    1. Request the UAP read the PPD result administered to the client 72 hours ago.
    2. Ask the UAP to obtain a urine specimen for the client having a urine drug screening.
    3. Tell the UAP to apply an ice pack to the client who slipped and has a sprained right ankle.
    4. Instruct the UAP to complete the incident report for the nurse who had a "dirty needle stick."

30. The nurse manager in the medical-surgical outpatient clinic is making assignments. Which task is most appropriate to delegate/assign to the UAP/LPN?
    1. Ask the LPN to administer the flu vaccine to the client.
    2. Tell the UAP to call the pharmacist to refill a prescription.
    3. Request the LPN to obtain the height and weight of the client.
    4. Instruct the UAP to empty the trashcans in the clients' rooms.

31. Which behavior warrants intervention by the clinical manager in the medical-surgical outpatient clinic?
    1. The UAP is discussing a client's condition in the waiting room.
    2. The LPN is talking to a client over the phone about laboratory tests.
    3. The RN is triaging phone messages during his or her lunch break.
    4. The UAP is taking vital signs for the client being placed in a room.

32. The UAP in the school nurse's office is listening to a female student who is pregnant and scared to tell her parents. Which action should the school nurse implement?
    1. Tell the UAP she cannot talk to the female student.
    2. Call the student's parents and tell them their daughter is pregnant.
    3. Do not take any action and allow the UAP to listen to the student.
    4. Ask the UAP to leave and continue to talk to the student.

33. The nurse observes an LPN discussing an intravenous pyleogram, a diagnostic test, with a client in the waiting room of the outpatient clinic. Which action should the nurse implement?
   1. Praise the LPN for talking to the client about the diagnostic test.
   2. Tell the LPN the nurse needs to talk to her in the office area.
   3. Go to the waiting room and tell the LPN not to discuss this there.
   4. Inform the HCP that the LPN was talking to the client in the waiting room.

34. The charge nurse in a large outpatient clinic notices the staff members are arguing and irritable with one other and the atmosphere has been very tense for the past week. Which action should the charge nurse take?
   1. Wait for another week to see whether the situation resolves itself.
   2. Write a memo telling all staff members to stop arguing.
   3. Schedule a meeting with the staff to discuss the situation.
   4. Tell the staff to stop arguing or they will be terminated.

35. The employee health nurse is obtaining a urine specimen for a pre-employment drug screen. Which action should the nurse implement first?
   1. Obtain informed consent for the procedure.
   2. Maintain the chain of custody for the specimen.
   3. Allow the client to go to any bathroom in the clinic.
   4. Take and record the client's tympanic temperature.

36. The client comes to the clinic reporting pain and burning on urination. Which action should the nurse implement first?
   1. Assess and document the client's vital signs.
   2. Determine whether the client has seen any blood in the urine.
   3. Request the client give a midstream urine specimen.
   4. Ask the client whether she wipes front to back after a bowel movement.

37. The nurse is working at the emergency health clinic in a disaster shelter. Which intervention is priority when initially assessing the client?
   1. Find out how long the client will be in the shelter.
   2. Determine whether the client has his or her routine medications.
   3. Document the client's health history in writing.
   4. Assess the client's vital signs, height, and weight.

38. The HCP orders an intravenous pyelogram for the 27-year-old male client diagnosed with R/O renal calculi. The client is diagnosed with schizophrenia and is delusional. Which action should the clinic nurse implement?
   1. Ask the client whether he is allergic to yeast.
   2. Request the client to sign a permit for the procedure.
   3. Obtain informed consent from the client's significant other.
   4. Discuss the local hospital's day surgery procedure with the client.

39. The home health (HH) aide tells the home health nurse one of the older male clients is taking an herbal supplement, saw palmetto, every day. Which statement is the nurse's best response?
   1. "Herbal supplements are dangerous and I will talk to the client."
   2. "Saw palmetto is used to treat benign prostatic hypertrophy. Let him take it."
   3. "I will notify the client's healthcare provider as soon as possible."
   4. "Many clients use herbal supplements. He has a right to take it."

40. The home health (HH) aide caring for the client who is postoperative kidney transplant asks the home health nurse, "Why is the physical therapist coming to visit the client?" Which statement is the home health nurse's best response?
   1. "The physical therapist will evaluate the client's swallowing difficulty."
   2. "The physical therapist will assist the client with fine motor coordination."
   3. "The physical therapist will assist with caregiver concerns and making referrals."
   4. "The physical therapist will work with the client on strengthening and endurance."

41. The home health (HH) nurse is admitting a female client diagnosed with end-stage renal disease who refuses to be placed on hemodialysis. The client is ready to die, but verbalizes having so many regrets in her life. Which intervention would be most appropriate for the nurse?
1. Contact the agency chaplain to come talk to the client.
2. Call her church pastor and discuss the client's concerns.
3. Ask the client whether or not she would like to pray with the nurse.
4. Determine whether or not the client has an advance directive.

42. The nurse is preparing to perform a dressing change on a female client who has end-stage renal disease. The nurse notes the client's husband is silently holding the client's hand and praying. Which action should the nurse implement first?
1. Continue to prepare for the dressing change in the room.
2. Call the chaplain to help the client and spouse pray.
3. Quietly leave the room and come back later for the dressing change.
4. Ask the husband whether or not he would like the nurse to join in the prayer.

43. The unit manager on the renal unit is evaluating the staff nurse. Which data should be included in the nurse's yearly evaluation?
1. The fact that the nurse clocked in late to work twice in the last year.
2. The complaint stating the nurse did not answer a call light during a code.
3. The number of times the nurse switched shifts with another nurse.
4. The appropriateness of the nurse's written documentation in the charts.

44. The hospice nurse is providing follow-up care with the family member of a client who died with chronic renal disease. Which intervention is priority?
1. Attend the client's funeral service or visitation.
2. Check on the family 1 to 2 months after the death of the client.
3. Make sure the arrangements are what the client wanted.
4. Help the family member dispose of the client's belongings as soon as possible.

45. The nurse is attempting to start an intravenous (IV) line in an elderly client who is dehydrated. After two unsuccessful attempts, which intervention should the nurse implement?
1. Keep trying to get a patent IV access.
2. Ask the HCP to order oral fluid replacement.
3. Ask a second nurse to attempt to start the IV.
4. Place cold packs on the client's arms for comfort.

46. The client diagnosed with chronic kidney disease (CKD), and who has a left forearm graft, is assigned to the nurse and unlicensed assistive personnel (UAP). Which action by the UAP requires immediate intervention by the nurse?
1. The UAP avoids using soap while bathing the client.
2. The UAP takes the BP on the client's left arm.
3. The UAP tells the client she should not eat chips.
4. The UAP measures a scant amount of urine in the BSC.

47. The nurse is on the day shift in a long-term care facility. Which medication should the nurse question administering to the 85-year-old client with chronic pyelonephritis and heart failure?

Client Name: Mr. C.D.	Account Number: 245 86 9		Allergies: NKDA	
Height: 65 inches	Weight in pounds: 165 Weight in kg: 75		Date of Birth: 02/10/1922	
Date: Today	Medication	2301–0700	0701–1500	1501–2300
	Lanoxin (digoxin) 0.125 mg PO daily		0900	
	Lasix 40 mg PO daily		0900	
	K Dur 20 mEq PO bid		0900	1800
	Dulcolax (bisacodyl) 5 mg PO daily		0900	
Signature/Initials		Night Nurse RN/NN	Day Nurse RN/DN	

1. Lanoxin.
2. Lasix.
3. K Dur.
4. Dulcolax.

48. The elderly patient diagnosed with heart failure is scheduled to receive a unit of packed red blood cells (PRBCs). The PRBCs are prepared in 350 mL of solution. At what rate should the nurse set the pump? _____

49. Which interventions should the nurse delegate to the unlicensed assistive personnel (UAP) when caring for the client who is 2 days postoperative open surgery of the kidney? **Select all that apply.**
1. Explain the procedure for using the patient-controlled analgesia (PCA) pump.
2. Check the client's flank surgical dressing for drainage.
3. Take and record the client's vital signs and pulse oximeter reading.
4. Empty the client's indwelling catheter bag at the end of the shift.
5. Assist the client to ambulate in the hallway three to four times a day.

50. The client with open surgery of the kidney has an AP 118 and B/P 88/58. Which intervention should the nurse implement first?
1. Obtain the client's pulse oximeter reading.
2. Check the client's last hemoglobin and hematocrit.
3. Notify the client's surgeon immediately.
4. Monitor the client's urine output.

51. The 88-year-old female client is complaining of urinary frequency and dribbling. Which nursing interventions should be implemented? Rank in order of performance.
1. Have the unlicensed assistive personnel (UAP) make "potty" rounds on the client every 2 hours.
2. Give the client perineal pads to place inside her underwear.
3. Place an absorbent pad on the client's bed.
4. Put a bedside commode at the client's bedside.
5. Instruct the client in providing a clean-catch urine specimen.

52. The nurse in the dialysis center is initiating the morning dialysis run. Which client should the nurse assess first?
   1. The client who has a hemoglobin of 9.0 mg/dL and hematocrit of 26%.
   2. The client who does not have a palpable thrill or auscultated bruit.
   3. The client who is reporting a 3.6 kg weight gain and is refusing dialysis.
   4. The client on peritoneal dialysis who is complaining of a hard, rigid abdomen.

53. The male client with chronic kidney disease has received the initial dose of erythropoietin, a biological response modifier, 1 week ago. Which data warrants the nurse to notify the healthcare provider?
   1. The client's pulse oximeter reading of 95%.
   2. The client has a platelet count of 155,000.
   3. The client has a blood pressure reading of 184/102.
   4. The client has a tympanic temperature of 99.8°F.

54. The nurse is developing a nursing care plan for the client diagnosed with chronic kidney disease. Which nursing problem should be addressed first?
   1. Self-care deficit.
   2. Knowledge deficit.
   3. Chronic pain.
   4. Excess fluid volume.

55. The client with chronic kidney disease is placed on a fluid restriction of 1,500 milliliters per day. On the 7 a.m. to 7 p.m. shift the client drank an 8-ounce cup of coffee, 8 ounces of juice, 16 ounces of tea, and 8 ounces of water with medications. What amount of fluid can the 7 p.m. to 7 a.m. nurse give to the client? _____

56. The client receiving dialysis is complaining of being dizzy and light-headed. Which priority intervention should the nurse implement?
   1. Place the client in the reverse Trendelenburg position.
   2. Decrease the volume of blood being removed from the client.
   3. Bolus the client 300 mL of 0.9% saline solution.
   4. Notify the healthcare provider as soon as possible.

57. The client is NPO and is receiving total parenteral nutrition (TPN) via a subclavian line. Which precautions should the nurse implement? **Select all that apply.**
   1. Place the client's TPN on a gravity intravenous line.
   2. Monitor the client's blood glucose every 24 hours.
   3. Weigh the client daily, first thing in the morning.
   4. Change the client's IV tubing with every TPN bag administered.
   5. Monitor the client's intake and output every shift.

58. The client has received IV solutions for 3 days through a 20-gauge IV catheter placed in the left cephalic vein. On morning rounds the nurse notes the IV site is tender to palpation, it is edematous, and a red streak has formed. Which interventions should the nurse implement? Rank in priority order.
   1. Start a new IV in the right hand.
   2. Discontinue the intravenous line.
   3. Complete an incident record.
   4. Place a warm washcloth over the site.
   5. Document the situation in the client's chart.

59. The nurse and unlicensed assistive personnel (UAP) are caring for a group of clients. Which nursing intervention should the nurse perform?
   1. Measure the client's output from the indwelling catheter.
   2. Record the client's intake and output on the I&O sheet.
   3. Instruct the client on appropriate fluid restrictions.
   4. Provide water for a client diagnosed with acute polynephritis.

QUESTIONS

60. The nurse emptied 2,340 mL from the drainage bag of a continuous irrigation of a client who had a transurethral resection of the prostate (TURP). The amount of irrigation in the hanging bag was 3,000 mL at the beginning of the shift. There was 1,550 mL left in the bag 8 hours later. What is the correct urine output at the end of the 8 hours? _____

61. Which nursing diagnosis is priority for the client who has undergone a transurethral resection of the prostate (TURP)?
    1. Potential for sexual dysfunction.
    2. Potential for altered urinary elimination.
    3. Potential for infection.
    4. Potential for hemorrhage.

62. The client is 1 day postoperative transurethral resection of the prostate (TURP). Which action by the unlicensed assistive personnel (UAP) warrants intervention by the nurse?
    1. The UAP increased the client's irrigation fluid to clear clots from the tubing.
    2. The UAP elevated the client's scrotum on a towel roll for support.
    3. The UAP emptied the client's indwelling urinary catheter bag.
    4. The UAP brought ice water to the client's bedside.

63. The male client diagnosed with renal calculi is admitted to the medical unit. Which intervention should the nurse implement first?
    1. Request the client to urinate in a urinal.
    2. Assess the client's pain.
    3. Increase the client's oral fluid intake.
    4. Strain the client's urine.

64. The female client with renal calculi is scheduled for a STAT kidney, ureter, bladder (KUB). Which statement by the client warrants intervention by the nurse?
    1. "I am allergic to shell fish and iodine."
    2. "I just had my lunch tray and ate all of it."
    3. "I have not had my period for 3 months."
    4. "I am having pain in my lower back."

65. The client diagnosed with renal calculi is scheduled for a 24-hour urine specimen collection. Which interventions should the nurse implement? **Select all that apply.**
    1. Keep the client NPO during the time the urine is being collected.
    2. Instruct the client to urinate, and include this urine when starting collection.
    3. Place client's urine in an appropriate specimen container for 24 hours.
    4. Insert an indwelling catheter in client after having the client empty the bladder.
    5. Post signs on the client's door alerting staff to save all of the client's urine output.

66. The client diagnosed with renal calculi is 1 hour post-procedure lithotripsy. Which task is most appropriate for the nurse to delegate to the unlicensed assistive personnel (UAP)?
    1. Tell the UAP to check the amount, color, and consistency of the client's urine output.
    2. Request the UAP to transcribe the client's healthcare provider's orders.
    3. Instruct the UAP to strain the client's urine and place any sediment in a sterile container.
    4. Ask the UAP to take the client's post-procedural vital signs.

67. The client had surgery to remove a kidney stone. Which of the following laboratory assessment data warrants intervention by the nurse?
    1. A serum potassium level of 5.2 mEq/L.
    2. A urinalysis showing blood in the urine.
    3. A creatinine level of 1.2 mg/100 mL.
    4. A white blood cell count of 9,500 mm/dL.

68. Which intervention should the nurse implement first for the client diagnosed with urinary incontinence?
1. Palpate the bladder after an incontinent episode.
2. Administer oxybutynin, an anticholinergic agent.
3. Ensure the client does not sit or lie in the urine.
4. Instruct the client to go to the bathroom every 2 hours.

69. The nurse is caring for an elderly female client who has an indwelling catheter. Which data warrants notifying the healthcare provider?
1. The client's vital signs are T 98, AP 90, RR 16, B/P 142/88.
2. The client has had a change in her mental status.
3. The client's urine is cloudy with sediment.
4. The client has no discomfort or pain.

70. The nurse is observing the unlicensed assistive personnel (UAP) provide care to a client with an indwelling catheter. Which action by the UAP warrants immediate intervention by the nurse?
1. The UAP does not secure the tubing to the client's leg with tape.
2. The UAP wears gloves when providing catheter care to the client.
3. The UAP positions the collection bag on the side of the client's bed.
4. The UAP cares for the client's catheter after washing his or her hands.

RENAL AND GENITOURINARY CLINICAL SCENARIO

Ms. Brenda is the clinical manager on a 20-bed renal unit. Today, Ms. Brenda is the charge nurse for the 7p-7a shift because the regular charge nurse is on emergency family leave. The staff for the shift includes two RNs (Mr. Ray and Ms. Mary), one LPN (Ms. Cindy), and two unlicensed assistive personnel (UAPs) (Ms. Debbie and Ms. Paula).

1. Ms. Mary, RN, and Ms. Debbie, the UAP, are caring for clients on the unit. Which nursing task would be most appropriate for Ms. Mary to delegate to Ms. Debbie?
   1. Assist the radiology technician with a portable chest x-ray.
   2. Evaluate the client's 8-hour intake and output.
   3. Perform an in and out catheterization for a sterile urine specimen.
   4. Administer a cation-exchange resin enema.

2. Mr. Ray is preparing to perform hemodialysis on the client diagnosed with end-stage renal disease. Which data warrants immediate intervention from Mr. Ray?
   1. A hemoglobin of 9.8 mg/dL and hematocrit of 30%.
   2. Inability to palpate thrill or auscultate a bruit.
   3. Complaints of being exhausted and unable to sleep.
   4. No urine output in the past 12 hours.

3. The client who is 1 day postoperative cystectomy has a nasogastric tube (NGT) in place and an IV running at 150 mL/hr via an IV pump. Which data should Ms. Mary report to the healthcare provider?
   1. The client's peripheral intravenous access is infiltrated.
   2. The client has hypoactive bowel sounds.
   3. The client has crackles bilaterally in the lower lobes.
   4. The client has 2+ bilateral pedal pulses.

4. The elderly client is diagnosed with chronic glomerulonephritis. Which lab value indicates the condition has gotten worse?
   1. The BUN is 18 mg/dL.
   2. The creatinine level is 1.0 mg/dL.
   3. The glomerular filtration rate is 60 mL/minute.
   4. The 24-hour creatinine clearance is 120 mL/minute.

5. Ms. Debbie emptied 3,000 mL from the drainage bag of a continuous bladder irrigation (CBI) of a client who had a transurethral resection of the prostate (TURP). The amount of irrigation in the bag hanging was 4,000 mL at the beginning of the shift. There was 2,000 mL left in the bag at 0700. What is the corrected urine output for the shift? _____

6. The client returned from surgery after having a TURP and has a P 96, R 20, B/P 110/70 and light pink urine draining in the indwelling urinary bag. Which interventions should Mr. Ray implement? **Select all that apply.**
   1. Assess the urine in the continuous irrigation drainage bag.
   2. Increase the irrigation fluid in the continuous irrigation catheter.
   3. Lower the head of the bed while raising the foot of the bed.
   4. Contact the surgeon to give an update in the client's condition.
   5. Monitor the client's postoperative hematocrit and hemoglobin.

7. The client diagnosed with renal calculi is admitted to the unit. Which intervention should Ms. Mary implement first?
   1. Complete the admission assessment documentation.
   2. Assess the client's pain and rule out complications.
   3. Increase the client's oral fluid intake.
   4. Transcribe the client's healthcare provider's orders.

8. The client diagnosed with renal calculi is scheduled for lithotripsy. Which post-procedure nursing task is most appropriate to delegate to Ms. Debbie, the UAP?
    1. Assess the amount, color, and consistency of urine output.
    2. Teach the client about care of the indwelling urinary catheter.
    3. Instruct Ms. Debbie to strain the client's urine.
    4. Maintain the client on strict bed rest.

9. Ms. Brenda is making rounds on clients. Which client should Ms. Brenda assess first?
    1. The client with end-stage renal disease on hemodialysis who has a palpable thrill.
    2. The client with acute glomerulonephritis who has hematuria and proteinuria.
    3. The client with bladder cancer who has painless urination with bright red urine.
    4. The client with an ileal conduit who has not had any drainage in the drainage bag.

10. Ms. Mary, the RN, and Ms. Cindy, the LPN, are caring for clients. Which intervention should Ms. Mary assign Ms. Cindy?
    1. Teach the client the home care of the suprapubic catheter.
    2. Monitor of the post-op client with a WBC of 22,000 mm/dL.
    3. Administer antineoplastic medications to the client with bladder cancer.
    4. Administer a narcotic analgesic to the client with renal calculi.

ANSWERS AND RATIONALES

The correct answer number and rationale for why it is the correct answer are given in **boldface type**. Rationales for why the other possible answer options are incorrect also are given, but they are not in boldface type.

1. 1. The nurse would expect the client with acute glomerulonephritis to have oliguria and periorbital edema. Acute glomerulonephritis is a disorder of the glomeruli (glomerulonephritis), or small blood vessels in the kidneys.
2. **The nurse would not expect the client with BPH to have oozing blood from the intravenous site. This may indicate disseminated intravascular coagulation (DIC), which is a potentially life-threatening complication and requires immediate intervention.**
3. The nurse would expect the client with renal calculi to have pain, but a level 5 pain indicates the pain is under control; therefore, this client does not need to be seen first.
4. The nurse would expect the client with nephrotic syndrome to have proteinuria (protein in the urine) and hypoalbuminemia (decreased protein in the blood). Nephrotic syndrome is a nonspecific disorder in which the kidneys are damaged, causing them to leak large amounts of protein into the urine.
   Content – Medical/Surgical: **Category of Health Alteration** *– Genitourinary:* **Integrated Processes** *– Nursing Process: Assessment:* **Client Needs** *– Physiological Integrity: Reduction of Risk Potential:* **Cognitive Level** *– Analysis*

MAKING NURSING DECISIONS: The nurse must determine which sign/symptom is not expected for the disease process. If the sign/symptom is not expected, or if it is an emergency situation, the nurse should assess the client first. This type of question is determining if the nurse is knowledgeable of signs/symptoms of a variety of disease processes.

2. 1. This is an appropriate question, but even clients with prostate problems can have an indwelling catheter inserted carefully.
2. **Betadine is included in the indwelling catheter kit; so another form of cleaning agent must be used when inserting the catheter. Therefore, this is the first intervention.**
3. This is appropriate, but not the first intervention.

4. Urine should be obtained in the catheter, but it is not the first intervention.
   Content – Medical/Surgical: **Category of Health Alteration** *– Genitourinary:* **Integrated Processes** *– Nursing Process: Implementation:* **Client Needs** *– Physiological Integrity: Reduction of Risk Potential:* **Cognitive Level** *– Application*

MAKING NURSING DECISIONS: When the question asks, "Which intervention should be implemented first?" it means all the options are things a nurse could implement, but only one should be implemented first. The nurse should use the nursing process and remember: If the client is in distress, do not assess; if the client is not in distress, the nurse should assess.

3. 1. The nurse should clamp the tubing to ensure the medication goes directly into the client and not retrograde up the tubing, but it is not the first administration.
2. The medication should be administered over 2 minutes, but it is not the first intervention.
3. The nurse should always ensure the medication is being administered to the correct client, but the nurse should first make sure the route of administration is safe.
4. **Ensuring the site is patent is the first intervention because even if it is the correct client, the medication should not be administered if the IV site is infiltrated.**
   Content – Medical/Surgical: **Category of Health Alteration** *– Genitourinary:* **Integrated Processes** *– Nursing Process: Implementation:* **Client Needs** *– Physiological Integrity: Pharmacological and Parenteral Therapies:* **Cognitive Level** *– Application*

MAKING NURSING DECISIONS: When the question asks, "Which intervention should be implemented first?" it means all the options are things a nurse could implement, but only one should be implemented first. The nurse should use the nursing process and remember: If the client is in distress, do not assess; if the client is not in distress, the nurse should assess.

4. 1. **The client who is in pain is priority. None of the other clients have a life-threatening condition. Pain is considered the fifth vital sign.**
2. Routine antibiotics are not priority over a client who has postoperative pain.
3. Risk for a stress ulcer is a potential, not an actual, problem, and proton-pump inhibitors

are administered routinely to help prevent stress ulcers.

4. The loop diuretic is a routine medication prescribed for a medical comorbid condition, not for surgical debridement.

Content – Medical/Surgical: Category of Health Alteration – Genitourinary: Integrated Processes – Nursing Process: Implementation: Client Needs – Physiological Integrity: Pharmacological and Parenteral Therapies: Cognitive Level – Application

MAKING NURSING DECISIONS: When the nurse is making a decision about prioritizing medication administration, client comfort takes priority over regularly scheduled medications.

5. 1. The unlicensed assistive personnel (UAP) can empty an indwelling catheter drainage bag because this does not require judgment.

2. **The client who received a narcotic analgesic 30 minutes ago is at risk for falling because of the effects of the medication; therefore, the UAP should not ambulate this client. The nurse should intervene.**

3. The UAP can provide juice to the client, and apple juice is part of the client's liquid diet.

4. Moisture barrier cream is not a medication; therefore, the UAP can apply such creams to an intact perianal area.

Content – Medical/Surgical: Category of Health Alteration – Genitourinary: Integrated Processes – Nursing Process: Planning: Client Needs – Safe and Effective Care Environment: Management of Care: Cognitive Level – Synthesis

MAKING NURSING DECISIONS: The nurse cannot delegate assessment, evaluation, teaching, administration of medications, or an unstable client to an unlicensed assistive personnel (UAP).

6. 1. The LPN can administer routine as well as some PRN medications; assigning the nurse to administer all PRN medications is not appropriate.

2. The housekeeping department, not the UAP, is assigned to clean recently vacated rooms.

3. **It is within an LPN's scope of practice to change an ileal conduit drainage bag; therefore, this would be the most appropriate assignment for the LPN.**

4. The nurse would be the most appropriate staff member to complete the admission assessment.

Content – Medical/Surgical: Category of Health Alteration – Genitourinary: Integrated Processes – Nursing Process: Planning: Client Needs – Safe and Effective Care Environment: Management of Care: Cognitive Level – Synthesis

MAKING NURSING DECISIONS: When the nurse is deciding which option is the most appropriate

task to delegate/assign, the nurse should choose the task that allows each staff member to function within their scope of practice. Remember, the nurse cannot delegate assessment, teaching, evaluation, medications, or an unstable client to the UAP and cannot assign assessment, teaching, evaluation, or an unstable client to the LPN.

7. 1. **The most experienced nurse should be assigned to the client who requires teaching prior to being discharged. Postoperative complications can occur, so the client must be knowledgeable of when to call the healthcare provider and how to take care of the surgical site.**

2. A less experienced nurse can talk to the client who is crying and upset. The most experienced nurse should care for a client who requires more knowledge.

3. A less experienced nurse can administer and monitor blood transfusion to the client.

4. Although the creation of an arteriovenous fistula requires assessment and teaching on the part of the most experienced nurse, this client is not being discharged home at this time.

Content – Medical/Surgical: Category of Health Alteration – Genitourinary: Integrated Processes – Nursing Process: Planning: Client Needs – Safe and Effective Care Environment: Management of Care: Cognitive Level – Synthesis

MAKING NURSING DECISIONS: The nurse must determine which client is the most unstable or requires extensive teaching. This client requires the most experienced nurse, thus making this type of question an "except" question. Three clients are either stable or have non–life-threatening conditions.

8. 1. If the HCP deems that the client can continue to take the herbal supplement, then an order must be written; however, this is not the first intervention.

2. The nurse could ask for clarification of the reason he is taking the herbal supplement, but this is not the first intervention. Many clients use herbal supplements for a variety of healthcare needs.

3. **According to the NSCBN NCLEX-RN® test plan, collaboration with interdisciplinary team members is part of the management of care. The nurse should first consult with the pharmacist to determine whether the client is taking any medications that could interact with the saw palmetto.**

4. The PDR is available to research medications, not herbal supplements.

*Content – Medical Surgical: **Category of Health
Alteration** – Complimentary Alternative Medicine:
Integrated Processes – Nursing Process: Planning:
Client Needs – Physiological Integrity: Pharmacological
and Parenteral Therapies: **Cognitive Level** – Synthesis*

MAKING NURSING DECISIONS: The nurse must
be knowledgeable of interventions when administering medications to clients undergoing surgery, such as, the client should not receive any
PO medications, the client should not receive
any medications that could increase bleeding,
or if the client is taking any complementary
alternative medications, such as herbs.

9. 1. **HIPAA does not apply in some situations,
      including the reporting of sexually trans-
      mitted diseases to the Public Health De-
      partment. The Public Health Department
      will attempt to notify any sexual partners
      the client reports.**
   2. This is a false statement. HIPAA does not
      apply in certain situations, and the nurse must
      be knowledgeable of HIPAA guidelines.
   3. The client should notify her sexual partners
      so they can be treated; however, in response
      to the client asking, "Does anyone have to
      know?" the nurse's best response is to
      provide facts.
   4. This is a therapeutic response aimed at en-
      couraging the client to verbalize feelings, but
      the nurse should provide factual information
      in this situation.
   *Content – Medical/Surgical: **Category of Health
   Alteration** – Genitourinary: **Integrated Processes** –
   Nursing Process: Planning: **Client Needs** – Health
   Promotion and Maintenance: **Cognitive Level** –
   Comprehension*

MAKING NURSING DECISIONS: There will be
management questions on the NCLEX-RN®.
In many instances, there is no test-taking
strategy for these questions; the nurse must be
knowledgeable of management issues. The
Health Insurance Portability and Accountability
Act (HIPAA) passed into law in 1996 to standardize exchange of information between
healthcare providers and to ensure patient
record confidentiality.

10. 1. **The unlicensed assistive personnel (UAP)
       can calculate intake and output for clients.
       The UAP cannot evaluate the numbers to
       determine if the treatment is effective, but
       the UAP can obtain the numbers.**
    2. Two nurses must double-check a unit of
       blood prior to infusing the blood; therefore,
       this task cannot be delegated.
    3. The surgeon or the nurse must change the
       surgical dressing for a kidney transplant.

This task cannot be delegated to personnel
with a lower level of expertise.
4. The UAP cannot transfer the unstable
   client from the renal unit to the intensive
   care unit.
*Content – Medical/Surgical: **Category of Health
Alteration** – Genitourinary: **Integrated Processes** –
Nursing Process: Planning: **Client Needs** – Safe and
Effective Care Environment: Management of Care:
Cognitive Level – Synthesis*

MAKING NURSING DECISIONS: An RN cannot
delegate assessment, teaching, evaluation,
medications, or an unstable client to a UAP.
Tasks that cannot be delegated are nursing
interventions requiring nursing judgment.

11. 1. Interstitial cystitis is a chronic, painful
       inflammatory disease of the bladder
       characterized by urgency/frequency and
       pain in the bladder and/or pelvis. Since the
       signs/symptoms are expected, the nurse
       would not assess this client first.
    2. The clinical manifestations of acute post–
       streptococcal glomerulonephritis are varied,
       including generalized body edema, hyperten-
       sion, oliguria, hematuria with a smoky or
       rusty appearance, and proteinuria. Since the
       signs/symptoms are expected, the nurse
       would not assess this client first.
    3. Goodpasture syndrome is a rare autoimmune
       disease seen primarily in young male smokers
       characterized by hematuria, weakness, pallor,
       anemia, and renal failure. Since the
       signs/symptoms are expected, the nurse
       would not assess this client first.
    4. **Nephrolithiasis, kidney stones, is charac-
       terized by pain and hematuria, but the
       nurse must assess the pain to determine
       whether a complication has occurred or it
       is the expected routine pain. Pain is the
       common priority of these four clients.**
    *Content – Medical/Surgical: **Category of Health
    Alteration** – Genitourinary: **Integrated Processes** –
    Nursing Process: Assessment: **Client Needs** – Physiological
    Integrity: Reduction of Risk Potential: **Cognitive
    Level** – Analysis*

MAKING NURSING DECISIONS: The nurse can
use Maslow's Hierarchy of Needs to determine
which client to assess first. Pain is a physiological
need.

12. 1. **The trough should be drawn before the
       aminoglycoside, vancomycin, antibiotic is
       hung. This requires intervention by the
       critical care charge nurse.**
    2. The LPN should change out a "sharps"
       container that is full; if not changed, then
       this consitutes an OSHA violation.

3. The LPN must have a narcotic wastage observed by another nurse.
4. The LPN can insert an indwelling urinary catheter in their scope of practice.

Content – Medical/Surgical: **Category of Health Alteration** *– Genitourinary:* **Integrated Processes** *– Nursing Process: Implementation:* **Client Needs** *– Physiological Integrity: Pharmacological and Parenteral Therapies:* **Cognitive Level** *– Application*

MAKING NURSING DECISIONS: The nurse must know the scope of practice for the LPN. The nurse must know the correct procedure for administering medications to the client and OSHA standards.

13. 1. The unlicensed assistive personnel (UAP) can take a specimen to the lab, but this is not the first intervention.
2. The findings should be documented in the nurse's notes, but it is not the first intervention.
3. **The nurse must first assess the UAP's findings and the client before taking any further action.**
4. The UAP can take the client's vital signs, but it is not the first intervention for the nurse.

Content – Medical/Surgical: **Category of Health Alteration** *– Genitourinary:* **Integrated Processes** *– Nursing Process: Assessment:* **Client Needs** *– Physiological Integrity: Reduction of Risk Potential:* **Cognitive Level** *– Analysis*

MAKING NURSING DECISIONS: A rule of thumb when answering test questions is this: If anyone gives the nurse information about a client, the nurse's first intervention is to assess the client. The nurse should always make decisions based on his or her assessment of the client.

14. 1. **Although cystectomy is a major surgical procedure, it has a predictable course, and no complications were identified. After removing the bladder, the client must have an ileal conduit. This is expected with this type of surgery, and the new graduate nurse could be assigned of this client.**
2. A client on continuous hemodialysis would require a nurse trained in this area of nursing; therefore, this client should be assigned to a more experienced nurse.
3. Renal trauma is unpredictable and requires continuous assessment. A more experienced nurse should be assigned to this client.
4. An eviscerated wound indicates the client's incision has opened and the bowels are out of the abdomen. This client is critically ill and should not be assigned to an inexperienced nurse.

Content – Medical/Surgical: **Category of Health Alteration** *– Genitourinary:* **Integrated Processes** *– Nursing Process: Planning:* **Client Needs** *– Safe and Effective Care Environment: Management of Care:* **Cognitive Level** *– Synthesis*

MAKING NURSING DECISIONS: When the test taker is deciding which client should be assigned to a new graduate, the most stable client should be assigned to the least experienced nurse.

15. 1. The charge nurse should have as many beds as possible available for any clients who must be transferred to the unit. The charge nurse should send a nurse to ED and then assess the bed situation.
2. This may need to be done, but it is not the first intervention, and the charge nurse could assign this to a staff member who is not providing direct client care.
3. **Most disaster policies require one nurse to be sent immediately from each area; therefore, this intervention should be implemented first. The charge nurse must determine which staff nurse would be most helpful in the ED without compromising the staffing in the ICU.**
4. The charge nurse should not request anyone leave the hospital. This is not typical protocol for a disaster.

Content – Medical/Surgical: **Category of Health Alteration** *– Genitourinary:* **Integrated Processes** *– Nursing Process: Implementation:* **Client Needs** *– Safe and Effective Care Environment: Safety and Infection Control:* **Cognitive Level** *– Application*

MAKING NURSING DECISIONS: The nurse must be knowledgeable of emergency preparedness. Employees receive this information in employee orientation and are responsible for implementing procedures correctly. The NCSBN NCLEX-RN® blueprint includes questions on safe and effective care environment.

16. 1. The nurse must diffuse the situation and remove the mother from the client's room because a seriously ill client does not need to be yelled at.
2. Hospital security does not need to be called unless the mother refuses to leave the client's room in the critical care unit.
3. **The nurse should remove the mother from the room and allow her to ventilate her feelings about the accident her son sustained while he was under the influence.**
4. The nurse should remove the mother because she is upset and let her ventilate. Telling the mother she must be quiet is

condescending, and when someone is upset, telling the person to be quiet is not helpful.

Content – Medical/Surgical: **Category of Health Alteration** *– Genitourinary:* **Integrated Processes** *– Nursing Process: Implementation:* **Client Needs** *– Psychosocial Integrity:* **Cognitive Level** *– Application*

MAKING NURSING DECISIONS: The NCLEX-RN® blueprint includes Therapeutic Community as a subcategory in Psychosocial Integrity. The nurse should allow clients and family to ventilate feelings.

17. 1. The nurse may need to administer an anti-spasmodic medication, but not before assessment of the client. Bladder spasms in a client who has had a TURP are usually caused by clots remaining in the bladder. A three-way indwelling catheter that is working properly will flush the clots from the bladder.
2. The nurse should calculate the client's urine output, but that is not the first intervention and will not address the client's pain.
3. The nurse could palpate the client's bladder for distention, but this will not help decrease the client's pain.
4. **The three-way indwelling catheter is placed during surgery to keep blood clots from remaining in the bladder and causing bladder spasms and increasing bleeding. The nurse should first assess the drainage system to make sure that it has not become obstructed with a clot.**

Content – Medical/Surgical : **Category of Health Alteration** *– Genitourinary:* **Integrated Processes** *– Nursing Process: Assessment:* **Client Needs** *– Physiological Integrity: Reduction of Risk Potential:* **Cognitive Level** *– Analysis*

MAKING NURSING DECISIONS: The test taker should use a systematic guide when deciding on a priority intervention. The nursing process is an excellent tool for the test taker to use in this question. Assessment is the first step of the nursing process.

18. 1. The client with polycystic kidney disease, the most common life-threatening genetic disease in the world, is expected to have hypertension along with hematuria and a feeling of heaviness in the back, side, or abdomen. The nurse should not assess this client first since the clinical manifestations are expected.
2. The clinical manifestation of bladder cancer is painless gross hematuria; therefore, the nurse would not assess this client first.
3. The nurse should check to determine whether the client has passed a stone, but this is a desired outcome and could wait until the

client with an emergency has been assessed and appropriate interventions initiated.
4. **The client with acute pyelonephritis, an inflammation of the renal parenchyma and collecting system, is not expected to get dehydrated; therefore, this client should be assessed first.**

Content – Medical/Surgical: **Category of Health Alteration** *– Genitourinary:* **Integrated Processes** *– Nursing Process: Assessment:* **Client Needs** *– Physiological Integrity: Reduction of Risk Potential:* **Cognitive Level** *– Analysis*

MAKING NURSING DECISIONS: The test taker must read all the options to determine whether an option contains a life-threatening situation. If an option contains information that is expected or within normal limits, that client does not have priority.

19. 1. Avoiding crowds may help the elderly client avoid getting a cold or the flu, but it is not the important intervention to help prevent getting sick during the winter months.
2. **The yearly flu shot is the best way to help prevent getting sick during the winter months, since the flu can cause serious illness, and even death, in the elderly. Alport syndrome is also known as chronic hereditary nephritis.**
3. Eating a well-balanced diet is helpful, but it will not ensure the elderly do not get sick during the winter months.
4. Dressing appropriately in the winter months is appropriate, but the flu vaccine provides the elderly with added immunity.

Content – Medical/Surgical: **Category of Health Alteration** *– Genitourinary:* **Integrated Processes** *– Nursing Process: Implementation:* **Client Needs** *– Physiological Integrity: Physiological Adaptation:* **Cognitive Level** *– Application*

MAKING NURSING DECISIONS: The nurse must be able to teach health promotion to clients. Immunizations are priority for children and the elderly.

20. 1. Hormone replacement therapy may be needed, but not due to vaginal dryness. The client should discuss this with her HCP, but it does not address the client's statement.
2. Many elderly are sexually active and sexual activity should be encouraged by the nurse, not discouraged.
3. **Vaginal lubricant will help with the vaginal dryness and help decrease pain during sexual intercourse.**
4. Vaginal dryness is common in the elderly, but the nurse should discuss ways to address the dryness, not explain that it is normal.

Content – Medical/Surgical: Category of Health Alteration – Genitourinary: Integrated Processes – Nursing Process: Implementation: Client Needs – Physiological Integrity: Physiological Adaptation: Cognitive Level – Application

MAKING NURSING DECISIONS: When the question asks for the priority intervention, it means one or more of the options could be something a nurse might discuss with the client. The test taker should select the option that answers the client's statement directly.

21. 1. Fosamax should be administered in the morning on an empty stomach to increase absorption, but it is not priority over the client's sitting up for 30 minutes. The client should remain upright for at least 30 minutes to prevent regurgitation into the esophagus and esophageal erosion.
2. The client with peptic ulcer disease may be more a risk for esophageal erosion, but the HCP should have assessed this prior to prescribing this medication for the client.
3. The client with osteoporosis should be encouraged to walk to increase bone density, but this is not pertinent when administering the medication.
4. **Fosamax should be administered on an empty stomach with a full glass of water to promote absorption of the medication. The client should remain upright for at least 30 minutes to prevent regurgitation into the esophagus and esophageal erosion.**
Content – Medical/Surgical: Category of Health Alteration – Drug Administration: Integrated Processes – Nursing Process: Implementation: Client Needs – Physiological Integrity: Pharmacological and Parenteral Therapies: Cognitive Level – Application

MAKING NURSING DECISIONS: The nurse must be aware of interventions that must be implemented when administering medications. The nurse must know which interventions will help prevent untoward complications when administering medications.

22. 1. **The LPN is qualified to perform a sterile procedure, such as inserting an indwelling catheter before surgery. This is an appropriate assignment.**
2. Turning and repositioning a client can be delegated to an unlicensed assistive personnel (UAP).
3. Emptying a client's bedside commode and recording the amount of urine can be delegated to a UAP.
4. The nurse should feed the client who choked during the last meal to assess the client's

ability to swallow. This client is unstable and cannot be assigned/delegated.
Content – Medical/Surgical: Category of Health Alteration – Genitourinary: Integrated Processes – Nursing Process: Planning: Client Needs – Safe and Effective Care Environment: Management of Care: Cognitive Level – Synthesis

MAKING NURSING DECISIONS: The nurse cannot delegate or assign assessment, teaching, evaluation, or an unstable client to an LPN. The LPN can transcribe HCP orders, can call HCPs on the phone to obtain orders for a client, and can perform sterile procedures.

23. 1. **The therapeutic PTT level should be 1.5 to 2 times the normal PTT of 39 seconds. The therapeutic levels of heparin are 58 and 78. With a PTT of 92, the client is at risk for bleeding, and the heparin drip should be held. The nurse should assess this client first.**
2. The client on peritoneal dialysis should have clear dialysate, so this client does not have to be assessed first.
3. The client on hemodialysis should have an audible bruit over the fistula, which indicates the fistula is patent.
4. Cystitis is inflammation of the urinary bladder, and burning on urination is an expected symptom.
Content – Medical/Surgical: Category of Health Alteration – Genitourinary: Integrated Processes – Nursing Process: Assessment: Client Needs – Physiological Integrity: Reduction of Risk Potential: Cognitive Level – Analysis

MAKING NURSING DECISIONS: The test taker must determine if any of the assessment data are normal or abnormal for the client's diagnosis. If the data are abnormal, then this client should be seen first.

24. 1. Digoxin can be administered later because it is a routine medication.
2. Lasix can be administered within the 1-hour leeway (30 minutes before and after); it does not need to be administered first.
3. Darvon is not due yet; the nurse should assess the client and determine whether non-pharmacological interventions to relieve pain can be implemented, but this medication cannot be administered for 2 hours.
4. **Tylenol is administered for mild-to-moderate pain. By the time the nurse obtains the medication and performs all of the steps to administer a medication correctly, it will be time for the client to receive the Tylenol. This medication should be administered first.**

Content – Medical/Surgical: **Category of Health Alteration** *– Genitourinary:* **Integrated Processes** *– Nursing Process: Implementation:* **Client Needs –** *Physiological Integrity: Pharmacological and Parenteral Therapies:* **Cognitive Level** *– Application*

MAKING NURSING DECISIONS: The nurse must be knowledgeable of how and when to administer medications.

25. 1. **Credé's maneuver is a method used for expressing urine by pressing the hand on the bladder, especially a paralyzed bladder. It is a non-invasive procedure and should be implemented first prior to catheterization, which is an invasive procedure.**
     2. Intermittent catheterization is an invasive procedure, which may lead to possible infection when done every 3 to 4 hours.
     3. The nurse could place the client on the bedside commode, but this is used for clients with an uninhibited bladder pattern.
     4. Drinking water prior to attempting to urinate will not help the client.

Content – Medical/Surgical: **Category of Health Alteration** *– Genitourinary:* **Integrated Processes** *– Nursing Process: Implementation:* **Client Needs –** *Physiological Integrity: Reduction of Risk Potential:* **Cognitive Level** *– Analysis*

MAKING NURSING DECISIONS: If the nurse was undecided between an invasive or a non-invasive procedure, the nurse should select the non-invasive procedure first.

26. 1. The client with pyelonephritis typically presents with costovertebral tenderness over the affected side; therefore, this is expected and the nurse would not assess this client first.
     2. **More than likely, this client has a urinary tract infection, which requires a midstream urinalysis. Of these four clients, this client should be seen first to have the test ordered.**
     3. The client with urethritis would present with these symptoms; therefore, the clinic nurse would not need to see this client first.
     4. Hesitancy, terminal dribbling, and intermittency are signs/symptoms of benign prostatic hypertrophy, which requires surgery; therefore, this client should not be seen prior to a client with a possible urinary tract infection.

Content – Medical/Surgical: **Category of Health Alteration** *– Genitourinary:* **Integrated Processes** *– Nursing Process: Assessment:* **Client Needs –** *Physiological Integrity: Reduction of Risk Potential:* **Cognitive Level** *– Analysis*

MAKING NURSING DECISIONS: When deciding which client to assess first, the test taker should

determine whether the signs/symptoms the client is exhibiting are normal for the client situation. After eliminating the expected options, the test taker should determine which situation can be cured, or which is more life threatening.

27. 1. The nurse should not delegate medication administration, including giving the client boxes of sample medications, to an unlicensed assistive personnel (UAP).
     2. Showing the client how to use a glucometer is teaching the client, and the nurse cannot delegate teaching.
     3. Triaging calls requires nursing judgment; this responsibility cannot be delegated to the UAP.
     4. **The UAP is trained to take vital signs on a client who is stable. This task could safely be delegated by the nurse.**

Content – Medical/Surgical: **Category of Health Alteration** *– Genitourinary:* **Integrated Processes** *– Nursing Process: Planning:* **Client Needs –** *Safe and Effective Care Environment: Management of Care:* **Cognitive Level** *– Synthesis*

MAKING NURSING DECISIONS: The nurse cannot delegate assessment, evaluation, teaching, administration of medications, or care of an unstable client to a UAP.

28. 1. **The unlicensed assistive personnel (UAP) can escort a client who is stable to the radiology department; therefore, this is the most appropriate task to delegate to the UAP.**
     2. The UAP cannot obtain a sterile specimen; therefore, this task cannot be delegated.
     3. The UAP cannot hang intravenous bags because they are medications, and medication administration cannot be delegated to a UAP.
     4. Discharge instructions are teaching, and teaching cannot be delegated to a UAP.

Content – Medical/Surgical: **Category of Health Alteration** *– Genitourinary:* **Integrated Processes** *– Nursing Process: Planning:* **Client Needs –** *Safe and Effective Care Environment: Management of Care:* **Cognitive Level** *– Synthesis*

MAKING NURSING DECISIONS: An RN cannot delegate assessment, teaching, evaluation, medications, or an unstable client to a UAP. Tasks that cannot be delegated are nursing interventions requiring nursing judgment.

29. 1. The unlicensed assistive personnel (UAP) cannot administer medication or evaluate the effectiveness of medication; therefore, this task cannot be delegated.
     2. This is a legal issue and should not be delegated to the UAP.

3. **The UAP can apply ice to the right ankle since the client is stable.**
4. The nurse should complete the incident report, not the UAP.
*Content – Medical/Surgical: **Category of Health Alteration** – Genitourinary: **Integrated Processes** – Nursing Process: Planning: **Client Needs** – Safe and Effective Care Environment: Management of Care: **Cognitive Level** – Synthesis*

MAKING NURSING DECISIONS: The nurse cannot delegate assessment, teaching, evaluation, medications, or an unstable client to the UAP. Remember, most forms should be completed by the individual whom the form is about, not completed by someone who is not aware of the situation.

30. 1. **The LPN can administer medication to the client; therefore, this is an appropriate assignment.**
2. The unlicensed assistive personnel (UAP) cannot call in prescription refills to the pharmacist.
3. The LPN can obtain the weight/height of a client, but the UAP can do this task, so it is more appropriate to delegate it to the UAP.
4. The UAP can empty the trashcans, but the custodian/housekeeper would be a more appropriate delegation of this task.
*Content – Medical/Surgical: **Category of Health Alteration** – Genitourinary: **Integrated Processes** – Nursing Process: Planning: **Client Needs** – Safe and Effective Care Environment: Management of Care: **Cognitive Level** – Synthesis*

MAKING NURSING DECISIONS: The nurse cannot delegate assessment, teaching, evaluation, medications, or an unstable client to the UAP. The nurse cannot assign assessment, teaching, evaluation, or an unstable client to the LVN. Remember to delegate/assign the task to the least educated person who can safely do the task.

31. 1. **The unlicensed assistive personnel (UAP) is violating HIPAA rules concerning confidentiality, so the clinical manager should intervene.**
2. The LPN can talk to the client over the phone about laboratory tests so this does not warrant intervention.
3. The RN can triage phone messages, so this does not warrant intervention.
4. The UAP can take vital signs on a client who is stable, and clients in an outpatient clinic are considered stable unless otherwise specified.
*Content – Medical/Surgical: **Category of Health Alteration** – Genitourinary: **Integrated Processes** – Nursing Process: Implementation: **Client Needs** – Safe*

*and Effective Care Environment: Management of Care: **Cognitive Level** – Analysis*

MAKING NURSING DECISIONS: The nurse is responsible for the actions and behavior of UAPs and LPNs working in the unit. The nurse must correct behavior as needed.

32. 1. The unlicensed assistive personnel (UAP) is a member of the healthcare team and should be able to listen to a student's concerns.
2. The nurse cannot violate the student's rights, even in the school nurse setting.
3. **The nurse should allow the UAP to continue to talk to the female student, and then the nurse can talk to the student after the UAP and student finish talking.**
4. The UAP has established a relationship with the student and should be allowed to talk to the student. If the student had wanted to talk to the school nurse, the student would have done so.
*Content – Medical/Surgical: **Category of Health Alteration** – Genitourinary: **Integrated Processes** – Nursing Process: Implementation: **Client Needs** – Psychosocial Integrity: **Cognitive Level** – Application*

MAKING NURSING DECISIONS: The nurse is responsible for the actions and behavior of UAPs in any healthcare setting. The nurse should know when to intervene and when not to intervene.

33. 1. This is a breach of confidentiality. The LPN should not discuss the client's health problem in the waiting room area where everyone can hear.
2. **The nurse should remove the LPN from the situation without embarrassing the LPN. Asking the LPN to come to the office area is the appropriate action for the nurse to take. The LPN's action is a violation of HIPAA.**
3. The nurse should not correct the LPN's behavior in front of the client. This is embarrassing to both the LPN and the client.
4. The nurse does not have to report this to the HCP. The nurse can talk to the LPN concerning this breach of confidentiality.
*Content – Medical/Surgical: **Category of Health Alteration** – Genitourinary: **Integrated Processes** – Nursing Process: Implementation: **Client Needs** – Safe and Effective Care Environment: Management of Care: **Cognitive Level** – Application*

MAKING NURSING DECISIONS: The nurse is responsible for knowing and complying with local, state, and federal standards of care. The LPN's discussion of a confidential matter in a public area is a violation of HIPAA.

34. 1. The charge nurse must address this situation because it has been going on for more than a week.
2. Writing a memo does nothing to discover the cause of the tense atmosphere.
3. **The charge nurse should call a meeting and attempt to determine what is causing the staff's behavior and the tense atmosphere. The charge nurse could then problem-solve, with the goal being to have a more relaxed atmosphere in which to work.**
4. This is threatening, which is not an appropriate way to resolve a staff problem.
   Content – *Medical/Surgical:* ***Category of Health Alteration*** *– Genitourinary:* ***Integrated Processes*** *– Nursing Process: Planning:* ***Client Needs*** *– Safe and Effective Care Environment: Management of Care:* ***Cognitive Level*** *– Synthesis*

MAKING NURSING DECISIONS: In any business, including a healthcare facility, arguing should not occur among staff of any level where the customers—in this case, the clients—can hear it or see it. The nurse should address the situation directly with the staff members.

35. 1. Obtaining a urine sample is not an invasive procedure and does not require informed consent.
2. **The urine specimen must adhere to a chain of custody, so the client cannot dispute the results.**
3. The bathroom for drug testing should not have access to any water via a sink, so that the client cannot dilute the urine specimen.
4. The tympanic temperature is taken in the client's ear and is not required for a urine drug sample.
   Content – *Medical/Surgical:* ***Category of Health Alteration*** *– Genitourinary:* ***Integrated Processes*** *– Nursing Process: Implementation:* ***Client Needs*** *– Physiological Integrity: Reduction of Risk Potential:* ***Cognitive Level*** *– Application*

MAKING NURSING DECISIONS: There are management questions on the NCLEX-RN®. In many instances, there is no test-taking strategy for these questions. The nurse must be knowledgeable of management issues, and know what must comply with local, state, and federal requirements.

36. 1. Any client seen in the clinic should have the vital signs taken, but given the signs/symptoms of the client, the nurse should first obtain a urinalysis.
2. The nurse should determine whether there has been blood in the urine, but it is not the

nurse's first intervention. The HCP needs a urinalysis to confirm the probable diagnosis.
3. **The client is verbalizing the classic signs/symptoms of a urinary tract infection, but it must be confirmed with a urinalysis. The nurse should first obtain the specimen so the results will be available by the time the HCP sees the client.**
4. The nurse should always teach the client and asking this question is appropriate, but it is not the clinic nurse's first intervention.
   Content – *Medical/Surgical:* ***Category of Health Alteration*** *– Genitourinary:* ***Integrated Processes*** *– Nursing Process: Assessment:* ***Client Needs*** *– Physiological Integrity: Reduction of Risk Potential:* ***Cognitive Level*** *– Analysis*

MAKING NURSING DECISIONS: The client's signs/symptoms often provide the nurse with the most likely problem, and the nurse should confirm the condition with a laboratory test, if possible. Clinic and emergency room nurses obtain tests so the HCP will have the results when seen.

37. 1. The nurse may need to know how long the client will be in the shelter, but this is not priority during the initial assessment of the client.
2. **During a disaster, the priority is to determine whether the client has routine medications that can be taken while in the shelter. If clients have life-sustaining medications, then obtaining the medications becomes priority. Remember, psychiatric medications are life sustaining.**
3. The client's health history is important, but no matter what the history is, if the client does not have life-sustaining medications, the client will end up in the hospital.
4. The client should be assessed, but unless the client has a specific complaint in this situation, assessment of vital signs, height, and weight is not priority.
   Content – *Medical/Surgical:* ***Category of Health Alteration*** *– Genitourinary:* ***Integrated Processes*** *– Nursing Process: Implementation:* ***Client Needs*** *– Safe and Effective Care Environment: Management of Care:* ***Cognitive Level*** *– Application*

MAKING NURSING DECISIONS: The nurse must be knowledgeable of emergency preparedness. This is part of hospital requirements since 9/11. The NCSBN NCLEX-RN® blueprint includes questions on safe and effective care environment.

38. 1. The nurse should ask whether the client is allergic to iodine, such as shellfish.
2. An incompetent client cannot sign the consent form. Because the client is diagnosed

with schizophrenia, asking him to sign a permit form is not an appropriate intervention.

3. **An incompetent client is an individual who is not autonomous and cannot give or withhold consent—for example, individuals who are cognitively impaired, mentally ill, neurologically incapacitated, or under the influence of mind-altering drugs. This client is diagnosed with schizophrenia, a mental illness, and is delusional; therefore, the client's significant other must sign for the procedure.**

4. This procedure is performed in the radiology department, not in a day surgery department.

Content – Medical/Surgical: ***Category of Health Alteration*** *– Genitourinary:* ***Integrated Processes*** *– Nursing Process: Diagnosis:* ***Client Needs*** *– Psychosocial Integrity:* ***Cognitive Level*** *– Application*

MAKING NURSING DECISIONS: The NCLEX-RN® blueprint includes questions on nursing care that is ruled by legal requirements. The nurse must be knowledgeable of these issues.

39. 1. Some herbal supplements can interact with prescribed medications and become dangerous, but saw palmetto is not one of them.

2. **Saw palmetto is recommended by many urologists and used to treat BPH; therefore, this is the most appropriate statement.**

3. The nurse should notify the client's HCP, but the best response is to support the client's use of saw palmetto for BPH.

4. This is a true statement, but the nurse should address the client taking the saw palmetto, not make a general statement.

Content – Medical/Surgical: ***Category of Health Alteration*** *– Complimentary Alternative Medicine:* ***Integrated Processes*** *– Nursing Process: Implementation:* ***Client Needs*** *– Physiological Integrity: Pharmacological and Parenteral Therapies:* ***Cognitive Level*** *– Application*

MAKING NURSING DECISIONS: The NCLEX-RN® tests complementary alternative medicine (CAM), so the nurse must be familiar with the common herbs used to treat disease processes.

40. 1. This is the role of the speech therapist, a member of the home care team.

2. This is the role of the occupational therapist, a member of the home care team.

3. This is the role of the social worker, a member of the home care team.

4. **This is the role of the physical therapist, a member of the home care team.**

Content – Medical/Surgical: ***Category of Health Alteration*** *– Genitourinary:* ***Integrated Processes*** *– Nursing Process: Implementation:* ***Client Needs*** *– Health*

Promotion and Maintenance: ***Cognitive Level*** *– Comprehension*

MAKING NURSING DECISIONS: The home health (HH) nurse must know the roles of the members of the home care team. The HH nurse must be able to make appropriate referrals.

41. 1. **The NCSBN NCLEX-RN® test blueprint includes referrals, under Management of Care. The client is in spiritual distress, and the chaplain is the member of the team who addresses spiritual needs.**

2. The nurse should not discuss the client's concerns with the client's pastor. The nurse should contact the agency chaplain, and then, if needed, the agency chaplain could talk to the client's pastor.

3. This is crossing professional boundaries. The nurse should not impose his or her religious beliefs on the client. If the client asks the nurse to pray, then the nurse could—but the nurse should not ask the client to pray.

4. The client is verbalizing thoughts about dying, not asking questions about living wills. This would not be an appropriate intervention.

Content – Medical/Surgical: ***Category of Health Alteration*** *– Genitourinary:* ***Integrated Processes*** *– Nursing Process: Implementation:* ***Client Needs*** *– Psychosocial Integrity:* ***Cognitive Level*** *– Application*

MAKING NURSING DECISIONS: The test taker must be knowledgeable of the roles of all members of the multidisciplinary healthcare team.

42. 1. This is a private moment between the client and spouse; the nurse should not impose on the situation.

2. The client and spouse did not ask for help; the nurse should not assume that help is needed.

3. **This is a private moment and should be respected by the nurse. The nurse should allow the client and spouse quiet time together.**

4. This is a private moment between the client and spouse; the nurse should not impose on the situation.

Content – Medical/Surgical: ***Category of Health Alteration*** *– Genitourinary:* ***Integrated Processes*** *– Nursing Process: Implementation:* ***Client Needs*** *– Psychosocial Integrity:* ***Cognitive Level*** *– Application*

MAKING NURSING DECISIONS: The nurse must be aware of spiritual needs and help to support the client's needs whenever possible.

43. 1. Clocking in late twice in a year's time is not a pattern of behavior.

2. The nurse involved in a code would not be able to leave the code to answer a call light.

3. The nurse has covered him- or herself, or may be changing to cover someone else. This action is assuming responsibility for the client care on the unit and does not require a mention in the evaluation, unless the nurse is changing at the request of management.

4. **The nurse's care is being evaluated, including the nurse's documentation. The completeness of documentation should be included in the evaluation.**

Content – Medical/Surgical: **Category of Health Alteration** *– Genitourinary:* **Integrated Processes** *– Nursing Process: Planning:* **Client Needs** *– Safe and Effective Care Environment: Management of Care:* **Cognitive Level** *– Synthesis*

MAKING NURSING DECISIONS: There will be management questions on the NCLEX-RN®. In many instances, there is no test-taking strategy for these questions; the nurse must be knowledgeable of management issues.

44. 1. This is a nice gesture, but the priority is to provide support when the family and friends have returned to their own lives.

2. **The family and friends will have returned to their own lives 1 to 2 months after a family member has died. This is when the next of kin needs support from the hospice nurse. Hospice will follow up with the significant other for up to 13 months.**

3. This is the family's responsibility, not that of the hospice nurse.

4. This is not the nurse's responsibility and should be discouraged for a short period of time. In the immediate grieving period, the significant other may get rid of possessions that later he or she may wish had been kept.

Content – Medical/Surgical: **Category of Health Alteration** *– Genitourinary:* **Integrated Processes** *– Nursing Process: Implementation:* **Client Needs** *– Psychosocial Integrity:* **Cognitive Level** *– Application*

MAKING NURSING DECISIONS: The test taker must be knowledgeable of the roles of all members of the multidisciplinary healthcare team. This knowledge will be tested on the NCLEX-RN® exam.

45. 1. The nurse should not continue to attempt IV access if there is another nurse available who may be able to insert the IV line successfully.

2. The client needs IV replacement at this time.

3. **After two attempts, the nurse should arrange for a second nurse to attempt the placement.**

4. Cold packs would cause the circulatory system to contract and make it more difficult to start an IV line. Hot packs dilate the blood vessels.

Content – Medical/Surgical: **Category of Health Alteration** *– Genitourinary:* **Integrated Processes** *– Nursing Process: Implementation:* **Client Needs** *– Physiological Integrity: Basic Care and Comfort:* **Cognitive Level** *– Application*

MAKING NURSING DECISIONS: The nurse must be able to perform skills safely. The nurse should not continue to inflict pain on the client after attempting invasive procedures more than twice.

46. 1. The unlicensed assistive personnel (UAP) should not use soap when bathing a client diagnosed with CKD. Soap is drying and the client diagnosed with CKD has altered skin integrity.

2. **The nurse should stop the UAP from using the arm with the graft. Pressure on the graft could occlude the graft.**

3. The UAP can tell the client not to eat contraband food. This is not teaching.

4. This is an appropriate action for the UAP; the nurse would not need to intervene.

Content – Medical/Surgical: **Category of Health Alteration** *– Genitourinary:* **Integrated Processes** *– Nursing Process: Assessment:* **Client Needs** *– Safe and Effective Care Environment: Safety and Infection Control:* **Cognitive Level** *– Analysis*

MAKING NURSING DECISIONS: "Delegation" means that the nurse is responsible for the UAP's actions and performance. The nurse must correct the UAP's performance to ensure the client is cared for safely, in the hospital or the home.

47. 1. Lanoxin is frequently ordered for elderly patients with a history of heart failure. The nurse should take an apical heart rate and hold the medication if the apical pulse is less than 60. This is a maintenance dose of the medication.

2. Lasix is a diuretic frequently prescribed for patients with a history of heart failure. The nurse should determine if the patient is having muscle cramping, which is a sign of potassium deficiency. The nurse would not question administering this medication without an indication of potassium deficiency.

3. K Dur is potassium, which is given to prevent potassium depletion when administering a diuretic.

4. **Dulcolax is a stimulant laxative. Overuse of stimulant laxatives can cause laxative dependency and colon obstruction. The nurse should contact the HCP and**

arrange for a bulk laxative if the client requires a daily laxative.

Content – Medical/Surgical: **Category of Health Alteration** *– Genitourinary:* **Integrated Processes** *– Nursing Process: Assessment:* **Client Needs** *– Physiological Integrity: Pharmacological and Parenteral Therapies:* **Cognitive Level** *– Analysis*

MAKING NURSING DECISIONS: This is an alternate type of question included in the NCLEX-RN® blueprint. The test taker must be able to read a medication administration record (MAR), be knowledgeable of medications, and be able to make an appropriate decision as to the nurse's most appropriate intervention.

48. **Answer: 88 mL per hour (350 divided by 4 hours = 87.5 mL per hour)**
The client is diagnosed with heart failure, which indicates the client is at high risk for fluid volume overload when administering any type of fluids. Blood must be administered within 4 hours.

Content – Medical/Surgical: **Category of Health Alteration** *– Drug Administration:* **Integrated Processes** *– Nursing Process: Implementation:* **Client Needs** *– Physiological Integrity: Pharmacological and Parenteral Therapies:* **Cognitive Level** *– Application*

MAKING NURSING DECISIONS: The NCLEX-RN® blueprint includes dosage calculations under Pharmacological and Parenteral Therapies. This category is included under Physiological Integrity, which promotes physical health and wellness by providing care and comfort, reducing client risk potential, and managing health alterations.

49. **3, 4, and 5 are correct.**
1. Teaching is the responsibility of the nurse and cannot be delegated to an unlicensed assistive personnel (UAP).
2. The word "check" indicates a step in the assessment process, and the nurse cannot delegate assessing to a UAP.
3. **The client is 2 days postoperative and vital signs should be stable so the UAP can take vital signs. The nurse must make sure the UAP knows when to immediately notify him/her of vital signs not within the guidelines the nurse provides to the UAP.**
4. **This action does not require judging, assessing, teaching, or evaluating on the part of the UAP. This task can be delegated to the UAP.**
5. **A client who is 2 days postoperative should be ambulating frequently. The UAP can perform this task.**

Content – Medical/Surgical: **Category of Health Alteration** *– Genitourinary:* **Integrated Processes** *– Nursing Process: Planning:* **Client Needs** *– Safe and Effective Care Environment: Management of Care:* **Cognitive Level** *– Synthesis*

MAKING NURSING DECISIONS: This is an alternate type of question included in the NCLEX-RN®. The nurse must be able to select all of the options that answer the question correctly. There are no partially correct answers.

50. 1. The nurse could obtain the client's pulse oximeter reading, but this client is hemorrhaging and the surgeon should be notified immediately.
2. Checking the client's last H&H could be done, but this client's AP and B/P are indicating hemorrhaging; therefore, the first intervention is to notify the client's surgeon.
3. **The client's apical pulse (AP) and blood pressure (B/P) indicate the client is hemorrhaging; therefore, the nurse should first notify the client's surgeon.**
4. The nurse could monitor the client's urine output, but it will not help the client's hemorrhaging; therefore, this is not the nurse's first intervention.

Content – Medical/Surgical: **Category of Health Alteration** *– Genitourinary:* **Integrated Processes** *– Nursing Process: Assessment:* **Client Needs** *– Physiological Integrity: Reduction of Risk Potential:* **Cognitive Level** *– Analysis*

MAKING NURSING DECISIONS: The test taker needs to read all of the options carefully before choosing the option that says, "Notify the HCP." If any of the options will provide information the HCP needs to know in order to make a decision, the test taker should choose that option. If, however, the HCP does not need any additional information to make a decision and the nurse suspects the condition is serious or life threatening, the priority intervention is to call the HCP.

51. Correct Answer: 4, 5, 2, 3, 1
4. **Safety should be the primary concern of the nurse. A bedside commode will provide the client with an option that is easier to get to than walking to the bathroom and prevent the client from slipping on urine that may be dribbled.**
5. **The nurse needs to obtain a urine culture, so antibiotic therapy can be initiated.**
2. **This will help the client stay dry and not soil his or her clothes, as well as allowing some independence in ambulation in the room and hallways.**

3. **This will protect the bed and the client from soiling.**
1. **Providing frequent assistance with toileting will prevent the client from having incontinence.**

Content – Medical/Surgical: ***Category of Health Alteration*** *– Genitourinary:* ***Integrated Processes*** *– Nursing Process: Assessment:* ***Client Needs*** *– Physiological Integrity: Reduction of Risk Potential:* ***Cognitive Level*** *– Analysis*

MAKING NURSING DECISIONS: This is an alternate type of question included in the NCLEX-RN® blueprint. The nurse must be able to implement interventions in the correct order.

52. 1. These laboratory findings are low, but would not require a blood transfusion. These laboratory findings are often expected in a client who is anemic secondary to chronic kidney disease.
2. This client's dialysis access is compromised and should be assessed, but this is not life threatening.
3. This client should be seen, but not prior to a potentially life-threatening situation.
4. **The client on peritoneal dialysis who has a hard, rigid abdomen has a potentially life-threatening complication; this client should be assessed first and then sent to the hospital.**

Content – Medical/Surgical: ***Category of Health Alteration*** *– Genitourinary:* ***Integrated Processes*** *– Nursing Process: Assessment:* ***Client Needs*** *– Physiological Integrity: Reduction of Risk Potential:* ***Cognitive Level*** *– Analysis*

MAKING NURSING DECISIONS: The test taker must determine if any of the assessment data are normal or abnormal for the client's diagnosis. If the data are abnormal, then this client should be seen first. If the data are normal, then a client with a psychosocial problem is the client the nurse should assess first.

53. 1. This pulse oximeter reading is above 93%; therefore, this information does not warrant notifying the healthcare provider.
2. The client's platelet count is within normal limits; therefore, this information does not warrant notifying the healthcare provider.
3. **After the initial administration of erythropoietin, a client's antihypertensive medications may need to be adjusted. Therefore, this elevated blood pressure warrants notifying the healthcare provider. Erythropoietin therapy is contraindicated in clients with hypertension that cannot be controlled.**

4. The client's tympanic temperature is within normal limits; therefore, this does not warrant notifying the healthcare provider.

Content – Medical/Surgical: ***Category of Health Alteration*** *– Genitourinary:* ***Integrated Processes*** *– Nursing Process: Assessment:* ***Client Needs*** *– Physiological Integrity: Pharmacological and Parenteral Therapies:* ***Cognitive Level*** *– Analysis*

MAKING NURSING DECISIONS: The test taker should select the option that is potentially life threatening, or a complaint that would require the medication to be adjusted or discontinued. The nurse should notify the HCP if the medication is causing an adverse effect, not an expected side effect.

54. 1. The stem of the question does not provide any information indicating the client has a self-care deficit, and it is not automatically suspected with a client diagnosed with chronic kidney disease.
2. Teaching is always an important part of the care plan, but it is not priority over a physiological problem.
3. Chronic pain may occur with a client diagnosed with chronic kidney disease, but would not be priority over excess fluid volume.
4. **Excess fluid volume is priority because of the stress placed on the heart and vessels, which could lead to heart failure, pulmonary edema, and death.**

Content – Medical/Surgical: ***Category of Health Alteration*** *– Genitourinary:* ***Integrated Processes*** *– Nursing Process: Planning:* ***Client Needs*** *– Physiological Integrity: Physiological Adaptation:* ***Cognitive Level*** *– Synthesis*

MAKING NURSING DECISIONS: The NCLEX-RN® integrates the nursing process throughout the Client Needs categories and subcategories. The nursing process is a scientific, clinical reasoning approach to client care that includes assessment, analysis, planning, implementation, and evaluation. The nurse will be responsible for identifying a nursing diagnosis for clients.

55. **Answer: 300 mL.** The nurse must add up how many milliliters of fluid the client drank on the 7 a.m. to 7 p.m. shift, then subtract that number from 1,500 mL to determine how much fluid the client can receive on the 7 p.m. to 7 a.m. shift. One ounce is equal to 30 mL. The client drank 26 ounces (8 + 8 + 16 + 8) of fluid, or 1,200 mL (40 × 30) of fluid. Therefore, the client can have 300 mL (1,500 – 1,200) of fluid on the 7 p.m. to 7 a.m. shift.
Content – Medical/Surgical: ***Category of Health Alteration*** *– Genitourinary:* ***Integrated***

Processes – Nursing Process: Implementation: **Client Needs** *– Physiological Integrity: Reduction of Risk Potential:* **Cognitive Level** *– Application*

MAKING NURSING DECISIONS: The NCLEX-RN® blueprint includes dosage calculations under Pharmacological and Parenteral Therapies. This category is included under Physiological Integrity, which promotes physical health and wellness by providing care and comfort, reducing client risk potential, and managing health alterations.

56. 1. Reverse Trendelenburg position has the nurse elevating the client's chair, which will not help the client's dizziness and light-headedness.
    2. Decreasing the volume of blood being re-moved is an appropriate intervention, but it will not help the client's dizziness and light-headedness as fast as will infusing normal saline.
    3. **Normal saline infusion increases the amount of volume in the bloodstream, which will decrease the client's light-headedness and dizziness.**
    4. Hypotension is an expected occurrence in clients receiving dialysis; therefore, the HCP does not need to be notified.

Content – Medical/Surgical: **Category of Health Alteration** *– Genitourinary:* **Integrated Processes** *– Nursing Process: Implementation:* **Client Needs** *– Physiological Integrity: Reduction of Risk Potential:* **Cognitive Level** *– Analysis*

MAKING NURSING DECISIONS: When the question asks, "Which intervention should be implemented first?" it means all the options are things a nurse could implement, but only one should be implemented first. The nurse should use the nursing process and remember: If the client is in distress, do not assess; if the client is not in distress, the nurse should assess.

57. 3, 4, and 5 are correct.
    1. TPN is a hypertonic solution that has enough calories, proteins, lipids, electrolytes, and trace elements to sustain life. It is admin-istered via a pump to prevent too rapid infu-sion. It should not be administered without a pump or via a gravity intravenous line.
    2. TPN contains 50% dextrose solution; there-fore, the client is monitored to ensure that the pancreas is adapting to the high glucose levels. The glucose level is checked every 6 hours, not every 24 hours.
    3. **The client is weighed daily in the same clothes and at the same time to monitor for fluid overload and evaluate daily weight.**

4. **The IV tubing is changed with every bag because the high glucose level can cause bacterial growth.**
5. **Intake and output are monitored to observe for fluid balance.**

Content – Medical/Surgical: **Category of Health Alteration** *– Drug Administration:* **Integrated Processes** *– Nursing Process: Implementation:* **Client Needs** *– Physiological Integrity: Pharmacological and Parenteral Therapies:* **Cognitive Level** *– Application*

MAKING NURSING DECISIONS: This is an alternate type of question included in the NCLEX-RN®. The nurse must be able to select all of the options that answer the question correctly. There are no partially correct answers.

58. **Correct Answer: 2, 1, 4, 5, 3**
    2. **The client has signs of phlebitis and the IV must be removed to prevent further complications.**
    1. **A new IV will be started in the right hand after the IV is discontinued.**
    4. **A warm washcloth placed on an IV site sometimes provides comfort to the client. If this is done, it should be done for 20 minutes four times a day.**
    5. **All pertinent situations should be documented in the client's chart.**
    3. **Depending on the healthcare facility, this may or may not be done, but client care comes before documentation.**

Content – Medical/Surgical: **Category of Health Alteration** *– Drug Administration:* **Integrated Processes** *– Nursing Process: Implementation:* **Client Needs** *– Safe and Effective Care Environment: Safety and Infection Control:* **Cognitive Level** *– Analysis*

MAKING NURSING DECISIONS: This is an alternate type of question included in the NCLEX-RN® blueprint. The nurse must be able to perform skills in the correct order. Documentation is always completed after direct client care.

59. 1. An unlicensed assistive personnel (UAP) can empty the catheter and measure the amount.
    2. The UAP can record intake and output on the I&O sheet.
    3. **The nurse cannot delegate teaching to the UAP.**
    4. The client has a disease, but all the UAP is being asked to do is take water to the client.

Content – Medical/Surgical: **Category of Health Alteration** *– Genitourinary:* **Integrated Processes** *– Nursing Process: Planning:* **Client Needs** *– Safe and Effective Care Environment: Management of Care:* **Cognitive Level** *– Synthesis*

MAKING NURSING DECISIONS: This is an "except" question. The nurse could determine which task is appropriate to delegate to the UAP; three options would be appropriate to delegate. The nurse should implement the task that is not appropriate to delegate. Remember, the nurse cannot delegate assessment, teaching, evaluation, medications, or an unstable client to the UAP.

60. **Answer: 890 mL.** First, determine the amount of irrigation fluid: 3,000 – 1,550 = 1,450 mL of irrigation fluid. Then, subtract 1,450 irrigation fluid from the drainage of 2,340 to determine the urine output: 2,340 – 1,450 = 890 mL of urine output

    Content – Medical/Surgical: **Category of Health Alteration** *– Genitourinary:* **Integrated Processes** *– Nursing Process: Implementation:* **Client Needs** *– Physiological Integrity: Pharmacological and Parenteral Therapies:* **Cognitive Level** *– Application*

MAKING NURSING DECISIONS: The NCLEX-RN® blueprint includes dosage calculations under Pharmacological and Parenteral Therapies. This category is included under Physiological Integrity, which promotes physical health and wellness by providing care and comfort, reducing client risk potential, and managing health alterations.

61. 1. TURPs may cause a sexual dysfunction, but if there were a sexual dysfunction, it is not priority over a physiological problem, such as hemorrhaging.
    2. This may be a possible nursing diagnosis, but is not priority over hemorrhaging, which is the priority nursing diagnosis.
    3. All postoperative clients have the risk of infection, but the client with a TURP priority nursing concern is hemorrhaging due to the surgical procedure.
    4. **This is a potential life-threatening nursing diagnosis and is the client's priority. This is the reason for the three-way continuous bladder irrigation.**

    Content – Medical/Surgical: **Category of Health Alteration** *– Genitourinary:* **Integrated Processes** *– Nursing Process: Planning:* **Client Needs** *– Physiological Integrity: Physiological Adaptation:* **Cognitive Level** *– Synthesis*

MAKING NURSING DECISIONS: The NCLEX-RN® integrates the nursing process throughout the Client Needs categories and subcategories. The nursing process is a scientific, clinical reasoning approach to client care that includes assessment, analysis, planning, implementation, and evaluation. The nurse will be responsible for identifying nursing diagnoses for clients.

62. 1. The unlicensed assistive personnel (UAP) cannot increase the irrigation fluid because this requires assessment and judgment. This behavior warrants intervention by the nurse.
    2. Elevating the scrotum on a towel for support is an intervention a UAP can implement. It does not require judgment and the client is stable; therefore, action does not warrant intervention by the nurse.
    3. The UAP can empty catheter bags, since this does not require any judgment. This action does not warrant intervention by the nurse.
    4. The client can bring ice water to the client's bedside, since the client is not NPO.

    Content – Medical/Surgical: **Category of Health Alteration** *– Genitourinary:* **Integrated Processes** *– Nursing Process: Assessment:* **Client Needs** *– Safe and Effective Care Environment: Management of Care:* **Cognitive Level** *– Analysis*

MAKING NURSING DECISIONS: "Delegation" means the nurse is responsible for the UAP's actions and performance. The nurse must correct the UAP's performance to ensure the client is cared for safely, in the hospital or the home.

63. 1. The client should use a urinal, so the nurse can strain the urine prior to placing it in the commode.
    2. **Assessment is the first part of the nursing process and is always priority. The intensity of the renal colic pain can be so intense it can cause a vasovagal response, with resulting hypotension and syncope.**
    3. Increased fluid increases urinary output, which will facilitate movement of the renal stone through the ureter and help decrease pain, but it is not the first intervention.
    4. The nurse should strain the client's urine to determine if the renal calculi have been passed via the urine.

    Content – Medical/Surgical: **Category of Health Alteration** *– Genitourinary:* **Integrated Processes** *– Nursing Process: Implementation:* **Client Needs** *– Physiological Integrity: Basic Care and Comfort:* **Cognitive Level** *– Application*

MAKING NURSING DECISIONS: When the question asks, "Which intervention should be implemented first?" it means that all the options are things a nurse could implement, but only one should be implemented first. The nurse should use the nursing process and remember: if the client is in distress, do not assess; if the client is not in distress, the nurse should assess.

64. 1. A KUB is an x-ray and does not include administering any type of contrast dye.
   2. Food, fluids, and ordered medication are not restricted prior to a KUB.
   3. An x-ray should not be completed on a client who may be pregnant. The x-rays could harm the fetus.
   4. The client with renal calculi is expected to have pain, depending on where the calculi are located, but this statement would not warrant intervention for the KUB.

   Content – Medical/Surgical: ***Category of Health Alteration*** *– Genitourinary:* ***Integrated Processes*** *– Nursing Process: Evaluation:* ***Client Needs*** *– Physiological Integrity: Physiological Adaptation:* ***Cognitive Level*** *– Synthesis*

MAKING NURSING DECISIONS: This question asks the nurse to identify which statement warrants intervention, which indicates three of the options are appropriate for the disease process or disorder but one is incorrect. This is an "except" question, but it does not say all the options are correct "except."

65. 3 and 5 are correct.
   1. The healthcare provider may order certain foods and medications when obtaining a 24-hour urine collection to evaluate for calcium oxalate or uric acid, but the client will not be NPO.
   2. When the collection begins, the client should completely empty the bladder and discard that urine. The first urine specimen should not be included.
   3. All urine for 24 hours should be saved and put in a container with a preservative, refrigerated, or put on ice, as indicated. Not following specific instructions will result in an inaccurate test result.
   4. The urine is obtained in some type of urine collection device such as a bedpan, bedside commode, or commode hat. The client is not catheterized.
   5. Posting signs will help ensure that all the urine is saved during the 24-hour period. If any urine is discarded, the test may result in inaccurate information or the need to start the test over.

   Content – Medical/Surgical: ***Category of Health Alteration*** *– Genitourinary:* ***Integrated Processes*** *– Nursing Process: Implementation:* ***Client Needs*** *– Physiological Integrity: Reduction of Risk Potential:* ***Cognitive Level*** *– Analysis*

MAKING NURSING DECISIONS: This is an alternate type of question included in the NCLEX-RN®. The nurse must be able to select all of the options that answer the question correctly. There are no partially correct answers.

66. 1. The urine must be assessed for bleeding and cloudiness. Initially, the urine is bright red, but the color soon diminishes, and cloudiness may indicate an infection. This assessment should not be delegated to an unlicensed assistive personnel (UAP).
   2. The UAP cannot transcribe a healthcare provider's orders.
   3. The UAP can strain the client's urine. This task does not require judgment or evaluation. Any sediment should be placed in a sterile container and sent to the laboratory for analysis.
   4. The kidney is highly vascular. Hemorrhaging and the resulting shock are potential complications of lithotripsy, so the nurse should not delegate vital signs post-procedure.

   Content – Medical/Surgical: ***Category of Health Alteration*** *– Genitourinary:* ***Integrated Processes*** *– Nursing Process: Planning:* ***Client Needs*** *– Safe and Effective Care Environment: Management of Care:* ***Cognitive Level*** *– Synthesis*

MAKING NURSING DECISIONS: The nurse cannot delegate assessment, teaching, evaluation, medications, or an unstable client to a UAP. Tasks that cannot be delegated are nursing interventions requiring nursing judgment.

67. 1. This potassium level is within normal limits, 3.5 to 5.5 mEq/L.
   2. Hematuria is not uncommon after removal of a kidney stone, but cause for further assessment by the nurse. It may indicate hemorrhaging, which is life threatening.
   3. A normal creatinine level is 0.8 to 1.2 mg/100 mL.
   4. This white blood cell count is elevated; normal is 5,000–10,000 mm.

   Content – Medical/Surgery: ***Category of Health Alteration*** *– Genitourinary:* ***Integrated Processes*** *– Nursing Process: Assessment:* ***Client Needs*** *– Physiological Integrity: Reduction of Risk Potential:* ***Cognitive Level*** *– Analysis*

MAKING NURSING DECISIONS: The nurse must be knowledgeable of normal laboratory values. These values must be memorized, and the nurse must be able to determine if the laboratory value is normal for the client's disease process or for medications the client is taking.

68. 1. The nurse should assess first to determine the etiology of the incontinence before the treatment plan can be formulated. By palpating the bladder after voiding, the nurse can determine if the incontinence was the result of overdistention of the bladder.

2. Medications—for instance, anticholinergic agents such as oxybutynin—can cause adverse effects. Non-pharmacological methods of treatment are preferred before medications are administered.

3. The nurse should ensure the client does not have skin breakdown secondary to urinary incontinence, but the first intervention is assessment.

4. The nurse should instruct the client to go to the bathroom every 2 hours to attempt to urinate, which may decrease the number of incontinent episodes.

*Content – Medical/Surgical: **Category of Health Alteration** – Genitourinary: **Integrated Processes** – Nursing Process: Implementation: **Client Needs** – Physiological Integrity: Reduction of Risk Potential: **Cognitive Level** – Analysis*

MAKING NURSING DECISIONS: When the question asks, "Which intervention should be implemented first?" it means that all the options are things a nurse could implement, but only one should be implemented first. The nurse should use the nursing process and remember: If the client is in distress, do not assess; if the client is not in distress, the nurse should assess.

69. 1. This vital signs are within normal limits and would not require further investigation.

2. **When an elderly client's mental status changes, the nurse should notify the HCP because it is not normal or expected. This could indicate a urinary tract infection secondary to an indwelling catheter. Elderly clients often do not present with classic signs and symptoms of infection.**

3. The client's urine should be clear and light yellow, but cloudy urine with sediment is not life threatening. The nurse would not need to notify the client's HCP.

4. The client should have no discomfort and pain; therefore, this would not warrant further investigation.

*Content – Medical/Surgical: **Category of Health Alteration** – Genitourinary: **Integrated Processes** – Nursing Process: Assessment: **Client Needs** – Physiological Integrity: Reduction of Risk Potential: **Cognitive Level** – Analysis*

MAKING NURSING DECISIONS: When the question asks, "Which data set warrants notifying the HCP?" it is an "except" question. Three of the data sets are expected with the client's disease process or condition, one is not expected and warrants notifying the HCP.

70. 1. **The client's catheter should be secured on the leg to prevent manipulation, which increases the risk for a urinary tract infection. This warrants immediate intervention by the nurse.**

2. The unlicensed assistive personnel (UAP) must adhere to Standard Precautions when providing care to the client; therefore, this doesn't warrant immediate intervention by the nurse.

3. The drainage bag should be kept below the level of the bladder to prevent reflux of urine into the renal system; therefore, this does not warrant intervention by the nurse.

4. Hand hygiene is important before and after handling any portion of the drainage system; therefore, this does not warrant intervention by the nurse.

*Content – Medical/Surgical: **Category of Health Alteration** – Genitourinary: **Integrated Processes** – Nursing Process: Assessment: **Client Needs** – Safe and Effective Care Environment: Safety and Infection Control: **Cognitive Level** – Analysis*

MAKING NURSING DECISIONS: When the question asks, "Which intervention warrants immediate intervention?" it is an "except" question. Three of the interventions indicate the UAP understands the appropriate care for the client, and one indicates the UAP does not understand the appropriate care.

CLINICAL SCENARIO ANSWERS AND RATIONALES

The correct answer number and rationale for why it is the correct answer are given in boldface type. Rationales for why the other possible answer options are incorrect also are given, but they are not in boldface type.

1. 1. **Ms. Debbie, the UAP, can assist the radiology technician with the portable chest x-ray. The RN cannot delegate assessment, teaching, evaluation, medications, or an unstable client. If Ms. Debbie is pregnant, then the nurse should not delegate this task.**
   2. Ms. Debbie can obtain the client's intake and output, but the nurse must evaluate the data to determine if interventions are needed or if interventions are effective.
   3. In some units, UAPs can perform urinary catheterization, but of the four options, the nurse should delegate the least invasive task.
   4. This is a medication enema, and Ms. Debbie cannot administer medications. Also, for this to be ordered, the client must be unstable with an excessively high serum potassium level.

2. 1. The laboratory findings are low, but would not require a blood transfusion. These laboratory findings are often expected in a client who is anemic secondary to ESRD.
   2. **The dialysis access is compromised; therefore, this client warrants intervention because Mr. Ray cannot perform hemodialysis.**
   3. It is not uncommon for a client undergoing dialysis to be exhausted and sleep through the treatment; therefore, this does not warrant intervention.
   4. The client in end-stage renal disease would not have urinary output; therefore, this does not warrant intervention from Mr. Ray.

3. 1. Ms. Mary can restart the client's IV access without notifying the healthcare provider.
   2. Hypoactive bowel sounds may be abnormal, but airway problems take priority over gastrointestinal distress. Remember Maslow's Hierarchy of Needs.
   3. **The client may be developing pneumonia or acute respiratory distress syndrome; therefore, Ms. Mary should notify the healthcare provider. This is a complication of surgery.**
   4. A 2+ pedal pulse is expected data; therefore, Ms. Mary does not need to notify the healthcare provider.

4. 1. Normal blood urea nitrogen levels are 7–18 mg/dL or 8–20 mg/dL for clients older than age 60 years.
   2. Normal creatinine levels are 0.6–1.2 mg/dL.
   3. **Glomerular filtration rate (GFR) is approximately 120 mL per minute. If the GFR is decreased to 60 mL per minute, the kidneys are functioning at about one-half filtration capacity.**
   4. Normal creatinine clearance is 85–125 mL per minute for males and 75–115 mL per minute for females.

5. Answer: 1,000 mL. First, determine the amount of irrigation fluid: 4,000 – 2,000 = 2,000 mL of irrigation fluid. Then, subtract 2,000 of irrigation fluid from the drainage of 3,000 to determine the urine output: 3,000 – 2,000 = 1,000 mL of urine output

6. 1 and 5 are correct.
   1. **The client is stable, but Mr. Ray should assess the drainage. The drainage should be light pink for a client who had a TURP.**
   2. The client is stable; therefore, Mr. Ray should not increase the irrigation fluid, unless the drainage is dark red.
   3. If the client is hypovolemic, the head of the bed should be lowered and the foot should be elevated to protect the brain. This client is stable.
   4. The surgeon needs to be notified if the client is unstable or experiencing a complication of surgery. This client is stable; therefore, Mr. Ray should not notify surgeon.
   5. **Mr. Ray should monitor the client's laboratory values for bleeding or infection.**

7. 1. Ms. Mary needs to complete the admission assessment, but the priority should always be the client's body; therefore, assessing pain is priority.
   2. **Assessment is the first part of the nursing process and is always priority. The intensity of the renal colic pain can be so intense it can cause a vasovagal response, with resulting hypotension and syncope.**
   3. Increased fluid increases urinary output, which will facilitate movement of the renal stone through the ureter and help decrease pain, but it is not the first intervention.
   4. The nurse should transcribe the client's HCP order, but not priority over the client's body—pain is priority. Ms. Brenda, the charge nurse, can check the HCP orders to determine if there is any priority order.

8. 1. The urine must be assessed for bleeding and cloudiness. Initially, the urine is bright red, but the color soon diminishes, and cloudiness may indicate an infection. This assessment should not be delegated to Ms. Debbie.

2. Teaching cannot be delegated to Ms. Debbie, and the client with renal calculi should not have an indwelling urinary catheter.

3. **The client's urine must be strained to determine if the renal stone was dissolved and is being passed out of the body. Straining the urine is not assessment, teaching, evaluation, medications, or an unstable client; therefore, this can be delegated to Ms. Debbie.**

4. The client is not on strict bed rest after lithotripsy; therefore, Ms. Debbie should not implement this intervention.

9. 1. The client with a palpable thrill is stable; therefore, Ms. Brenda would not need to see this client first.

2. The client with acute glomerulonephritis is expected to have hematuria and proteinuria; therefore, Ms. Brenda should not assess this client first.

3. The sign/symptom of bladder cancer is painless hematuria; therefore, Ms. Brenda would not need to see this client first.

4. **An ileal conduit is a procedure that diverts urine from the bladder and provides an alternate cutaneous pathway for urine to exit the body. Urinary output should always be at least 30 mL per hour. This client should be assessed to make sure that the stents placed in the ureters have not become dislodged, or to ensure that edema of the ureters is not occurring.**

10. 1. Teaching cannot be assigned to an LPN, no matter how knowledgeable the LPN.

2. This client has the laboratory symptoms of an infection; therefore, Ms. Mary cannot assign an unstable client to the LPN.

3. Antineoplastic medication can only be administered by a qualified registered nurse.

4. **The LPN can administer narcotic analgesics to a client; therefore, this would be an appropriate assignment.**

Neurological Management

7

To be effective and organized, the nurse must continually prioritize what must be done.

—Ray A. Hargrove-Huttel

QUESTIONS

1. The charge nurse has received laboratory data for clients in the medical department. Which client would require intervention by the charge nurse?
   1. The client diagnosed with a stroke who has a platelet level of 250,000 µ/L.
   2. The client with a seizure disorder who has a divalproex (Depakote) level of 75 µg/mL.
   3. The client with multiple sclerosis on prednisone who has a glucose level of 208 mg/dL.
   4. The client receiving the anticonvulsant phenytoin (Dilantin) who has serum levels of 24 mg/dL.

2. The nurse is administering medications for clients on a neurological unit. Which medication should the nurse administer first?
   1. A pain medication to a client complaining of a headache rated an 8 on 1 to 10 pain scale.
   2. A steroid to the client experiencing an acute exacerbation of multiple sclerosis.
   3. An anticholinesterase medication to a client diagnosed with myasthenia gravis.
   4. An antacid to a client with pyrosis who has called several times over the intercom.

3. The nurse has just received the shift report. Which client should the nurse assess first?
   1. The client with Guillain-Barré syndrome who has ascending paralysis to the knees.
   2. The client with a C-6 spinal cord injury who has autonomic dysreflexia.
   3. The client with Parkinson's disease who is experiencing "pill rolling."
   4. The client with Huntington's disease who has writhing, twisting movements of the face.

4. The nurse and unlicensed assistive personnel (UAP) are caring for a client with right-sided paralysis. Which action by the UAP requires the nurse to intervene?
   1. The UAP places the gait belt around the client's waist prior to ambulating.
   2. The UAP places the client on the abdomen with the client's head to the side.
   3. The UAP places her hand under the client's right axilla to help the client move up in bed.
   4. The UAP praises the client for performing activities of daily living independently.

5. The charge nurse is making client assignments for a neuro-medical floor. Which client should be assigned to the most experienced nurse?
   1. The elderly client who is experiencing a stroke in evolution.
   2. The client diagnosed with a transient ischemic attack 48 hours ago.
   3. The client diagnosed with Guillain-Barré syndrome who complains of leg pain.
   4. The client with Alzheimer's disease who is wandering in the halls.

173

6. The client diagnosed with a cerebrovascular accident (CVA) has residual right-sided hemiparesis and difficulty swallowing, but is scheduled for discharge. Which referral is most appropriate for the case manager to make at this time?
   1. Inpatient rehabilitation unit.
   2. Home healthcare agency.
   3. Long-term care facility.
   4. Outpatient therapy center.

7. The nurse and LPN are caring for a client diagnosed with a stroke. Which intervention should the nurse assign to the LPN?
   1. Feed the client who is being allowed to eat for the first time.
   2. Administer the client's anticoagulant subcutaneously.
   3. Check the client's neurological signs and limb movement.
   4. Teach the client to turn the head and tuck the chin to swallow.

8. The nurse is caring for a client diagnosed with Alzheimer's disease. Which nursing tasks should **not** be delegated to the unlicensed assistive personnel (UAP)? **Select all that apply.**
   1. Check the client's skin under the restraints.
   2. Administer the client's antipsychotic medication.
   3. Perform the client's morning hygiene care.
   4. Ambulate the client to the bathroom.
   5. Obtain the client's routine vital signs.

9. The nurse on the surgical unit is working with an unlicensed assistive personnel (UAP). Which task is most appropriate for the nurse to delegate to the UAP?
   1. Change an abdominal dressing on a client who is 2 days postoperative.
   2. Check the client's IV insertion site on the right arm.
   3. Monitor vital signs on a client who has just returned from surgery.
   4. Escort a client who has been discharged to the client's vehicle.

10. Which client should the charge nurse assess first after receiving the change-of-shift report?
    1. The client with a C-6 SCI who is complaining of dyspnea and has a respiratory rate of 12 breaths/minute.
    2. The client with an L-4 SCI who is frightened about being transferred to the rehabilitation unit.
    3. The client with an L-2 SCI who is complaining of a headache and feeling very hot all of a sudden.
    4. The client with a C-4 SCI who is on a ventilator and has a pulse oximeter reading of 98%.

11. The client with a C-6 spinal cord injury (SCI) comes to the emergency department complaining of a throbbing headache and has a B/P of 200/120. Which intervention should the nurse implement first?
    1. Place the client on a telemetry unit.
    2. Complete a neurological assessment.
    3. Insert an indwelling urinary catheter.
    4. Request a STAT CT scan on the head.

12. The intensive care unit nurse and unlicensed assistive personnel (UAP) are caring for a client with right-sided paralysis secondary to a cerebrovascular accident. Which action by the UAP requires the nurse to intervene?
    1. The UAP performs passive range-of-motion (ROM) exercises for the client.
    2. The UAP places the client on the abdomen with the head to the side.
    3. The UAP uses a lift sheet when moving the client up in bed.
    4. The UAP praises the client for attempting to feed him- or herself.

13. The critical care charge nurse is making client assignments for the shift. Which client should the charge nurse assign to the graduate nurse who just completed the orientation?
   1. The client with amyotrophic lateral sclerosis on a ventilator who is dying and whose family is at the bedside.
   2. The client who has a closed head injury and has increasing intracranial pressure receiving intravenous osmitrol (Mannitol).
   3. The client with a C-5 spinal cord injury who is experiencing spinal shock and is on the vasoconstrictor dopamine.
   4. The client with a seizure disorder who has been experiencing status epilepticus for the past 24 hours.

14. The critical care nurse is caring for a client with a head injury secondary to a motorcycle accident who, on morning rounds, is responsive to painful stimuli and assumes decorticate posturing. Two hours later, which data would warrant immediate intervention by the nurse?
   1. The client has purposeful movement when the nurse rubs the sternum.
   2. The client extends the upper and lower extremities in response to painful stimuli.
   3. The client is aimlessly thrashing in the bed when a noxious stimulus is applied.
   4. The client is able to squeeze the nurse's hand on a verbal request.

15. The charge nurse is making rounds and notices that the sharps container in the client's room is above the fill line. Which action should the charge nurse implement?
   1. Complete an adverse occurrence report.
   2. Discuss the situation with the primary nurse.
   3. Instruct the UAP to change the sharps container.
   4. Notify the infection control nurse immediately.

16. The wife of a client diagnosed with a brain tumor tells the nurse, "I don't know how I will make it if something happens to my husband. I love him so much." Which statement is most appropriate for the nurse?
   1. "I will call the chaplain to come and talk to you."
   2. "Do you have any family support to be with you?"
   3. "You don't know how you will make it if something happens."
   4. "Do not worry, everything will be all right. You are a strong woman."

17. Which priority client problem should be included in the care plan for the client diagnosed with Guillain-Barré syndrome who is admitted to the critical care unit?
   1. Decreased cardiac output.
   2. Fear and anxiety.
   3. Complications of immobility.
   4. Ineffective breathing pattern.

18. To which collaborative healthcare team member should the critical care nurse refer the client in the late stages of myasthenia gravis (MG)?
   1. Occupational therapist.
   2. Physical therapist.
   3. Social worker.
   4. Speech therapist.

19. The nurse caring for a client is accidentally stuck with the stylet used to start an IV infusion. The nurse flushes the skin with water and tries to get the area to bleed. Which action should the nurse implement next?
   1. Have the laboratory draw the client's blood.
   2. Notify the charge nurse and complete the incident report.
   3. Contact the employee health nurse to start prophylactic medication.
   4. Follow up with the employee health nurse to have lab work drawn.

20. The nurse is caring for clients in a long-term care facility. Which client should the nurse assess first after receiving the morning report?
1. The client diagnosed with Parkinson's disease who began to hallucinate during the night.
2. The client diagnosed with congestive heart failure who has 3+ pitting edema of both feet.
3. The client diagnosed with Alzheimer's disease who was found wandering in the hall at 0200.
4. The client diagnosed with terminal cancer who has lost 8 pounds since the last weight taken 4 weeks ago.

21. The nurse in a long-term care facility is administering medications to a group of clients. Which medication should the nurse administer first?
1. Acetylsalicylic acid (aspirin) to a client diagnosed with cerebrovascular disease.
2. Neostigmine (Prostigmin) to a client diagnosed with myasthenia gravis.
3. Cephalexin (Keflex) to a client diagnosed with an acute urinary tract infection.
4. Acyclovir (Zovirax) to a client diagnosed with Bell's palsy.

22. The nurse in a long-term care facility is developing the plan of care for a client diagnosed with end-stage Alzheimer's disease. Which client problem is priority for this client?
1. Inability to do activities of daily living.
2. Increased risk for injury.
3. Potential for constipation.
4. Ineffective family coping.

23. The clinic nurse is providing discharge instructions to an elderly client diagnosed with cataracts. Which intervention is most important for the nurse to implement?
1. Teach the client to increase the light in the home.
2. Encourage the client to wear dark glasses outside.
3. Discuss the need to have the cataracts removed.
4. Tell the family not to rearrange furniture in the home.

24. A wife tells the clinic nurse her husband had been fine and is now confused, doesn't know where he is, and is not acting like his usual self. Which intervention should the nurse implement first?
1. Perform a neurological assessment.
2. Notify the client's healthcare provider.
3. Ask the wife to explain more about the behavior.
4. Determine when the client last had something to eat.

25. The charge nurse observes the client's nurse telling the unlicensed assistive personnel (UAP) to feed an elderly client diagnosed with a cerebrovascular accident (CVA). Which question should the charge nurse ask the client's nurse?
1. "How does the client swallow the medications?"
2. "Did you complete your head to toe assessment?"
3. "Does the client have some Thick-It in the room?"
4. "Why would you delegate feeding to a UAP?"

26. The client diagnosed with a cerebrovascular accident (CVA) is confined to a wheelchair for most of the waking hours. Which intervention is priority for the nurse to implement?
1. Encourage the client to move the buttocks every 2 hours.
2. Order a high-protein diet to prevent skin breakdown.
3. Get a pressure-relieving cushion to place in the wheelchair.
4. Refer the client to physical therapy for transfer teaching.

27. The nurse enters the room, and the client is beginning to have a tonic-clonic seizure. Which action should the nurse implement first?
1. Identify the first area that began seizing.
2. Note the time the client's seizure began.
3. Pad the siding of the client's bed rails.
4. Provide the client with privacy during the seizure.

28. The rehabilitation nurse tells the unlicensed assistive personnel (UAP) to assist the client recovering from Guillain-Barré syndrome with a.m. care. Which action by the UAP warrants immediate intervention?
1. The UAP closes the door and cubicle curtain.
2. The UAP massages the client's back with lotion.
3. The UAP checks the temperature of the bathing water.
4. The UAP puts the side rails up when bathing the client.

29. The client diagnosed with a right-sided cerebral vascular accident (CVA), or brain attack, is admitted to the rehabilitation unit. Which interventions should be included in the nursing care plan? **Select all that apply.**
1. Position the client to prevent shoulder adduction.
2. Refer the client to occupational therapy daily.
3. Encourage the client to move the affected side.
4. Perform quadriceps exercises five times a day.
5. Instruct the client to hold the fingers in a fist.

30. The nurse is the first person on the scene of a motor vehicle accident. The driver is in the driver's seat unconscious. Which action should the nurse implement first?
1. Stabilize the driver's cervical spine.
2. Do not move the client from the accident.
3. Ensure the driver has a patent airway.
4. Control any external bleeding.

31. The clinic nurse is making assignments for the large family practice clinic. Which task should be assigned to the staff nurse who is 4 months pregnant?
1. Have the staff nurse answer the telephone calls from clients.
2. Instruct the staff nurse to work in the radiology department.
3. Tell the staff nurse to work in the front desk triage area.
4. Assign the staff nurse to work in the oncology clinic.

32. Which task is most appropriate for the clinic nurse to delegate to the unlicensed assistive personnel (UAP)?
1. Request the UAP to ride in the ambulance with a client.
2. Ask the UAP to escort the client in a wheelchair to the car.
3. Instruct the UAP to show the client how to use crutches.
4. Tell the UAP to call the pharmacy to refill a prescription.

33. The employee health nurse is caring for an employee who fell off a ladder and is complaining of low back pain radiating down both legs. Which intervention should the nurse implement first?
1. Refer the client to an HCP for further evaluation.
2. Complete the workers' compensation documentation.
3. Investigate the cause of the fall off the ladder.
4. Notify the employee's supervisor of the incident.

34. The employee health nurse is caring for a male employee who reports tripping and is complaining of right knee pain. There is no visible injury, and the client has a normal neurovascular assessment. Which intervention should the nurse implement?
1. Request the employee to return to work.
2. Obtain a urine specimen for a drug screen.
3. Send the client to the emergency department.
4. Place a sequential compression device on the leg.

35. The community health nurse is triaging victims at the site of a disaster. Which client should the nurse categorize as black, priority 4?
1. The client who is alert and has a sucking chest wound.
2. The client who cannot stop crying and can't answer questions.
3. The client whose abdomen is hard and tender to the touch.
4. The client who has full thickness burns over 60% of the body.

36. The home health (HH) nurse enters the home of an 80-year-old female client who had a cerebrovascular accident (CVA), or "brain attack," 2 months ago. The client is complaining of a severe headache. Which intervention should the nurse implement first?
    1. Determine what medication the client has taken.
    2. Assess the client's pain on a pain scale of 1 to 10.
    3. Ask whether the client has any acetaminophen (Tylenol).
    4. Tell the client to sit down, and take her blood pressure.

37. A client has been diagnosed with rule out bacterial meningitis, and a nurse is assisting the healthcare provider with a lumbar puncture. Which intervention should the nurse implement first?
    1. Have the client lie in the lateral recumbent position.
    2. Tell the client to empty the bladder.
    3. Encourage the client to complete an advance directive.
    4. Keep the client NPO prior to the procedure.

38. The home health (HH) nurse is scheduling visits for the day. Which client should the nurse visit first?
    1. The client with an L-4 SCI who is complaining of a severe, pounding headache.
    2. The client with amyotrophic lateral sclerosis (ALS) who is depressed and wants to die.
    3. The client with Parkinson's disease who is walking with a short, shuffling gait.
    4. The client with a C-5 SCI who reports redness and drainage at the Halo vest sites.

39. The clinic nurse is triaging client's telephone calls. Which client should the nurse call first?
    1. The client diagnosed with AIDS who has developed Kaposi's sarcoma.
    2. The client diagnosed with dementia who is having difficulty dressing himself.
    3. The client with trigeminal neuralgia who is having lightening-like shock to the cheeks.
    4. The client whose friend has botulism who has vomiting and abdominal cramping pain.

40. The home health (HH) nurse is caring for a 22-year-old female client who sustained an L-5 spinal cord injury 2 months ago. The client says, "I will never be happy again. I can't walk, I can't drive, and I had to quit college." Which intervention should the nurse implement first?
    1. Allow the client to ventilate her feelings of powerlessness.
    2. Refer the client to the home healthcare agency social worker.
    3. Recommend contacting the American Spinal Cord Association.
    4. Ask the client whether she has any friends who come and visit.

41. The client being admitted with transient ischemic attack is complaining of a headache. The client is allergic to morphine, iodine, and codeine. Which healthcare provider order should the nurse question?
    1. Schedule for CT scan with contrast in a.m.
    2. Administer acetaminophen 2 PO for headache.
    3. Take client's vital signs per protocol.
    4. Provide the client with a low-fat, low-cholesterol diet.

42. The home health (HH) nurse is admitting a female client diagnosed with myasthenia gravis. The client tells the nurse, "Even with my medication I get exhausted when I do anything." Which intervention should the nurse implement?
    1. Talk to the client's husband about helping around the house more.
    2. Contact the HH occupational therapist to discuss the client's concern.
    3. Allow the client to verbalize her feelings of being exhausted.
    4. Recommend the client make an appointment with her HCP.

43. The nurse is caring for clients in the emergency department. Which client should the nurse assess first?
    1. The client with an epidural hematoma.
    2. The client who had a seizure who is in the postictal state.
    3. The client diagnosed with R/O encephalitis who has a headache.
    4. The client with multiple sclerosis who has scanning speech.

44. The nurse in the neurological clinic is triaging phone calls. Which client should the nurse contact first?
    1. The client with a tension headache who is reporting nausea and vomiting.
    2. The client with a migraine headache who is reporting bilateral throbbing pain.
    3. The client with a cluster headache who is reporting a sharp and stabbing pain.
    4. The client with hypertension who is reporting pressure type pain in the back of head.

45. A client sustained a severe head injury, and his wife is concerned about what to do if he has a seizure when they go home. Which statement indicates the wife understands the most important action to take if her husband has a seizure?
    1. "I should check to see if my husband urinates on himself."
    2. "I will move all the furniture out of his way."
    3. "I will call 911 as soon as the seizure begins."
    4. "I will make sure he rests after the seizure is over."

46. The multidisciplinary team is meeting to discuss a client with right-sided weakness who has developed a Stage 2 pressure ulcer over the sacral area that is not healing. Which priority intervention should the client's home health (HH) nurse recommend?
    1. Recommend the client get a hospital bed with a trapeze bar.
    2. Recommend a home health aide provide care 7 days a week for the client.
    3. Recommend the client be transferred to a skilled nursing unit.
    4. Recommend a referral to the home healthcare agency wound care nurse.

47. The home health (HH) aide tells the nurse the client diagnosed with multiple sclerosis is having problems getting out of the bed to the chair, and is now having problems getting into the shower. Which intervention should the nurse implement?
    1. Ask the HH aide whether the bathroom has grab bars.
    2. Assess the client's ability to transfer in the home.
    3. Instruct the HH aide to give the client a bed bath.
    4. Contact the agency physical therapist about the situation.

48. The nurse is teaching the client with tension-type headaches. Which statement indicates the client needs more teaching?
    1. "I will do some type of exercise every day."
    2. "I am going to do yoga techniques when I get a headache."
    3. "Cold packs to the back of my neck will help my headache."
    4. "Foods containing amines like cheese and chocolate can cause headaches."

49. The client in a multiple car crash dies in the emergency department. Which priority intervention should the emergency department nurse implement when addressing the needs of the client's family?
    1. Ask if the client wanted to be a tissue donor.
    2. Give the family the client's personal belongings.
    3. Escort the family to a private room to grieve.
    4. Determine which funeral home should be contacted.

50. The neurologist has explained to the family of a 22-year-old client with a traumatic brain injury placed on a ventilator after a motor vehicle accident that the client does not have any brain function. Which referral is appropriate at this time?
    1. A local funeral director.
    2. A hospice agency.
    3. A home health nurse.
    4. A tissue and organ bank.

51. The nurse is caring for clients in an ophthalmology clinic. Which client warrants intervention by the nurse?
    1. The client with cataracts who reports decreased vision and abnormal color perception.
    2. The client with a retinal detachment who reports a painless loss of peripheral vision.
    3. The client with an external hordeolum who reports reddened tender area under eye.
    4. The client with primary open angle glaucoma who reports excruciating eye pain.

52. The nurse is at a park and observes a client fall and a stick become impaled into the right eye. Which intervention should the nurse implement first?
    1. Tell someone to call 911 immediately.
    2. Stabilize the stick in the client's eye.
    3. Apply direct pressure to the right eye.
    4. Use a non-toxic liquid and irrigate the eye.

53. The nurse and unlicensed assistive personnel (UAP) are caring for a minimally responsive client diagnosed with multiple sclerosis who weighs more than 400 pounds. Which action is priority when moving the client in the bed?
    1. Obtain a lifting device made for lifting heavy clients.
    2. Do not attempt to move the client because of the weight.
    3. Get another UAP to help move the client in the bed.
    4. Tell the family that the client must assist in moving in the bed.

54. The terminally ill client diagnosed with ALS (Lou Gehrig's disease) has a DNR order in place and is currently complaining of "pain all over." The nurse notes the client has shallow breathing and a P 67, R 8, B/P 104/62. Which intervention should the nurse implement?
    1. Administer the narcotic pain medication IVP.
    2. Turn and reposition the client for comfort.
    3. Refuse to administer pain medication.
    4. Notify the HCP of the client's vital signs.

55. The nurse in a rehabilitation facility is evaluating the progress of a female client who sustained a C-6–C-7 spinal cord injury. Which outcome indicates the client is improving?
    1. The client can maneuver the automatic wheelchair into the hallway.
    2. The client states she will be able to return to work in a few weeks.
    3. The client uses eye blinks to communicate yes and no responses.
    4. The client's husband built a wheelchair ramp onto their house.

56. The nurse is triaging phone calls in a neurosensory clinic. Which client should the nurse contact first?
    1. The client with Méniére's disease who is complaining of vertigo and tinnitus.
    2. The client with otitis media with effusion complaining of feeling of fullness in the ear.
    3. The client with external otitis who has serosanguineous drainage and otalgia.
    4. The client with otoclersosis who has bilateral hearing loss.

57. The nurse is planning care for the client diagnosed with Parkinson's disease (PD). Which client problem is priority?
    1. Altered nutrition.
    2. Altered mobility.
    3. Altered elimination.
    4. Altered body image.

58. A client comes to the emergency department after having bleach splash in the eyes. Which intervention should the nurse implement first?
    1. Cover both the eyes with sterile patches.
    2. Assess the client's visual acuity.
    3. Irrigate the eyes with sterile solution.
    4. Elevate head of bed 45 degrees.

59. The 24-year-old client diagnosed with a traumatic brain injury is being transferred to a rehabilitation unit. Which healthcare provider order should the nurse question?
    1. Physical therapy to work on lower extremity strength daily.
    2. Occupational therapy to work on cognitive functioning bid.
    3. A soft diet with mechanical ground meats and thickening agent in fluids.
    4. Methylprednisolone (Solu-Medrol), a steroid, IVP q 6 hours.

60. The rehabilitation nurse is planning the discharge of a 68-year-old client whose status post–subarachnoid hemorrhage includes residual speech and balance deficits. Which referral should the nurse initiate at this time?
    1. Referral to a hospice organization.
    2. Referral to the speech therapist.
    3. Referral to the physical therapist.
    4. Referral to a home health agency.

61. The client is postoperative a right eye enucleation. Which statement indicates the client needs more discharge teaching?
    1. "It will be approximately 2 weeks before I can get a prosthetic eye."
    2. "I can show you how to insert the conformer in the socket in case it falls out."
    3. "I should insert the eye drops into the lower conjunctiva of my eye."
    4. "If I develop an increased temperature I should call my healthcare provider."

62. The nurse is caring for a client newly diagnosed with multiple sclerosis. Which referral is appropriate at this time?
    1. To a social worker to apply for disability.
    2. To a dietician for a nutritional consult.
    3. To a psychological counselor for therapy.
    4. To a chaplain to discuss spiritual issues.

63. The nurse and LPN have been assigned to care for clients on a neurology unit. Which nursing task is most appropriate to assign to the LPN?
    1. Administer the adrenocorticotropic hormone to the client with multiple sclerosis.
    2. Take the vital signs for the client who is experiencing status epilepticus.
    3. Assist the client with Parkinson's disease to ambulate to the bathroom.
    4. Assess the client newly admitted who has pneumonia and restless legs syndrome.

64. The nurse is administering medications on a neurological unit. Which medication should the nurse administer first?
    1. The osmotic diuretic to the client with a closed head injury.
    2. The morning medications to the client scheduled for physical therapy.
    3. The narcotic pain medication to a client with increased intracranial pressure.
    4. The anticonvulsant gabapentin (Neurontin) to the client with restless legs syndrome.

65. The charge nurse observes the new graduate nurse delegating tasks to the unlicensed assistive personnel (UAP) and the UAP appears to be ignoring the graduate nurse. Which action should the charge nurse implement first?
    1. Wait and observe how the graduate nurse handles the situation.
    2. Tell the UAP to get busy and complete the assigned tasks.
    3. Discuss learning to assert authority with the new graduate.
    4. Informally counsel the UAP about the response to the nurse.

66. The nurse is on the day shift of a rehabilitation unit. Given the medication administration record (MAR) below, which medication should the nurse administer first?

Client Name: D. F.	Account Number: 9 25 645		Allergies: Penicillin	
Height: 69 inches	Weight in pounds: 178 Weight in kg: 80.9		Date of Birth: 05/07/1955	
Date: Today	Medication	2301–0700	0701–1500	1501–2300
	Synthroid 0.75 mcg PO daily			
	MS Contin (morphine sulfate) 30 mg PO bid			
	Fleets enema per rectum Q day			
	Metformin (Glucophage) 850 mg PO bid			
Signature/Initials		Night Nurse RN/NN	Day Nurse RN/DN	

1. Administer the Synthroid.
2. Administer the MS Contin.
3. Administer the Fleets enema.
4. Administer the metformin.

67. The client on the rehabilitation unit post–motor vehicle accident has been prescribed 50 mg of Baclofen (Lioresol) per dose orally for muscle spasms. Baclofen comes in 10-mg, 20-mg, and 75-mg tablets. How many tablets should the nurse administer and in which quantity? _____

68. The 19-year-old client is in the rehabilitation unit following a traumatic brain injury. Which intervention should the nurse delegate to the unlicensed assistive personnel (UAP)? **Select all that apply.**
1. Make safety rounds hourly.
2. Refer the client to a college and career counselor.
3. Assist the client with meals.
4. Clamp and unclamp the indwelling catheter every 2 hours.
5. Discuss discharge placement with the parents.

69. The 69-year-old client post–right cerebral vascular accident (CVA) is on the rehab unit with left-sided weakness. Where should the nurse place the quadriplex cane when assisting the client to ambulate?

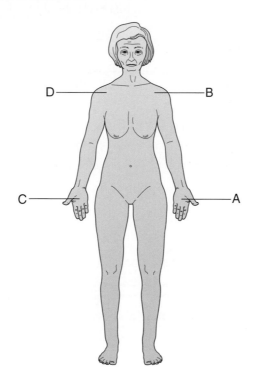

1. A
2. B
3. C
4. D

70. The male client is in the emergency department after a fall, resulting in a closed head injury. The admitting nurse notes the client responds by opening his eyes and pushing the nurse's arm away when painful stimuli is applied, but does not make any verbal response. Which rating on the Glasgow Coma Scale should be documented by the nurse?

Glasgow COMA Scale

Appropriate Stimulus	Response	Score
Eyes Open		
*Approach to bedside	Spontaneous response	4
*Verbal Command	Opens eyes to name on command	3
*Pain	Lack of opening of eyes to previous stimuli but opens to pain	2
	Lack of opening of eyes to any stimulus	1
	Untestable	0
Best Verbal Response		
Verbal questioning with maximum arousal	Oriented to person, place, time, and events	5
	Confusion, conversant but disoriented	4
	Disorganized use of words	3
	Incomprehensible words, groaning	2
	Lack of sound even with painful stimuli	1
	Untestable	0
Best Motor Response		
Verbal Command	Follows verbal command	6
Pain (pressure on proximal nail bed)	Localizes pain, attempts to remove offending stimulus	5
	Flexion withdrawal of arm in response to pain without abnormal posturing	4
	Abnormal flexion, flexing of arm at elbow and pronation, making a fist	3
	Abnormal extension, extension of arm at elbow with adduction, and internal rotation of arm at shoulder	2
	Lack of response	1
	Untestable	0

1. Client scored a 12 on the Glasgow Coma Scale.
2. Client scored a 10 on the Glasgow Coma Scale.
3. Client scored an 8 on the Glasgow Coma Scale.
4. Client scored a 6 on the Glasgow Coma Scale.

NEUROLOGICAL CLINICAL SCENARIO

Mr. Leo is the head nurse on the 10-bed Neurological Intensive Care Unit and 20-bed Neurological Step-Down unit. He supervises 15 nurses in the ICU, along with 30 nurses and 15 UAPs.

1. Elizabeth, who is the day staff nurse, and the UAP are caring for a client with a right-sided cerebrovascular accident (CVA) with hemi-paralysis. Which action by the UAP requires Elizabeth to intervene?
   1. The UAP places the call light on the client's left side.
   2. The UAP assists the client to eat the breakfast meal.
   3. The UAP uses the draw sheet to move the client up in bed.
   4. The UAP places a small pillow under the client's left shoulder.

2. The client diagnosed with a right-sided cerebrovascular accident (CVA) is complaining of a severe headache. Which intervention should Elizabeth implement first?
   1. Administer acetaminophen, a narcotic analgesic.
   2. Prepare for STAT computed tomography (CT) scan.
   3. Notify the client's healthcare provider.
   4. Assess the client's neurological status.

3. Courtney is caring for the following clients on the Neurological Intensive Care unit. Which client should Courtney assess first?
   1. The client with a C-6 SCI who is complaining of dyspnea and has crackles in the lungs.
   2. The client with Guillain-Barré syndrome who is complaining ascending paralysis.
   3. The client with traumatic brain injury who has a Glasgow Coma Scale score of 6.
   4. The client diagnosed with a cerebrovascular accident (CVA) who has expressive aphasia.

4. The ICU unit is very busy and Mr. Leo is transcribing the healthcare provider's admission orders for a client with a closed head injury. Which medication order should Mr. Leo question?
   1. A subcutaneous anticoagulant.
   2. An intravenous osmotic diuretic.
   3. An intravenous anticonvulsant.
   4. An intravenous proton-pump inhibitor.

5. Jessie is caring for a client who had a C-6 SCI 2 years ago and is admitted for Stage IV pressure ulcers in the coccyx area. The client is complaining of a severe headache and the B/P is 190/110. Which intervention should Jessie implement first?
   1. Insert a urinary catheter into the client.
   2. Complete a neurological assessment.
   3. Put the client in Trendelenburg position.
   4. Palpate the client's bladder.

6. Mr. Leo is making rounds and as he enters the room the client is having tonic-clonic seizure. Which priority intervention should Mr. Leo implement?
   1. Place the client on the side.
   2. Call the Rapid Response Team.
   3. Determine if the client is incontinent of urine.
   4. Provide the client with privacy during the seizure.

7. The UAP is attempting to put an oral airway in the mouth of a client having a tonic-clonic seizure. Which intervention should Mr. Leo take first?
   1. Complete an adverse occurrence report.
   2. Instruct the UAP to stop inserting the oral airway.
   3. Assist the UAP to insert the oral airway.
   4. Note the time of the seizure and observe seizure.

8. Mr. Leo is telling one of his graduate nurses the correct procedure for assisting the healthcare provider with a lumbar puncture to R/O meningitis. Which interventions should Mr. Leo discuss with the graduate nurse? **Select all that apply.**
   1. Obtain an informed consent from the client or significant other.
   2. Determine if the client is allergic to iodine or shellfish.
   3. Place the client in the supine position with the foot of the bed elevated.
   4. Instruct the client to relax and breathe normally.
   5. Explain to the client what to expect during the procedure.

9. Mr. Leo is making shift assignments. Which client should be assigned to the most experienced nurse?
   1. The client diagnosed with bacterial meningitis who is experiencing photophobia.
   2. The client with an L-4 SCI who has spastic muscle spasms of the lower extremities.
   3. The client diagnosed with Parkinson's who has a mask-like face and has pill rolling.
   4. The client amyotrophic lateral sclerosis (ALS) who is having respiratory distress.

10. The nurse is caring for clients on a Neurological Intensive Care unit. Which client should be assessed first?
    1. The client with increased intracranial pressure whose Glasgow Coma Scale went from 11 to 14.
    2. The client diagnosed with a C-6 SCI who has bradycardia, hypotension, and hyperflexia.
    3. The client with a brain stem herniation whose big toe moves toward the top surface of the foot and the other toes fan out after the sole of the foot has been firmly stroked.
    4. The client diagnosed with West Nile virus who has a temperature of 101.2°F and generalized body aches.

ANSWERS AND RATIONALES

The correct answer number and rationale for why it is the correct answer are given in **boldface type.** Rationales for why the other possible answer options are incorrect also are given, but they are not in boldface type.

1. 1. The serum platelet level is within the normal range of 150,000 to 400,000 mL; therefore, this laboratory does not warrant intervention by the charge nurse.
2. A therapeutic Depakote level is 50 to 100 ug/mL; therefore, this laboratory result does not warrant action by the nurse.
3. Steroids, such as prednisone, elevate a client's blood glucose level; therefore, this does not warrant intervention by the nurse.
4. **The therapeutic range for Dilantin is 10–20 mg/dL. This client's higher level warrants intervention because the serum level is above therapeutic range.**

Content – Medical/Surgical: *Category of Health Alteration* – Neurological: *Integrated Processes* – Nursing Process: Assessment: *Client Needs* – Safe and Effective Care Environment: Management of Care: *Cognitive Level* – Analysis

MAKING NURSING DECISIONS: The nurse must be knowledgeable of normal laboratory values. These values must be memorized and the nurse must be able to determine if the laboratory value is normal for the client's disease process or medications the client is taking.

2. 1. A pain medication is important to administer in a timely manner, but its administration is not priority over a medication that must be administered on time to prevent respiratory complications.
2. A steroid medication is not priority over a client who may experience respiratory difficulty. Steroids must be given to prevent adrenal sufficiency but it does not have to be administered first.
3. **Anticholinesterase medications administered for myasthenia gravis must be administered on time to preserve muscle functioning, especially the functioning of the muscles of the upper respiratory tract. This is the priority medication.**
4. Clients who have called for medications should be attended to, but this client would not receive an antacid for heartburn before the client diagnosed with myasthenia gravis or the client in pain.

Content – Medical/Surgical: *Category of Health Alteration* – Neurological: *Integrated Processes* – Nursing Process: Implementation: *Client Needs* – Physiological Integrity: Pharmacological and Parenteral Therapies: *Cognitive Level* – Analysis

MAKING NURSING DECISIONS: The nurse must be aware of expected actions of medications, and assess data indicating whether the medication is effective or the medication is causing a side effect or an adverse effect.

3. 1. The nurse would expect the client with Guillain-Barré syndrome to have ascending paralysis and the problem has just reached the knees, so the nurse should not need to assess this client first.
2. **The client with a C-6 SCI is expected to have autonomic dysreflexia but it is an emergency situation; therefore, the nurse should assess this client first.**
3. "Pill rolling," a hand tremor wherein the thumb and forefinger appear to move in a rotary fashion as if rolling a pill, is an expected clinical manifestation of Parkinson's; therefore, the nurse would not assess this client first.
4. The client with Huntington's disease has chorea, which includes abnormal and excessive involuntary movements; therefore, this client would not be assessed first.

Content – Medical/Surgical: *Category of Health Alteration* – Neurological: *Integrated Processes* – Nursing Process: Assessment: *Client Needs* – Safe and Effective Care Environment: Management of Care: *Cognitive Level* – Comprehension

MAKING NURSING DECISIONS: The nurse must determine which sign/symptom is not expected for the disease process. If the sign/symptom is not expected or it is an emergency situation, then the nurse should assess the client first. This type of question is determining if the nurse is knowledgeable of signs/symptoms of a variety of disease processes.

4. 1. Placing a gait belt prior to ambulating is an appropriate action for safety and would not require the nurse to intervene.
2. Placing the client in a prone position helps promote hyperextension of the hip joints, which is essential for normal gait and helps prevent knee and hip flexion contractures; therefore, this would not require the nurse to intervene.

3. This action is inappropriate and would require intervention by the nurse because pulling on a flaccid shoulder joint could cause shoulder dislocation; the client should be pulled up by placing the arm underneath the client's back or using a lift sheet.

4. The client should be encouraged and praised for attempting to perform any activities independently, such as combing hair or brushing teeth.

Content – Medical/Surgical: **Category of Health Alteration** *– Neurological:* **Integrated Processes** *– Nursing Process: Implementation:* **Client Needs** *– Safe and Effective Care Environment: Management of Care:* **Cognitive Level** *– Application*

MAKING NURSING DECISIONS: The nurse must ensure the UAP can perform any tasks that are delegated. It is the nurse's responsibility to demonstrate and/or teach the UAP how to perform the task, and evaluate the task.

5. 1. **Because the client is having an evolving stroke, the client is experiencing a worsening of signs/symptoms over several minutes to hours; thus, the client is at risk for dying and should be cared for by the most experienced nurse.**

2. A transient ischemic attack by definition lasts less than 24 hours; thus, this client should be stable at this time.

3. Pain is expected in clients with Guillain-Barré syndrome, and symptoms typically occur on the lower half of the body, which wouldn't affect the airway. Therefore, a less experienced nurse could care for this client.

4. The charge nurse could assign this client to an unlicensed assistive personnel (UAP).

Content – Medical/Surgical: **Category of Health Alteration** *– Neurological:* **Integrated Processes** *– Nursing Process: Planning:* **Client Needs** *– Safe and Effective Care Environment: Management of Care:* **Cognitive Level** *– Synthesis*

MAKING NURSING DECISIONS: When the nurse is deciding which client should be assigned to the most experienced nurse, the most critical and unstable client should be assigned to the most experienced nurse.

6. 1. **This client should be referred to an inpatient rehabilitation facility for intensive therapy before deciding on long-term placement (home with home healthcare or a long-term care facility). The initial rehabilitation a client receives can set the tone for all further recuperation. This is the appropriate referral at this time.**

2. A home healthcare agency may be needed when the client returns home, but the most

appropriate referral is to a rehabilitation center where intensive therapy can take place.

3. A long-term care facility may be needed at some point, but the client should be given the opportunity to regain as much lost ability as possible at this time.

4. The outpatient center would be utilized when the client is ready for discharge from the inpatient center.

Content – Medical/Surgical: **Category of Health Alteration** *– Neurological:* **Integrated Processes** *– Nursing Process: Planning:* **Client Needs** *– Physiological Integrity: Physiological Adaptation:* **Cognitive Level** *– Synthesis*

MAKING NURSING DECISIONS: The nurse must be knowledgeable of the role of all members of the multidisciplinary healthcare team, as well as HIPAA rules and regulations. These will be tested on the NCLEX-RN® exam.

7. 1. The nurse should be the first one to feed the client in order for the nurse to evaluate the client's ability to swallow and not aspirate.

2. **The LPN could administer routine parenteral medications. This is the best task to assign to the LPN.**

3. This involves assessing the client; therefore, the nurse should not delegate this assignment to the LPN.

4. Teaching is the responsibility of the RN.

Content – Medical/Surgical: **Category of Health Alteration** *– Neurological:* **Integrated Processes** *– Nursing Process: Planning:* **Client Needs** *– Safe and Effective Care Environment: Management of Care:* **Cognitive Level** *– Synthesis*

MAKING NURSING DECISIONS: The nurse cannot assign assessment, teaching, evaluation, or an unstable client to a LPN. The LPN can transcribe HCP orders and can call HCPs on the phone to obtain orders for a client.

8. 1 and 2 are correct.

1. **Checking the client's skin involves assessment; therefore, the nurse cannot delegate this assignment to the UAP.**

2. **The nurse cannot delegate medication administration to a UAP.**

3. The UAP can perform routine hygiene care. The nurse must then make the time to assess the client's skin.

4. The UAP can ambulate a client to the bathroom.

5. The UAP can take routine vital signs.

Content – Management of Care: **Category of Health Alteration** *– Neurological:* **Integrated Processes** *– Nursing Process: Planning:* **Client Needs** *– Safe and Effective Care Environment: Management of Care:* **Cognitive Level** *– Synthesis*

MAKING NURSING DECISIONS: This is a type of alternate question included in the NCLEX-RN®. The nurse must be able to select all the options that answer the question correctly. There are no partial correct answers.

9. 1. The UAP cannot change abdominal dressings because the incision must be assessed for healing.
   2. The UAP cannot check the client's IV site. Remember, check is "assess."
   3. The nurse must monitor the vital signs on a client recently returned from surgery to determine whether the client is stable; the UAP can take vital signs and report results to the nurse.
   4. **The UAP can escort the client to the vehicle after discharge.**
   Content – Management of Care: ***Category of Health Alteration*** *– Neurological:* ***Integrated Processes –*** *Nursing Process: Planning:* ***Client Needs*** *– Safe and Effective Care Environment: Management of Care:* ***Cognitive Level*** *– Synthesis*

MAKING NURSING DECISIONS: A nurse cannot delegate assessment, teaching, evaluation, medications, or an unstable client to a UAP. Tasks that cannot be delegated are nursing interventions requiring nursing judgment.

10. 1. **This client with dyspnea and a respiration rate of 12 has signs/symptoms of a respiratory complication and should be assessed first because ascending paralysis at the C-6 level could cause the client to stop breathing.**
   2. This is a psychosocial need and should be addressed, but it is not priority over a physiological problem.
   3. A client with a lower SCI would not be at risk for autonomic dysreflexia; therefore, a complaint of headache and feeling hot would not be priority over an airway problem.
   4. The client with a pulse oximeter reading greater than 93% is receiving adequate oxygenation.
   Content – Medical/Surgical: ***Category of Health Alteration*** *– Neurological:* ***Integrated Processes –*** *Nursing Process: Assessment:* ***Client Needs*** *– Safe and Effective Care Environment: Management of Care:* ***Cognitive Level*** *– Analysis*

MAKING NURSING DECISIONS: When deciding which client to assess first, the test taker should determine whether the signs/symptoms the client is exhibiting are normal or expected for the situation. After eliminating the expected options, the test taker should determine which situation is more life threatening.

11. 1. The client is experiencing autonomic dysreflexia, a complication of SCI above the T6,

and the most common cause is a full bladder. Placing the client on telemetry is not the nurse's first intervention.
   2. Completing a neurological assessment is an intervention a nurse could implement, but it should not be the first for a client experiencing autonomic dysreflexia.
   3. **Autonomic dysreflexia is a life-threatening condition and can be considered a medical emergency requiring immediate attention. The nurse should not assess but should intervene, and the most common cause is a full bladder.**
   4. A CT scan of the head would be appropriate if the elevated B/P was secondary to a CVA, not due to a complication of a SCI.
   Content – Medical/Surgical: ***Category of Health Alteration*** *– Neurological:* ***Integrated Processes –*** *Nursing Process: Assessment:* ***Client Needs*** *– Physiological Integrity: Reduction of Risk Potential:* ***Cognitive Level*** *– Analysis*

MAKING NURSING DECISIONS: When the test question asks the test taker to determine which intervention should be implemented first, it means that all the options are something a nurse could implement. The test taker should apply the nursing process: If the client is in distress then do not assess; the nurse should do something to help the client.

12. 1. It would be appropriate for the UAP to perform ROM exercises to help prevent contractures; therefore, this action would not require the nurse to intervene.
   2. **This is not an appropriate intervention because the client is at risk for increased intracranial pressure (ICP); therefore, the client should not be placed on the stomach. The prone position helps promote hyperextension of the hip joints, which is essential for normal gait and helps prevent knee and hip flexion contractures, and done in rehabilitation.**
   3. The client should be pulled up in bed by placing the arm underneath the back or using a lift sheet; therefore, the nurse would not need to intervene.
   4. The client should be encouraged and praised for attempting to perform any activities independently, such as combing hair, brushing teeth, or feeding him- or herself. The nurse would not need to intervene.
   Content – Medical/Surgical: ***Category of Health Alteration*** *– Neurological:* ***Integrated Processes –*** *Nursing Process: Implementation:* ***Client Needs*** *– Physiological Integrity: Reduction of Risk Potential:* ***Cognitive Level*** *– Analysis*

MAKING NURSING DECISIONS: The nurse must ensure the UAP can perform any tasks that are delegated. It is the nurse's responsibility to demonstrate and/or teach the UAP how to perform the task, and evaluate the task.

13. 1. **The less experienced nurse could care for the client on a ventilator and console the family as needed. This client is not in a life-threatening situation and is stable for the condition.**
    2. A client with increased intracranial pressure requires a more experienced critical care nurse.
    3. This client is unstable and requires a more experienced critical care nurse.
    4. Status epilepticus is a state of continuous seizure activity and is the most serious complication of epilepsy. This is a neurological emergency. This client should be assigned to a more experienced nurse.

    Content – *Medical/Surgical:* **Category of Health Alteration** – *Neurological:* **Integrated Processes** – *Nursing Process: Planning:* **Client Needs** – *Safe and Effective Care Environment: Management of Care:* **Cognitive Level** – *Synthesis*

MAKING NURSING DECISIONS: The most stable client should be assigned to the graduate nurse. The more critical clients should be assigned to the more experienced nurses.

14. 1. Purposeful movement following painful stimuli would indicate an improvement in the client's condition and would not warrant intervention by the nurse.
    2. **Extension of the upper and lower extremities is assuming a decerebrate posture, which indicates the client's intracranial pressure (ICP) is increasing. This would warrant immediate intervention by the nurse.**
    3. Aimless thrashing would indicate an improvement in the client's condition and would not warrant intervention by the nurse.
    4. If the client is able to follow simple commands, then the client's condition is improving and would not warrant intervention by the nurse.

    Content – *Medical/Surgical:* **Category of Health Alteration** – *Neurological:* **Integrated Processes** – *Nursing Process: Assessment:* **Client Needs** – *Safe and Effective Care Environment: Management of Care:* **Cognitive Level** – *Synthesis*

MAKING NURSING DECISIONS: The test taker should ask, "Are the assessment data normal?" for the disease process. If they are normal for the disease process, then the nurse would not need

to intervene; if they are not normal for the disease process, then this warrants intervention by the nurse.

15. 1. An adverse occurrence report is completed for incidents occurring to clients.
    2. The nurse should talk to the primary nurse, but the sharps container should be changed immediately.
    3. **The UAP can change a sharps container. This must be done because a sharps container above the fill line is a violation of Occupational Safety Health Administration (OSHA) rules and can result in a financial fine.**
    4. The infection control nurse does not need to be notified of this situation.

    Content – *Legal:* **Category of Health Alteration** – *Neurological:* **Integrated Processes** – *Nursing Process: Implementation:* **Client Needs** – *Safe and Effective Care Environment: Safety and Infection Control:* **Cognitive Level** – *Application*

MAKING NURSING DECISIONS: The nurse is responsible for knowing and complying with local, state, and federal standards of care.

16. 1. **The nurse should address the client's comment and not "pass the buck" to someone else.**
    2. The nurse should address the client's statement and not attempt to problem-solve at this point in the conversation.
    3. The nurse is reflecting the client's comments, which will encourage the client to ventilate her feelings. This is the most appropriate response.
    4. This is false reassurance and an inappropriate response to the client's statement.

    Content – *Medical/Surgical:* **Category of Health Alteration** – *Oncology:* **Integrated Processes** – *Nursing Process: Implementation :* **Client Needs** – *Psychosocial Integrity:* **Cognitive Level** – *Application*

MAKING NURSING DECISIONS: The NCLEX-RN® blueprint includes Therapeutic Communication as a subcategory of Psychosocial Integrity. The nurse should allow clients and family to ventilate feelings.

17. 1. The client with Guillain-Barré syndrome is at risk for airway compromise resulting from the ascending paralysis. Cardiac output is not a priority.
    2. The client's psychological needs are important, but psychosocial problems are not priority.
    3. Complications of immobility are pertinent but do not take priority over the airway.

4. Guillain-Barré syndrome produces ascending paralysis that will cause respiratory failure; therefore, breathing pattern is priority.
Content – Medical/Surgical: **Category of Health Alteration** *– Neurological:* **Integrated Processes** *– Nursing Process: Planning:* **Client Needs** *– Physiological Integrity: Reduction of Risk Potential:* **Cognitive Level** *– Comprehension*

MAKING NURSING DECISIONS: The NCLEX-RN® integrates the nursing process throughout the Client Needs categories and subcategories. The nursing process is a scientific, clinical reasoning approach to client care that includes assessment, analysis, planning, implementation, and evaluation. The nurse will be responsible for identifying nursing problems for clients.

18. 1. The occupational therapist addresses assisting the client with ADLs, but with MG the client will have no problems with ADLs if the client takes the medication correctly, 30 minutes prior to performing ADLs.
2. A physical therapist addresses transfer and movement issues with the client, but this would not be priority in the critical care unit.
3. The social worker assists the client with discharge issues or financial issues, but this would not be appropriate for the client in the critical care unit.
4. **Speech therapists address swallowing problems, and clients with MG are dysphagic and are at risk for aspiration; the speech therapist can help match food consistency to the client's ability to swallow and thus help enhance client safety. This referral would be appropriate in the critical care unit.**
Content – Medical/Surgical: **Category of Health Alteration** *– Neurological:* **Integrated Processes** *– Nursing Process: Planning:* **Client Needs** *– Safe and Effective Care Environment: Management of Care:* **Cognitive Level** *– Comprehension*

MAKING NURSING DECISIONS: The NCLEX-RN® integrates the nursing process throughout the Client Needs categories and subcategories. The nursing process is a scientific, clinical reasoning approach to client care that includes assessment, analysis, planning, implementation, and evaluation. The nurse will be responsible for identifying nursing diagnoses for clients.

19. 1. This should be done but not prior to notifying the charge nurse and reporting the incident.
2. **The nurse should notify the charge nurse first so the hospital protocol can be followed, including notifying the infection**

control nurse, completing an incident report, obtaining blood from the client, and starting prophylactic medication if warranted.
3. This should be done within 4 hours of the stick, but the charge nurse should be notified first so that proper hospital protocol can be initiated.
4. This is done at 3 months and 6 months.
Content – Medical/Surgical: **Category of Health Alteration** *– Neurological:* **Integrated Processes** *– Nursing Process: Implementation:* **Client Needs** *– Safe and Effective Care Environment: Safety and Infection Control:* **Cognitive Level** *– Application*

MAKING NURSING DECISIONS: The NCLEX-RN® blueprint includes nursing care that is ruled by legal requirements as well as the Joint Commission, Centers for Medicare & Medicaid Services, the Centers for Disease Control and Prevention, and Occupational Safety and Health Administration rules and regulations. The nurse must be knowledgeable of these standards.

20. 1. **The client diagnosed with Parkinson's disease who has begun to hallucinate may be experiencing an adverse reaction to one of the medications used to treat the disease. The nurse should assess this client first.**
2. Peripheral edema is expected in a client diagnosed with heart failure. This client does not need to be assessed first.
3. Wandering and lack of sleeping are expected in a client diagnosed with Alzheimer's disease. This client does not need to be assessed first.
4. Weight loss in a client diagnosed with terminal cancer is expected. The nurse should review the client's intake, food preferences, and pain control before making an intervention. Weight loss does not occur in a matter of minutes to hours, and this client's needs do not merit assessment before the client with a new problem.
Content – Management of Care: **Category of Health Alteration** *– Neurological:* **Integrated Processes** *– Nursing Process: Assessment:* **Client Needs** *– Safe and Effective Care Environment: Management of Care:* **Cognitive Level** *– Analysis*

MAKING NURSING DECISIONS: The nurse should determine whether a new problem is occurring or whether the problem is expected for the disease process. If the symptom is expected for the disease process and it is not life threatening, then that client does not have priority.

21. 1. A daily aspirin is not a priority medication. This medication can be administered within

30 minutes before or 30 minutes after the scheduled time.

2. **Prostigmin promotes muscle function in clients diagnosed with myasthenia gravis. This medication should always be administered on time to prevent loss of muscle tone, especially the muscles of the upper respiratory tract. This is the priority medication to administer at this time.**

3. An oral antibiotic can be administered within 30 minutes before or after the scheduled time frame.

4. Acyclovir (Zovirax) alone or in combination with predisone may be used to treat Bell's palsy but this medication is not a priority medication.

Content – Adult Health, Pharmacology: **Category of Health Alteration** *– Neurological:* **Integrated Processes** *– Nursing Process: Implementation:* **Client Needs** *– Physiological Integrity: Pharmacological and Parenteral Therapies:* **Cognitive Level** *– Analysis*

MAKING NURSING DECISIONS: When the nurse is deciding on a priority medication, the test taker must first decide on the expected response of the client. If the expected response prevents or treats an emergency situation, then that medication becomes the priority medication to administer.

22. 1. Clients diagnosed with Alzheimer's disease may have problems with completing activities of daily living, but this is not the client's priority problem.

2. **Safety is the highest priority for clients diagnosed with end-stage Alzheimer's disease because the client is unaware of his or her own surroundings and can easily wander from an area of safety.**

3. The client in end-stage disease may have an increased risk for constipation, but this is not priority over safety of the client.

4. The client's family is often distraught over seeing their loved one deteriorate because of Alzheimer's, but it is not priority over the safety of the client.

Content – Management of Care: **Category of Health Alteration** *– Neurological:* **Integrated Processes** *– Nursing Process: Planning:* **Client Needs** *– Physiological Integrity: Physiological Adaptation:* **Cognitive Level** *– Synthesis*

MAKING NURSING DECISIONS: The test taker can use Maslow's Hierarchy of Needs to determine the correct answer. On the pyramid of needs, beginning at the bottom, physiological needs have priority, followed by safety.

23. 1. Cataracts cause less light to be filtered through an opaque lens to the retina.

The client should have as much light as possible in the home to prevent falls.

2. Dark glasses protect the eyes from the sun's rays when outside, as they do for anyone, but this client needs more light indoors.

3. This is the responsibility of the HCP, not the nurse.

4. The furniture in the client's house should not be moved. If the furniture is left in its usual position, the client will be less likely to fall or stumble. However, the priority intervention is safety when walking; therefore, increasing light in the home is priority.

Content – Geriatrics: **Category of Health Alteration** *– Neurological:* **Integrated Processes** *– Nursing Process: Planning:* **Client Needs** *– Physiological Integrity: Reduction of Risk Potential:* **Cognitive Level** *– Synthesis*

MAKING NURSING DECISIONS: This question requires the test taker to use knowledge of the disease process and Maslow's Hierarchy of Needs. Cataracts cause opacity of the lens of the eye, and safety is a high priority according to Maslow.

24. 1. **The nurse should first assess the client's neurological status. It is not normal for an elderly person to have a change in behavior; this is cause for assessment.**

2. The nurse may need to notify the HCP but not prior to completing a neurological assessment.

3. The nurse should first assess the client prior to further interviewing the client's wife.

4. The nurse could determine the last time the client ate, since the confusion could be due to hypoglycemia, but the first intervention is to complete a neurological assessment.

Content – Medical/Surgical: **Category of Health Alteration** *– Neurological:* **Integrated Processes** *– Nursing Process: Implementation:* **Client Needs** *– Safe and Effective Care Environment: Management of Care:* **Cognitive Level** *– Analysis*

MAKING NURSING DECISIONS: Any time the nurse receives information about a client who may be experiencing a complication, the nurse must assess the client. The nurse should not make decisions about the client's needs based on another staff member's information.

25. 1. **This question will determine whether the nurse has assessed the client's ability to swallow. The nurse cannot delegate unstable clients, and a client newly diagnosed with a CVA may be unstable and have difficulty swallowing.**

2. This question does not address the client's ability to swallow.

3. Thick-It might be needed if the client has difficulty swallowing, but the charge nurse has not established that the client has swallowing difficulty.
4. A UAP can feed clients who are stable and do not require nursing judgment during the process.
*Content – Medical/Surgical: **Category of Health Alteration** – Neurological: **Integrated Processes** – Nursing Process: Analysis **Client Needs** – Safe and Effective Care Environment: Safety and Infection Control: **Cognitive Level** – Analysis*

MAKING NURSING DECISIONS: The nurse cannot delegate assessment, evaluation, teaching, administering medications, or the care of an unstable client to a UAP.

26. 1. The client should be encouraged to move the buttocks to increase blood circulation to the area, but a wheelchair cushion used every time the client is in the wheelchair will help prevent pressure ulcers.
2. A high-protein diet will assist with maintaining a positive nitrogen balance that will support wound healing, but it will not prevent pressure from causing a breakdown of the skin.
3. **All clients remaining in a wheelchair for extended periods of time should have a wheelchair cushion that relieves pressure to prevent skin breakdown.**
4. The more the client can move from the wheelchair to a chair to the bed, the more it will help decrease the possibility of a pressure ulcer, but a wheelchair cushion helps relieve pressure continuously.
*Content – Medical/Surgical: **Category of Health Alteration** – Neurological: **Integrated Processes** – Nursing Process: Implementation: **Client Needs** – Physiological Integrity: Basic Care and Comfort: **Cognitive Level** – Comprehension*

MAKING NURSING DECISIONS: The nurse must be knowledgeable of expected medical treatment for the client. This is a knowledge-based, or comprehension, question.

27. 1. Identifying the first area that began seizing will provide information and clues as to the location of the seizure origin in the brain, but it is not the nurse's first intervention.
2. **The nurse should first look at his or her watch and time the seizure. Assessment is the first intervention because there is no action the nurse can implement to stop or intervene with the seizure.**
3. The client's bed rails should be padded, but this is not the first intervention when walking into a room where the client is beginning

to have a seizure. The nurse should first assess the seizure and then pad the side rails if there is time. The seizure may be over by the time the nurse can pad the side rails.
4. The client should be protected from onlookers, but the nurse should always assess and care for the client first.
*Content – Medical/Surgical: **Category of Health Alteration** – Neurological: **Integrated Processes** – Nursing Process: Implementation: **Client Needs** – Safe and Effective Care Environment: Safety and Infection Control: **Cognitive Level** – Analysis*

MAKING NURSING DECISIONS: The nurse should always apply the nursing process when answering a question requiring the nurse to "determine which intervention to implement first." The first part of the nursing process is to assess.

28. 1. Closing the door and cubicle curtain protects the client's privacy and would not warrant immediate intervention from the nurse.
2. Providing a back massage is a wonderful action to take and would not warrant intervention by the nurse.
3. Checking the temperature of the bathwater prevents scalding the client with water that is too hot or making the client uncomfortable with water that is too cold. This action would not warrant immediate intervention.
4. **The client is recovering from a potentially debilitating disease, and in the rehabilitation unit the client should be out of the bed as much as possible. Bathing the client in bed would warrant intervention by the nurse.**
*Content – Medical/Surgical: **Category of Health Alteration** – Neurological: **Integrated Processes** – Evaluation: **Client Needs** – Physiological Integrity: Reduction of Risk Potential: **Cognitive Level** – Synthesis*

MAKING NURSING DECISIONS: Delegation means the nurse is responsible for the UAP's actions and performance. The nurse must correct the UAP's performance to ensure the client is cared for safely in the hospital, the rehabilitation unit, or the home.

29. 1, 2, 3, and 4 are correct.
1. **Placing a small pillow under the shoulder will prevent the shoulder from adducting toward the chest and developing a contracture.**
2. **The client should be referred to occupational therapy for assistance with performing activities of daily living (ADLs).**
3. **The client should not ignore the paralyzed side, and the nurse must encourage the client to move it as much as possible;**

a written schedule may assist the client in exercising.

4. **These exercises should be done at least five times a day for 10 minutes at a time to help strengthen the muscles used for walking.**

5. The fingers should be positioned so that they are barely flexed, to prevent contracture.

Content – Medical/Surgical: **Category of Health Alteration** *– Neurological:* **Integrated Processes** *– Nursing Process: Planning:* **Client Needs** *– Health Promotion and Maintenance:* **Cognitive Level** *– Synthesis*

MAKING NURSING DECISIONS: This is an alternate type of question included in the NCLEX-RN®. The nurse must be able to select all the options that answer the question correctly. There are no partially correct answers.

30. 1. The nurse should stabilize the client's cervical spine to help prevent a spinal cord injury or the patient's spine can sustain irreparable damage during movement.

2. Unless the driver is in danger (car on fire or in water) the nurse should not move the driver.

3. **The nurse should first ensure a patent airway. According to Maslow's Hierarchy of Needs, airway is always priority.**

4. The nurse should control external bleeding but the first intervention is airway.

Content – Medical/Surgical: **Category of Health Alteration** *– Neurological:* **Integrated Processes** *– Nursing Process: Implementation:* **Client Needs** *– Physiological Integrity: Reduction of Risk Potential:* **Cognitive Level** *– Analysis*

MAKING NURSING DECISIONS: The test taker should use some tool as a reference to guide in the decision-making process. In this situation, Maslow's Hierarchy of Needs should be applied.

31. 1. **This would be the most appropriate assignment because the nurse would not be exposed to any contagious diseases or dangerous radiological procedures.**

2. The pregnant nurse should not be exposed to x-rays, which could endanger the fetus.

3. Working in the front desk triage area would allow the pregnant nurse to be exposed to any type of contagious or infectious disease. This is not an appropriate assignment.

4. The oncology clinic will have clients receiving chemotherapeutic agents that may endanger the fetus; this would not be the most appropriate assignment. Even if the nurse is not administering the medication, the most appropriate assignment is to assign the nurse to an area that poses no danger to the fetus.

Content – Medical/Surgical: **Category of Health Alteration** *– Neurological:* **Integrated Processes** *– Nursing Process: Implementation:* **Client Needs** *– Safe*

and Effective Care Environment: Management of Care: **Cognitive Level** *– Application*

MAKING NURSING DECISIONS: Pregnant nurses should not and can refuse to perform duties that could harm the fetus. Most medications and many diagnostic tests and treatments can harm the fetus.

32. 1. If the client must be transferred from the clinic to the hospital, then the client is unstable and therefore should not be assigned to a UAP.

2. **The client is stable because he or she is being sent home; therefore, the UAP could safely complete this task.**

3. Showing the client how to walk with crutches is teaching, and the nurse cannot delegate teaching to the UAP.

4. The UAP should not be calling a pharmacy because this is not within the scope of practice of unlicensed personnel. The HCP is responsible for delegating this task.

Content – Management of Care: **Category of Health Alteration** *– Neurological:* **Integrated Processes** *– Nursing Process: Planning:* **Client Needs** *– Safe and Effective Care Environment: Management of Care:* **Cognitive Level** *– Synthesis*

MAKING NURSING DECISIONS: A nurse cannot delegate assessment, teaching, evaluation, medications, or an unstable client to a UAP. Tasks that cannot be delegated are nursing interventions requiring nursing judgment.

33. 1. **The nurse should first care for the client and refer the client to an HCP for possible x-rays, pain medication, and further treatment. The employee health nurse's responsibility is to ensure the employee is safe to work, and this client is not.**

2. This information should be completed because any injury on the job must be covered by workers' compensation insurance so that all costs will be covered for the client. Documentation is never priority over caring for the client.

3. The employee health nurse should determine whether there are unsafe areas in the workplace or whether the employee was negligent, but this is not the nurse's first intervention.

4. The employee's supervisor does need to be notified, but this is not the nurse's first intervention. The safety of the client is always first.

Content – Medical/Surgical: **Category of Health Alteration** *– Neurological:* **Integrated Processes** *– Nursing Process: Assessment:* **Client Needs** *– Physiological Integrity: Reduction of Risk Potential:* **Cognitive Level** *– Analysis*

MAKING NURSING DECISIONS: When the question asks which intervention should be

implemented first, it means all the options are something a nurse could implement, but only one should be implemented first. The test taker should use the nursing process to determine the appropriate action: If the client is in distress do not assess; if the client is not in distress then the nurse should assess.

34. 1. If a client is complaining of pain, the nurse should not ask the client to return to work. If nothing else, the client should be allowed to stay in the clinic until the pain subsides.
2. **The employee must submit to a urine drug screen anytime there is an injury. This is standard practice by many employers to help determine whether the employee was under the influence during the time of the accident. Workers' compensation will not be responsible if the employee is under the influence of alcohol or drugs.**
3. Because there are no visible injuries and the neurovascular assessment is normal, a referral to the emergency department is not warranted. The employee health nurse could send the employee home with further instructions. None of the complaints warrants the employee's needing an x-ray.
4. A sequential compression device is used to help prevent deep vein thrombosis for clients on bed rest. This is not an appropriate intervention.
*Content – Medical/Surgical: **Category of Health Alteration** – Neurological: **Integrated Processes** – Nursing Process: Implementation: **Client Needs** – Safe and Effective Care Environment: Management of Care: **Cognitive Level** – Application*

MAKING NURSING DECISIONS: The NCLEX-RN® blueprint includes nursing care that is ruled by legal requirements as well as the Joint Commission, Centers for Medicare & Medicaid Services, Centers for Disease Control and Prevention, and Occupational Safety and Health Administration rules and regulations. The nurse must be knowledgeable of these standards.

35. 1. An alert client with a sucking chest wound should be categorized as red, priority 1, which means the injury is life threatening but survivable with minimal intervention. These clients can deteriorate rapidly without treatment.
2. A client who cannot stop crying and cannot answer questions should be categorized as green, priority 3, which means the injury is minor and treatment can be delayed hours to days. These clients should be moved away from the main triage area. Clients with behavioral and psychological problems are included in this category.

3. A client whose abdomen is hard and tender should be categorized as a yellow, priority 2, which means the injury is significant and requires medical care but can wait hours without threat to life or limb. Clients in this category receive treatment only after immediate casualties are treated.
4. **This client should be categorized as black, priority 4, which means the injury is extensive and chances of survival are unlikely even with definitive care. Clients should receive comfort measures and be separated from other casualties, but not abandoned.**
*Content – Medical/Surgical: **Category of Health Alteration** – Neurological: **Integrated Processes** – Nursing Process: Assessment: **Client Needs** – Safe and Effective Care Environment: Management of Care: **Cognitive Level** – Analysis*

MAKING NURSING DECISIONS: The NCLEX-RN® blueprint includes questions on disaster management. The nurse needs to be aware of triaging clients, nursing care, and procedures and protocols during disasters.

36. 1. The nurse should determine what medication the client has taken, but the nurse should first attempt to determine whether the headache is secondary to high blood pressure.
2. No matter what number the client identifies on the pain scale in the home setting, the nurse must attempt to determine the cause. One way to try to determine the cause or to eliminate a possible cause is to take the client's blood pressure.
3. If the client's blood pressure is not elevated, the client could take the non-narcotic analgesic acetaminophen (Tylenol), but if the client's blood pressure is elevated, the Tylenol will not help.
4. **The number 1 risk factor for a CVA is arterial hypertension. Because the client has a history of a CVA and is complaining of a severe headache, which is a symptom of hypertension, the nurse should first take the client's blood pressure. If it is elevated, the client needs to be taken to the emergency department. In the home setting, asking about the pain scale would not affect the care the nurse provides.**
*Content – Medical/Surgical: **Category of Health Alteration** – Neurological: **Integrated Processes** – Nursing Process: Implementation: **Client Needs** – Physiological Integrity: Reduction of Risk Potential: **Cognitive Level** – Analysis*

MAKING NURSING DECISIONS: When the question asks which intervention should be implemented

first, it means that all the options are something a nurse could implement, but only one should be implemented first. The test taker should use the nursing process to determine the appropriate action: If the client is in distress do not assess; if the client is not in distress then the nurse should assess.

37. 1. The nurse should assist the client to lie in the "C" position with the back as near as possible to the edge of the bed, but it is not the first intervention.
   2. **The first intervention is to empty the client's bladder prior to the procedure.**
   3. All clients should have an advance directive, but it is not mandated by law, and clients can decide not to have one.
   4. The client does not have to be NPO for this procedure.
   *Content – Medical/Surgical: **Category of Health Alteration** – Neurological: **Integrated Processes** – Nursing Process: Implementation: **Client Needs** – Safe and Effective Care Environment: Management of Care: **Cognitive Level** – Analysis*

MAKING NURSING DECISIONS: The nurse must be knowledgeable of normal diagnostic tests pre- and post-procedure. These interventions must be memorized and the nurse must be able to determine if the client is able to have the diagnostic procedure and post-procedure care to ensure the client is safe.

38. 1. A severe, pounding headache would be priority for a client with a T-6 or above spinal cord injury (SCI) because it could be autonomic dysreflexia, but not in a client with a lower-level lesion.
   2. The client's psychosocial need is not priority over clients with physiological problems. This client should not be visited first.
   3. The client with Parkinson's disease is expected to have a short, shuffling gait; therefore, this client does not need to be seen first.
   4. **The client is reporting an infection at insertion sites into the bone, which can lead to osteomyelitis. This client is exhibiting a potentially life-threatening condition and should be seen first.**
   *Content – Medical/Surgical: **Category of Health Alteration** – Neurological: **Integrated Processes** – Nursing Process: Assessment: **Client Needs** – Safe and Effective Care Environment: Management of Care: **Cognitive Level** – Analysis*

MAKING NURSING DECISIONS: When deciding which client to assess first, the test taker should determine whether the signs/symptoms the

client is exhibiting are normal or expected for the client situation. After eliminating the expected option, the test taker should determine which situation is more life threatening.

39. 1. A client with AIDS would be expected to have Kaposi's sarcoma; therefore, this client would not need to be visited first.
   2. A client with dementia would be expected to have difficulty dressing; therefore, this client would not need to be visited first.
   3. The classic feature of trigeminal neuralgia is excruciating pain described as a burning, knife-like, or lightning-like shock in the lips, upper or lower gums, cheek, forehead, or side of the nose. The nurse would not return this call first since the client is experiencing the normal signs/symptoms for the disease process.
   4. **Botulism is the most serious type of food poisoning and the client is exhibiting signs/symptoms of it; therefore, the nurse should return this phone call first.**
   *Content – Medical/Surgical: **Category of Health Alteration** – Neurological: **Integrated Processes** – Nursing Process: Assessment: **Client Needs** – Safe and Effective Care Environment: Management of Care: **Cognitive Level** – Analysis*

MAKING NURSING DECISIONS: When deciding which client to assess first, the nurse should determine whether the signs/symptoms the client is exhibiting are normal or expected for the client situation. After eliminating the expected options, the test taker should determine which situation is more dangerous for the client.

40. 1. **Therapeutic communication addresses the client's feelings and attempts to allow the client to verbalize feelings. The client is still grieving over her loss, and the nurse should let her vent feelings.**
   2. The social worker may be able to help the client with driving and going back to college, but this is not the nurse's first intervention.
   3. The American Spinal Cord Association is an excellent resource for clients with spinal cord injuries, but the client is still grieving, and the nurse should allow the client to express her feelings.
   4. Attempting to help identify a support system for the client is an appropriate intervention, but the first intervention is to allow the client to vent her feelings.
   *Content – Medical/Surgical: **Category of Health Alteration** – Neurological: **Integrated Processes** – Nursing Process: Implementation: **Client Needs** – Psychosocial Integrity: Therapeutic Communication: **Cognitive Level** – Analysis*

MAKING NURSING DECISIONS: The NCLEX-RN® blueprint includes Therapeutic Communication as a subcategory of Psychosocial Integrity. The nurse should allow clients and family to ventilate feelings.

41. 1. **The client is allergic to iodine; therefore, the client cannot have the CT scan with contrast because it is iodine. The nurse should question this HCP order.**
    2. The client is not allergic to Tylenol; therefore, this order should not be questioned.
    3. The client should have vital signs taken; therefore, this order should not be questioned.
    4. A low-fat, low-cholesterol diet would be appropriate for this client.
    *Content – Medical/Surgical: **Category of Health Alteration** – Neurological: **Integrated Processes** – Nursing Process: Analysis: **Client Needs** – Physiological Integrity: Reduction of Risk Potential: **Cognitive Level** – Analysis*

MAKING NURSING DECISIONS: When the stem asks the nurse to determine which healthcare provider's order to question, the test taker should realize this is an "except" question. Three of the options are appropriate for the HCP to prescribe and one is not appropriate for the client's disease process or procedure.

42. 1. The client has a chronic illness. The nurse should empower the client to deal with her disease process, not put more responsibility on her husband.
    2. **The occupational therapist could assist the client in identifying ways to save energy when performing activities of daily living. Myasthenia gravis is a neurological condition that causes skeletal muscle weakness.**
    3. The HH nurse should realize that exhaustion is a symptom of her disease process and should utilize any member of the home healthcare team who could help the client. Allowing the client to verbalize her feelings about exhaustion is an appropriate therapeutic intervention, but this client needs specific advice on how to handle her exhaustion.
    4. If the client is taking her medication, she does not need to be referred to her HCP. Myasthenia gravis is a chronic illness, and muscle weakness is the primary symptom.
    *Content – Medical/Surgical: **Category of Health Alteration** – Neurological: **Integrated Processes** – Nursing Process: Implementation: **Client Needs** – Physiological Integrity: Physiological Adaptation: **Cognitive Level** – Analysis*

MAKING NURSING DECISIONS: The test taker must be knowledgeable of the role of all members of the multidisciplinary healthcare team as well as HIPAA rules and regulations. These will be tested on the NCLEX-RN® exam.

43. 1. **An epidural hematoma results from bleeding between the dura and the inner surface of the skull, and is a medical emergency. This client should be seen first.**
    2. Postictal state is a sleepy state the client has after having a seizure. This client is stable; therefore, this client does not have to be assessed first.
    3. The client with encephalitis may have fever, headache, nausea, and vomiting. The client needs to be assessed but not prior to a head injury with active arterial bleeding.
    4. The client with multiple sclerosis is expected to have scanning speech; therefore, the nurse should not assess this client first.
    *Content – Medical/Surgical: **Category of Health Alteration** – Neurological: **Integrated Processes** – Nursing Process: Assessment: **Client Needs** – Safe and Effective Care Environment: Management of Care: **Cognitive Level** – Analysis*

MAKING NURSING DECISIONS: The test taker should use some tool as a reference to guide in the decision-making process. In this situation, Maslow's Hierarchy of Needs should be applied.

44. 1. **The tension headache does not involve nausea or vomiting but may involve photophobia or phonophobia. Since the nausea and vomiting are not expected, the nurse should return this phone call first.**
    2. The migraine headache is a recurring headache characterized by unilateral or bilateral throbbing pain; therefore, this client should not be contacted first.
    3. The pain of cluster headaches is sharp and stabbing, which is not like the pulsing pain of a migraine headache. This client does not need to be contacted first.
    4. This is the typical type of pain clients with hypertension experience; therefore, this client does not need to be contacted first.
    *Content – Medical/Surgical: **Category of Health Alteration** – Neurological: **Integrated Processes** – Nursing Process: Assessment: **Client Needs** – Safe and Effective Care Environment: Management of Care: **Cognitive Level** – Analysis*

MAKING NURSING DECISIONS: The test taker must determine which sign/symptom is not expected for the disease process. If the sign/symptom is not expected then the nurse should assess the client first. This type of question is determining if the nurse is knowledgeable of signs/symptoms of a variety of disease processes.

ANSWERS

45. 1. The wife should check to determine whether the client is incontinent of urine, but the client's safety is priority.

2. The most important action the wife can take if her husband has a seizure is to make sure he does not get injured during the seizure. Moving all the furniture out of the way will help ensure the client's safety.

3. Seizures are not life threatening. If the wife calls 911, the ambulance will probably arrive after the client's seizure has ended. Seizures lasting longer than 4 to 5 minutes warrant calling 911.

4. The client should be allowed to rest after the seizure when he is in the postictal state, but it is not the most important action to take. Safety of the client during the seizure is priority.

Content – Medical/Surgical: **Category of Health Alteration** *– Neurological:* **Integrated Processes** *– Nursing Process: Evaluation; Teaching/Learning:* **Client Needs** *– Physiological Integrity: Physiological Adaptation:* **Cognitive Level** *– Analysis*

MAKING NURSING DECISIONS: The nurse must be knowledgeable of the expected medical treatment for the client's condition. Safety is priority for the client, especially when the client is at home.

46. 1. The client may benefit from a hospital bed, but this is not the priority intervention to address the client's non-healing pressure ulcer.

2. HH care agencies do not provide care 7 days a week. Even if the client could have an HH aide 7 days a week, it is not the priority intervention to address the client's non-healing pressure ulcer.

3. The client does not need to be transferred to a skilled nursing unit. The wound care nurse should attempt to heal the pressure ulcer in the home first.

4. The wound care nurse's primary role is to address non-healing pressure ulcers. This referral is the priority intervention.

Content – Medical/Surgical: **Category of Health Alteration** *– Integumentary:* **Integrated Processes** *– Nursing Process: Planning:* **Client Needs** *– Physiological Integrity: Reduction of Risk Potential:* **Cognitive Level** *– Synthesis*

MAKING NURSING DECISIONS: The test taker must be knowledgeable of the role of all members of the multidisciplinary healthcare team as well as HIPAA rules and regulations. These will be tested on the NCLEX-RN® exam.

47. 1. Grab bars address safety issues, but the client is having transfer difficulty, which requires the help of the physical therapist.

2. In most situations, the nurse should assess the client prior to taking action, but the HH aide has the ability and knowledge to determine if the client is having problems getting out of the bed and into the shower. The nurse should allow the physical therapist to assess the client's transfer ability.

3. The goal of HH nursing is to keep the client as independent as possible, and having the client receive a bed bath is increasing the client's dependency on the HH aide.

4. The physical therapist is the member of the healthcare team who is responsible for helping the client with mobility issues.

Content – Management of Care: **Category of Health Alteration** *– Neurological:* **Integrated Processes** *– Nursing Process: Implementation:* **Client Needs** *– Safe and Effective Care Environment: Management of Care:* **Cognitive Level** *– Application*

MAKING NURSING DECISIONS: The test taker must be knowledgeable of the role of all members of the multidisciplinary healthcare team as well as HIPAA rules and regulations. These will be tested on the NCLEX-RN® exam.

48. 1. Daily exercise, relaxation periods, and socializing are encouraged because each can help decrease the occurrence of headaches. This statement indicates the client understands the teaching.

2. Alternative ways of handling the pain of a headache include techniques such as relaxation, meditation, yoga, and self-hypnosis. This statement indicates the client understands the teaching.

3. Massage and moist hot packs to the neck and head can help a client with tension-type headaches. This statement indicates the client needs more teaching.

4. Foods containing amines (cheese, chocolate), nitrites (hot dogs), vinegar, onions, caffeine, and alcohol (especially red wine) can trigger a headache. The statement indicates the client understands the teaching.

Content – Medical/Surgical: **Category of Health Alteration** *– Neurological:* **Integrated Processes** *– Nursing Process: Evaluation; Teaching/Learning:* **Client Needs** *– Physiological Integrity: Physiological Adaptation:* **Cognitive Level** *– Analysis*

MAKING NURSING DECISIONS: This question asks the nurse to identify which statement indicates the client understands the teaching, indicating that three of the options are appropriate for the teaching, but one is incorrect. This is an "except" question, even though it does not say all the options are correct "except."

49. 1. The nurse should ask if the client wishes to be a tissue donor but the priority intervention is to address the family's grieving.
2. The nurse should give the client's personal belongings to the family but the priority intervention is to address the family's grieving.
3. **The nurse's priority intervention should be to address the grieving process of the family.**
4. The client's body will have to be sent to a funeral home but it is not the nurse's priority intervention.
*Content – End-of-Life: **Category of Health Alteration** – Neurological: **Integrated Processes** – Nursing Process: Implementation: **Client Needs** – Psychosocial Integrity: **Cognitive Level** – Analysis*

MAKING NURSING DECISIONS: The nurse must address all areas of the client's death, but the priority intervention is to address the client's family. Helping the client's family initially after the death with the grieving process should be the nurse's priority.

50. 1. The family should designate a funeral home of their choice. The nurse does not make this referral.
2. Hospice is for clients who are dying, but this client is considered brain dead.
3. A home health nurse cannot help this client or family.
4. **A 22-year-old client who experienced a traumatic brain death may be a good candidate for organ donation. Most tissue and organ banks prefer to be the ones to approach the family. This is the best referral.**
*Content – End-of-life: **Category of Health Alteration** – Neurological: **Integrated Processes** – Nursing Process: Planning: **Client Needs** – Physiological Integrity: Physiological Adaptation: **Cognitive Level** – Application*

MAKING NURSING DECISIONS: The NCLEX-RN® blueprint includes nursing care that is ruled by legal requirements as well as The Joint Commission, Centers for Medicare & Medicaid Services, Centers for Disease Control and Prevention, and Occupational Safety and Health Administration rules and regulations. The nurse must be knowledgeable of these standards.

51. 1. The client with cataracts is expected to have decreased vision and abnormal color perception, and will need surgery but it is elective surgery. Therefore, this client does not warrant intervention.
2. Loss of peripheral vision is an expected symptom of a retinal detachment and should be seen because the client needs surgery;

without surgery, the condition could lead to blindness. But this does not warrant intervention over the client having pain.
3. A hordeolum is a "sty," which is an infection of the sebaceous glands in the lid margin. It is not an emergency and is treated with warm, moist compresses to the eye four times a day.
4. **The client with primary open-angle glaucoma reports no symptom of pain or pressure, so a client reporting eye pain warrants intervention by the nurse.**
*Content – Medical/Surgical: **Category of Health Alteration** – Neurological: **Integrated Processes** – Nursing Process: Assessment: **Client Needs** – Physiological Integrity: Reduction of Risk Potential: **Cognitive Level** – Analysis*

MAKING NURSING DECISIONS: The test taker must determine which sign/symptom is not expected for the disease process. If the sign/symptom is not expected then the nurse should assess the client first. This type of question is determining if the nurse is knowledgeable of signs/symptoms of a variety of disease processes.

52. 1. Someone should call 911 because the client needs to go to the emergency department, but the nurse should first take care of the client.
2. **The nurse should first stabilize the foreign object to help prevent further damage. The stick should not be removed because it will cause more damage and possibly enucleate the eye.**
3. The nurse should not apply direct pressure to the eye. The nurse should stabilize the foreign object and not apply pressure, which could cause further damage.
4. The eye should be irrigated for a chemical exposure, not an impaled object.
*Content – Medical/Surgical: **Category of Health Alteration** – Neurological: **Integrated Processes** – Nursing Process: Implementation: **Client Needs** – Physiological Integrity: Reduction of Risk Potential: **Cognitive Level** – Analysis*

MAKING NURSING DECISIONS: The nurse should remember that if a client is in distress and the nurse can do something to relieve the distress, that action should be done first, before assessment. The nurse should select an intervention that directly helps the client's condition or prevents further damage.

53. 1. **The nurse and the UAP should protect themselves from injury. A lifting device should be used before attempting to move the client.**
2. The nurse and the UAP should provide the best care possible, including turning the client every 2 hours.

3. One other person may not be enough to turn or move the client adequately without injuring the staff.

4. The client is not responsive enough to assist in movement.

*Content – Medical/Surgical: **Category of Health Alteration** – Neurological: **Integrated Processes** – Nursing Process: Implementation: **Client Needs** – Safe and Effective Care Environment: Safety and Infection Control: **Cognitive Level** – Application*

MAKING NURSING DECISIONS: The NCLEX-RN® blueprint includes nursing care that is ruled by legal requirements as well as the Joint Commission, Centers for Medicare & Medicaid Services, Centers for Disease Control and Prevention, and Occupational Safety and Health Administration rules and regulations. The nurse must be knowledgeable of these standards.

54. 1. **The nurse should administer the IVP narcotic pain medication even if the client has shallow breathing, with respirations of 8. A nurse should never administer a medication with the intent of hastening the client's death, but medicating a dying client to achieve a peaceful death is an appropriate intervention.**

2. Repositioning the client would not be effective for "pain all over."

3. This is cruel to do to a client who is dying and has made himself or herself a DNR.

4. The HCP has all the orders needed in place. There is no reason to notify the HCP.

*Content – End-of-life: **Category of Health Alteration** – Neurological: **Integrated Processes** – Nursing Process: Implementation: **Client Needs** – Physiological Integrity: Basic Care and Comfort: **Cognitive Level** – Application*

MAKING NURSING DECISIONS: The NCLEX-RN® addresses questions concerned with end-of-life care. This is included in the Psychosocial Integrity section of the test blueprint. If unsure of the correct option, selecting an intervention addressing an individual is a better choice.

55. 1. **The client's ability to maneuver a wheelchair indicates that the client has progressed in therapy.**

2. This statement indicates the client is in denial about the prognosis of the injury.

3. Eye blinks may be used for communication in a client with a higher-level injury.

4. The building of a wheelchair ramp indicates the husband is preparing for the client's return home, not that the client is progressing in therapy.

*Content – Medical/Surgical: **Category of Health Alteration** – Neurological: **Integrated Processes** – Nursing*

*Process: Evaluation: **Client Needs** – Physiological Integrity: Physiological Adaptation: **Cognitive Level** – Analysis*

MAKING NURSING DECISIONS: The NCLEX-RN® integrates the nursing process throughout the Client Needs categories and subcategories. The nursing process is a scientific, clinical reasoning approach to client care that includes assessment, analysis, planning, implementation, and evaluation. The nurse will be responsible for determining if goals are being met or are not met.

56. 1. Méniére's disease, an excessive accumulation of endolymph in the membranous labyrinth, is characterized by episodic vertigo, tinnitus, fluctuating sensorineural hearing loss, and aural fullness. This client does not need to be contacted first.

2. Otitis media with effusion is an inflammation of the middle ear in which a collection of fluid is present in the middle ear space, resulting in a feeling of fullness of the ear and decreased hearing. This is expected; therefore, the nurse does not need to contact this client first.

3. **This client needs to be contacted so culture and sensitivity (C&S) can be done and mild analgesics prescribed. The ear canal has to be cleansed and antibiotic eardrops administered to the ear. Otalgia is ear pain. This client should be contacted for treatment.**

4. Otosclerosis is an autosomal disease, the fixation of the footplate of the stapes of the oval window, and results in conductive hearing loss; therefore, this client does not need to be notified.

*Content – Medical/Surgical: **Category of Health Alteration** – Neurological: **Integrated Processes** – Nursing Process: Assessment: **Client Needs** – Physiological Integrity: Reduction of Risk Potential: **Cognitive Level** – Analysis*

MAKING NURSING DECISIONS: The test taker must determine which sign/symptom is not expected for the disease process. If the sign/symptom is not expected then the nurse should assess the client first. This type of question is determining if the nurse is knowledgeable of signs/symptoms of a variety of disease processes.

57. 1. Altered nutrition is a physiological problem but is not priority over safety.

2. **Altered mobility is a problem experienced by clients diagnosed with Parkinson's disease. It leads to many other concerns, including the risk for falls resulting from the client's shuffling gait. This is the priority problem.**

3. Altered elimination is a problem that the client's altered mobility can cause. This is not, however, the priority problem.
4. Altered body image is a psychological problem and is not priority.
   Content – Mental Health: **Category of Health Alteration –** *Neurological:* **Integrated Processes –** *Nursing Process: Planning:* **Client Needs –** *Physiological Integrity: Reduction of Risk Potential:* **Cognitive Level –** *Synthesis*

MAKING NURSING DECISIONS: The NCLEX-RN® integrates the nursing process throughout the Client Needs categories and subcategories. The nursing process is a scientific, clinical reasoning approach to client care that includes assessment, analysis, planning, implementation, and evaluation. The nurse will be responsible for identifying nursing diagnoses for clients.

58. 1. The nurse must irrigate the eyes, not patch the eyes.
    2. The client is in distress and the nurse needs to flush the client's eyes, not assess the visual acuity.
    3. **For chemical injuries, the nurse should begin ocular irrigation with sterile, pH-balanced, physiological solution.**
    4. The nurse should elevate the head of bed but it is not the nurse's first intervention.
       Content – Medical/Surgical: **Category of Health Alteration –** *Neurological:* **Integrated Processes –** *Nursing Process: Implementation:* **Client Needs –** *Physiological Integrity: Reduction of Risk Potential:* **Cognitive Level –** *Analysis*

MAKING NURSING DECISIONS: The nurse should remember that if a client is in distress, and the nurse can do something to relieve the distress, it should be done first, before assessment. The nurse should select an option that directly helps the client's condition.

59. 1. The client admitted to a rehabilitation unit is expected to participate in therapy for at least 3 hours each day. The nurse would not question this order.
    2. The client admitted to a rehabilitation unit is expected to participate in therapy for at least 3 hours each day. The nurse would not question this order.
    3. Clients with neurological deficits may have trouble swallowing. The nurse would not question this order.
    4. **A client in a rehabilitation unit for a brain injury should not require IV medications. The nurse should question this order.**
       Content – Medical/Surgical: **Category of Health Alteration –** *Neurological:* **Integrated Processes –** *Nursing Process: Assessment:* **Client Needs –** *Safe and*

Effective Care Environment: Management of Care: **Cognitive Level –** *Analysis*

MAKING NURSING DECISIONS: When the stem asks the nurse to determine which healthcare provider's order to question, the test taker needs to realize this is an "except" question. Three of the options are appropriate for the HCP to prescribe, and one is not appropriate for the client's disease process or procedure.

60. 1. A hospice organization is designed for terminally ill clients. The client is not terminally ill.
    2. The speech therapist helps clients regain speech and swallowing abilities. This therapy should have been occurring while the client was in the rehab facility.
    3. The physical therapist assists the client with gait and muscle strengthening. This therapy should have been occurring while the client was in the rehab facility.
    4. **The client is being discharged. The nurse should plan for continuity of care by arranging for a home health agency to follow the client at home.**
       Content – Management of Care: **Category of Health Alteration –** *Neurological:* **Integrated Processes –** *Nursing Process: Planning:* **Client Needs –** *Physiological Integrity: Physiological Adaptation:* **Cognitive Level –** *Synthesis*

MAKING NURSING DECISIONS: The test taker must be knowledgeable of the role of all members of the multidisciplinary healthcare team as well as HIPAA rules and regulations. These will be tested on the NCLEX-RN® exam.

61. 1. It will take approximately 6 weeks for the wound to sufficiently heal prior to being fitted for a prosthetic eye.
    2. The nurse should ensure the client can insert the conformer in the eye socket and the client should be able to demonstrate this to the client. The client does not need more teaching.
    3. Eye drops must be placed in the lower conjunctiva; therefore, the client does not need more discharge teaching.
    4. The client is at risk for infection and should call the HCP if an elevation in temperature occurs. The client does not need more discharge teaching.
       Content – Medical/Surgical: **Category of Health Alteration –** *Neurological:* **Integrated Processes –** *Nursing Process: Evaluation; Teaching/Learning:* **Client Needs –** *Physiological Integrity: Physiological Adaptation:* **Cognitive Level –** *Analysis*

MAKING NURSING DECISIONS: This question asks the nurse to identify which statement supports the notion that the client needs more teaching, indicating three of the statements are appropriate for the disease process or disorder, but one is incorrect. This is an "except" question even though it does not say all the options are correct "except."

62. 1. The client may be able to maintain the ability to work for several years before needing to apply for disability. The stem does not suggest the client is disabled.
2. The client is newly diagnosed; nutrition would not be a problem at this time.
3. **The client should be referred to a psychological counselor to develop skills for coping with the long-term chronic illness.**
4. The chaplain may need to see the client, but the stem did not indicate the client was having a problem with spiritual distress.
   Content – Management of Care: **Category of Health Alteration** – Neurological: **Integrated Processes** – Nursing Process: Planning: **Client Needs** – Physiological Integrity: Physiological Adaptation: **Cognitive Level** – Synthesis

MAKING NURSING DECISIONS: The test taker must be knowledgeable of the role of all members of the multidisciplinary healthcare team as well as HIPAA rules and regulations. These will be tested on the NCLEX-RN® exam.

63. 1. **The LPN can administer medications to clients; therefore, this task is appropriate for the nurse to assign to the LPN.**
2. The client experiencing status epilepticus is an unstable client and the nurse should not assign this task to the LPN.
3. The UAP could assist the client to the bathroom. Remember to assign/delegate tasks based on his or her education and job description.
4. The nurse cannot assign assessment to the LPN.
   Content – Medical/Surgical: **Category of Health Alteration** – Neurological: **Integrated Processes** – Nursing Process: Planning: **Client Needs** – Safe and Effective Care Environment: Management of Care: **Cognitive Level** – Synthesis

MAKING NURSING DECISIONS: When the test taker is deciding which option is the most appropriate task to delegate/assign, the test taker should choose the task that allows each staff member to function within his or her full scope of practice. Do not assign a task to a staff member that falls outside the staff member's or volunteer's expertise. Remember: The nurse cannot delegate assessment, teaching, evaluation, or the care of an unstable client to the LPN.

64. 1. **The client with a closed head injury is at risk for increased intracranial pressure and the osmotic diuretic is a priority medication.**
2. The nurse should administer the medications to the client prior to leaving the unit but the client with a physiological, potentially life-threatening complication is priority.
3. Before administering a narcotic, the nurse must first assess the client to make sure that administering the medication is not going to mask symptoms.
4. This is a routine medication and can be administered 30 minutes before or after the routine scheduled time. This is not a priority medication.
   Content – Medical/Surgical: **Category of Health Alteration** – Neurological: **Integrated Processes** – Nursing Process: Analysis: **Client Needs** – Physiological Integrity: Pharmacological and Parenteral Therapies: **Cognitive Level** – Analysis

MAKING NURSING DECISIONS: The test taker should know which medications are priority medications such as those indicated in life-threatening situations. These must be administered first.

65. 1. **The charge nurse will not always be available to intercede for the new graduate. The charge nurse should wait and see whether the new graduate is capable of handling the situation before intervening.**
2. The charge nurse should wait to allow the new graduate to deal with the UAP.
3. The charge nurse should wait to allow the new graduate to deal with the UAP.
4. The charge nurse should wait to allow the new graduate to deal with the UAP.
   Content – Management of Care: **Category of Health Alteration** – Neurological: **Integrated Processes** – Teaching/Learning: **Client Needs** – Safe and Effective Care Environment: Management of Care: **Cognitive Level** – Application

MAKING NURSING DECISIONS: There will be management questions on the NCLEX-RN®. In many instances, there is no test-taking strategy; the nurse must be knowledgeable of management issues.

66. 1. Synthroid is a daily medication.
2. **MS Contin is a narcotic analgesic in sustained release form. Patients experiencing pain are unlikely to be able to participate fully in the treatment program. The patient should be medicated to ensure the ability to comply with the treatment regimen.**

3. The Fleets enema is utilized daily to assist the patient in regaining control of the bowels. This should be administered sometime during the evening hours since administering it during the day would interfere with other therapies such as physical or occupational therapy. Most therapy is completed during the daytime hours.
4. Metformin should be administered with meals to prevent nausea and could be the second medication administered.

   Content – Medical/Surgical: **Category of Health Alteration** *– Neurological:* **Integrated Processes** *– Nursing Process: Analysis:* **Client Needs** *– Physiological Integrity: Pharmacological and Parenteral Therapies:* **Cognitive Level** *– Analysis*

MAKING NURSING DECISIONS: This is an alternate type of question included in the NCLEX-RN® blueprint. The test taker must be able to read a medication administration record (MAR), be knowledgeable of medications, and be able to make an appropriate decision as to the nurse's most appropriate intervention.

67. **Answer: Two 20-mg tablets and one 10-mg tablet.**
    20 + 20 + 10 = 50 mg
    The nurse cannot split a 75-mg tablet into 2/3 of a tablet, so the patient must receive multiple tablets.

    Content – Adult Health, Pharmacology: **Category of Health Alteration** *– Neurological:* **Integrated Processes** *– Nursing Process: Implementation:* **Client Needs** *– Physiological Integrity: Pharmacological and Parenteral Therapies:* **Cognitive Level** *– Application*

MAKING NURSING DECISIONS: This is an alternate type of question included in the NCLEX-RN®. The nurse must know how to solve math questions.

68. **1, 3, and 4 are correct.**
    1. **The UAP can make hourly rounds on the client, taking the client to the bathroom, giving the client a drink of water, checking to make sure the client is not climbing out of bed, etc.**
    2. This is the responsibility of the registered nurse or the social worker.
    3. **This client is in rehab and should be stable so that the UAP can set up the tray or feed the patient.**
    4. **The UAP can clamp and unclamp an indwelling catheter in a rehab area. This is a non-invasive skill that can be taught to the UAP. It does not require judgment.**

5. This is the responsibility of the registered nurse or the social worker.

   Content – Medical/Surgical: **Category of Health Alteration** *– Neurological:* **Integrated Processes** *– Nursing Process: Planning:* **Client Needs** *– Safe and Effective Care Environment: Management of Care:* **Cognitive Level** *– Synthesis*

MAKING NURSING DECISIONS: This is an alternate type of question included in the NCLEX-RN®. The nurse must be able to select all the options that answer the question correctly. There are no partially correct answers.

69. 1. The left hand is weak and cannot be depended on to hold a cane.
    2. The shoulder is not appropriate for a cane.
    3. **The right hand is the strongest hand and should be the one holding the cane. A right-sided CVA results in damage to the left side of the body.**
    4. The shoulder is not appropriate for a cane.

    Content – Medical/Surgical: **Category of Health Alteration** *– Neurological:* **Integrated Processes** *– Physiological Integrity: Physiological Adaptation:* **Client Needs** *– Safe and Effective Care Environment: Safety and Infection Control:* **Cognitive Level** *– Application*

MAKING NURSING DECISIONS: This is an alternate type of question on the NCLEX-RN® called "hot spot," which asks the nurse to identify the area with the computer arrow.

70. 1. The client has a much lower score than 12 on the Glasgow Coma Scale.
    2. The client has a lower score than 10 on the scale.
    3. **The client received 2 points for lack of opening of eyes to previous stimuli but opens to pain; the client receives 1 point for lack of sound even with painful stimuli; 5 points for localizing pain, attempts to remove offending stimulus. This is a total of 8 points.**
    4. The client has a higher score than 6.

    Content – Medical/Surgical: **Category of Health Alteration** *– Neurological:* **Integrated Processes** *– Nursing Process: Assessment:* **Client Needs** *– Safe and Effective Care Environment: Management of Care:* **Cognitive Level** *– Analysis*

MAKING NURSING DECISIONS: This is an alternate type of question included in the NCLEX-RN® blueprint. The test taker must be able to read a chart, be able to assess the client, and be able to make an appropriate decision as to the nurse's most appropriate action.

CLINICAL SCENARIO ANSWERS AND RATIONALES

The correct answer number and rationale for why it is the correct answer are given in boldface type. Rationales for why the other possible answer options are incorrect also are given, but they are not in boldface type.

1. 1. **The client with a right-sided CVA has left-sided paralysis, so placing the call light on the left side is inappropriate. The client would not be able to use the call light since the left side is paralyzed; Elizabeth should intervene.**
   2. The UAP should assist the client with meals since the client is unable to use the right arm.
   3. Using a draw sheet is an appropriate way to move the client up in bed.
   4. Placing a small pillow under the shoulder will prevent the shoulder from adducting toward the chest and developing a contracture, so this action does not require Elizabeth to intervene.

2. 1. The client may need acetaminophen for the pain but the nurse should first assess the client to determine whether this is a headache or whether the client has an evolving CVA, which would require notifying the healthcare provider.
   2. The client may need a CT scan but that cannot be determined until Elizabeth assesses the client to determine if the headache is indicative of an evolving stroke.
   3. Elizabeth must assess the client to obtain data that will be needed when notifying the healthcare provider; therefore, this is not Elizabeth's first intervention.
   4. **Elizabeth must first assess the client to determine whether the client's neurological status is deteriorating, which requires notifying the HCP; or, if the headache is expected, then it would require a narcotic analgesic.**

3. 1. The client may be developing pneumonia and needs to be assessed but not prior to a client with a Glasgow Coma Scale of 6 which is life threatening.
   2. Ascending paralysis is a symptom of Guillain-Barré syndrome; therefore, Courtney would not need to assess this client first.
   3. **A 15 on the Glasgow Coma Scale indicates the client is neurologically intact, and a 6 indicates the client is not neurologically intact; therefore, Courtney should see this client first.**
   4. Courtney should expect a client diagnosed with a CVA (stroke) to have some sequelae of the problem, including the inability to speak.

4. 1. **This medication could possibly cause bleeding; therefore, this medication should be questioned by Mr. Leo.**
   2. An osmotic diuretic is the medication of choice used to treat increased intracranial pressure which can occur with a closed head injury.
   3. Any client with a head injury will be on prophylactic anticonvulsants to prevent seizure activity so Mr. Leo would not question this order.
   4. Clients in the ICU are administered proton-pump inhibitors to help prevent stress ulcers; therefore, Mr. Leo would not question this order.

5. 1. If the client's bladder is full, Jessie needs to insert a urinary catheter, which will relieve the head. The client may be experiencing autonomic dysreflexia, but Jessie will need to palpate the bladder first.
   2. The client is in distress; therefore, the nurse should not assess the client first.
   3. The client should be put in the Trendelenburg position for hypovolemia not for autonomic dysreflexia.
   4. **The nurse should first palpate the client's bladder to determine if the client is experiencing autonomic dysreflexia, which is what Jessie should consider first with the client's signs/symptoms.**

6. 1. **Placing the client on the side to maintain patent airway is Mr. Leo's priority intervention.**
   2. The Rapid Response Team is called when the client is alive but the nurse thinks the client is a potentially life-threatening situation. This is a possible intervention but it is not priority as Mr. Leo walks in the room.
   3. Mr. Leo should determine if the client is incontinent of urine or stool and assess the client's seizure for type of activity—are the client's eyes rolling, or is the client making guttural sounds?—but it is not priority over maintaining patent airway.
   4. The client should have privacy but it is not priority over maintaining patent airway.

7. 1. An adverse occurrence report may need to be completed, but it is not Mr. Leo's first intervention.

2. Mr. Leo's first intervention is to stop the UAP from inserting the oral airway. Once the seizure has started, there should be no attempts to insert anything in the mouth. At times an oral airway could be inserted if the client has an aura and prior to the seizure, but not once the seizure has started.

3. Once a seizure has started nothing should be inserted in the client's mouth.

4. Mr. Leo should observe the time the seizure started and the seizure activity but it is not the first intervention.

8. 1, 3, 4, and 5 are correct.

1. A lumbar puncture is an invasive procedure; therefore, an informed consent is required.

2. A lumbar puncture does not insert dye into the client; therefore, this is not an appropriate intervention.

3. The client should be in the side-lying position with the back arched. This position increases the space between the vertebrae, which allows the HCP easier entry into the spinal column.

4. The client is encouraged to relax and breathe normally; the client should feel some pressure in the back but there should be no pain.

5. The nurse should always explain to the client what is happening prior to and during a procedure.

9. 1. The client with bacterial meningitis would be expected to have photophobia so the most experienced nurse would not need to be assigned to this client.

2. The client with an L-4 SCI could have spastic muscle spasms and is not a complication; therefore, a less experienced nurse could care for this client.

3. A less experienced nurse would be assigned the client with Parkinson's disease because these symptoms are expected for this client.

4. The client with ALS has deteriorating respiratory distress, which is expected, but with these four clients the most experienced nurse should be assigned to the client who has respiratory distress. Maslow's Hierarchy of Needs identifies airway as a priority.

10. 1. A Glasgow Coma Scale of 15 indicates intact neurological status so an increase from 11 to 14 is good and the nurse would not need to see this client first.

2. These signs/symptoms indicate spinal shock; therefore, this client should be assessed first and appropriate medications administered.

3. This is the sign of a positive Babinski, which is expected in a client with a brain stem herniation, so this client would not need to be assessed first.

4. These are expected signs/symptoms of West Nile virus; therefore, the nurse would not need to assess this client first.

Endocrine Management

Intuition will tell the thinking mind where to look next.

—John Salk

QUESTIONS

1. After receiving the shift report, the 7:00 p.m. to 7:00 a.m. nurse is reviewing the medication administration record (MAR) of the client diagnosed with type 2 diabetes. Which intervention should the nurse implement?

Client's Name:	Account Number: 123456	Allergies: NKDA	
Height: 70 inches	**Weight:** 265 lbs		
Date / **Medication**	**2301–0700**	**0701–1500**	**1501–2300**
Regular Insulin by bedside glucose subcu ac & hs			
<60 notify HCP 150 0 units 151–200 2 units		0730 DNBG 42 0 units	
201–250 4 units 251–300 6 units		1130 DNBG 245 4 units	
301–350 8 units 351–400 10 units >400 notify HCP			1630 DNBG 398 10 units
Humulin N 48 units bid subcu ac		0730 DN	1630 DN
Signature/Initials	**Day Nurse** **RN/DN**	**Night Nurse** **RN/NN**	

   1. Make sure the client receives a snack at bedtime.
   2. Check the client's blood glucose level immediately.
   3. Have the unlicensed assistive personnel (UAP) give the client some orange juice.
   4. Teach the client about the symptoms of diabetic ketoacidosis (DKA).

2. Which task is most appropriate for the medical nurse to delegate to the unlicensed assistive personnel (UAP)?
   1. Request the UAP to take the diabetic client's HS snack to the client.
   2. Ask the UAP to escort the client on the PCA pump to the bathroom.
   3. Tell the UAP to witness the client's advance directive.
   4. Ask the UAP to show the client how to take the client's radial pulse.

3. Which task is most appropriate for the charge nurse to assign to the licensed practical nurse (LPN)?
   1. Tell the LPN to change the client's subclavian dressing.
   2. Request the LPN to obtain the client's daily weight.
   3. Assign the LPN to care for the client in myxedema coma.
   4. Ask the LPN to complete discharge teaching to the client.

4. The new graduate nurse on the endocrine unit is having difficulty completing the workload in a timely manner. Which suggestion could the preceptor make to help the new graduate become more organized?
   1. Suggest the new nurse take a break whenever the nurse feels overwhelmed with tasks.
   2. Tell the new nurse to start the shift with a work organization sheet for the assigned clients.
   3. Instruct the new nurse to take five deep breaths at the beginning of the shift, and then begin.
   4. Review each day's assignments for the new nurse and organize the work for the new nurse.

5. The rehabilitation nurse is caring for a client diagnosed with type 2 diabetes who is 1 week postoperative for left carotid endarterectomy. The client's 11:30 a.m. bedside glucometer reading is 408 mg/dL. Based on the medication administration record (MAR), which intervention should the nurse implement first?

Client's Name:	Account Number: 123456	Allergies: NKDA		
Height: 69 inches	Weight: 165 pounds			
Date Medication	2301–0700	0701–1500	1501–2300	
Regular insulin by bedside glucose subcu ac & hs				
<60 notify HCP 150 0 units		0730 DNBG 142 0 units		
151–200 2 units				
201–250 4 units				
251–300 6 units				
301–350 8 units				
351–400 10 units				
>400 notify HCP				
Signature/Initials	Day Nurse RN/DN			

1. Notify the healthcare provider.
2. Administer 10 units regular insulin.
3. Notify the laboratory to draw a serum glucose level.
4. Recheck the bedside glucometer reading.

6. The charge nurse on the endocrine surgical unit is making assignments. Which task should be delegated/assigned to the team members?
   1. Request the licensed practical nurse (LPN) assess the client who is hypoglycemic.
   2. Ask the unlicensed assistive personnel (UAP) to assist feeding the client with an adrenalectomy who has a paralytic ileus.
   3. Instruct the UAP to insert a nasogastric (N/G) tube into the client who has had a thyroidectomy.
   4. Tell the LPN to perform an in and out catheterization for the client diagnosed with acromegaly.

7. Which task is most appropriate for the nurse to delegate/assign when caring for clients on a surgical unit?
   1. Instruct the licensed practical nurse (LPN) to feed the client who is 1 day post-operative unilateral thyroidectomy.
   2. Ask another nurse to administer an IVP pain medication to a postoperative client in severe pain.
   3. Request the unlicensed assistive personnel (UAP) to check the client whose vital signs are AP 112, RR 26, BP 92/58.
   4. Instruct the licensed practical nurse (LPN) to obtain the pre-transfusion assessment on a postoperative client.

8. The client diagnosed with Addison's disease is being prepared for emergency surgery and is asking to complete an advance directive. Which type of advance directive should the nurse recommend the client complete at this time?
   1. Power of attorney.
   2. Living will.
   3. Do not resuscitate (DNR) order.
   4. Durable power of attorney for healthcare.

9. The nurse is caring for clients in the post-anesthesia care unit (PACU). Which client requires immediate intervention by the PACU nurse?
   1. The client who had a bilateral adrenalectomy who is exhibiting masseter rigidity.
   2. The client who had a subtotal thyroidectomy who has not urinated since surgery.
   3. The client who had general anesthesia who is sleepy but arouses easily to verbal stimuli.
   4. The client who had a pituitary tumor removed and has hypoactive bowel sounds.

10. The charge nurse on a busy 20-bed endocrinology unit must send one staff member to the nursery. Which staff member is most appropriate to send to the nursery?
    1. The nurse who has worked on the endocrinology unit for 4 years.
    2. The graduate nurse who has been on the endocrinology unit for 6 months.
    3. The licensed practical nurse (LPN) who has worked in a newborn nursery at another facility.
    4. The unlicensed assistive personnel (UAP) who has six small children of her own.

11. The nurse is working in an endocrinology unit. Which client warrants immediate intervention by the nurse?
    1. The client with acromegaly who has club-like fingertips and large feet.
    2. The client with syndrome of inappropriate antidiuretic hormone who has decreased urine output.
    3. The client with Cushing's syndrome who has truncal obesity and thin, fragile skin.
    4. The client with pheochromocytoma who has a severe pounding headache and chest pain.

12. The night nurse enters the client's room and finds the client crying. The client asks the nurse, "Am I dying? I think something is terribly wrong with me, but no one is telling me." The nurse knows the client has pancreatic cancer and has less than 6 months to live. Which response is an example of the ethical principle of veracity?
    1. "You are concerned no one is telling you something is wrong."
    2. "Your diagnosis is pancreatic cancer."
    3. "If you feel something is wrong you should speak with your doctor in the morning."
    4. "What makes you think there is something wrong and you are dying?"

13. The critical care nurse has just received the a.m. shift report on a client diagnosed with heart failure and who has pre-existing type 2 diabetes. The client has the following medication administration record (MAR). Which medication should the nurse administer first?

Client's Name:	Account Number: 123456		Allergies: Penicillin	
Height: 67 inches	Weight: 148 pounds			
Date	Medication	2301–0700	0701–1500	1501–2300
	Metformin (Glucophage) 100 mg PO bid		0800	2000
	70/30 insulin 24 units subcu		0730	
	Digoxin 0.125 mg IVP qd		0800	
	Rocephin 100 mg IVPB	0700		
Signature/Initials		Day Nurse RN/DN	Night Nurse RN/NN	

   1. Administer metformin (Glucophage) 100 mg PO.
   2. Administer digoxin 0.125 mg IVP.
   3. Administer Rocephin (ceftriaxone) 100 mg IVPB.
   4. Administer 70/30 insulin subcutaneously.

14. Which client should the charge nurse on a medical unit assign to a nurse who is 3 months pregnant?
    1. The client who is receiving chemotherapy who is immunosuppressed.
    2. The client with postoperative hyperparathyroidism who has shingles (herpes zoster).
    3. The client with hyperthyroidism who is receiving radioactive iodine I-131.
    4. The client diagnosed with AIDS who has a cytomegalovirus infection.

15. The client with hypothyroidism and a diagnosis of myxedema coma is admitted to the critical care unit. Which assessment data warrants immediate intervention by the nurse?
    1. The client's blood glucose level is 74 mg/dL.
    2. The client's temperature is 96.2°F; AP, 54; R, 12; and BP, 90/58.
    3. The client's ABG values are pH, 7.33; PaO_2, 78; $PaCO_2$, 48; HCO_3, 25.
    4. The client is lethargic and sleeps all the time.

16. The nurse is preparing to administer morning medications. Which medication should the nurse administer first?
    1. The levothyroxine (Synthroid), a thyroid hormone, to a client diagnosed with hypothyroidism.
    2. The Humulin N insulin, a pancreatic hormone, to a client diagnosed with type 2 diabetes.
    3. The prednisone, a glucocorticoid, to a client diagnosed with Addison's disease.
    4. The tiotropium (Spiriva) inhaler, a bronchodilator, to a client diagnosed with chronic asthma.

17. The nurse is working on an endocrinology unit. Which client should the nurse assess first?
1. The client diagnosed with diabetes insipidus who has polyuria and polydipsia.
2. The client who is 1 day postoperative thyroidectomy who has neck edema.
3. The client who has hypoparathyroidism who has painful muscle cramps and irritability.
4. The client diagnosed with Addison's who has weakness, fatigue, and anorexia.

18. The client is admitted to the endocrinology unit newly diagnosed with an acute exacerbation of central diabetes insipidus (DI). Which intervention is the priority nursing intervention?
1. Obtain the client's baseline weight.
2. Administer desmopressin acetate (DDAVP) intranasally.
3. Administer intravenous hypotonic saline.
4. Monitor the client's intake and output.

19. The unlicensed assistive personnel (UAP) tells the nurse the client who had a thyroidectomy has a T 104°F, P 128, RR 26, B/P 164/88. Which intervention should the nurse implement first?
1. Prepare to administer the beta-adrenergic blocker propranolol (Inderal).
2. Notify the healthcare provider immediately.
3. Assess the client's vital signs and surgical dressing.
4. Administer acetaminophen (Tylenol) PO STAT.

20. The unlicensed assistive personnel (UAP) tells the nurse that a client is crying and upset because she has been told her husband has just died. Which intervention should the nurse implement?
1. Tell the UAP to go and sit with the client.
2. Make a referral for the chaplain to see the client.
3. Ask the HCP to prescribe a mild sedative.
4. Leave the client alone in the room to grieve.

21. At 1000, the client diagnosed with type 1 diabetes is complaining of being jittery, having a headache, and being dizzy. Which intervention should the nurse implement first?
1. Give the client glucose tablets.
2. Provide the client with the lunch meal.
3. Request the laboratory to draw a serum glucose level.
4. Determine the last time the client received insulin.

22. An elderly client diagnosed with thyroid cancer frequently makes statements that are inappropriate for the situation, and is not oriented to place, time, or date. The HCP has ordered a magnetic resonance imaging (MRI) scan of the client's brain. Which intervention should the nurse implement?
1. Administer a mild sedative to prevent claustrophobia.
2. Order a vest restraint for use by the client during the MRI.
3. Make sure the client does not have a pacemaker.
4. Ask a family member to stay with the client while the test is performed.

23. An elderly female client is admitted from the long-term care facility with hyperglycemic hyperosmolar nonketotic coma. The client does not have any family or friends present. Which resource(s) should the admission nurse utilize to obtain information about the client?
1. The nurse should wait until a significant other can be contacted.
2. The verbal report from the ambulance workers and STAT lab work.
3. The transfer form from the nursing home and old hospital records.
4. The healthcare provider's telephone orders about care needed.

24. The nurse administering medications to clients on a medical unit discovers the wrong medication was administered to a client, Mrs. Jones. Mrs. Jones had replied she was Mrs. Smith when the nurse asked her name from the MAR. Which step in medication administration did the nurse violate when administering the medication?
    1. Asking the client to repeat her name.
    2. Verifying the client's armband with the MAR.
    3. Checking the medication against the MAR.
    4. Documenting the medication on the MAR.

25. The female client diagnosed with type 2 diabetes has frequent urinary tract infections (UTIs). Which priority intervention should the nurse implement?
    1. Encourage the client to empty her bladder regularly and completely.
    2. Instruct the client to drink 8 ounces of cranberry or lingonberry juice a day.
    3. Explain the importance of taking oral hypoglycemic medications.
    4. Discuss the importance of taking all the antibiotics.

26. Which laboratory data should the nurse monitor for the client receiving the intravenous Solu-Medrol?
    1. Potassium level.
    2. Sodium level.
    3. Liver enzymes.
    4. Glucose level.

27. The nurse is working in an outpatient clinic triaging phone calls. Which client warrants notifying the healthcare provider?
    1. The client with type 2 diabetes receiving hemodialysis who has gained 6 pounds since the last dialysis treatment.
    2. The client with type 1 diabetes who has early stage chronic renal disease and reports having to go to the bathroom several times at night.
    3. The client with syndrome of inappropriate antidiuretic hormone who is very upset because no one has returned the previous phone call.
    4. The client with type 1 diabetes who had a kidney transplant and reports decreased urine output and flu-like symptoms.

28. Which client should the endocrinology nurse assess first after receiving the shift report?
    1. The client who is 1 day postoperative transsphenoidal hypophysectomy who has clear drainage from the nose.
    2. The client diagnosed with Grave's disease who has exophthalmos and bruits over the thyroid gland.
    3. The client with hyperparathyroidism who is complaining of weakness, loss of appetite, and constipation.
    4. The client with Addison's disease who has orthostatic hypotension, nausea, and vomiting.

29. Which client is priority to be assigned to a case manager in the outpatient clinic so that care can be achieved?
    1. The client with renal calculi who is 2 weeks post–lithotripsy procedure.
    2. The client who has type 2 diabetes and coronary artery disease (CAD).
    3. The client who is diagnosed with hypothyroidism receiving radiation treatment.
    4. The client with Addison's disease who is on corticosteroid therapy.

30. Which client is most appropriate for the parish nurse to care for?
    1. The post-gestational diabetic client who had triplets and is a single parent.
    2. The Presbyterian client who is confined to the home due to severe arthritis.
    3. The obese client with Cushing's syndrome who is requesting help with losing weight.
    4. The client with chronic renal disease who is being cared for in the home by the wife.

31. Which task should the ambulatory care nurse delegate to the unlicensed assistive personnel (UAP)?
1. Ask the UAP to remove the trash from the room of the client who received radioactive iodine with hyperthyroidism.
2. Instruct the UAP to escort the client outside who is asking to smoke a cigar.
3. Request the UAP check the surgical dressing on the client with an ileal conduit.
4. Tell the UAP to take the glucometer reading on the client about to go to surgery.

32. The nurse is hanging 1,000 mL of IV fluids to run for 8 hours. The intravenous tubing is a microdrip. At how many gtt/min should the IV rate be set? _____

33. The clinic nurse is caring for clients using complementary alternative medicine (CAM). Which is not an example of CAM?
1. The client with hypothyroidism who takes *Centella asiatica*.
2. The type 2 diabetic client who takes cinnamon daily.
3. The client with coronary artery disease (CAD) who takes a daily baby aspirin.
4. The client who uses acupuncture to help quit smoking cigarettes.

34. Which statement is an example of community-oriented, population-focused nursing?
1. The nurse cares for an elderly client living in the community who has had a kidney transplant.
2. The nurse develops an educational program for the type 2 diabetics in the community.
3. The nurse refers a client with Cushing's syndrome to the registered dietician.
4. The nurse provides pamphlets to the client with chronic renal disease.

35. Which priority intervention should the nurse implement when teaching the client with type 2 diabetes about glucometer checks?
1. Instruct the client to keep a written record of the glucometer readings.
2. Recommend the client check the glucometer reading in the morning.
3. Have the client demonstrate how to correctly perform the glucometer reading.
4. Tell the client to dispose of the lancets and strips appropriately.

36. Which client would most benefit from acupressure, a traditional Chinese medicine, which is considered complementary alternative medicine (CAM)?
1. The client with thyroid cancer who has chemotherapy induced nausea.
2. The client with type 2 diabetes diagnosed with chronic renal disease.
3. The postpartum client who is diagnosed with Sheehan syndrome.
4. The client diagnosed with arterial hypertension.

37. The Home Health Director of Nurses hears a nurse and the occupational therapist loudly disagreeing about the care of a newly admitted client while they are sitting in an area that is accessible to anyone coming into the office. Which action should the Director of Nurses implement first?
1. Ask the staff members to move the argument to another room.
2. Request both individuals to come into the director's office.
3. Call the secretary with instructions for the staff to quit arguing.
4. Tell the staff members that arguing is not allowed in the office.

38. Which client should the nurse on the endocrinology unit assess first?
1. The client with hypothyroidism whose vital signs are T 94.2, AP 48, RR 14, B/P 90/68.
2. The client with hypoparathyroidism who has a positive Chvostek's sign.
3. The client who is 1 day postoperative thyroidectomy who is hoarse.
4. The client with diabetes insipidus who is drinking large amounts of water.

39. Which activities are examples of home healthcare nurse responsibilities when caring for clients with endocrine disorders? **Select all that apply.**
1. Complete nutritional counseling and teaching for a client on a high-fiber diet.
2. Discuss preoperative teaching for the client having a total right hip replacement.
3. Manage oxygen therapy for a client with chronic obstructive pulmonary disease (COPD).
4. Teach the client and family about administration and side effects of medications.
5. Draw blood for studies related to monitoring disease processes and therapy.

40. The unlicensed assistive personnel (UAP) has just taken the blood pressure of a client who had a thyroidectomy. The UAP tells the nurse that the client's hand turned into a claw when the blood pressure was taken. Which intervention should the nurse implement first?
1. Prepare to administer intravenous calcium gluconate.
2. Assess the client for signs/symptoms of hypoparathyroidism.
3. Request the UAP to elevate the client's head of the bed.
4. Notify the client's healthcare provider immediately.

41. The client diagnosed with type 2 diabetes who has chronic renal disease asks the nurse, "How can I qualify for home healthcare when I go home?" Which statement is the nurse's best response?
1. "You must need constant skilled care by the nurse."
2. "You must have a family member living with you."
3. "You must be homebound to receive home healthcare."
4. "You must be referred by the hospital social worker."

42. The nurse is providing complementary alternative medicine (CAM) by teaching the client with hyperthyroidism to focus attention, increase self-awareness, and increase concentration on an object. Which type of mind-body intervention is the nurse teaching?
1. Meditation.
2. Imagery.
3. Aromatherapy.
4. Acupressure.

43. Which priority intervention should the nurse implement for the client diagnosed with syndrome of inappropriate antidiuretic hormone (SIADH)?
1. Maintain the prescribed daily fluid restriction.
2. Position the client's head of bed with no more than 10 degrees of elevation.
3. Turn and reposition the client every 2 hours while on bed rest.
4. Provide frequent oral hygiene every 2 hours for the client.

44. The home health (HH) agency Chief Nursing Officer (CNO) is making assignments for the nurses. Which client should be assigned to the new graduate nurse who just completed orientation?
1. The client diagnosed with Cushing's syndrome who is dyspneic and confused.
2. The client who does not have the money to get prescriptions filled.
3. The client with full-thickness burns on the arm who needs a dressing change.
4. The client complaining of pain who is diagnosed with diabetic neuropathy.

45. The nurse on the endocrinology unit is caring for clients, assisted by an unlicensed assistive personnel (UAP). Which task is most appropriate to delegate to the UAP?
1. Feed the client who is 1 day postoperative transsphenoidal hypophysectomy.
2. Obtain a urine specimen for the client diagnosed with diabetes insipidus.
3. Take the vital signs for the client diagnosed with myxedema coma.
4. Assess the pulse oximeter reading of the client with an Addisonian crisis.

46. The clinical nurse manager on the endocrine unit overhears the staff nurses upset and arguing over how the clients are being assigned by the charge nurse. Which statement indicates a democratic leadership style by the clinical nurse manager?
1. "My charge nurse makes the assignments and I support how she does it."
2. "As long as there are no complaints from the clients I will not interfere."
3. "I appreciate you telling me about the situation and I will handle it."
4. "I will schedule a meeting and we will all sit down and discuss the situation."

47. The hospice nurse is writing a care plan for a client diagnosed with type 2 diabetes mellitus who has peripheral neuropathy. Which client problem has priority for the client?
1. Altered glucose metabolism.
2. Anticipatory grieving.
3. Alteration in comfort.
4. Spiritual distress.

48. The unlicensed assistive personnel (UAP) tells the nurse the client with thyroid cancer who is terminally ill is having deep-rapid breathing, but then doesn't breathe for about a minute. Which intervention should the nurse implement first?
1. Explain the client is having Cheyne-Stokes respirations.
2. Notify the hospital chaplain to come to the client's room.
3. Go to the client's room immediately and assess the client.
4. Contact the client's family that the client's death is near.

49. Which interventions should the nurse implement for the client diagnosed with hyperthyroidism? **Select all that apply.**
1. Establish a supportive and trusting relationship to help the client cope.
2. Assist with exercises involving large muscle groups.
3. Instruct the unlicensed assistive personnel (UAP) to apply multiple blankets to the bed
4. Explain that the caregiver should not leave the client alone.
5. Place the client in a cool room away from high-traffic areas.

50. Which statement by the client experiencing exophthalmos indicates the client needs more teaching by the endocrinology nurse?
1. "I will use artificial tears to moisten my eyes."
2. "I need to wear dark glasses to prevent irritation."
3. "I should not move my eyes unless absolutely necessary."
4. "I should lightly tape my eyes shut when I sleep"

51. Which action by the unlicensed assistive personnel (UAP) warrants intervention by the nurse caring for the client with type 2 diabetes with chronic renal disease who is on hemodialysis?
1. The UAP times the client's activities to help conserve energy.
2. The UAP applies a lubricant to the lips and oral mucous membranes.
3. The UAP ties a sheet around the client sitting in the chair.
4. The UAP uses a fan to facilitate movement of cool air.

52. The nurse supervisor in the home health (HH) office is assigning tasks for the day. Which task is most appropriate for the nurse supervisor to assign the licensed practical nurse (LPN)?
1. Tell the LPN to complete the admission assessment for the client with Cushing's disease.
2. Request the LPN to evaluate the client's response to the new pain medication regime.
3. Request the LPN perform the wound care for the client with a Stage 4 pressure ulcer.
4. Instruct to the LPN to visit the client with type 2 diabetes who is stable and needs a hospital bed.

53. The charge nurse is checking the morning laboratory results for the clients. Which laboratory results require notifying the client's healthcare provider?
    1. The client with hypoparthyroidism who has a decreased serum calcium level.
    2. The client with Cushing's disease who has a decreased urine cortisol level.
    3. The client with diabetes insipidus who has a low urine specific gravity.
    4. The client with hyperthyroidism who has an increased TSH level.

54. The nurse on the medical unit is preparing to administer 0900 medications. Which medication should the nurse question administering?
    1. The hormone levothyroxine (Synthroid) to the client diagnosed with hypothyroidism.
    2. The metformin (Glucophage) to the type 2 diabetic who just had a CT scan with dye.
    3. The Humulin N insulin to the client with type 1 diabetes who is no longer NPO.
    4. The steroid prednisone to a client diagnosed with Addison's disease.

55. The nurse and unlicensed assistive personnel (UAP) are caring for clients on an endocrinology unit. Which task should not be delegated to the UAP?
    1. Ambulate the client who had a unilateral adrenalectomy.
    2. Change the linens on the client with acute thyrotoxicosis who is diaphoretic.
    3. Bring ice-cold water to the client diagnosed with diabetes insipidus.
    4. Take the vital signs of a client who has just returned from the post-anesthesia care unit (PACU).

56. The unit manager of an endocrinology unit is overbudget for the year and must transfer one staff member to another unit. Which option is the best action for the unit manager to take before deciding which staff member to transfer?
    1. Assess each staff member's abilities.
    2. Choose the last staff member hired.
    3. Ask for input from the staff members.
    4. Request the transfer documentation form.

57. The clinic nurse is caring for a 10-year-old client diagnosed with diabetes mellitus type 2. Which client problem is priority?
    1. Altered nutrition, excessive intake.
    2. Risk for low self-esteem.
    3. Hypoglycemia.
    4. Risk for loss of body part.

58. The overhead page has just announced a Code Red, actual fire, on a unit two floors below the unit where the nurse is working. Which action should the nurse implement first?
    1. Turn off the oxygen supply to the rooms.
    2. Evacuate the clients to a lower floor.
    3. Close all of the doors to the clients' rooms.
    4. Make a list of clients to discharge.

59. The nurse is preparing to administer medications for clients on a medical unit. The client diagnosed with hypothyroidism is complaining of being hot all the time, feeling palpations, and being jittery. Which intervention should the nurse implement first?
    1. Check the client's serum thyroid levels.
    2. Assess the client for diarrhea.
    3. Document the finding in the chart.
    4. Hold the client's thyroid medication.

60. The nurse is administering medications on an endocrinology unit. Which medication should the nurse question administering?
1. The propylthiouracil (PTU) to the client diagnosed with hyperthyroidism.
2. The desmopressin acetate (DDAVP) to the client diagnosed with diabetes insipidus.
3. The somatropin (Genotropin) to the client diagnosed with hypopituitarism.
4. The propranolol (Inderal) to the client diagnosed with hypothyroidism.

61. The hospice nurse caring for a client diagnosed with diabetes mellitus type 2 observes the client eating a bowl of ice cream. Which intervention should the nurse implement first?
1. Allow the client to enjoy the ice cream.
2. Check the client's blood glucose.
3. Remind the client not to eat ice cream.
4. Suggest the client eat low-fat sweets.

62. The nurse is caring for the client who is 1 day postoperative transsphenoidal hypophysectomy. Which action by the unlicensed assistive personnel (UAP) warrants intervention by the nurse?
1. The UAP places the client with the HOB 30 degrees elevated.
2. The UAP tells the client not to cough vigorously.
3. The UAP is helping the client splint the incision.
4. The UAP is taking the client's vital signs.

63. The charge nurse of a surgical unit has been notified of an external disaster with multiple casualties. Which client should the charge nurse request to be discharged from the hospital to make room for clients from the disaster?
1. The client scheduled for a bilateral adrenalectomy in the morning whose preoperative teaching has not been started.
2. The client who had a total abdominal hysterectomy 2 days ago and PCA machine has been discontinued.
3. The client who is postoperative bilateral thyroidectomy who has a hemoglobin of 7 mg/dL and a hematocrit of 22.1%.
4. The client with type 2 diabetes who has just had a kidney transplant and is experiencing fever and pain at the surgical site.

64. For which client's laboratory data should the charge nurse notify the HCP?
1. The potassium level of 3.6 mEq/L in a client diagnosed with heart failure who is taking the loop diuretic furosemide (Lasix).
2. The PTT level of 78 in the client diagnosed with pulmonary embolism who is receiving IV heparin.
3. The blood urea nitrogen (BUN) of 84 mg/dL in a client diagnosed with end-stage renal disease (ESRD) and peripheral edema.
4. The blood glucose level of 543 mg/dL in a client diagnosed with uncontrolled diabetes mellitus type 1.

65. Which nursing intervention is priority for the intensive care nurse to implement when caring for a client diagnosed with diabetic ketoacidosis (DKA)?
1. Assess for a fruity breath odor.
2. Check blood glucose levels ac and hs.
3. Monitor the client's pulse oximeter readings.
4. Maintain the regular insulin IV rate on an infusion pump.

66. The client diagnosed with diabetes mellitus type 2 has a hemoglobin A1C of 11 mg/dL. Which intervention should the nurse implement first?
1. Check the client's current blood glucose level.
2. Assess the client for neuropathy and retinopathy.
3. Teach the client about the effects of uncontrolled hyperglycemia.
4. Monitor the client's BUN and creatinine levels.

67. The nurse is working in an outpatient clinic reviewing lab data. Which client should the nurse notify the HCP first?

Patient Name: F G	Account Number: 55 689 25	Gender: Male
Laboratory Test	Patient Values	Normal Values
White blood cell	14.3	5–10 (10^3)
Red blood cell	4.3	Female 3.8–5.1 (10^6) Male 4.2–5.7 (10^6)
Hemoglobin	13.3	Female 11.7–16 g/dL Male 13.2–17.3 g/dL
Hematocrit	39.6	Female 35%–47% Male 39%–50%
Platelet	149	150–400 (10^3)

Patient Name: J K	Account Number: 44 895 78	Gender: Female
Laboratory Test	Patient Values	Normal Values
White blood cell	5.3	5–10 (10^3)
Red blood cell	3.9	Female 3.8–5.1 (10^6) Male 4.2–5.7 (10^6)
Hemoglobin	12.0	Female 11.7–16 g/dL Male 13.2–17.3 g/dL
Hematocrit	36.9	Female 35%–47% Male 39%–50%
Platelet	150	150–400 (10^3)

Patient Name: L M	Account Number: 68 79 25	Gender: Female
Laboratory Test	Patient Values	Normal Values
Sodium	140	135–145 mEq/L
Potassium	4.9	3.5–5.0 mEq/L
Glucose	125	70–120 g/dL

Patient Name: O R	Account Number: 25 89 54	Gender: Male
Laboratory Test	Patient Values	Normal Values
Sodium	136	135–145 mEq/L
Potassium	5.1	3.5–5.0 mEq/L
Glucose	98	70–120 g/dL

68. The client diagnosed with type 1 diabetes is receiving regular insulin, a pancreatic hormone, by sliding scale. The client's glucometer reading is 249. The order reads blood glucose level:
<150 0 units
151–200 5 units
201–250 8 units
251–300 12 units
>301 Contact healthcare provider
How much insulin should the nurse administer to the client? _____

69. The nurse in the outpatient clinic is working with an unlicensed assistive personnel (UAP). Which tasks are most appropriate for the nurse to delegate to the UAP? **Select all that apply.**
1. Take the client to the examination room and take the vital signs.
2. Weigh the client and document the weight in the client's chart.
3. Clean the room and set it up for the next client.
4. Discuss the prescriptions prescribed by the healthcare provider.
5. Call the pharmacy to authorize a refill on a client's prescription.

70. The nurse in an outpatient clinic is returning telephone calls. Rank the calls in the order they should be returned, with the highest priority call first.
1. The call from a husband who states his wife started on an antidepressant and now will not wake up.
2. The call from a client who states the medication that was prescribed for her diabetes mellitus type 2 is too expensive.
3. The client with hypothyroidism who is reporting feeling hot, having hand tremors, and having diarrhea.
4. The call from the pharmacist wanting an authorization to change a medication from a trade name to a generic name drug.
5. The call from the client who had a magnetic resonance imaging (MRI) scan 2 days ago and has not received the results.

QUESTIONS

ENDOCRINE CLINICAL SCENARIO

1. Mr. Larry, a 24-year-old client diagnosed with type 1 diabetes mellitus, called the office nurse, Mr. John, to report nausea and vomiting. Which of the following interventions should Mr. John implement? **Select all that apply.**
    1. Ask Mr. Larry if he has vomited and if so how many times.
    2. Determine Mr. Larry's blood glucose level.
    3. Find out what medications the client has taken for the nausea.
    4. Tell the patient to drink diet sodas to keep from being dehydrated.
    5. Make sure the client does not take his insulin.
    6. Tell Mr. Larry to monitor his urine ketones.
    7. Have Mr. Larry go immediately to the emergency department of his local hospital.
    8. Request Mr. Larry to call 911.
    9. Have Mr. Larry call the healthcare provider if he is showing ketones in his urine.
    10. Discuss trying to intake carbohydrates equal to his usual caloric intake.

2. Mr. Larry does not improve and is seen in the Emergency Department of a local hospital and is diagnosed with diabetes ketoacidosis (DKA). He is admitted to the Intensive Care Unit. List five interventions his nurse, Ms. Leslie, should implement at this time.

3. Mr. Larry recovers from the DKA and is being discharged from the medical unit. His nurse, Mr. Justin, is preparing the discharge information. Which information should Mr. Justin include in the discharge instructions?

ANSWERS AND RATIONALES

The correct answer number and rationale for why it is the correct answer are given in **boldface type.** Rationales for why the other possible answer options are incorrect also are given, but they are not in boldface type.

1. 1. **The client received an intermediate-acting insulin at 1630 plus the sliding-scale insulin dose to lower the client's blood glucose level. This client should receive a bedtime snack to make sure the client does not experience a hypoglycemic reaction during the night. Intermediate insulin generally peaks 6 to 8 hours after administration, 2230 to 0030 for this client.**
   2. The nurse should check the client's blood glucose at 2100 hours, not at the current time.
   3. Nothing indicates the client needs an intervention for hypoglycemia at this time.
   4. The client with type 2 diabetes would experience hyperglycemic hyperosmolar nonketotic coma (HHNC) syndrome, not DKA.
   Content – *Medical/Surgical:* **Category of Health Alteration** – *Endocrine:* **Integrated Processes** – *Nursing Process: Implementation:* **Client Needs** – *Physiological Integrity: Pharmacological and Parenteral Therapies:* **Cognitive Level** – *Application*

MAKING NURSING DECISIONS: This is an alternate type of question included in the NCLEX-RN® blueprint. The test taker must be able to read a medication administration record (MAR), be knowledgeable of medications, and be able to make a decision as to the nurse's most appropriate intervention.

2. 1. **The UAP can take food to the client since this is not a medication and the client is stable.**
   2. The client on a PCA pump is under the influence of narcotic analgesics and should be on bed rest, not ambulated to the bathroom.
   3. None of the hospital employees should witness the client's advance directive.
   4. The nurse cannot delegate teaching to the UAP.
   Content – *Medical/Surgical:* **Category of Health Alteration** – *Endocrine:* **Integrated Processes** – *Nursing Process: Implementation:* **Client Needs** – *Safe and Effective Care Environment: Management of Care:* **Cognitive Level** – *Analysis*

MAKING NURSING DECISIONS: The nurse should not delegate assessment, teaching, evaluation, medications, or an unstable client to the UAP.

3. 1. **The LPN can change sterile dressings according to his or her scope of practice.**
   2. The UAP can obtain the client's weight; therefore, it should not be assigned to the LPN.
   3. The client in myxedema coma is not a stable client and should be assigned to the nurse, not the LPN.
   4. Teaching should not be assigned to the LPN, only to the nurse.
   Content – *Medical/Surgical:* **Category of Health Alteration** – *Endocrine:* **Integrated Processes** – *Nursing Process: Implementation:* **Client Needs** – *Safe and Effective Care Environment: Management of Care:* **Cognitive Level** – *Analysis*

MAKING NURSING DECISIONS: The RN should not assign assessment, teaching, evaluation, or the care of an unstable client to an LPN. If any task can be assigned to a UAP, then it should not be assigned to an LPN.

4. 1. The new graduate cannot take a break whenever he or she becomes overwhelmed because the work may never get done. The new graduate should schedule breaks throughout the shift, not when he or she wants to take them.
   2. **The preceptor should recommend that the new graduate use some tool to organize the work so important tasks, such as medication administration and taking vital signs, are not missed.**
   3. Encouraging the new graduate to calm him or herself down (five deep breaths) before beginning work is good, but it will not help the new graduate with time management.
   4. The new graduate must find the best way to organize him- or herself. Doing the organizing for the new graduate will not help him or her.
   Content – *Medical/Surgical:* **Category of Health Alteration** – *Endocrine:* **Integrated Processes** – *Nursing Process: Implementation:* **Client Needs** – *Safe and Effective Care Environment: Management of Care:* **Cognitive Level** – *Synthesis*

MAKING NURSING DECISIONS: There will be management questions on the NCLEX-RN®. Concepts of Management is included under the category Safe and Effective Care Environment and the subcategory Management of Care.

5. 1. The HCP should be notified when the glucose level is verified by the laboratory.
   2. The sliding scale indicates that a blood glucose level of 351 to 400 mg/dL requires 10 units of

regular insulin. There is no insulin dosage administered for 408 mg/dL.

3. This should be done, but not until the nurse rechecks the blood glucose level at the bedside.

4. **The nurse should first recheck the blood glucose level at the bedside prior to taking any further action.**

Content – Medical/Surgical: **Category of Health Alteration** *– Endocrine:* **Integrated Processes** *– Nursing Process: Implementation:* **Client Needs** *– Physiological Integrity: Reduction of Risk Potential: Diagnostic Tests:* **Cognitive Level** *– Analysis*

MAKING NURSING DECISIONS: The test taker needs to read all of the options carefully before choosing the option that says, "Notify the HCP." If any of the options will provide information the HCP needs to know in order to make a decision, the test taker should choose that option. Assessment is the first step in the nursing process.

6. 1. The LPN is not licensed to assess the client who is hypoglycemic, nor should the nurse assign or delegate an unstable client. This client is unstable and requires the nurse's assessment skills.

2. The client with a paralytic ileus is NPO and should not have any food.

3. The UAP does not have the skill or training to insert a nasogastric tube.

4. **The LPN can perform a sterile procedure such as completing an in and out catheterization.**

Content – Medical/Surgical: **Category of Health Alteration** *– Endocrine:* **Integrated Processes** *– Nursing Process: Implementation:* **Client Needs** *– Safe and Effective Care Environment: Management of Care:* **Cognitive Level** *– Synthesis*

MAKING NURSING DECISIONS: The test taker must not only know which tasks should be delegated or assigned to the UAP and LPN, the nurse must also know which interventions are appropriate for the client's condition.

7. 1. This would be an inappropriate assignment because the UAP, not the LPN, could feed this stable client.

2. **The nurse could request that another nurse administer pain medication so that the client obtains immediate pain relief.**

3. This client's vital signs indicate that the client is unstable; therefore, the nurse should check on this client and not delegate the assessment to a UAP.

4. The client who requires a blood transfusion is unstable. The nurse should complete the pre-transfusion assessment. The RN, not the LPN, assesses.

Content – Medical/Surgical: **Category of Health Alteration** *– Endocrine:* **Integrated Processes** *– Nursing Process: Implementation:* **Client Needs** *– Safe and Effective Care Environment: Management of Care:* **Cognitive Level** *– Synthesis*

MAKING NURSING DECISIONS: A nurse cannot delegate assessment, teaching, evaluation, medications, or an unstable client to a UAP. The nurse cannot assign assessment, teaching, evaluation, or an unstable client to an LPN. The nurse can assign a task to another nurse.

8. 1. A power of attorney is a legal document authorizing an individual to conduct business for the client. The nurse should not recommend this type of document for a healthcare situation.

2. The living will usually requests the client's refusal of life-sustaining treatment. General anesthesia requires the client to be intubated and placed on a ventilator; therefore, the client's request to deny this type of life-sustaining effort will not be honored in the OR. The nurse should not recommend this type of advance directive.

3. A DNR order must be written in the client's chart by the HCP and may reflect the client's wishes, but it is not an advance directive.

4. **This document would be most appropriate for the nurse to recommend because it names an individual to be responsible in the event the client cannot make healthcare decisions for himself or herself.**

Content – Management: **Category of Health Alteration** *– Endocrine:* **Integrated Processes** *– Nursing Process: Planning:* **Client Needs** *– Safe and Effective Care Environment: Management of Care:* **Cognitive Level** *– Analysis*

MAKING NURSING DECISIONS: Questions on advance directives are included in the NCLEX-RN®. This content is included under the category Safe and Effective Care Environment and the subcategory Management of Care.

9. 1. **Masseter rigidity is a sign of malignant hyperthermia, which is a life-threatening complication of surgery. The client will also exhibit tachycardia (a heart rate greater than 150 bpm), hypotension, decreased cardiac output, and oliguria. It is a rare muscle disorder chemically induced by anesthesia.**

2. The client was NPO after midnight and during surgery; therefore, not urinating since surgery does not warrant immediate intervention.

3. The client who received general anesthesia is expected to be sleepy after surgery and easy to

arouse; therefore, this client does not warrant immediate intervention.

4. As long as the client has bowel sounds after surgery, hypoactive or hyperactive, then this client does not warrant immediate intervention.

Content – Medical/Surgical: **Category of Health Alteration** *– Endocrine:* **Integrated Processes** *– Nursing Process: Assessment:* **Client Needs** *– Physiological Integrity:* **Cognitive Level** *– Analysis*

MAKING NURSING DECISIONS: When deciding which client to assess first, the test taker should determine whether the signs/symptoms the client is exhibiting are normal or expected for the client situation. After eliminating the expected option, the test taker should determine which situation is more life threatening.

10. 1. The nurse who has worked on the unit for 4 years should not be sent because the nurse's expertise is needed on the unit.

2. The graduate nurse, while knowledgeable of the endocrinology unit with 6 months of experience, would not be sent because he or she does not have experience in the maternal child area.

3. **The LPN with maternal child area experience would be most helpful to the nursery.**

4. The charge nurse should not make assignments based on a staff member's personal life.

Content – Management: **Category of Health Alteration** *– Endocrine:* **Integrated Processes** *– Nursing Process: Implementation:* **Client Needs** *– Safe and Effective Care Environment: Management of Care:* **Cognitive Level** *– Analysis*

MAKING NURSING DECISIONS: There will be management questions on the NCLEX-RN®. Charge nurse responsibilities are included under the category Safe and Effective Care Environment and the subcategory Supervision.

11. 1. Acromegaly, an excessive secretion of growth hormone, results in overgrowth of the bones and soft tissues. Clubbed fingertips and large feet are expected; therefore, this client doesn't warrant intervention.

2. The client with SIADH, due to sustained secretion of antidiuretic hormone (ADH), would be expected to have a low urinary output. This client does not warrant intervention by the nurse.

3. The client with Cushing's syndrome would have truncal obesity and thin, fragile skin; therefore, this client does not warrant intervention by the nurse. Cushing's syndrome is caused by excess secretion of glucocorticoids by the adrenal gland.

4. **The client diagnosed with pheochromocytoma, a tumor of the adrenal medulla that produces excessive catecholamine, is expected to have a severe pounding headache and chest pain; but of these four clients this client is having pain, which is priority. This client warrants intervention by the nurse.**

Content – Medical/Surgical: **Category of Health Alteration** *– Endocrine:* **Integrated Processes** *– Nursing Process: Assessment:* **Client Needs** *– Physiological Integrity:* **Cognitive Level** *– Analysis*

MAKING NURSING DECISIONS: The test taker should use some tool as a reference to guide in the decision-making process. In this situation, Maslow's Hierarchy of Needs should be applied. Pain is priority even if it is expected.

12. 1. This statement is a therapeutic response, but it is not telling the client the truth.

2. **The ethical principle of veracity is the duty to tell the truth.**

3. This statement is "passing the buck," which the nurse should not do if at all possible.

4. This is attempting to obtain more information about the situation, but it is not telling the truth.

Content – Management: **Category of Health Alteration** *– Endocrine:* **Integrated Processes** *– Nursing Process: Implementation:* **Client Needs** *– Safe and Effective Care Environment: Management of Care:* **Cognitive Level** *– Comprehension*

MAKING NURSING DECISIONS: The NCLEX-RN® blueprint includes nursing care addressing ethical principles, including autonomy, beneficence, justice, and veracity, to name a few.

13. 1. After the a.m. shift report, the priority medication should be the insulin prior to the breakfast meal, not Lasix.

2. After the a.m. shift report, the priority medication should be the insulin prior to the breakfast meal, not digoxin.

3. An antibiotic IVPB is a routine, scheduled medication and should have been administered by the night nurse; there's also a 1-hour leeway when administering this medication. The nurse would have to see whether the IVPB apparatus was hanging at the client's bedside or contact the night nurse before administering this medication.

4. **Insulin is a medication that must be administered prior to the meal; therefore, this medication is priority.**

Content – Medical/Surgical: **Category of Health Alteration** *– Endocrine:* **Integrated Processes** *– Nursing*

*Process: Implementation: **Client Needs** – Physiological Integrity: Pharmacological and Parenteral Therapies: **Cognitive Level** – Synthesis*

MAKING NURSING DECISIONS: The test taker should know which medications are priority medications such as life-threatening medications, insulin, and medications that have specific requirements for effectiveness, such as mucosal barrier agents (Carafate). These medications should be administered first by the nurse.

14. 1. **The pregnant nurse can administer antineoplastic medications to clients. The nurse should not be exposed to antineoplastic agents outside of the administration bags and tubing. The pregnant nurse can care for a client who is immunosuppressed.**

 2. Shingles (herpes zoster) is a painful, blistering skin rash due to the varicella-zoster virus, the virus that causes chicken-pox. The pregnant nurse should not be assigned this client.

 3. The client receiving radioactive iodine should not be around pregnant women or young children; therefore, the nurse who is pregnant should not care for this client.

 4. The client has the cytomegalovirus, which crosses the placental barrier. Therefore, a pregnant nurse should not be assigned this client. Any client with a communicable disease that crosses the placental barrier should not be assigned to a nurse who is pregnant.

 *Content – Medical/Surgical: **Category of Health Alteration** – Endocrine: **Integrated Processes** – Nursing Process: Implementation: **Client Needs** – Safe and Effective Care Environment: Management of Care: Supervision: **Cognitive Level** – Analysis*

MAKING NURSING DECISIONS: There will be management questions on the NCLEX-RN®. Charge nurse responsibilities are included under the category Safe and Effective Care Environment and subcategory Supervision.

15. 1. This is within the normal range of 70 to 120 mg/dL. Hypoglycemia is expected in a client with myxedema; therefore, a 74 mg/dL blood glucose level would be expected.

 2. The client's metabolism is slowed in myxedema coma, which would result in these vital signs.

 3. **These ABGs indicate respiratory acidosis (ph <7.35, Paco$_2$ >45) and hypoxemia (O$_2$ <80); therefore, this client would warrant immediate intervention by the nurse. Untreated respiratory acidosis**

can result in death if not treated immediately.

 4. Lethargy is an expected symptom in a client diagnosed with myxedema; therefore, this would not warrant immediate intervention.

 *Content – Medical/Surgical: **Category of Health Alteration** – Endocrine: **Integrated Processes** – Nursing Process: Assessment: **Client Needs** – Physiological Integrity, Disease Process: **Cognitive Level** – Analysis*

MAKING NURSING DECISIONS: The nurse must be knowledgeable of expected medical treatment for the client. This is a knowledge-based question. The nurse must be knowledgeable of normal laboratory values. These values must be memorized and the nurse must be able to determine if the laboratory value is normal for the client's disease process or medications the client is taking.

16. 1. Synthroid is a daily medication and can be administered within the 1-hour time frame (30 minutes before and 30 minutes after the dosing time).

 2. **Insulin should be administered before a meal for best effects. This medication should be administered first.**

 3. Prednisone is a routine medication and can be administered within the 1-hour time frame (30 minutes before and 30 minutes after the dosing time).

 4. Spiriva is a routine daily medication and can be administered within the 1-hour time frame (30 minutes before and 30 minutes after the dosing time).

 *Content – Medical/Surgical: **Category of Health Alteration** – Endocrine: **Integrated Processes** – Nursing Process: Implementation: **Client Needs** – Physiological Integrity, Pharmacological and Parenteral Therapies: **Cognitive Level** – Synthesis*

MAKING NURSING DECISIONS: The test taker should know what medications are priority medications such as life-threatening medications, insulin, and medications with specific requirements for effectiveness, such as mucosal barrier agents (Carafate). These medications should be administered first by the nurse.

17. 1. The client with diabetes insipidus, a deficiency in the production of the antidiuretic hormone, will have an increase in thirst and urination. The nurse should not assess this client first.

 2. **The nurse should assess the client with a thyroidectomy for hemorrhaging every 2 hours. Neck edema, irregular breathing, and frequent swelling are signs of hemorrhaging; therefore, the nurse should assess this client first.**

3. The client with hypofunction of the parathyroid gland is expected to have muscle cramps and irritability; therefore, the nurse should not assess this client first. Bleeding and loss of airway are priority over an expected symptom of the disease process, which is not as immediately life threatening.

4. Addison's disease, hypofunction of the adrenal gland, causes the client weakness, fatigue, and anorexia. These signs/symptoms are expected; therefore, the nurse should not assess this client first.

Content – Medical/Surgical: **Category of Health Alteration** *– Endocrine:* **Integrated Processes** *– Nursing Process: Assessment:* **Client Needs** *– Physiological Integrity: Safety:* **Cognitive Level** *– Synthesis*

MAKE NURSING DECISIONS: The test taker must determine which sign/symptom is not expected for the disease process. If the sign/symptom is not expected, then the nurse should assess the client first. This type of question is determining if the nurse is knowledgeable of signs/symptoms of a variety of disease processes.

18. 1. The nurse should obtain the client's baseline weight but it is not the priority intervention over restoring the client's circulatory status.

2. Desmopressin acetate (DDAVP), an analog of the antidiuretic hormone, is the hormone replacement of choice for central DI. It is not the first intervention because restoring circulatory volume is priority.

3. **In acute DI, hypotonic saline is administered intravenously and is titrated to replace urinary output. Restoring circulatory volume is the priority intervention. Remember Maslow's Hierarchy of Needs; physiological needs are priority.**

4. Monitoring the client's intake and output is an appropriate nursing intervention but not priority over restoring circulatory volume.

Content – Medical/Surgical: **Category of Health Alteration** *– Endocrine:* **Integrated Processes** *– Nursing Process: Implementation:* **Client Needs** *– Physiological Integrity: Pharmacological and Parenteral Therapies:* **Cognitive Level** *– Synthesis*

19. 1. Beta-adrenergic blockers are used to treat relief of thyrotoxicosis, a thyroid storm, but it is not the nurse's first intervention.

2. The nurse should notify the healthcare provider of this rare condition, thyrotoxic crisis, but the nurse should first assess the client prior to calling HCP.

3. **Since the UAP gave the nurse this information, the nurse must assess the client prior to taking any further action.**

4. The nurse should administer acetaminophen (Tylenol) PO STAT to help decrease the fever, but the nurse should first assess the client since the UAP gave the nurse the information.

Content – Medical/Surgical: **Category of Health Alteration** *– Endocrine:* **Integrated Processes** *– Nursing Process: Assessment:* **Client Needs** *– Physiological Integrity: Pharmacological and Parenteral Therapies:* **Cognitive Level** *– Analysis*

MAKING NURSING DECISIONS: Any time a nurse receives information from another staff member about a client who may be experiencing a complication, the nurse must assess the client. A nurse should not make decisions about the client's needs based on another staff member's information.

20. 1. The UAP cannot sit for an extended period of time with a grieving client.

2. **A chaplain is a spiritual adviser who can stay with the client until a family member or the client's personal spiritual adviser can come to the hospital to be with the client.**

3. The client should not be sedated. Grieving is a natural process that must be worked through. Sedating the client will delay the grieving process. The nurse should allow the client to ventilate her feelings to foster the grieving process, not numb the client.

4. The client may request to be left alone, but the nurse should refer the client for spiritual support first and not assume the client wants to be left alone. Most clients feel the need for someone's presence.

Content – Medical/Surgical: **Category of Health Alteration** *– Endocrine:* **Integrated Processes** *– Nursing Process: Implementation:* **Client Needs** *– Safe and Effective Care Environment: Management of Care; Supervision:* **Cognitive Level** *– Cognitive*

MAKING NURSING DECISIONS: The test taker must be knowledgeable of the role of all members of the multidisciplinary healthcare team as well as HIPAA rules and regulations. These will be tested on the NCLEX-RN® exam.

21. 1. **The client is exhibiting signs of hypoglycemia; therefore, the nurse should treat the client's symptoms with a simple carbohydrate, such as glucose tablets. This is the first intervention.**

2. The nurse should provide the client with complex carbohydrates so another episode of hypoglycemia will not occur.

3. The nurse could obtain a glucometer reading at the bedside, but having the laboratory

draw a serum blood glucose level should not be the nurse's first intervention.

4. The nurse should determine the last time the client received insulin but it is not the first intervention. Remember: The nurse should not assess if the client is in distress.

Content – Medical/Surgical: **Category of Health Alteration** – Endocrine: **Integrated Processes** – Nursing Process: Implementation: **Client Needs** – Physiological Integrity: Pharmacological and Parenteral Therapies: **Cognitive Level** – Analysis

MAKING NURSING DECISIONS: When the question asks which intervention should be implemented first, it means all the options are something a nurse could implement, but only one should be implemented first. The test taker should use the nursing process to determine the appropriate response: If the client is in distress do not assess; if the client is not in distress then the nurse should assess.

22. 1. The client has not complained of claustrophobia. The client has some type of neurological abnormality.

    2. A vest restraint will not keep the client's head still during the MRI.

    3. **The nurse should make sure that the client does not have any medical device implanted that could react with the magnetic field created by the MRI scanner. An implanted ECG device could prevent the client from having an MRI, depending on the age of the pacemaker and the material with which it was made.**

    4. Family members are requested to stay outside of the area where the MRI is performed.

    Content – Medical/Surgical: **Category of Health Alteration** – Endocrine: **Integrated Processes** – Nursing Process: Assessment: **Client Needs** – Safe and Effective Management of Care; Diagnostic Examinations: **Cognitive Level** – Analysis

MAKING NURSING DECISIONS: The nurse must be knowledgeable of normal diagnostic tests pre- and postprocedure. These interventions must be memorized and the nurse must be able to determine if the client is able to have the diagnostic procedure and post-procedure care to ensure the client is safe.

23. 1. The nurse needs as much information as possible in order to provide care for the client. The client may or may not have a significant other to be contacted. This is not the best way to try to get information on the client.

    2. The ambulance workers will only be able to give a cursory report based on the limited

information that was provided to them. This is not the best place to try to get information on the client.

3. **The nursing home should send a transfer form with the client that details current medications and diagnoses as well as hygiene needs. Previous hospital records will include a history and physical examination and a discharge summary. This is the best place to start to glean information regarding the client.**

4. The HCP orders may contain a current diagnosis but will not contain any information about the client's medical history. This is not the best place to try to get information on the client.

Content – Medical/Surgical: **Category of Health Alteration** – Endocrine: **Integrated Processes** – Nursing Process: Assessment: **Client Needs** – Safe and Effective Care Environment: Management of Care: **Cognitive Level** – Synthesis

MAKING NURSING DECISIONS: Assessment is the first step of the nursing process, and the test taker should use the nursing process or some other systematic process to assist in determining priorities. The nurse should access documentation that has objective data about the client's condition.

24. 1. The nurse asked the client her name, and the client replied that she was a different person.

    2. **The step the nurse did not take was to verify the client's armband against the MAR. Checking the identification band against the MAR would have prevented the error.**

    3. This is not the step that was overlooked.

    4. This is not the step that was missed.

    Content – Medical/Surgical – Medication: **Category of Health Alteration** – Drug Administration: **Integrated Processes** – Nursing Process: Implementation: **Client Needs** – Physiological Integrity: Pharmacological and Parenteral Therapies: **Cognitive Level** – Comprehension

MAKING NURSING DECISIONS: The NCLEX-RN® blueprint includes the category Medication Administration under Physiological Integrity: Pharmacological and Parenteral Therapies. This is a knowledge-based question.

25. 1. Health promotion activities that help prevent UTIs include emptying the bladder. Bacteria can grow in stagnated urine in the bladder and emptying the bladder will help prevent this. The client is diagnosed with a UTI and antibiotic therapy is the priority nursing intervention.

    2. Enzymes found in cranberries inhibit attachment of urinary pathogens (especially *E. coli*)

to the bladder epithelium. Daily cranberry juice helps prevent UTIs but the priority nursing intervention is taking antibiotic therapy.

3. Women with diabetes are two to three times more likely to have bacteria in their bladders than women without diabetes. Taking hypoglycemic medication is important, but when the UTI is diagnosed, antibiotic therapy is priority.

4. **Antibiotic therapy is the priority intervention for the client with a diagnosed UTI. None of the health promotion activities will treat the UTI, though they will help prevent further UTIs.**

Content – Medical/Surgical: ***Category of Health Alteration*** *– Endocrine:* ***Integrated Processes*** *– Nursing Process: Implementation:* ***Client Needs*** *– Physiological Integrity: Pharmacological and Parenteral Therapies:* ***Cognitive Level*** *– Comprehension*

MAKING NURSING DECISIONS: The test taker needs to be aware of adjectives in the stem of the question. The word "diagnosed" should guide the nurse as to the correct answer. Health promotion activities do not treat infections. Antibiotic therapy treats the infection and is the priority intervention.

26. 1. Steroids do not affect the client's potassium level.
    2. Glucocorticoids do not affect the client's sodium level.
    3. Steroids do not affect the client's liver enzymes.
    4. **Steroids are excreted as glucocorticoids from the adrenal gland and are responsible for insulin resistance by the cells, which may cause hyperglycemia; therefore, the nurse should monitor the glucose level.**

Content – Medical/Surgical: ***Category of Health Alteration*** *– Endocrine:* ***Integrated Processes*** *– Nursing Process: Implementation:* ***Client Needs*** *– Physiological Integrity: Pharmacological and Parenteral Therapies:* ***Cognitive Level*** *– Synthesis*

MAKING NURSING DECISIONS: The nurse must be knowledgeable of laboratory values affected by medication. These values must be memorized and the nurse must be able to determine if the laboratory value is normal for the client's disease process or medications the client is taking.

27. 1. A 6-pound weight gain between dialysis treatments is expected; therefore, the nurse would not need to notify the client's HCP.
    2. In the early stage of renal insufficiency, polyuria results from the inability of the kidneys to concentrate urine, which most

often happens at night (nocturia). The nurse would not notify the client's HCP.

3. The nurse should call this client, but psychosocial problems do not take priority over physiological, potentially life-threatening problems.

4. **These are signs of an acute transplant rejection, which is potentially a life-threatening problem; therefore, the nurse should notify the healthcare provider about this client.**

Content – Medical/Surgical: ***Category of Health Alteration*** *– Endocrine:* ***Integrated Processes*** *– Nursing Process: Assessment:* ***Client Needs*** *– Physiological Integrity: Reduction of Risk Potential:* ***Cognitive Level*** *– Synthesis*

MAKING NURSING DECISIONS: The nurse should ask, "Are the assessment data normal?" for the disease process. If they are normal for the disease process then the nurse would not need to intervene; if they are not normal for the disease process then this warrants intervention by the nurse.

28. 1. **This client should be seen first because clear nasal drainage could be cerebrospinal fluid (CSF), which is a potentially life-threatening complication from surgery. The nurse needs to determine if the drainage has glucose. If it does, it is CSF and the surgeon needs to be notified.**
    2. The client with Grave's disease has exophthalmos (protruding eyes) and bruits (swishing sound) over the thyroid gland so the nurse would not assess this client first.
    3. The client with hyperparathyroidism is expected to have weakness, loss of appetite, and constipation; therefore, the nurse would not assess this client first.
    4. The client with Addison's disease is expected to have orthostatic hypotension, nausea, and vomiting; therefore, the nurse would not assess this client first.

Content – Medical/Surgical: ***Category of Health Alteration*** *– Endocrine:* ***Integrated Processes*** *– Nursing Process: Assessment:* ***Client Needs*** *– Physiological Integrity: Reduction of Risk Potential:* ***Cognitive Level*** *– Synthesis*

MAKE NURSING DECISIONS: The test taker must determine which sign/symptom is not expected for the disease process. If the sign/symptom is not expected, then the nurse should assess the client first. This type of question is determining if the nurse is knowledgeable of signs/symptoms of a variety of disease processes.

29. 1. A case manager is assigned to a client with a chronic illness; therefore, a client with a renal calculi who had lithotripsy would not be appropriate for a case manager.
2. **It would be appropriate to assign this client to a case manager since this client has two chronic illnesses, often having multiple hospitalizations and chronic complications and requires long-term healthcare.**
3. Hypothyroidism is not a disease process resulting in multiple hospitalizations or chronic complications.
4. A client with Addison's disease on corticosteroid therapy would not be a client referred to a case manager.
Content – Medical/Surgical: **Category of Health Alteration** *– Endocrine:* **Integrated Processes** *– Nursing Process: Evaluation:* **Client Needs** *– Safe and Effective Care Environment: Management of Care; Supervision:* **Cognitive Level** *– Synthesis*

MAKING NURSING DECISIONS: Diabetes and CAD are well-known chronic disease processes and should make the test taker look at this option as the correct answer. Postoperative clients, for the most part, return to their normal life, which would not require a case manager.

30. 1. This client would benefit from a home health nurse but not a parish nurse.
2. **A parish nurse (PN) is a registered nurse with a minimum of 2 years of experience who works in a faith community, addressing health issues of its members as well as those in the broader community or neighborhood. The client is a Presbyterian so that is the reason the parish nurse should care for this client.**
3. This option has no faith base; therefore, the parish nurse should not be assigned this client.
4. The client with chronic renal disease and the caregiver need assistance in the home, but the parish nurse does not need to offer it.
Content – Medical/Surgical: **Category of Health Alteration** *– Endocrine:* **Integrated Processes** *– Nursing Process: Implementation:* **Client Needs** *– Safe and Effective Care Environment: Management of Care; Cultural Effectiveness:* **Cognitive Level** *– Analysis*

MAKING NURSING DECISIONS: The nurse must be knowledgeable of the roles and responsibilities of different nurses working in different areas of the hospital and the community.

31. 1. The UAP should not remove anything from the room. The nuclear medicine personnel will check the waste from the room for radioactivity prior to the removal and if radioactive will arrange for disposal in a way that protects the environment.
2. The UAP is hired to care for clients in the ambulatory care unit, not to take a client out to smoke. Clients in ambulatory care should not be smoking prior to or after surgery or procedure.
3. The UAP cannot assess the client's surgical dressing.
4. **The UAP can obtain a glucometer reading on a client who is stable, and clients in the ambulatory care unit are stable.**
Content – Medical/Surgical: **Category of Health Alteration** *– Endocrine:* **Integrated Processes** *– Nursing Process: Implementation:* **Client Needs** *– Safe and Effective Care Environment: Management of Care: Delegation:* **Cognitive Level** *– Application*

MAKING NURSING DECISIONS: The nurse cannot delegate assessment, teaching, evaluation, medications, or an unstable client to the UAP.

32. **Answer: 125 gtt/min.** A microdrip delivers 60 gtt/mL. The formula for this dosage problem is as follows:
1,000 mL divided by 8 = 125 mL per hour
125 times 60 = 7,500 gtt per hour
7,500 divided by 60 minutes = 125 gtts per minute
Content – Adult Health, Pharmacology: **Category of Health Alteration** *– Endocrine:* **Integrated Processes** *– Nursing Process: Implementation:* **Client Needs** *– Physiological Integrity: Pharmacological and Parenteral Therapies:* **Cognitive Level** *– Application*

MAKING NURSING DECISIONS: This is an alternate type of question included in the NCLEX-RN®. The nurse must know how to perform math calculations.

33. 1. Some herbal remedies commonly recommended for hypothyroid conditions include: *Equisetum arvense, Avena sativa, Centella asiatica, Coleus forskohlii,* and *Fucus vesiculosus.* This is an example of an herbal CAM, a healing practice that does not fall within the realm of conventional medicine.
2. Cinnamon is a popular spice and flavoring that has shown considerable evidence of lowering blood sugar. This is an example of a CAM, a healing practice that does not fall within the realm of conventional medicine.
3. **Daily baby aspirin is a medically accepted practice and prescribed by medical doctors. This is not an example of a CAM.**
4. This is an example of a CAM, a healing practice that does not fall within the realm of conventional medicine. Acupuncture is a type of traditional Chinese medicine.

*Content – Medical/Surgical: **Category of Health Alteration** – Complementary and Alternative Therapy: **Integrated Processes** – Nursing Process: Implementation: **Client Needs** – Physiological Integrity: Pharmacological and Parenteral Therapies: **Cognitive Level** – Analysis*

**MAKING NURSING DECISIONS: The NCLEX-RN®
tests candidates on complementary alternative
medicine, so the test taker should be knowledgeable of types of CAMs. Many clients use these
along with conventional medical interventions.**

34. 1. This is an example of community-based
       nursing wherein nurses care for an individual
       client living in the community.
    2. **Community-oriented, population-focused
       nursing practice involves the engagement
       of nursing in promoting and protecting
       the health of populations, not individuals
       in the community. Therefore, this is
       an example of community-oriented,
       population-focused nursing.**
    3. This is an example of community-based
       nursing wherein nurses care for an individual
       client living in the community.
    4. This is an example of community-based
       nursing wherein nurses care for an individual
       client living in the community.

    *Content – Community Health: **Category of Health Alteration** – Endocrine: **Integrated Processes** – Nursing Process: Assessment: **Client Needs** – Safe and Effective Care Environment: **Cognitive Level** – Comprehension*

**MAKING NURSING DECISIONS: The test taker
should note options 1, 3, and 4 all address an
individual client, but option 2 is the "odd man
out" and addresses a group of clients; this should
cause the test taker to select this option as the
correct answer.**

35. 1. The client should keep a written record of
       the results but it is not priority.
    2. The glucometer readings should be done
       in the morning when the client has not
       had anything to eat, but it can be done
       several times a day. This is not a priority.
    3. **Have the client demonstrate the skill to
       ensure the client can correctly perform
       the glucometer reading. This is the prior-
       ity when teaching about glucometer
       checks.**
    4. Proper disposal of lancets and strips with
       blood on them is important, but not
       priority over the client demonstrating
       the skill.

    *Content – Medical/Surgical: **Category of Health Alteration** – Endocrine: **Integrated Processes** – Nursing Process: Implementation: **Client Needs** – Physiological Integrity: Pharmacological and Parenteral Therapies: **Cognitive Level** – Analysis*

**MAKING NURSING DECISIONS: In questions that
ask the nurse to identify a priority intervention, all
the options are plausible. The priority intervention when teaching the client any skill is having
the client perform the skill in front of the nurse.**

36. 1. **Acupressure applies pressure along
       the body's energy meridian. Applying
       pressure on the medial forearm helps
       decrease the client's feeling of nausea.**
    2. This client must have medical interventions
       and would not benefit from acupressure.
    3. Sheehan syndrome is a postpartum condition
       of pituitary necrosis and hypopituitarism that
       occurs after circulatory collapse from uterine
       hemorrhaging. This client would not be
       treated with acupressure.
    4. The client with hypertension needs medica-
       tions and would not benefit from acupressure.

    *Content – Medical/Surgical: **Category of Health Alteration** – Complementary and Alternative Medicine: **Integrated Processes** – Nursing Process: Implementation: **Client Needs** – Physiological Integrity: Pharmacological and Parenteral Therapies: **Cognitive Level** – Analysis*

**MAKING NURSING DECISIONS: The NCLEX-RN®
tests complementary alternative medicine (CAM),
so the nurse must be familiar with the different
types of activities and therapies used for clients.**

37. 1. Moving the staff members to another room
       will just allow the argument to continue.
       This is not the director's first intervention.
    2. **The nursing supervisor should intervene
       and listen to both staff members' con-
       cerns and attempt to help resolve the
       disagreement. This is the director's first
       intervention.**
    3. The director should not ask another staff
       member to intervene in the argument. The
       director should address the professional staff
       about unprofessional behavior.
    4. The director should not act unprofessionally
       and correct the staff in front of everyone in
       the office. This should be done in private.

    *Content – Medical/Surgical: **Category of Health Alteration** – Management: **Integrated Processes** – Nursing Process: Implementation: **Client Needs** – Safe and Effective Care Environment: Management of Care: Supervision: **Cognitive Level** – Synthesis*

**MAKING NURSING DECISIONS: In any business,
arguments should not occur among staff of any
level where the customers or other staff can hear
or see it.**

38. 1. **These are signs of myxedema coma, which
       is characterized by subnormal temperature,
       hypotension, and hypoventilation. This
       client should be seen first by the nurse.**

2. The client with hypoparathyroidism is expected to have a positive Chvostek's sign; therefore, the nurse should not assess this client first.

3. Hoarseness is expected for 3 to 4 days after surgery because of edema; therefore, the nurse should not assess this client first.

4. The client with diabetes insipidus has polyuria and compensates for the fluid loss by drinking great amounts of water; therefore, the nurse should not assess this client first.

Content – *Medical/Surgical:* **Category of Health Alteration** – *Endocrine:* **Integrated Processes** – *Nursing Process: Assessment:* **Client Needs** – *Physiological Integrity: Pharmacological and Parenteral Therapies:* **Cognitive Level** – *Analysis*

MAKE NURSING DECISIONS: The test taker must determine which sign/symptom is not expected for the disease process. If the sign/symptom is not expected then the nurse should assess the client first. This type of question is determining if the nurse is knowledgeable of signs/symptoms of a variety of disease processes.

39. **1, 3, 4, and 5 are correct.**
    1. **This is an example of an activity the home health nurse would implement in the home.**
    2. Preoperative teaching is not an activity the home health nurse performs in the home. This is usually completed by the preoperative nurse.
    3. **This is an example of an activity the home health nurse would implement in the home.**
    4. **This is an example of an activity the home health nurse would implement in the home.**
    5. **This is an example of an activity the home health nurse would implement in the home.**

Content – *Medical/Surgical:* **Category of Health Alteration** – *Endocrine:* **Integrated Processes** – *Nursing Process: Assessment:* **Client Needs** – *Safe and Effective Care Environment:* **Cognitive Level** – *Analysis*

MAKING NURSING DECISIONS: This is an alternate type of question included in the NCLEX-RN®. The nurse must be able to select all the options that answer the question correctly. There are no partially correct answers.

40. 1. The client is exhibiting Trousseau's sign indicating hypoparathyroidism and is treated with IV calcium gluconate, but it is not the nurse's first intervention. The nurse must first assess the client prior to taking any action.
    2. **When the UAP gives information to the nurse about a client, the nurse must**

first assess the client prior to taking any action.

3. The client is exhibiting signs/symptoms of hypoparathyroidism, which makes this client unstable, and the nurse should not delegate any task to the UAP for the client who is unstable.

4. The nurse will need to notify the HCP, but not prior to assessing the client first.

Content – *Medical/Surgical:* **Category of Health Alteration** – *Endocrine:* **Integrated Processes** – *Nursing Process: Assessment:* **Client Needs** – *Physiological Integrity: Pharmacological and Parenteral Therapies:* **Cognitive Level** – *Synthesis*

MAKING NURSING DECISIONS: Any time a nurse receives information from another staff member about a client who may be experiencing a complication, the nurse must assess the client. A nurse should not make decisions about the client's needs based on another staff member's information.

41. 1. The client must need intermittent professional skilled care (such as nursing) not constant care.
    2. The client does not have to have a family member living in the home to be eligible for home healthcare.
    3. **The client must be confined to the home or require a considerable and taxing amount of effort to leave the home for brief periods to be eligible for home healthcare.**
    4. The client can be referred directly from a healthcare provider's office or a long-term care facility, and clients may also request home healthcare for themselves.

Content – *Medical/Surgical:* **Category of Health Alteration** – *Endocrine:* **Integrated Processes** – *Nursing Process: Planning:* **Client Needs** – *Physiological Integrity: Illness Management:* **Cognitive Level** – *Analysis*

MAKING NURSING DECISIONS: The nurse must be knowledgeable of the areas of nursing, and how and why the client would qualify for the care. The nurse must be a resource and advocate for the client.

42. 1. **This is an example of meditation.**
    2. Imagery uses the client's mind to generate images to help have a calming effect on the body.
    3. Aromatherapy, a biologically based therapy, involves the use of plants' essential oils for their beneficial effect.
    4. Acupressure is a manipulative and body-based method applying finger and hand pressure to specific areas of the body.

*Content – Medical/Surgical: **Category of Health Alteration** – Complementary and Alternative Medicine: **Integrated Processes** – Nursing Process: Implementation: **Client Needs** – Physiological Integrity: Reduction of Risk Potential: Therapeutic Procedures: **Cognitive Level** – Comprehension*

MAKING NURSING DECISIONS: The NCLEX-RN® tests complementary alternative medicine (CAM), so the nurse must be familiar with the different types of activities and therapies used for clients.

43. 1. **The priority intervention is to restrict fluids to help prevent weight gain, edema, or a serum sodium decline.**
2. This position enhances venous return to the heart and increases left atrial filling pressure, reducing ADH release, but it is not priority over fluid restriction.
3. The edematous skin is fragile and at risk for skin breakdown, and turning every 2 hours is a pertinent intervention but it is not priority over fluid retention.
4. The client needs oral hygiene, but it is not priority over fluid restriction.

*Content – Medical/Surgical: **Category of Health Alteration** – Endocrine: **Integrated Processes** – Nursing Process: Implementation: **Client Needs** – Physiological Integrity: Reduction of Risk Potential: Potential for Alterations in Body Systems: **Cognitive Level** – Analysis*

MAKING NURSING DECISIONS: Physiological problems have the highest priority when deciding on a course of action. The nurse should use Maslow's Hierarchy of Needs, and fluid and electrolyte balance is the priority.

44. 1. Dyspnea and confusion are not expected in a client diagnosed with Cushing's syndrome; therefore, this client would warrant a more experienced nurse to assess the reason for the complications.
2. The client with financial problems should be assigned to a social worker, not to a nurse.
3. A full-thickness (third-degree) burn is the most serious burn and requires excellent assessment skills to determine whether complications are occurring. This client should be assigned to a more experienced nurse.
4. **The client diagnosed with diabetic neuropathy would be expected to have pain; therefore, this client could be assigned to a nurse new to home health nursing. The client is not exhibiting a complication or an unexpected sign/symptom.**

*Content – Medical/Surgical: **Category of Health Alteration** – Endocrine: **Integrated Processes** – Nursing Process: Assessment: **Client Needs** – Physiological*

*Integrity: Reduction of Risk Potential: **Cognitive Level** – Analysis*

MAKE NURSING DECISIONS: When the test taker is deciding which client should be assigned to a new graduate, the most stable client should be assigned to the least experienced nurse.

45. 1. The client who is 1 day postoperative transsphenoidal hypophysectomy is able to feed him- or herself; therefore, this task should not be delegated.
2. **The UAP is able to obtain a urine specimen from the client. This task is not assessment, teaching, evaluation, medications, or the care of an unstable client.**
3. The client with myxedema coma is unstable; therefore, this task cannot be delegated.
4. The UAP cannot assess, and the client with an Addisonian crisis is not stable; therefore, this task cannot be delegated.

*Content – Medical/Surgical: **Category of Health Alteration** – Management: **Integrated Processes** – Nursing Process: Implementation: **Client Needs** – Safe and Effective Care Environment: Management of Care: Delegation: **Cognitive Level** – Application*

MAKING NURSING DECISIONS: This is an "except" question. The test taker could ask which task is appropriate to delegate to the UAP; three options would be appropriate to delegate and one would not be. Remember: The nurse cannot delegate assessment, teaching, evaluation, medications, or an unstable client to the UAP.

46. 1. This statement does not allow the nurses to have any input into the assignments; therefore, this is the statement of an autocratic manager. These managers use an authoritarian approach to direct the activities of others.
2. Laissez-faire managers maintain a permissive climate with little direction or control. Allowing the assistants to have total control is laissez-faire management. Supporting the assistants in front of the charge nurse is an appropriate action, but it does not address the needs of the field nurses.
3. This statement does not support a democratic leadership style. It is more autocratic: The director is going to take care of the problem.
4. **Democratic managers are people oriented and emphasize efficient group functioning. The environment is open, and communication flows both ways. Meetings to discuss concerns illustrate a democratic leadership style.**

*Content – Medical/Surgical: **Category of Health Alteration** – Management: **Integrated Processes** – Nursing Process: Evaluation: **Client Needs** – Safe and Effective Care Environment: Management of Care: **Cognitive Level** – Synthesis*

MAKING NURSING DECISIONS: There will be management questions on the NCLEX-RN®. Concepts of Management is included under the category Safe and Effective Care Environment and the subcategory Management of Care.

47. 1. The client may be diagnosed with diabetes, but at the end of life this is not the priority nursing diagnosis. In fact, as a comfort measure, many clients are allowed to eat whatever they wish occasionally without regard to carbohydrates.
    2. This is a psychosocial diagnosis and not a priority over the physiological problems.
    3. **The client has peripheral neuropathy, which produces shooting pain in the extremities. The priority at the end of life is to keep the client comfortable.**
    4. This is a psychosocial diagnosis and not a priority over the physiological problems.

    *Content – End of Life: **Category of Health Alteration** – Endocrine: **Integrated Processes** – Nursing Process: Assessment: **Client Needs** – Physiological Integrity: Physiological Adaptation: Illness Management: **Cognitive Level** – Synthesis*

MAKING NURSING DECISIONS: The test taker must be aware of the setting, which dictates the appropriate intervention. The "hospice nurse" tells the test taker that this client has a prognosis of less than 6 months to live. Comfort measures are very important at the end of life.

48. 1. This type of breathing is called Cheyne-Stokes respirations, a pattern of breathing characterized by alternating periods of apnea and deep-rapid breathing. This is not the nurse's first intervention.
    2. The nurse should notify the chaplain but it is not the nurse's first intervention.
    3. **The nurse must first assess the client since the UAP gave the nurse the information.**
    4. The family should be contacted but not prior to assessing the client.

    *Content – End of Life: **Category of Health Alteration** – Endocrine: **Integrated Processes** – Nursing Process: Assessment: **Client Needs** – Physiological Integrity: Physiological Adaptation: Illness Management: **Cognitive Level** – Synthesis*

MAKING NURSING DECISIONS: Whenever any other person gives the nurse information about a client the nurse must first assess the client prior to taking any other action.

49. 1, 2, and 5 are correct.
    1. **This is an intervention the nurse should establish with every client.**
    2. **Exercises with large muscles allow the release of nervous tension and restlessness. Tremors can interfere with small-muscle coordination.**
    3. The UAP should use light coverings not heavy covering because the client with hyperthyroidism feels hot.
    4. The client with hyperthyroidism is not terminal and there is no reason the caregiver cannot leave the client's bedside.
    5. **A calm, quiet, cool room should be provided because increased metabolism causes sleep disturbances and the feeling of being hot.**

    *Content – Medical/Surgical: **Category of Health Alteration** – Endocrine: **Integrated Processes** – Nursing Process: Implementation: **Client Needs** – Physiological Integrity: Physiological Adaptation: Pathophysiology: **Cognitive Level** – Analysis*

MAKING NURSING DECISIONS: The test taker will have alternate types of questions on the NCLEX-RN®. The test taker must select all the correct options to get the question correct.

50. 1. This statement indicates the client understands the teaching and the client does not need more teaching. The exophthalmos that occurs with the disease allows the eyes to dry out, making them uncomfortable, and exposes the client to a risk of sclera damage.
    2. The client should wear dark glasses; therefore, the client understands the teaching.
    3. **To maintain flexibility, the client should exercise the intraocular muscles several times a day by turning the eyes in the complete range of motion. This statement indicates the client needs more teaching.**
    4. The client should tape the eyes shut; therefore, this client understands the client teaching.

    *Content – Medical/Surgical: **Category of Health Alteration** – Endocrine: **Integrated Processes** – Nursing Process: Implementation: **Client Needs** – Physiological Integrity, Pharmacological and Parenteral Therapies: **Cognitive Level** – Analysis*

MAKING NURSING DECISIONS: This is an "except" question. Three of the comments indicate the client understands the teaching and one indicates the client does not understand the teaching. These are occasionally found on the NCLEX-RN® and are worded in this manner. The test taker must realize that the reverse of the usual is in place. A hint: If the test taker is sure more than one option is correct, then the

test taker should re-read to make sure that a word or words such as "inappropriate" or "needs more teaching" have not been overlooked.

51. 1. Conserving the energy of the client who is dying is an appropriate intervention and does not warrant intervention by the hospice nurse.
     2. Applying lubricant to the client's dry lips and mouth is an appropriate intervention and does not warrant intervention by the hospice nurse.
     3. **This is a form of restraint, and the UAP cannot restrain the client in the home or in the acute care setting. This behavior warrants intervention by the nurse.**
     4. This is an appropriate action to help with shortness of breath or dyspnea. This action would not warrant intervention by the nurse.
     Content – Medical/Surgical: ***Category of Health Alteration*** *– Endocrine:* ***Integrated Processes*** *– Nursing Process: Implementation:* ***Client Needs*** *– Safe and Effective Care Environment; Management of Care:* ***Cognitive Level*** *– Comprehension*

MAKING NURSING DECISIONS: The nurse must ensure the UAP can perform any tasks delegated. It is the nurse's responsibility to demonstrate and/or teach the UAP how to perform the task, and then evaluate the task.

52. 1. The LPN cannot perform assessments on new admissions.
     2. The nurse cannot assign evaluation of the client's medical regime to the LPN.
     3. The wound care nurse should perform care for a Stage 4 pressure ulcer, not the LPN.
     4. **The LPN can contact medial supply companies and request durable medical equipment (DME); therefore, this is the most appropriate task to assign the LPN.**
     Content – Medical/Surgical: ***Category of Health Alteration*** *– Management:* ***Integrated Processes*** *– Nursing Process: Implementation:* ***Client Needs*** *– Safe and Effective Care Environment: Management of Care: Delegation:* ***Cognitive Level*** *– Synthesis*

MAKING NURSING DECISIONS: The nurse cannot assign assessment, teaching, evaluation, or an unstable client to the LPN in the home or in the acute care setting.

53. 1. The client with hypoparathyroidism is expected to have decreased serum calcium level; therefore, the nurse would not contact the client's HCP.
     2. The client with Cushing's syndrome is expected to have a urine cortisol level of 50 to 100 mcg/day; therefore, the nurse would not notify the client's HCP.
     3. The client with diabetes insipidus is expected to have a low urine specific gravity (<1.005);

therefore, the nurse would not notify the client's HCP.
     4. **The client diagnosed with hyperthyroidism should have a decreased TSH level; therefore, the nurse should notify the client's HCP.**
     Content – Medical/Surgical: ***Category of Health Alteration*** *– Endocrine:* ***Integrated Processes*** *– Nursing Process: Assessment:* ***Client Needs*** *– Physiological Integrity: Reduction of Risk Potential; Laboratory Values:* ***Cognitive Level*** *– Analysis*

MAKING NURSING DECISIONS: The nurse must be knowledgeable of normal laboratory values. These values must be memorized and the nurse must be able to determine if the laboratory value is normal for the client's disease process or medications the client is taking.

54. 1. The nurse would expect to administer a thyroid hormone to the client diagnosed with hypothyroidism.
     2. **Metformin must be held 24 hours after a client has received any type of contrast dye, since it can cause renal failure. This medication should be questioned by the nurse.**
     3. The client with DM should receive their prescribed insulin as soon as they are no longer NPO.
     4. The client with Addison's would be receiving prednisone; therefore, the nurse would not question administering this medication.
     Content – Medical/Surgical: ***Category of Health Alteration*** *– Endocrine:* ***Integrated Processes*** *– Nursing Process: Implementation:* ***Client Needs*** *– Physiological Integrity: Pharmacological and Parenteral Therapies:* ***Cognitive Level*** *– Synthesis*

MAKING NURSING DECISIONS: The nurse must be aware of interventions that must be implemented prior to administering medications. The nurse must know what to monitor prior to administering medications because untoward reactions and possibly death can occur.

55. 1. The client with a unilateral adrenalectomy should be ambulated to prevent postoperative complications. This task could be delegated to the UAP.
     2. The UAP can change linens for a client. Acute thyrotoxicosis is not a life-threatening condition.
     3. The client with DI is very thirsty and craves ice water; therefore, this task can be delegated to the UAP.
     4. **The client just returning from surgery and the PACU should be assessed immediately by the nurse. The UAP is not qualified to identify an unstable situation.**

Content – Medical/Surgical: **Category of Health Alteration** – *Endocrine:* **Integrated Processes** – *Nursing Process: Management:* **Client Needs** – *Safe and Effective Care Environment: Management of Care: Supervision:* **Cognitive Level** – *Analysis*

MAKING NURSING DECISIONS: The nurse must ensure the UAP can perform any tasks that are delegated. It is the nurse's responsibility to demonstrate and/or teach the UAP how to perform the task, and evaluate the task.

56. 1. **The manager should assess the abilities of each staff member for the needs of the unit before deciding which staff member to transfer.**
    2. This may be the method used by many managers, but the best action is to evaluate the needs of the unit and the abilities of the staff.
    3. In many instances, the unit manager must make hard decisions without consulting the staff members. Asking for the staff members' input could cause tension among the staff; therefore, this is not an appropriate intervention.
    4. This will be completed after the decision has been made and the staff member notified.

Content – Medical/Surgical: **Category of Health Alteration** – *Management:* **Integrated Processes** – *Nursing Process: Evaluation:* **Client Needs** – *Safe and Effective Care Environment: Management of Care: Supervision:* **Cognitive Level** – *Comprehension*

MAKING NURSING DECISIONS: There will be management questions on the NCLEX-RN®. Concepts of Management is included under the category Safe and Effective Care Environment and subcategory Management of Care.

57. 1. **Children are being diagnosed with type 2 diabetes mellitus because of excessive intake of calories and lack of exercise. This is the priority problem. Many states are performing screening activities to identify children at risk for developing type 2 DM so that interventions can be made to delay or prevent the child being diagnosed with type 2 DM. Acanthosis nigricans (hyperinsulinemia) can be identified with simple, non-invasive screening.**
    2. The client has a risk of low self-esteem because of the excess weight, but if the client and parents adhere to the recommended treatment regimen for weight control, diet, and exercise, the client's self-esteem should improve.
    3. The client's problem is hyperglycemia, not hypoglycemia.

4. Amputation is a chronic problem associated with diabetes and occurs after years of uncontrolled blood glucose levels. This is not the priority problem at this time.

Content – Medical/Surgical: **Category of Health Alteration** – *Endocrine:* **Integrated Processes** – *Nursing Process: Evaluation:* **Client Needs** – *Health Promotion and Maintenance: Health Promotion/Disease Prevention:* **Cognitive Level** – *Synthesis*

MAKING NURSING DECISIONS: The NCLEX-RN® integrates the nursing process throughout the Client Needs categories and subcategories. The nursing process is a scientific, clinical reasoning approach to client care that includes assessment, analysis, planning, implementation, and evaluation. The nurse will be responsible for identifying nursing diagnoses for clients.

58. 1. On a floor not directly affected by the fire, the oxygen is turned off only at the instruction of the administrative supervisor or plant operations director.
    2. The clients are safer on the floor where they are, not in an area closer to the fire.
    3. **The first action in a Code Red (actual fire) is to Rescue (R) the clients in immediate danger, followed by confine (C), closing the doors. Doors in a hospital must be fire rated to confine a blaze for an hour and a half.**
    4. This could be done, but it is a charge nurse's responsibility that is not called for at this time.

Content – Medical/Surgical: **Category of Health Alteration** – *Management:* **Integrated Processes** – *Nursing Process: Implementation:* **Client Needs** – *Safe and Effective Care Environment: Management of Care: Supervision:* **Cognitive Level** – *Synthesis*

MAKING NURSING DECISIONS: The nurse must be knowledgeable of emergency preparedness. Employees receive this information in employee orientation and are responsible for implementing procedures correctly. The NCSBN NCLEX-RN® blueprint includes questions on promoting a Safe and Effective Care Environment.

59. 1. The nurse should check the laboratory tests to determine the thyroid levels, but this is not the first intervention.
    2. Assessing the client for diarrhea could be done, but it is more important not to worsen the problem, and, therefore, the nurse should hold the thyroid medication first.
    3. Documentation of client complaints is always important, but it is not the first intervention.
    4. **The client is describing symptoms of hyperthyroidism. Because the client is**

diagnosed with hypothyroidism, has been prescribed thyroid hormone replacement, and now has symptoms of hyperthyroidism, it can be assumed that the client now has an excess of thyroid hormone. Therefore, the nurse should hold the thyroid medication and check the client's thyroid profile.

Content – Medical/Surgical: **Category of Health Alteration** *– Endocrine:* **Integrated Processes** *– Nursing Process: Evaluation:* **Client Needs** *– Physiological Integrity: Pharmacological and Parenteral Therapies:* **Cognitive Level** *– Synthesis*

MAKING NURSING DECISIONS: The nurse must be aware of expected actions of medications. The nurse must be aware of assessment data indicating whether the medication is effective or whether the medication is causing a side effect or an adverse effect.

60. 1. PTU blocks peripheral conversion of T_4 to T_3 and is prescribed for the client diagnosed with hyperthyroidism. The nurse would not question administering this medication.
    2. DDAVP is the treatment of choice for the client diagnosed with central diabetes insipidus.
    3. Genotropin, a growth hormone, is the treatment of choice for clients with hypofunction of the pituitary gland.
    4. **The client with hypothyroidism has a decreased pulse rate; therefore, the nurse should not administer a beta blocker, which could further decrease pulse rate. The client with thyrotoxicosis (hyperthyroidism) would receive Inderal. The nurse should question administering this medication.**

    Content – Medical/Surgical: **Category of Health Alteration** *– Endocrine:* **Integrated Processes** *– Nursing Process: Assessment:* **Client Needs** *– Physiological Integrity: Pharmacological and Parenteral Therapies:* **Cognitive Level** *– Analysis*

MAKING NURSING DECISIONS: The nurse must be aware of medications prescribed for specific conditions and disease processes. The nurse is the last person who ensures the client receives the correct medications.

61. 1. **A terminally ill client should be allowed comfort measures even when the activity would normally not be encouraged or allowed. The client can receive sliding-scale insulin, if needed, to cover the ice cream.**
    2. The nurse could do this after the ice cream has been metabolized to determine whether an insulin injection is needed.

3. The nurse should tell the client that food such as ice cream may be consumed in moderation and with the appropriate coverage.
4. Low-fat sweets may be a good substitute for some of the foods the client may want to eat.

Content – End of Life: **Category of Health Alteration** *– Endocrine:* **Integrated Processes** *– Nursing Process: Implementation:* **Client Needs** *– Physiological Integrity: Pharmacological and Parenteral Therapies:* **Cognitive Level** *– Synthesis*

MAKING NURSING DECISIONS: The NCLEX-RN® addresses questions concerned with end-of-life care. This is included in the Psychosocial Integrity section of the test blueprint. Supporting the client's choice is an appropriate option when working with clients who are dying.

62. 1. The HOB should be elevated 30-degrees because the elevation avoids pressure on the sella turcica and decreases headaches, a frequent postoperative problem.
    2. A hypophysectomy is surgery that removes the pituitary gland by making an incision in the inner aspect of the upper lip and gingival. The client should avoid vigorous coughing, sneezing, and straining at stool.
    3. **A hypophysectomy is surgery that removes the pituitary gland by making an incision in the inner aspect of the upper lip and gingival. The sella turicica is entered through the floor of the nose and sphenoid sinuses. There are no visual incisions and the nose cannot be splinted.**
    4. The UAP can take the client's vital signs. This would not warrant intervention by the nurse.

    Content – Medical/Surgical: **Category of Health Alteration** *– Endocrine:* **Integrated Processes** *– Nursing Process: Evaluation:* **Client Needs** *– Safe and Effective Care Environment: Management of Care: Supervision:* **Cognitive Level** *– Analysis*

MAKING NURSING DECISIONS: The nurse must ensure the UAP can perform any tasks that are delegated. It is the nurse's responsibility to demonstrate and/or teach the UAP how to perform the task, and evaluate the task performed.

63. 1. The client needs preoperative teaching and the charge nurse should not request a discharge for a client having surgery in the morning.
    2. **This client is stable and could be prescribed oral pain medication. She could be discharged home and followed by home health nursing if needed. This client is the most appropriate client for the charge nurse to request to be discharged.**

3. This client is experiencing a complication of surgery and is hemorrhaging; the Hgb/Hct is very low. Therefore, this client cannot be discharged home.

4. This client may be showing signs of acute rejection; therefore, this client cannot be discharged home.

Content – Medical/Surgical: **Category of Health Alteration** *– Endocrine:* **Integrated Processes** *– Nursing Process: Implementation:* **Client Needs** *– Safe and Effective Care Environment: Management of Care: Delegation:* **Cognitive Level** *– Analysis*

MAKING NURSING DECISIONS: When the nurse is deciding which client should be discharged home, the most stable client should be discharged.

64. 1. This is a normal potassium level, and the HCP does not need to be notified.

2. This level is within therapeutic range, and the HCP does not need to be notified.

3. A BUN of 84 mg/dL is an abnormal lab value, but it would be expected in a client diagnosed with ESRD. The HCP does not need to be notified.

4. **This is a very high blood glucose level, and the client diagnosed with type 1 diabetes will be catabolizing fats at this level and is at risk for diabetic ketoacidosis (DKA) coma.**

Content – Medical/Surgical: **Category of Health Alteration** *– Endocrine:* **Integrated Processes** *– Nursing Process: Evaluation:* **Client Needs** *– Physiological Integrity: Reduction of Risk Potential: Laboratory Values:* **Cognitive Level** *– Analysis*

MAKING NURSING DECISIONS: The nurse must be knowledgeable of normal laboratory values. These values must be memorized and the nurse must be able to determine if the laboratory value is normal for the client's disease process or medications the client is taking.

65. 1. The client with DKA would have fruity breath; therefore, this nursing intervention does not have priority.

2. Glucose levels are monitored at least every hour.

3. The pulse oximeter reading is not priority for a client in DKA.

4. **The client will be on a regular insulin drip, which must be maintained at the prescribed rate on an intravenous pump device. Decreasing the client's blood glucose level is the priority nursing intervention.**

Content – Medical/Surgical: **Category of Health Alteration** *– Endocrine:* **Integrated Processes** *– Nursing Process: Assessment:* **Client Needs** *– Physiological*

Integrity: Physiological Adaptation: Illness Management: **Cognitive Level** *– Analysis*

MAKING NURSING DECISIONS: The nurse should remember if a client is in distress and the nurse can do something to relieve the distress, it should be done first, before assessment. The test taker should select an option that directly helps the client's condition.

66. 1. The client's hemoglobin A_{1C} is a test that reveals the average blood glucose for the previous 2 to 3 months. The current blood glucose level may or may not be in the desired range, but the client's diabetes with this level of hemoglobin A_{1C} is not controlled.

2. The nurse should assess for complications of diabetes, but this is not the first intervention. Getting the client to realize the meaning of a high hemoglobin A_{1C} is the priority at this time.

3. **The client must be taught the long-term effects of hyperglycemia. A hemoglobin A_{1C} of 11 indicates an average blood glucose of 310 mg/dL. Over time, a level higher than 120 to 140 mg/dL can lead to damage to many body systems.**

4. Monitoring blood work is not priority over teaching the client about complications of diabetes when having such a high A_{1C}.

Content – Medical/Surgical: **Category of Health Alteration** *– Endocrine:* **Integrated Processes** *– Nursing Process: Implementation:* **Client Needs** *– Physiological Integrity: Pharmacological and Parenteral Therapies:* **Cognitive Level** *– Analysis*

MAKING NURSING DECISIONS: The nurse must be knowledgeable of normal laboratory values. These values must be memorized and the nurse must be able to determine if the laboratory value is normal for the client's disease process or medications the client is taking.

67. 1. **This client has an elevated WBC count, which could indicate an infection. The HCP should be made aware of this client first.**

2. These are normal lab values.

3. These are normal lab values.

4. These are normal lab values.

Content – Medical/Surgical: **Category of Health Alteration** *– Endocrine:* **Integrated Processes** *– Nursing Process: Evaluation:* **Client Needs** *– Physiological Integrity: Reduction of Risk Potential: Laboratory Values:* **Cognitive Level** *– Analysis*

MAKING NURSING DECISIONS: This is an alternate type of question included in the NCLEX-RN® blueprint. The test taker must be able to read a

chart, be knowledgeable of laboratory data, and make decisions concerning the nurse's most appropriate action.

68. The nurse should administer 8 units of regular insulin, since 249 is between 201 and 250.
*Content – Medical/Surgical: **Category of Health Alteration** – Endocrine: **Integrated Processes** – Nursing Process: Implementation: **Client Needs** – Physiological Integrity: Pharmacological and Parenteral Therapies: **Cognitive Level** – Comprehension*

MAKING NURSING DECISIONS: A fill-in-the-blank question is an alternate type of question included in the NCLEX-RN®. The test taker must use the number keyboard to answer fill-in-the-blank questions.

69. 1, 2, and 3 are correct.
  1. The UAP can escort the patient to the examination room and take the initial vital signs.
  2. The UAP can weigh the patient and document the weight.
  3. The UAP can clean the room and prepare it for the next patient.
  4. Discussing prescriptions is teaching and the nurse cannot delegate teaching.
  5. Calling the pharmacy requires knowledge of medications and medication administration. This task cannot be delegated to a UAP.
  *Content – Medical/Surgical: **Category of Health Alteration** – Management: **Integrated Processes** – Nursing Process: Implementation: **Client Needs** – Safe and Effective Care Environment: Management of Care: Supervision: **Cognitive Level** – Analysis*

MAKING NURSING DECISIONS: This is an alternate type of question included in the NCLEX-RN®. The nurse must be able to select all the options that answer the question correctly. There are no partially correct answers. The nurse cannot delegate assessment, teaching, evaluation, medications, or an unstable client to the UAP.

70. Correct Answer: 1, 3, 4, 2, 5
  1. This client may have overdosed accidently or on purpose. This is a physiological

problem and the nurse must determine which intervention is required next. This is a potentially life-threatening situation, so the nurse should return this phone call first.
  3. The client with hypothyroidism is reporting signs of hyperthyroidism, indicating the client is overdosing on the thyroid hormone replacement and needs to be seen in the clinic. This is a physiological problem; therefore, the nurse should call this client second.
  4. The pharmacist needs to know if the substitution can be made in order to fill this prescription. This call should be returned third.
  2. The nurse needs to discuss the prescribed medication with the HCP to see if a different, less expensive medication would work as well for the client, or if there is an alternative medication program that could be discussed with the client. This phone call should be returned fourth.
  5. The nurse must first determine where the breakdown in the communication of the results of the MRI occurred, then obtain the results and provide them to the HCP prior to returning the call. This phone call can be returned last.
  *Content – Medical/Surgical: **Category of Health Alteration** – Endocrine: **Integrated Processes** – Nursing Process: Assessment: **Client Needs** – Physiological Integrity: Pharmacological and Parenteral Therapies: **Cognitive Level** – Synthesis*

MAKING NURSING DECISIONS: This is an alternate type of question that requires the nurse to assess clients in order of priority. This requires the nurse to evaluate each client's situation and determine which situations are life threatening, which situations are expected for the client's situation, and which client has a psychosocial problem.

CLINICAL SCENARIO ANSWERS AND RATIONALES

The correct answer number and rationale for why it is the correct answer are given in **boldface type.** Rationales for why the other possible answer options are incorrect also are given, but they are not in boldface type.

1. **1, 2, 3, 6, 9, and 10 are correct.**
   1. **This is an assessment question and is needed to determine the extent of the current situation.**
   2. **Knowing the blood glucose level is important for the nurse to determine if the client is at risk for diabetes ketoacidosis (DKA).**
   3. **This will determine what has been tried and what the next step will be.**
   4. The client should drink liquids that will provide calories, since for glucose control Mr. Larry will still need to take his insulin and he could experience a hypoglycemic reaction if he does not have some form of caloric intake.
   5. Without insulin Mr. Larry's body will begin to break down fats. A by-product of fat catabolism is acid. The buildup of acid in the body will result in diabetic ketoacidosis (DKA), which can lead to coma and death.
   6. **Mr. Larry should monitor his urine ketones. The body usually does not spill ketones in the urine until after the blood glucose levels reach 240 and above. Urine ketones indicate the client's, Mr. Larry's, body will begin to breakdown fats and ketones are the by-product of fat metabolism.**
   7. At this time Mr. Larry should try to practice "Sick Day Rules" for clients diagnosed with diabetes mellitus. It is the responsibility of Mr. John to teach the client how to manage the disease process during times of illness.

8. The Emergency Medical System should not be called until it is determined that Mr. Larry cannot manage the virus symptoms without further medical intervention.
9. **If Mr. Larry is "spilling" ketones in his urine, then the healthcare provider will need to adjust his insulin dosage.**
10. **In order to prevent DKA, Mr. Larry must continue to take his insulin. To prevent hypoglycemia he should attempt to ingest calories to balance the insulin. The antidote for insulin is food.**

2. 1. **Ms. Leslie should assess the client for dehydration and electrolyte imbalance.**
   2. **Ms. Leslie should perform bedside glucose checks at least every hour.**
   3. **Initiate an intravenous drip of NS and regular insulin.**
   4. **Perform oral care.**
   5. **Monitor electrolyte levels, potassium, and sodium levels.**

3. 1. **Review "Sick Day Rules" with Mr. Larry and have Mr. Larry verbalize the information back to the nurse, Mr. Justin.**
   2. **Let Mr. Larry know when the HCP wants to see him in the office.**
   3. **Refer Mr. Larry to a Clinical Diabetes Educator.**
   4. **Review diabetes care with Mr. Larry to include self-monitoring, foot care, and eye care.**

9

Integumentary Management

If something comes in life in others because of you, then you have made an approach to immortality.

—Norman Cousins

QUESTIONS

1. The nurse received the a.m. shift report on the following clients. Which client should the nurse assess first?
   1. The client with a right total knee replacement who wants to be removed from the continuous passive motion (CPM) machine.
   2. The client diagnosed with chronic low back pain who is crying and upset about being discharged home.
   3. The client who is 1 week postoperative for right total hip replacement (THR) who has a temperature of 100.4°F.
   4. The client who has full-thickness burns who needs to be medicated before being taken to whirlpool.

2. The nurse is working in an orthopedic unit. Which client should the nurse assess first?
   1. The client who is 2 weeks postoperative open reduction and external fixation (ORIF) of the right hip who is complaining of pain when ambulating.
   2. The client who is 10 days postoperative for left total knee replacement (TKR) who is refusing to use the continuous passive motion (CPM) machine.
   3. The client who is 1 week postoperative for L3–L4 laminectomy who is complaining of numbness and tingling of the feet.
   4. The client who is being admitted to the rehabilitation unit from the orthopedic surgical unit after a motor vehicle accident (MVA).

3. The client is 1 week postoperative for right below-the-knee amputation secondary to arterial occlusive disease. The nurse is unable to assess a pedal pulse in the left foot. Which intervention should the nurse implement first?
   1. Assess for paresthesia and paralysis.
   2. Utilize the Doppler device to auscultate the pulse.
   3. Place the client's leg in the dependent position.
   4. Wrap the client's left leg in a warm blanket.

4. The male client who has a history of cerebrovascular accident (CVA) is admitted to the orthopedic unit with a fractured right hip. The client is complaining of bleeding when brushing his teeth. The nurse reviews the client's medication administration record (MAR). Which intervention should the nurse implement first?

Client's Name:		Account Number: 123456	Allergies: NKDA
Height: 72 inches		**Weight:** 240 pounds	
Date	**Medication**	**0701–1900**	**1901–0659**
	Levothyroxine (Synthroid) 1 tablet PO qd	0900 DN	
	Atenolol (Tenormin) 50 mg PO qd	0900 DN AP 72	
	Warfarin (Coumadin) 5 mg PO 1700	1700 DN	
	Hydrocodone 5 mg/ 500 mg PO q 4–6 hours PRN for pain		
Signature/Initials		**Day Nurse RN/DN**	

    1. Prepare to administer AquaMephyton (vitamin K).
    2. Determine whether the client is using a soft-bristle toothbrush.
    3. Check the client's apical pulse and blood pressure.
    4. Request the laboratory to draw a STAT INR.

5. The nurse is preparing to administer morning (a.m.) medications to the following clients. Which medication should the nurse administer first?
    1. The NSAID to the client diagnosed with osteoarthritis.
    2. The intravenous antibiotic to the client with cellulitis.
    3. The antiviral agent to the client with herpes zoster (shingles).
    4. The antihistamine to the client with urticaria and pruritus.

6. The client tells the nurse, "I have a mole on my back which is darker and getting larger." Which intervention should the nurse implement first?
    1. Tell the client to use corticosteroid cream on the area.
    2. Recommend the client use SPF 15 when in the sun.
    3. Instruct the client to notify his or her healthcare provider immediately.
    4. Encourage the client to wear dark, woven clothing when outside.

7. The nurse is at a local playground and her 10-year-old son falls and complains of his left ankle and foot hurting. Which intervention should the nurse implement first at the scene of the accident?
    1. Instruct her son not to move the left leg.
    2. Elevate the left leg on two rolled towels.
    3. Apply an ice pack to the left ankle.
    4. Check her son's pedal pulse bilaterally.

8. The nurse is preparing to change a dressing on an 82-year-old client with a Stage III pressure ulcer. Which intervention should the nurse implement first?
    1. Obtain the needed equipment to perform the procedure.
    2. Remove the client's old dressing with nonsterile gloves.
    3. Explain the procedure to the client in understandable terms.
    4. Check to determine whether the client has received pain medication.

9. Which client should the charge nurse on the rehabilitation unit assess first after receiving the a.m. shift report?
    1. The client diagnosed with an open reduction and external fixation (ORIF) of the right hip who has a hemoglobin and hematocrit (H&H) of 8/24.
    2. The client diagnosed with rheumatoid arthritis who has a positive rheumatoid factor (RF).
    3. The client diagnosed with a Stage IV pressure ulcer who has a white blood cell (WBC) count of 14,000.
    4. The client diagnosed with systemic allergies on prednisone dose pack who has a glucose level of 189 mg/dL.

10. The client ambulating down the orthopedic hallway unassisted fell to the floor. Which action should the nurse implement first?
    1. Complete an adverse occurrence report.
    2. Notify the clinical manager on the unit.
    3. Determine whether the client has any injuries.
    4. Ask why the client was in the hall alone.

11. The nurse and the unlicensed assistive personnel (UAP) are caring for clients on a rehabilitation unit. Which nursing task is most appropriate for the nurse to delegate to the UAP?
    1. Flush the triple-lumen lines on a central venous catheter.
    2. Demonstrate for the client how to ambulate with a walker.
    3. Assist with bowel training by escorting the client to the bathroom.
    4. Apply corticosteroid cream to the client with allergic dermatitis.

12. The unlicensed assistive personnel (UAP) tells the nurse the client with a right above-the-knee amputation has a large amount of bright red blood on the right leg residual limb. Which action should the nurse implement?
    1. Assess the client's residual limb dressing.
    2. Tell the UAP to take the client's pulse and blood pressure.
    3. Remove the dressing to assess the incision.
    4. Request the UAP to reinforce the dressing.

13. Which action by the unlicensed assistive personnel (UAP) warrants immediate intervention by the nurse?
    1. The UAP tied the confused client to a chair with a sheet.
    2. The UAP escorted the client downstairs to smoke a cigarette.
    3. The UAP bought the client a carbonated beverage from the cafeteria.
    4. The UAP assisted the client to ambulate to the dayroom area.

14. The charge nurse, a licensed practical nurse (LPN), and two unlicensed assistive personnel (UAPs) are caring for clients. Which action is most appropriate for the charge nurse to assign/delegate?
    1. Ask the UAP to apply warm compresses to the client with tinea corporis.
    2. Request the LPN to apply antifungal cream to the client with tinea pedis.
    3. Tell the UAP to remove the toenail of the client with onychomycosis.
    4. Instruct the LPN to administer accutane to the client who is pregnant.

15. The nurse in the rehabilitation unit is caring for clients along with an unlicensed assistive personnel (UAP). Which action by the UAP warrants immediate intervention?
    1. The UAP assists a client 1 week postoperatively to eat a regular diet.
    2. The UAP calls for assistance when taking a client to the shower.
    3. The UAP is assisting the client who weighs 181 kg to the bedside commode.
    4. The UAP places the call light within reach of the client who is sitting in the chair.

16. The unlicensed assistive personnel (UAP) on the rehabilitation unit is placing the client with a left above-the-knee amputation in the prone position. Which action should the nurse implement?
    1. Tell the UAP to place the client on the back.
    2. Praise the UAP for positioning the client prone.
    3. Report this action verbally to the charge nurse.
    4. Explain to the UAP that the client should not be placed on the stomach.

17. The unlicensed assistive personnel (UAP) is applying elastic compression stockings to the client. Which action by the UAP indicates to the nurse the UAP understands the correct procedure for applying the elastic compression stockings?
    1. The UAP applies the stockings while the client is sitting in a chair.
    2. The UAP is unable to insert two fingers under the proximal end of the stocking.
    3. The UAP had the client elevate the legs prior to putting on the stockings.
    4. The UAP places the toe opening of the elastic stocking on top of the client's foot.

18. The charge nurse on the acute care rehabilitation unit is making assignments for the shift. Which client should the charge nurse assign to the most experienced nurse?
    1. The client with a full-thickness burn who is refusing to go to therapy.
    2. The client with osteomyelitis who has bone pain and a fever.
    3. The client with fractured tibia who has deep, unrelenting pain.
    4. The client with low back pain radiating down the left leg.

19. The charge nurse on the busy 36-bed rehabilitation unit must send one staff member to the emergency department (ED). Which staff member is the most appropriate person to send?
    1. The LPN who has worked on the rehabilitation unit for 3 years.
    2. The RN who has been employed on the rehabilitation unit for 8 years.
    3. The UAP who is completing the 4-week orientation to the rehabilitation unit.
    4. The RN who transferred to the rehabilitation unit from the medical unit.

20. Which task should the rehabilitation nurse delegate to the unlicensed assistive personnel (UAP)?
    1. Tell the UAP to show the client how to perform self-catheterization.
    2. Ask the UAP to place the newly confused client in the inclusion bed.
    3. Request the UAP give the client 30 mL of Maalox, an antacid.
    4. Encourage the UAP to attend the multidisciplinary team meeting.

21. The client is 8 hours postoperative spinal surgery. Which priority intervention should the nurse implement?
    1. Evaluate how much pain medication the client is using via the patient-controlled analgesia (PCA) pump.
    2. Logroll the client with three staff members when turning the client side to side.
    3. Assist the client to ambulate to the bathroom using an elevated commode seat.
    4. Place pillows under the thighs of each leg when the client is in supine position.

22. The elderly wife of a client with a total hip replacement who is being discharged home tells the nurse, "I am really worried about taking my husband home. I don't know how I will be able to take care of him." Which intervention is most appropriate for the nurse?
    1. Refer the client to the home health nurse.
    2. Discuss the possibility of placing her husband in a nursing home.
    3. Request the client's healthcare provider to talk to the wife.
    4. Allow the client's wife to ventilate her feelings about the situation.

23. The male nurse who has been told by the female nurse on previous occasions not to talk to her about her body says, "You really look hot in that scrub suit. You have a great-looking body." Which action should the female nurse take next?
    1. Document the comment in writing and file a formal grievance.
    2. Tell the male nurse this makes her feel very uncomfortable.
    3. Notify the clinical manager of the sexual harassment.
    4. Discuss the male nurse's behavior with the hospital lawyer.

24. The client who was admitted to the rehabilitation unit because of a debilitative state asks the nurse, "Why do I have to go to physical therapy every day?" Which statement is the nurse's best response?
   1. "The physical therapy will help you become more independent in caring for yourself."
   2. "You must have at least 3 hours of therapy a day to be able to stay in this rehab unit."
   3. "The multidisciplinary team determined that you should be in physical therapy daily."
   4. "The physical therapist will help you with exercises to improve your muscle strength."

25. The client diagnosed with a fractured right ankle needs to be instructed on crutch walking. Which member of the multidisciplinary team should address this problem?
   1. The physical therapist.
   2. The social worker.
   3. The occupational therapist.
   4. The rehabilitation physician.

26. The client with bilateral amputations tells the nurse, "I was told I can't go back to my job because they do not have handicap accessible bathrooms or ramps." Which action by the nurse is most helpful to the client?
   1. Discuss the situation with the multidisciplinary healthcare team.
   2. Explain the Americans with Disabilities Act (ADA) to the client.
   3. Contact the client's employer via telephone and discuss the situation.
   4. Encourage the client to hire an attorney and sue the employer.

27. Which action by the female primary nurse would warrant immediate intervention by the charge nurse on the rehabilitation unit?
   1. The primary nurse tells the unlicensed assistive personnel (UAP) to escort a client to the swimming pool.
   2. The primary nurse evaluates the client's plan of care with the family member.
   3. The primary nurse asks another nurse to administer an injection she prepared.
   4. The primary nurse requests another nurse to watch her clients for 30 minutes.

28. The client in a motor vehicle accident (MVA) is in critical condition with a pelvic fracture, flail chest, bilateral arm fractures, and a left hip fracture. The client tells the nurse, "I just want to die. I can't feed myself or clean myself." Which statement is the nurse's best response?
   1. "I know this must be hard for you but you can have a life."
   2. "I can see you must feel helpless; I am here to listen."
   3. "Have you thought about killing yourself?"
   4. "You are in shock but in time things will get better."

29. The nurse on the surgical unit is being sent to the neonatal intensive care unit (NICU) to work because the unit is short staffed. The nurse has never worked in the NICU. Which response by the nurse supports the ethical principle of nonmalfeasance?
   1. The nurse requests not to be floated to the NICU.
   2. The nurse accepts the assignment to the NICU.
   3. The nurse asks why another nurse can't go to the NICU.
   4. The nurse talks another nurse into going to the NICU.

30. The client's husband is frustrated and tells the nurse, "Everyone is telling me something different as to when my wife is going to be able to go home. I don't know whom to believe." Which statement is the rehabilitation nurse's best response?
   1. "I can see you are frustrated. Would you like to talk about how you feel?"
   2. "I will contact the case manager and have her talk to you as soon as possible."
   3. "Do not worry. Your wife won't go home until you and she are both ready."
   4. "Your wife's healthcare provider should be able to give you that information."

31. The client with an upper extremity amputation tells the nurse, "I do everything with my right hand and now it is gone. I have no idea what I am going to do after I get discharged. How will I support my family? I will need to get a new job." Which statement is the nurse's best response?
1. "With time you will be able to use your left hand now."
2. "The state rehabilitation commission will help retrain you."
3. "You should ask the social worker about applying for disability."
4. "You are worried about how you will be able to support your family."

32. The client tells the nurse, "I do not like my doctor and I want another doctor." Which statement is the nurse's best response?
1. "You should tell your doctor you are not happy with his care."
2. "Can you tell me what you don't like about your doctor's care?"
3. "I will notify my nursing supervisor and report your concern."
4. "I am sorry, but you really must keep this doctor until you are discharged."

33. The nurse and the unlicensed assistive personnel (UAP) are caring for a 74-year-old client who is 3 days postoperative right total hip replacement (THR). Which nursing task should be delegated to the UAP?
1. Place the abductor pillow between the client's legs.
2. Ensure the client stays on complete bed rest.
3. Feed the client the evening meal.
4. Check the client's right hip surgical dressing.

34. The nurse tells the unlicensed assistive personnel (UAP) to assist the client who is 1 day postoperative spinal surgery with a.m. care. Which action by the UAP warrants immediate intervention?
1. The UAP closes the door and cubicle curtain.
2. The UAP requests the client to turn to the side.
3. The UAP checks the temperature of the bathing water.
4. The UAP puts the side rails up when bathing the client.

35. The client with a right below-the-knee amputation who also has impetigo is admitted to a rehabilitation unit. Which interventions should be included in the nursing care plan? **Select all that apply.**
1. Elevate the client's right leg on two pillows.
2. Refer the client to occupational therapy daily.
3. Encourage the client to push the residual limb against a pillow.
4. Use warm soap and water to remove the crusts secondary to impetigo.
5. Ensure all staff members wear gloves when caring for client.

36. The overhead page has issued a Code Black, indicating a tornado in the area. Which intervention should the charge nurse implement?
1. Instruct the hospital staff to assist the clients and visitors to the cafeteria.
2. Request the client and visitors go into the bathroom in the client's room.
3. Have the clients and visitors remain in the hallway with the doors closed.
4. Tell the client and any visitors to remain in the client's room with the door open.

37. The male client is placed in a double hip spica cast for 3 months. The client's wife tells the nurse, "My husband said we are supposed to talk to his case manager. What is a case manager?" Which statement is the nurse's best response?
1. "A case manager discusses the cost and insurance issues concerning the rehabilitation."
2. "The case manager is responsible for the medical treatment regimen for your husband."
3. "The case manager is a member of the team who will assist your husband in finding another job."
4. "The case manager is a nurse who will coordinate the rehabilitation team and keep you informed."

38. The 28-year-old male client who sustained traumatic bilateral amputations secondary to a motor vehicle accident (MVA) is being discharged home to live with his wife and 3-year-old son. Which priority psychosocial intervention should the rehabilitation nurse discuss with the client?
1. Ask the client whether he has any sexual concerns he needs to discuss.
2. Determine whether the home is safe for ambulating with prosthetic devices.
3. Discuss the procedure for obtaining a specially equipped car.
4. Explain the importance of getting psychological counseling.

39. The primary nurse overhears the unlicensed assistive personnel (UAP) telling a family member of a client, "One of the clients will be going to prison because that person was charged with vehicular manslaughter. Two people in the motor vehicle accident died." Which action should the primary nurse implement first?
1. Apologize to the family member for the UAP's comments.
2. Tell the UAP that the comment is a violation of HIPAA.
3. Allow the UAP to complete the conversation and then discuss the situation.
4. Interrupt the conversation and tell the UAP to go to the nurse's station.

40. The clinical manager has verbally warned a female staff nurse about being late to work on two previous occasions. The nurse was 35 minutes late for today's shift. Which action should the charge nurse take?
1. Ask the staff nurse why she was late again today.
2. Notify the human resources department in writing.
3. Initiate the hospital policy for unacceptable behavior.
4. Do not allow the staff nurse to work on the unit today.

41. The charge nurse on the rehabilitation unit is making assignments for the day shift. Which assignment would be most appropriate for the licensed practical nurse (LPN)?
1. Have the LPN call the HCP to obtain an order for a diet change.
2. Instruct the LPN to complete the admission assessment.
3. Ask the LPN to teach the client about a high-fiber diet.
4. Request the LPN to obtain the intake and output for the clients.

42. The charge nurse received laboratory data on the following clients. Which client warrants immediate intervention by the charge nurse?
1. The client with COPD who has ABGs of pH, 7.35; PaO_2, 77; $PaCO_2$, 57; HCO_3, 24.
2. The client diagnosed with bilateral TKR who has a WBC count of 10,400.
3. The client on antibiotic therapy who has a serum potassium level of 3.3 mEq/L.
4. The client receiving TPN who has a glucose level of 145 mg/dL.

43. The client tells the primary nurse, "I just finished completing my living will and I need you to witness my signature." Which action should the nurse implement?
1. Witness the client's living will using an ink pen.
2. Explain that the nurse cannot witness this document.
3. Tell the client the document does not need a witness's signature.
4. Offer to have the hospital attorney to come notarize the form.

44. The nurse is preparing to ambulate the client with full-thickness burns on the lower extremities down the hall. Which priority intervention should the nurse implement?
1. Place rubber-soled shoes on the client.
2. Put a gait belt around the client's waist.
3. Explain the procedure to the client.
4. Provide a clear path for the client to walk.

45. The client in the rehabilitation unit tells the nurse, "I will not go to physical therapy again because it hurts so much when I do the exercises." Which statement supports the nurse's role as a client advocate?
1. "You do not have to go to physical therapy if it causes you pain."
2. "I will talk to the physical therapist (PT) about the exercises that cause you pain."
3. "Let me check and see if you can receive pain medication before therapy."
4. "I will discuss your concerns at the next multidisciplinary team meeting."

46. The rehabilitation nurse enters the client's room and the client is talking on the phone. The client asks the nurse to talk to his wife because she has some questions. Which action should the nurse take?
    1. Explain that HIPAA regulations prevent the nurse from talking to the wife.
    2. Tell the client it would be best for the nurse to talk to the wife in person.
    3. Request the client's wife to come to the weekly team meeting to ask questions.
    4. Honor the client's request and answer any questions the wife has on the phone.

47. The school nurse notes the child has impetigo. Which interventions should the nurse implement? Select all that apply.
    1. Administer an antibiotic ointment four times a day.
    2. Instruct the parents to keep the child at home until lesions crust over.
    3. Tell the parents to use separate towels for the child.
    4. Do not remove the crusts from the skin lesions.
    5. Tell the parents to have the child wear non-latex sterile gloves over both hands until no crusting is present.

48. Which action by the primary nurse requires immediate intervention by the charge nurse?
    1. The nurse is teaching the client how to use a glucometer.
    2. The nurse leaves the computer screen open at the nurse's station.
    3. The nurse is discussing a client situation on the phone with the HCP.
    4. The nurse contacts the chaplain to come and talk to a client.

49. The nurse is triaging phone calls in a dermatological clinic. Which client warrants the nurse making an appointment immediately?
    1. The client reports having white spots on both of the hands.
    2. The client reports redness and itching on the hands.
    3. The client reports a cherry angioma on the right lower leg.
    4. The client reports red patches on one side of the body.

50. The client has an area on the skin the dermatologist thinks may be basal cell carcinoma. Which intervention will the nurse implement to confirm the diagnosis?
    1. Refer the client for the magnetic resonance imaging (MRI).
    2. Explain how to obtain a washing of the abnormal skin area.
    3. Prepare the client for a biopsy of the abnormal skin growth.
    4. Tell the client there is no way to definitively confirm the diagnosis.

51. The nurse is assisting the client to use a cane when ambulating. Rank in order of performance the interventions the nurse would take.
    1. Request the client to move the cane forward.
    2. Move the weaker leg one step forward.
    3. Ensure the client places the cane in the strong hand.
    4. Move the stronger leg one step forward.
    5. Apply a gait's belt around the client's waist.

52. Which priority intervention should the nurse implement to help prevent pressure ulcers in the client who is on strict bed rest?
    1. Provide adequate skin care for the client.
    2. Turn the client every 2 hours or more often.
    3. Ensure sufficient nutritional intake.
    4. Use pressure-relieving devices such as waterbeds.

53. Which intervention should the nurse implement first for the client with a fractured femur who is suspected of having a fat embolism?
    1. Assess the client's bilateral breath sounds.
    2. Encourage the client to cough and deep breathe.
    3. Administer oxygen via nasal cannula.
    4. Prepare to administer intravenous heparin therapy.

54. The client with an electrical burn is brought to the emergency department (ED). The entrance wound is on the right hand and the exit wound is on the left foot. Which intervention should the nurse implement first?
    1. Place sterile gauze on the entrance and exit wounds.
    2. Assess the client's vital signs.
    3. Monitor the client's pulse oximetry.
    4. Place the client on cardiac telemetry.

55. The nurse is using an electric patient "Hoyer" lift to transfer the client from the bed to a stretcher. Which priority intervention should the nurse implement?
    1. Have two staff members assist when using the lift.
    2. Ensure the client is correctly placed in the lift prior to moving.
    3. Lift the client slowly off the bed when turning on the lift.
    4. Ensure the stretcher is in the correct position and locked.

56. The nurse is assessing the functional ability of a client using the Katz Index of Activities of Daily Living (ADLs). Which assessment grade would require the nurse to delegate feeding, bathing, and toileting to the unlicensed assistive personnel (UAP)?
    1. Katz Index of ADLs grade A.
    2. Katz Index of ADLs grade C.
    3. Katz Index of ADLs grade E.
    4. Katz Index of ADLs grade G.

57. The client has cellulitis on the right lower leg. Which intervention should the nurse implement?
    1. Place the client's right arm in the dependent position.
    2. Apply warm moist heat to the affected area.
    3. Wash the affected area with antistaphylococcal soap.
    4. Wrap the right arm with ACE bandages.

58. The unlicensed assistive personnel (UAP) is transferring the client from the bed to the chair. Which interventions should the nurse ensure the UAP implements during this procedure? Rank in order of priority.
    1. Assist the client to sit when the client's legs touch the edge of the chair.
    2. Place the wheelchair at an angle on the client's strong side.
    3. Assist the client to stand and put strong hand on the wheelchair armrest.
    4. Keep the client's weight forward and pivot the client.
    5. Lock the wheelchair brakes and secure the chair position.

59. The charge nurse on the rehabilitation unit is assigning/delegating tasks to the unlicensed assistive personnel (UAP) and licensed practical nurse (LPN). Which task is most appropriate for the nurse to delegate/assign?
    1. Tell the UAP to elevate client's residual limb above the heart.
    2. Instruct the LPN to give the diabetic clients their HS snacks.
    3. Request the UAP to insert an indwelling urinary catheter.
    4. Ask the LPN to assess the client who may have herpes zoster.

60. The nurse is caring for a client diagnosed with a full-thickness burn over the right lower extremity. Which task should the nurse delegate to the UAP?
    1. Instruct the UAP to check the client's right dorsalis pedal pulse.
    2. Ask the UAP to cleanse the client's dentures and place in the container.
    3. Request the UAP to perform passive range-of-motion (ROM) exercises.
    4. Tell the UAP to keep the client's right leg in the dependent position.

61. The client is admitted to the emergency department (ED) with a third-degree burn over the front of both legs. Which priority intervention should the nurse implement?
    1. Maintain sterile environment when caring for the client.
    2. Insert two large-bore intravenous access routes.
    3. Administer intravenous antibiotic therapy.
    4. Assess the client's pain level on a 1 to 10 pain scale.

62. The day nurse is preparing to administer medications to the client who is complaining of light-headedness when getting out of bed. Which medication should the day nurse question administering?

Client's Name: Smith		Account Number: 132456	
Height: 72 inches		Weight: 75 kg	
Date	Medication	0700–1900	1900–0700
	Atenolol (Tenormin) 50 mg PO qd	0900	
	Ceftriaxone (Rocephin) 150 mg IVBP q 12 hours	0900	
	Bisacodyl (Ducolax) 2 PO PRN constipation		
	Hydrocodone 5 mg/ 500 mg PO q 4–6 hours PRN for pain		
Signature/Initials		Day Nurse RN/DN	

    1. Atenolol (Tenormin) 50 mg.
    2. Ceftriaxone (Rocephin) 150 mg IVPB.
    3. Bisacodyl (Ducolax) 2 PO.
    4. Administer all medications as ordered.

63. The nurse is discussing alternative medication (CAM) with a client on the rehabilitation unit. Which therapies should the nurse discuss with the client? **Select all that apply.**
    1. Acupuncture.
    2. Guided imagery.
    3. Compression sequential devices.
    4. Music therapy.
    5. Muscle-strengthening exercises.

64. The nurse tells the client, "I am going to refer you to the vocational counselor." The client asks the nurse, "Why are you making this referral?" Which statement is the nurse's best response?
    1. "The counselor will assist you with job placement, training, or further education."
    2. "The counselor specializes in rehabilitative medicine and will help you get better."
    3. "The counselor will help develop your fine motor skills to help perform ADLs."
    4. "The counselor will help you continue or develop hobbies or interests."

65. The nurse is assessing the client's daily schedule and habits. Which question is most appropriate for the nurse to ask the client?
    1. "Do you have a family member who can assist you when you go home?"
    2. "What time do you prefer bathing and do you take a tub bath or a shower?"
    3. "Do you have insurance to help with the cost of rehabilitation?"
    4. "Do you have concerns about the care you are receiving here?"

66. The nurse is administering medication to the client with a third degree burn on the chest area. Which medication required a laboratory test?

Client Name: A.M.		Account Number: 12223		Allergies: NKDA
Height: 68 inches		Weight in pounds: 140 Weight in kg: 63.63		Date of Birth: 05/09/1941
Date	Medication	2301–0700	0701–1500	0501–2300
	Vancomycin IVPB 500 mg qd			
	Protonix 40 mg IVPB qd			
	Silvadene topical ointment to burn tid			
	Morphine 2–5 mg IVP PRN pain			
Signature/Initials		Night Nurse RN/NN		Day Nurse RN/DN

1. The vancomycin medication.
2. The Protonix medication.
3. The Silvadene topical antibiotic.
4. The morphine analgesic.

67. The home health (HH) nurse is arranging for the significant other (SO) of an elderly client diagnosed with heart failure to administer the routine diuretic medication furosemide (Lasix). The medication is to be administered 20 mg on Monday/Wednesday/Friday and 40 mg on Sunday/Tuesday/Thursday/Saturday. The prescription is for 40 mg scored tablets. How many tablets should the nurse teach the SO to administer on Sundays? _____

68. The home health (HH) nurse has arranged for a home health aide (HHA) to assist a 79-year-old client diagnosed with Alzheimer's disease. Which interventions should the nurse delegate to the HHA? **Select all that apply.**
1. Weigh the client once a week and document the weight on the patient record.
2. Stay with the client twice a week while the significant other (SO) goes out to run errands.
3. Take and record the client's vital signs.
4. Take the client to the bank and store to perform personal business.
5. Listen to the client's heart sounds and notify the HCP if abnormal sounds are heard.

69. The nurse is at the local mall and a young woman starts having shortness of breath, has hives on her face and arms, and is complaining of itching. Which intervention should the nurse implement first?
1. Tell a by-stander to call 911 immediately.
2. Ask the woman if she has an EpiPen.
3. Check the client for a medical alert bracelet.
4. Place a soft cushion under the client's head.

70. The home health (HH) nurse is planning to make rounds for the day. List the order the clients should be seen by priority.
1. The 29-year-old client diagnosed with spinal cord injury (SCI) post–motor vehicle accident (MVA) who needs a dressing changed on a Stage IV pressure area.
2. The 56-year-old client diagnosed with breast cancer who needs an injection of filgrastim (Neupogen) subcutaneously.
3. The 67-year-old client diagnosed with emphysema who called to report that the sputum is a rusty color this morning.
4. The 80-year-old client diagnosed with Alzheimer's disease who is confused and wandering around the house.
5. The 72-year-old client diagnosed with atrial fibrillation who needs a prothrombin time performed and called to the HCP.

INTEGUMENTARY CLINICAL SCENARIO

Ms. Glada is the charge nurse on the 7p to 7a shift for the 10-bed burn unit. There are three RNs (Mr. George, Mr. Rob, and Ms. Helen) along with four UAPs. There are no LVNs in the burn unit but there are burn techs—specially trained paraprofessionals who maintain the whirlpool baths.

1. The male client is admitted to the burn unit after a boiling pot of hot water accidentally spilled on his lower legs. The assessment reveals blistered, mottled red skin, and both feet are edematous. Which depth of burn should Mr. George document?
   1. Superficial partial thickness.
   2. Deep partial thickness.
   3. Full thickness.
   4. First degree.

2. Mr. Rob is caring for a client who experienced a full-thickness burn to 65% of the body 12 hours ago. After establishing a patent airway, which nursing intervention is priority for the client?
   1. Replace the client's fluids and electrolytes.
   2. Prevent the client from developing Curling's ulcers.
   3. Implement interventions to prevent infection.
   4. Prepare to assist with an escharotomy.

3. Ms. Glada is developing a nursing care plan for a client who experienced a full-thickness burn and deep partial-thickness burns over half the body 4 days ago. Which client problem should Ms. Glada make priority?
   1. High risk for infection.
   2. Pain.
   3. Impaired physical mobility.
   4. Fluid and electrolyte imbalance.

4. Which nursing interventions should be included for the client who has full-thickness and deep partial-thickness burns to 50% of the body? **Select all that apply.**
   1. Perform meticulous hand hygiene.
   2. Screen visitors for infections.
   3. Provide a low-cholesterol, low-protein diet.
   4. Change invasive lines once a week.
   5. Administer prophylactic antibiotics as prescribed.

5. Which nursing task should Ms. Kathy, the RN, delegate to a UAP for the client with full-thickness burns over the right leg?
   1. Instruct the UAP to take the client's pulse oximeter reading.
   2. Tell the UAP to change the dressing on the right leg.
   3. Ask the UAP to apply mafenide acetate, Sulfamylon, to the right leg.
   4. Request the UAP to complete the admission assessment.

6. Mr. Rob is caring for a client with deep partial-thickness and full-thickness burns to the chest area. Which of the following assessment data warrant notifying the healthcare provider?
   1. The client is complaining of pain rated 9 on 1 to 10 pain scale.
   2. The client's pulse oximeter reading is 90%.
   3. The client has a T 100.4°F, P 100, R 24, and BP 102/60.
   4. The client's urinary output is 150 mL in 4 hours.

7. Ms. Glada is teaching a group of community members about fire safety. A participant asks, "What should I do if I get hot grease burns on my hand?" Which statement is Ms. Glada's best response?
   1. "Apply an ice pack directly to the hand."
   2. "Place the hand under cool tap water."
   3. "Put burn ointment on the hand."
   4. "Go immediately to the doctor's office."

8. Ms. Glada is teaching a group of new UAPs about burn care. Which information regarding skin care should Ms. Glada emphasize?
   1. Keep the skin moist by leaving the skin damp after the bath.
   2. Ensure the client is pre-medicated prior to whirlpool.
   3. Tell the UAPs to turn the client from side to side at least every 2 hours.
   4. Instruct the UAPs to not implement any interventions regarding skin care.

9. Which action by the UAP warrants intervention by Ms. Glada?
   1. The UAP decreases the IV rate of the client whose total parenteral nutrition is almost empty.
   2. The UAP elevates the head of the bed for a client who is receiving a continuous tube feeding.
   3. The UAP assists the client with full-thickness burns to the upper extremities to eat a high-protein meal.
   4. The UAP mixes Thick-It into the glass of water for a client who has difficulty swallowing.

10. Ms. Glada is caring for clients on the burn unit. After the shift report which client should Ms. Glada assess first?
    1. The client with full and deep partial-thickness burns who has pain rated 8 on a 1 to 10 pain scale.
    2. The client with full-thickness burns who has a urinary output of 120 mL in the past 8 hours.
    3. The client with full-thickness burns on the chest who is having difficulty breathing.
    4. The client who has full-thickness burns to the right leg with no palpable pedal pulse.

ANSWERS AND RATIONALES

The correct answer number and rationale for why it is the correct answer are given in **boldface type**. Rationales for why the other possible answer options are incorrect also are given, but they are not in boldface type.

1. 1. This client needs assistance being removed from the CPM machine but it is not priority over a client who needs pain medication prior to a very painful procedure. Equipment is not priority over the client's body.
   2. This is a psychosocial need and should be addressed, but it is not priority over a physiological need.
   3. This temperature is elevated and the client should be seen, but the nurse should medicate the client going to whirlpool first then assess this client. Pain is priority over an elevated temperature.
   4. **The client must be medicated with a narcotic medication prior to being taken to whirlpool, which is a physiological need; therefore, the nurse should see this client first.**
   *Content – Medical/Surgical: **Category of Health Alteration** – Musculoskeletal: **Integrated Processes** – Nursing Process: Assessment: **Client Needs** – Physiological Integrity: Management of Care: **Cognitive Level** – Analysis*

MAKING NURSING DECISIONS: When deciding which client to assess first, the nurse should utilize Maslow's Hierarchy of Needs, in which physiological needs are priority over psychosocial needs. The alleviation of pain, actual or potential, is a priority need.

2. 1. The client having pain when ambulating after an ORIF of the hip is expected; this client would not need to be assessed first.
   2. The client should be ambulating and moving the left leg while in bed and would not need to be in the CPM machine 10 days postoperatively.
   3. **Numbness and tingling of the legs are signs of possible neurovascular compromise. This client should be assessed first.**
   4. The client being transferred should be assessed but would be considered stable; therefore, this client would not be assessed before a client experiencing possible neurovascular compromise.
   *Content – Medical/Surgical: **Category of Health Alteration** – Musculoskeletal: **Integrated Processes** – Nursing Process: Assessment: **Client Needs** – Physiological Integrity: Reduction of Risk Potential **Cognitive Level** – Analysis*

MAKING NURSING DECISIONS: The nurse must determine which sign/symptom is not expected for the disease process or surgical procedure. If the sign/symptom is not expected, then the nurse should assess the client first. This type of question is determining if the nurse is knowledgeable of the signs/symptoms of a variety of disease processes.

3. 1. **An absent pulse is not uncommon in a client diagnosed with arterial occlusive disease. If the client can move the toes and denies tingling or numbness, then no further action should be taken.**
   2. To identify the location of the pulse, the nurse should use a Doppler device to amplify the sound, but this is not the first intervention if the client is able to move the toes and denies numbness and tingling.
   3. Placing the client's leg in a dependent position will increase blood flow and may help the nurse palpate the pulse, but it is not the nurse's first intervention.
   4. Warming will dilate the arteries and may help the nurse to find the pedal pulse, but this is not the first intervention. (Cooling, in contrast, causes vasoconstriction and decreases the ability to palpate the pulse.)
   *Content – Medical/Surgical: **Category of Health Alteration** – Musculoskeletal: **Integrated Processes** – Nursing Process: Implementation: **Client Needs** – Physiological Integrity: Reduction of Risk Potential: **Cognitive Level** – Application*

MAKING NURSING DECISIONS: When the question asks which intervention should be implemented first, it means all the options are something a nurse could implement, but only one should be implemented first. The nurse should use the nursing process to determine the appropriate intervention: If the client is in distress, do not assess; if the client is not in distress, then the nurse should assess.

4. 1. If the client's International Normalized Ratio (INR) is elevated, the antidote for the oral anticoagulant warfarin (Coumadin) is vitamin K, but this is not the nurse's first intervention.
   2. The client should be using a soft-bristle toothbrush, but this is not the nurse's first intervention.
   3. The nurse can always check the client's vital signs, but it is not the first intervention when addressing the client's complaint of gums bleeding.

4. The nurse should first check the client's INR to determine whether the bleeding is secondary to an elevated INR level—above 3.
Content – Medical/Surgical: Category of Health Alteration – Drug Administration: Integrated Processes – Nursing Process: Assessment: Client Needs – Physiological Integrity: Pharmacological and Parenteral Therapies: Cognitive Level – Analysis

MAKING NURSING DECISIONS: This is an alternate type of question included in the NCLEX-RN® blueprint. The test taker must be able to read a medication administration record (MAR), be knowledgeable of medications, and be able to make an appropriate decision as to the nurse's most appropriate intervention.

5. 1. The nonsteroidal anti-inflammatory drug (NSAID) is a routine medication and is not a priority medication.
2. The client needs to receive the IV antibiotic but is not priority over the client who is complaining of an acute problem, itching, and hives.
3. The client should receive the antiviral agent but not prior to a client who is exhibiting hives and itching, which is an acute problem.
4. **The client with urticaria (hives) and pruritus (itching) is having some type of allergic reaction and should receive the antihistamine first.**
Content – Medical/Surgical: Category of Health Alteration – Drug Administration: Integrated Processes – Nursing Process: Implementation: Client Needs – Physiological Integrity: Pharmacological and Parenteral Therapies: Cognitive Level – Application

MAKING NURSING DECISIONS: The client who is exhibiting an acute reaction and/or problem should receive medical treatment first. Routine scheduled medications are not priority over medications addressing acute client needs.

6. 1. Corticosteroid cream will not treat potential melanoma, which is what the client is explaining to the nurse.
2. SPF 15 is recommended to help prevent skin cancer but it will not help treat a melanoma.
3. **A client should consult his or her HCP immediately if a mole or lesion shows any signs of melanoma—asymmetry, border irregularity, color change/variation, and diameter of 6 mm or more (ABCD).**
4. Dark, woven clothing helps prevent skin cancer but it will not do anything for a change in a mole.
Content – Medical/Surgical: Category of Health Alteration – Integumentary: Integrated Processes – Nursing Process: Implementation: Client Needs – Health Promotion and Maintenance: Cognitive Level – Application

MAKING NURSING DECISIONS: The test taker needs to read all of the options carefully before choosing the option that says, "Notify the HCP." If any of the options will provide information the HCP needs to know in order to make a decision, the test taker should choose that option. If, however, the HCP does not need any additional information to make a decision and the nurse suspects the condition is serious or life threatening, the priority intervention is to call the HCP.

7. 1. **The nurse should implement the first intervention, ensuring the client does not move the leg, because doing so may cause further injury. The client should not attempt to move or stand on the injured extremity.**
2. The client should elevate the leg to decrease edema but it is not the first intervention—remember to do no harm.
3. The application of ice will help decrease edema and pain but the first intervention is to do no harm.
4. Assessment is usually the first intervention, but when at the scene of an accident, the nurse should ensure the client does not cause further injury prior to assessing the client.
Content – Medical/Surgical: Category of Health Alteration – Musculoskeletal: Integrated Processes – Nursing Process: Implementation: Client Needs – Safe and Effective Care Environment: Safety and Infection Control: Cognitive Level – Application

MAKING NURSING DECISIONS: The nurse should use the nursing process when answering questions that ask which intervention to implement first. Assessment is the first step in the nursing process, but in an emergency situation, remember the nurse should ensure the client does not further injure himself or herself.

8. 1. The nurse should obtain the needed equipment, but that is not the first intervention.
2. The nurse should remove the old dressing with nonsterile gloves, but not before determining whether the client has been premedicated.
3. The nurse should explain the procedure prior to performing the dressing change, but that is not the first intervention.
4. **Dressing changes for a Stage III pressure ulcer will be painful for the client and the nurse should make sure the client has received pain medication at least 30 minutes prior to the procedure. This is showing client advocacy.**
Content – Medical/Surgical: Category of Health Alteration – Integumentary: Integrated Processes – Nursing Process: Implementation: Client Needs – Physiological Integrity: Basic Care and Comfort: Cognitive Level – Application

MAKING NURSING DECISIONS: There will be management questions on the NCLEX-RN® addressing client advocacy. A client advocate acts as a liaison between clients and healthcare providers to help improve or maintain a high quality of healthcare.

9. 1. **The H&H is low, which requires the nurse to assess this client first. The nurse must take the client's vital signs, check the surgical dressing, and determine whether the client is symptomatic for hypovolemia.**
   2. The client with rheumatoid arthritis should have a positive rheumatoid factor (RF). The positive RF factor confirms the diagnosis of this disease process.
   3. A client with a Stage IV pressure ulcer would frequently have an infection; therefore, the nurse would expect an elevated white blood cell (WBC) count.
   4. Corticosteroids elevate the client's glucose level; therefore, the nurse would not assess this client first.

   Content – Medical/Surgical: **Category of Health Alteration** *– Musculoskeletal:* **Integrated Processes** *– Nursing Process: Assessment:* **Client Needs** *– Physiological Integrity: Reduction of Risk Potential:* **Cognitive Level** *– Analysis*

MAKING NURSING DECISIONS: The nurse must be knowledgeable of normal laboratory values. These values must be memorized and the nurse must be able to determine if the laboratory value is normal for the client's disease process or medications the client is taking.

10. 1. The nurse should complete a report documenting the client's fall, but this is not the first intervention.
    2. The nurse should notify the clinical manager, but this is not the nurse's first intervention.
    3. **The nurse must first determine whether the client has any injuries before taking any other action. This is the first intervention the nurse must implement prior to moving the client.**
    4. The nurse should determine why the client was ambulating alone, but it is not the priority nursing intervention. Determining whether the client has any injuries is the most important intervention.

    Content – Medical/Surgical: **Category of Health Alteration** *– Musculoskeletal:* **Integrated Processes** *– Nursing Process: Assessment:* **Client Needs** *– Physiological Integrity: Reduction of Risk Potential:* **Cognitive Level** *– Analysis*

MAKING NURSING DECISIONS: Assessment is the first step of the nursing process, and the test

taker should use the nursing process or some other systematic process to assist in determining priorities.

11. 1. The triple-lumen lines should be flushed with 100 units/mL of heparin solution, and this task should not be delegated to a UAP.
    2. This is teaching, and the nurse should not delegate teaching to the client.
    3. **The UAP can assist the client to the bathroom as part of the bowel training; the nurse is responsible for the training, but the nurse can delegate this task.**
    4. Corticosteroid cream is a medication and the nurse cannot delegate medication to a UAP.

    Content – Medical/Surgical: **Category of Health Alteration** *– Musculoskeletal:* **Integrated Processes** *– Nursing Process: Planning:* **Client Needs** *– Safe and Effective Care Environment: Management of Care:* **Cognitive Level** *– Synthesis*

MAKING NURSING DECISIONS: The nurse cannot delegate assessment, evaluation, teaching, administering medications, or an unstable client to a UAP.

12. 1. Because the UAP is informing the nurse of pertinent information, the nurse should assess the client to determine which action to take.
    2. The client may be hemorrhaging; therefore, the nurse cannot delegate assessing vital signs on an unstable client.
    3. The nurse should not remove the dressing. The nurse should reinforce the dressing and notify the HCP if bleeding does not stop or if the client is showing signs of hypovolemia. Reinforcing the dressing would help decrease bleeding, but the nurse must assess first.
    4. **The client is potentially unstable; therefore, the nurse should not delegate any care to the UAP.**

    Content – Medical/Surgical: **Category of Health Alteration** *– Musculoskeletal:* **Integrated Processes** *– Nursing Process: Implementation:* **Client Needs** *– Physiological Integrity: Reduction of Risk Potential:* **Cognitive Level** *– Application*

MAKING NURSING DECISIONS: Any time the nurse receives information from another staff member about a client who may be experiencing a complication, the nurse must assess the client. The nurse should not make decisions about a client's needs based on another staff member's information.

13. 1. Tying a client to a chair is a form of restraint, and the client cannot be restrained without an HCP order; therefore, the nurse should immediately free the client. This is a legal issue.

2. The UAP is not hired to smoke with the client and the nurse should talk to the UAP, but this does not warrant an immediate response. The client being illegally restrained warrants immediate intervention.

3. Bringing a beverage to the client would not warrant immediate intervention.

4. The UAP can assist the client to ambulate.

Content – Medical/Surgical: **Category of Health Alteration** *– Management:* **Integrated Processes –** *Nursing Process: Implementation:* **Client Needs –** *Physiological Integrity: Safety and Infection Control:* **Cognitive Level** *– Application*

MAKING NURSING DECISIONS: Delegation means the nurse is responsible for the UAP's actions and performance. The nurse must correct the UAP's performance to ensure the client is cared for safely and legally in the hospital or the home.

14. 1. Tinea corporis is commonly known as "ringworm" and should have cool compresses applied, not warm compresses.

 2. **The LPN can apply medication to the client's athlete's foot; therefore, this is an appropriate assignment for the LPN.**

 3. Onychomycosis is a fungal infection of the toenails (crumbly, discolored, and thickened nails); the HCP, not the UAP, should remove the toenail.

 4. Isotretinoin (Accutane) used to treat acne is contraindicated in women who are pregnant or who are intending to become pregnant while on the drug.

Content – Medical/Surgical: **Category of Health Alteration** *– Integumentary:* **Integrated Processes –** *Nursing Process: Planning:* **Client Needs –** *Safe and Effective Care Environment: Management of Care:* **Cognitive Level** *– Synthesis*

MAKING NURSING DECISIONS: When the test taker is deciding which option is the most appropriate task to delegate/assign, the test taker should choose the task that allows each member of the staff to function within his or her full scope of practice. Do not assign a task to a staff member that requires a higher level of expertise than the staff member has.

15. 1. The UAP can assist a client to eat a regular meal; this would not warrant immediate action.

 2. The UAP's request for assistance is appropriate because it is ensuring client safety. This action would not warrant immediate intervention.

 3. **The UAP is attempting to move a client who weighs 400 pounds to the bedside commode. The UAP should request assistance to ensure client safety as well as**

to protect the UAP's back. This is a dangerous situation and requires intervention by the nurse.

4. This action ensures client safety and does not require immediate intervention by the nurse.

Content – Medical/Surgical: **Category of Health Alteration** *– Musculoskeletal:* **Integrated Processes –** *Nursing Process: Implementation:* **Client Needs –** *Safe and Effective Care Environment: Management of Care:* **Cognitive Level** *– Application*

MAKING NURSING DECISIONS: Delegation means the nurse is responsible for the UAP's actions and performance. The nurse must correct the UAP's performance to ensure the client is cared for safely and legally in the hospital or the home.

16. 1. The client with a lower extremity amputation should be placed in the prone position to prevent contractures.

 2. **The nurse should praise the UAP for taking the initiative and placing the client in the prone position. The prone position will help prevent contractures of the residual limb, which will make it easier to apply a prosthetic device.**

 3. This action is appropriate and should not be reported to the charge nurse. The nurse should first praise the UAP, and then report this behavior to the charge nurse to reward the UAP for appropriate behavior.

 4. The client with a lower extremity amputation presents one of the few times a client should be placed on the stomach, the prone position.

Content – Medical/Surgical: **Category of Health Alteration** *– Musculoskeletal:* **Integrated Processes –** *Nursing Process: Implementation:* **Client Needs –** *Physiological Integrity: Reduction of Risk Potential:* **Cognitive Level** *– Application*

MAKING NURSING DECISIONS: Delegation means the nurse is responsible for the UAP's actions and performance. The nurse should praise the UAP's action when warranted or must correct the UAP's performance to ensure the client is cared for safely and legally in the hospital or the home.

17. 1. Stockings should be applied after the legs have been elevated for a period of time when the amount of blood in the leg vein is at its lowest. Applying the stockings when the client is sitting in a chair indicates that the UAP does not understand the correct procedure for applying the elastic compression stockings.

 2. The top of stocking should not be too tight. The UAP should be able to insert two to three fingers under the proximal end of the stocking. Not allowing this much space

indicates the UAP does not understand the correct procedure for applying compression stockings.

3. **Stockings should be applied after the legs have been elevated for a period of time when the amount of blood in the leg vein is at its lowest. Having the client elevate the legs before placing the stockings on the legs indicates that the UAP understands the procedure for applying the elastic compression stockings.**

4. The toe opening should be positioned on the bottom of the foot; therefore, this indicates the client does not understand the correct procedure for applying the elastic compression stockings.

Content – *Medical/Surgical:* **Category of Health Alteration** – *Musculoskeletal:* **Integrated Processes** – *Nursing Process: Assessment:* **Client Needs** – *Physiological Integrity: Basic Care and Comfort:* **Cognitive Level** – *Analysis*

MAKING NURSING DECISIONS: Delegation means the nurse is responsible for evaluating the UAP's actions and performance. The nurse should praise the UAP's action when warranted or must correct the UAP's performance to ensure the client is cared for safely and legally in the hospital or the home.

18. 1. The client needs told the importance of therapy, but is not the most critical client; therefore, this client does not need to be assigned to the nurse.

2. Bone pain and fever are expected clinical manifestations of the client with osteomyelitis, so this client is stable and does not need to be assigned to the most experienced nurse.

3. **Deep, unrelenting pain is a sign of compartment syndrome, an acute, potentially life-threatening complication, in a client with a fracture; therefore, this client should be assigned to the most experienced nurse.**

4. The client with low back pain and radiating pain should be assessed, but this is not a sign of an acute complication; therefore, this client does not need to be assigned to the most experienced nurse.

Content – *Medical/Surgical:* **Category of Health Alteration** – *Musculoskeletal:* **Integrated Processes** – *Nursing Process: Planning:* **Client Needs** – *Safe and Effective Care Environment: Management of Care:* **Cognitive Level** – *Synthesis*

MAKING NURSING DECISIONS: The test taker must determine which client is the most

unstable and would require the most experienced nurse, thus making this type of question an "except" question. Three clients are either stable or have non-life-threatening conditions.

19. 1. The LPN should not be sent to the emergency department because the LPN's expertise is needed to care for the clients on the busy rehabilitation unit.

2. The RN has 8 years of experience on the rehabilitation unit, and the charge nurse does not want to send a nurse who is a vital part of the rehabilitation team.

3. The UAP who is completing orientation should stay on the unit, and a UAP would not be able to do as much in the emergency department as a licensed nurse.

4. **The RN with medical unit experience would be the most appropriate nurse to send to the emergency department because this nurse has experience that would be helpful in the ED. The nurse is also an RN, who would be more helpful in the ED than a UAP or an LPN.**

Content – *Medical/Surgical:* **Category of Health Alteration** – *Musculoskeletal:* **Integrated Processes** – *Nursing Process: Planning:* **Client Needs** – *Safe and Effective Care Environment: Management of Care:* **Cognitive Level** – *Synthesis*

MAKING NURSING DECISIONS: The charge nurse must be able to determine which staff member is most appropriate to float to another unit. The charge nurse does not want to leave his/her unit unsafe by sending the most experienced nurse, but wants to send the staff member who will be most helpful on the other unit.

20. 1. The UAP cannot teach the client; therefore, this task cannot be delegated.

2. The client is confused and should be assessed prior to being placed in an inclusion bed, which is used when a client wanders. The client should be assessed, and assessment cannot be delegated.

3. The UAP cannot administer medications; therefore, this task cannot be delegated.

4. **The UAP is a vital part of the healthcare team and should be encouraged to attend the multidisciplinary team meeting and provide input into the client's care.**

Content – *Medical/Surgical:* **Category of Health Alteration** – *Musculoskeletal:* **Integrated Processes** – *Nursing Process: Planning:* **Client Needs** – *Safe and Effective Care Environment: Management of Care:* **Cognitive Level** – *Synthesis*

MAKING NURSING DECISIONS: The test taker must be knowledgeable of the role of all members

of the multidisciplinary healthcare team as well as HIPAA rules and regulations. These will be tested on the NCLEX-RN® exam.

21. 1. The nurse should monitor the PCA pump but remember that equipment is not priority over the client's body.
   2. **Logrolling clients when turning is essential and priority to maintain proper body alignment.**
   3. The client with spinal surgery is on bed rest until the first postoperative day; therefore, this is not a priority intervention.
   4. The nurse can place pillows under the client's thighs but the priority postoperative intervention is to prevent postoperative complications; this means ensuring the client is logrolled when turning.
   Content – Medical/Surgical: **Category of Health Alteration** *– Musculoskeletal:* **Integrated Processes –** *Nursing Process: Implementation:* **Client Needs –** *Physiological Integrity: Physiological Adaptation:* **Cognitive Level** *– Application*

MAKING NURSING DECISIONS: When answering questions about a specific type of surgery and/or procedure the nurse should identify an intervention that is specific to the surgery/procedure.

22. 1. **This client would benefit from a home healthcare nurse's evaluation of the client's home and the wife's ability to care for the client.**
   2. The nurse should help the client care for her husband in the home. Placing him in a nursing home may be a possibility if she is unable to care for him, but the most appropriate response would be trying to help the wife care for her husband in the home.
   3. The HCP can talk to the wife but will not be able to address her concerns of taking care of her husband when he is discharged home.
   4. The nurse could allow the wife to ventilate feelings, but the first intervention is to address her concerns and do something to alleviate her concern.
   Content – Management of Care: **Category of Health Alteration** *– Musculoskeletal:* **Integrated Processes –** *Nursing Process: Implementation:* **Client Needs –** *Psychosocial Integrity:* **Cognitive Level** *– Application*

MAKING NURSING DECISIONS: The test taker must be knowledgeable of the role of all members of the multidisciplinary healthcare team as well as HIPAA rules and regulations. These will be tested on the NCLEX-RN® exam.

23. 1. This is a formal step in filing a grievance, but the nurse's next action should be to follow the chain of command and place an informal complaint with the clinical manager.
   2. The female nurse has already told the male nurse this makes her feel uncomfortable; therefore, this action is not appropriate.
   3. **If a direct request to the perpetrator does not stop the comments, then an informal complaint may be effective, especially if both parties realize a problem exists. The female nurse should utilize the chain of command and notify the clinical manager.**
   4. The female nurse should follow the chain of command and notify the clinical manager as the next action.
   Content – Legal: **Category of Health Alteration –** *Musculoskeletal:* **Integrated Processes –** *Nursing Process: Implementation:* **Client Needs –** *Safe and Effective Care Environment: Management of Care:* **Cognitive Level** *– Application*

MAKING NURSING DECISIONS: The nurse is responsible for knowing and complying with local, state, and federal standards of care, especially sexual harassment.

24. 1. Assisting the client to become independent in self-care is the role of the occupational therapist.
   2. The client must be in therapy at least 3 hours a day, but the 3-hour period includes all types of therapy, not just physical therapy. This is a true statement, but it does not answer the client's question.
   3. A multidisciplinary team decides which therapy the client should be receiving, but this does not answer the client's question.
   4. **The physical therapist will assist in improving the circulation, strengthening muscles, and ambulating and transferring the client from a bed to a chair. This is the nurse's best response to explain why the client goes to physical therapy daily.**
   Content – Medical/Surgical: **Category of Health Alteration –** *Musculoskeletal:* **Integrated Processes –** *Nursing Process: Implementation:* **Client Needs –** *Health Promotion and Maintenance:* **Cognitive Level** *– Application*

MAKING NURSING DECISIONS: The test taker must be knowledgeable of the role of all members of the multidisciplinary healthcare team as well as HIPAA rules and regulations. These will be tested on the NCLEX-RN® exam.

25. 1. **The physical therapist addresses crutch walking, how to use a walker, gait training, or transferring techniques. This is the most appropriate team member to address the problem.**

2. The social worker addresses the client's concerns that are usually outside the acute care arena, such as financial concerns or referrals.

3. The occupational therapist addresses the upper extremity activities of daily living, not walking difficulties.

4. The HCP can order the physical therapist to see the client to teach the client about crutch walking but would not be the one doing the instruction.

*Content – Medical/Surgical: **Category of Health Alteration** – Musculoskeletal: **Integrated Processes** – Nursing Process: Implementation: **Client Needs** – Health Promotion and Maintenance: **Cognitive Level** – Comprehension*

MAKING NURSING DECISIONS: The test taker must be knowledgeable of the role of all members of the multidisciplinary healthcare team as well as HIPAA rules and regulations. These will be tested on the NCLEX-RN® exam.

26. 1. The nurse can discuss this situation with the healthcare team, but the most helpful intervention is to explain the rights of the disabled according to the ADA.

2. **The ADA was passed in 1990 and ensures that a client with a disability has a right to be employed. Employers must make "reasonable accommodations," such as equipment or access ramps to facilitate employment of a person with a disability.**

3. The nurse should not interfere and contact the client's employer. The nurse should empower clients to care independently for themselves.

4. This client might be able to do this, but the most helpful intervention is to contact the ADA. The employer is violating the 1990 Americans with Disabilities Act.

*Content – Legal: **Category of Health Alteration** – Musculoskeletal: **Integrated Processes** – Nursing Process: Implementation: **Client Needs** – Safe and Effective Management of Care: Safety and Infection Control: **Cognitive Level** – Application*

MAKING NURSING DECISIONS: The nurse is responsible for knowing and complying with local, state, and federal standards of care.

27. 1. The UAP can escort clients to the different rehabilitation therapies. This action would not warrant immediate intervention.

2. The family members/significant others are an integral part of the healthcare team. This action would not warrant intervention by the charge nurse.

3. **The primary nurse cannot ask another nurse to administer medication that he or she prepared. The nurse preparing the injection must administer the medication. This action requires the charge nurse to intervene.**

4. Making sure someone watches the nurse's assigned clients is an appropriate action and would not require intervention by the charge nurse.

*Content – Medical/Surgical: **Category of Health Alteration** – Musculoskeletal: **Integrated Processes** – Nursing Process: Implementation: **Client Needs** – Safe and Effective Care Environment: Management of Care: **Cognitive Level** – Application*

MAKING NURSING DECISIONS: There will be management questions on the NCLEX-RN®. Concepts of Management is included under the category Safe and Effective Care Environment and subcategory Management of Care.

28. 1. This response does not address the client's fears and concerns.

2. **This statement will allow the client to ventilate feelings of helplessness and fear. It is the nurse's best response.**

3. The client is not verbalizing that he will kill himself; therefore, this is not the nurse's best response.

4. This is negating the client's feelings; the client has a C-6 SCI so the situation may not improve much. Therefore, this is not the nurse's best response.

*Content – Medical/Surgical: **Category of Health Alteration** – Musculoskeletal: **Integrated Processes** – Nursing Process: Implementation: **Client Needs** – Psychosocial Integrity: Therapeutic Communication: **Cognitive Level** – Application*

MAKING NURSING DECISIONS: The NCLEX-RN® blueprint includes Therapeutic Communication as a subcategory under Psychosocial Integrity. The nurse should allow clients and family to ventilate feelings.

29. 1. **Nonmalfeasance is the duty to prevent or avoid doing harm. The nurse asking not to be assigned to the NICU because of lack of experience in caring for critically ill infants is supporting the ethical principle of nonmalfeasance.**

2. The NICU is a very specialized unit requiring the nurse to be knowledgeable of equipment and caring for critically ill infants. Accepting the assignment may cause harm to one of the neonates.

3. This is challenging the charge nurse's assignment, and this does not support the ethical principle of nonmalfeasance.

4. This is blatantly violating the charge nurse's authority and does not support the ethical principle of nonmalfeasance.
   *Content – Nursing Ethics: **Category of Health Alteration** – Musculoskeletal: **Integrated Processes** – Nursing Process: Planning: **Client Needs** – Safe and Effective Care Environment: Management of Care: **Cognitive Level** – Comprehension*

MAKING NURSING DECISIONS: The NCLEX-RN® blueprint includes nursing care addressing ethical principles, including autonomy, beneficence, justice, and veracity, to name a few.

30. 1. This is a therapeutic response that encourages the husband to ventilate feelings, but the client's husband needs specific information.
    2. **According to the NCSBN, case management is content included in the management of care. The case manager is responsible for collaborating with and coordinating the services provided by all members of the healthcare team, including the home healthcare nurse who will be responsible for directing the client's care after discharge from the rehabilitation unit. This is the nurse's best response.**
    3. This is not addressing the husband's concern, and sometimes the client is discharged when the family and client are not ready in the client's opinion. This is a false reassurance and is not the nurse's best response.
    4. In rehabilitation, the HCP is part of the team and is not the only team member to determine the discharge date. This is not the nurse's best response.
    *Content – Management of Care: **Category of Health Alteration** – Musculoskeletal: **Integrated Processes** – Nursing Process: Implementation: **Client Needs** – Physiological Integrity: Basic Care and Comfort: **Cognitive Level** – Application*

MAKING NURSING DECISIONS: The test taker must be knowledgeable of the role of all members of the multidisciplinary healthcare team as well as HIPAA rules and regulations. These will be tested on the NCLEX-RN® exam.

31. 1. The nurse's comment does not address the client's question and concern. This is not an appropriate response.
    2. **The rehabilitation commission of each state will help evaluate and determine whether the client can receive training or education for another occupation after injury.**
    3. This client is not asking about disability. The client is concerned about employment. The nurse needs to refer the client to the appropriate agency.

4. This does not address the client's concern about gainful employment. This is a therapeutic response that will allow the client to ventilate feelings, but the client is asking for information.
   *Content – Medical/Surgical: **Category of Health Alteration** – Musculoskeletal: **Integrated Processes** – Nursing Process: Implementation: **Client Needs** – Psychosocial Integrity: **Cognitive Level** – Comprehension*

MAKING NURSING DECISIONS: There will be management questions on the NCLEX-RN®. In many instances, there is no test-taking strategy. The nurse must be knowledgeable of management issues and must comply with local, state, and federal requirements.

32. 1. The client is confiding in the nurse about a doctor, and the nurse should address the client's concern, not tell the client to talk to the doctor. Many clients do not feel comfortable talking to a doctor.
    2. **The nurse should determine what is concerning the client. It could be a misunderstanding or a real situation in which the client's care is unsafe or inadequate.**
    3. After the nurse determines whether the client's concern warrants a new doctor, the nurse should talk to the nursing supervisor and help the client get a second opinion. The nurse is the client's advocate.
    4. The choice of doctor is ultimately the client's, and the client has a right to another doctor.
    *Content – Medical/Surgical: **Category of Health Alteration** – Musculoskeletal: **Integrated Processes** – Nursing Process: Implementation: **Client Needs** – Safe and Effective Care Environment: Management of Care: **Cognitive Level** – Application*

MAKING NURSING DECISIONS: The nurse should always try and support the client or the family's request if it does not violate any local, state, or federal rules and regulations. The client has a right to request a second opinion if the client does not like the healthcare provider's care.

33. 1. **An abductor pillow is used for a client with a THR to help prevent hip dislocation and the UAP can place the pillow between the client's legs. This task is appropriate to delegate.**
    2. The client should be out of bed and ambulating by the third day post-op to help prevent complications secondary to immobility, such as deep vein thrombosis (DVT) or pneumonia.
    3. Just because the client is elderly does not mean the client must be fed. There is nothing in the stem of the question that would indicate the client could not feed him- or

herself. The nurse should encourage independence as much as possible and delegate feeding the client to a UAP only when it is necessary.

4. The nurse cannot delegate assessment to the UAP; therefore, checking the surgical dressing is not appropriate delegation.

Content – Medical/Surgical: **Category of Health Alteration** *– Musculoskeletal:* **Integrated Processes** *– Nursing Process: Planning:* **Client Needs** *– Safe and Effective Care Environment: Management of Care:* **Cognitive Level** *– Synthesis*

MAKING NURSING DECISIONS: A nurse cannot delegate assessment, teaching, evaluation, medications, or an unstable client to a UAP. Tasks that cannot be delegated are nursing interventions requiring nursing judgment.

34. 1. Closing the door and cubicle curtain protects the client's privacy and would not warrant immediate intervention from the nurse.

2. **The client with spinal surgery should be logrolled with at least two if not three staff members assisting with the turning from side to side. Logrolling the client ensures proper body alignment. Asking the client to turn would warrant intervention by the nurse.**

3. Checking the temperature of the bathwater prevents scalding the client with water that is too hot or making the client uncomfortable with water that is too cold. This action would not warrant immediate intervention.

4. The UAP must perform the skill safely; putting the side rails in an upright position ensures client will not fall out of the bed.

Content – Medical/Surgical: **Category of Health Alteration** *– Musculoskeletal:* **Integrated Processes** *– Nursing Process: Implementation:* **Client Needs** *– Physiological Integrity: Basic Care and Comfort:* **Cognitive Level** *– Application*

MAKING NURSING DECISIONS: The nurse must ensure the UAP can perform any tasks that are delegated. It is the nurse's responsibility to demonstrate and/or teach the UAP how to perform the task, and then evaluate the task performed.

35. 3, 4, and 5 are correct.
1. The right leg should not be elevated in the rehabilitation unit because it can cause a contracture of the right leg, which can lead to the prosthetic leg not fitting properly. The leg should be elevated the first 48 hours to decrease edema and then kept straight.

2. The occupational therapist addresses the client's activities of daily living and upper extremity problems, not lower extremity problems.

3. Pushing the residual limb against a pillow will help toughen the end of the limb, which is needed when wearing a prosthetic limb.

4. The expected treatment for a client with impetigo is warm saline followed by soap and water for removal of crusts, followed by topical antibiotic cream.

5. Impetigo is very contagious, so wearing gloves and meticulous hygiene is essential when caring for this client.

Content – Medical/Surgical: **Category of Health Alteration** *– Musculoskeletal:* **Integrated Processes** *– Nursing Process: Implementation:* **Client Needs** *– Physiological Integrity: Reduction of Risk Potential:* **Cognitive Level** *– Application*

MAKING NURSING DECISIONS: This is an alternate type of question included in the NCLEX-RN®. The nurse must be able to select all the options that answer the question correctly. There are no partially correct answers.

36. 1. The procedure for tornados is to have all clients, staff, and visitors stay in the hallway and close the doors to all the rooms. This will help prevent any flying debris or glass from hurting anyone.

2. This may be recommended for individuals in the home, but it is not the hospital protocol for tornados.

3. **The procedure for tornados is to have all clients, staff, and visitors stay in the hallway and close the doors to all the rooms. This will help prevent any flying debris or glass from hurting anyone.**

4. The client and visitors should be in the client's room with the door closed for a fire, but this is not the correct procedure for a tornado.

Content – Management of Care: **Category of Health Alteration** *– Musculoskeletal:* **Integrated Processes** *– Nursing Process: Implementation:* **Client Needs** *– Safe and Effective Care Environment: Safety and Infection Control:* **Cognitive Level** *– Comprehension*

MAKING NURSING DECISIONS: The nurse must be knowledgeable of emergency preparedness. Employees receive this information during employee orientation and are responsible for implementing procedures correctly. The NCSBN NCLEX-RN® blueprint includes questions on a Safe and Effective Care Environment.

37. 1. The finance office is responsible for discussing the cost and insurance issues with the client.

2. The physiatrist is a medical healthcare provider who cares for clients in the rehabilitation area.

3. The vocational counselor would assist the client with employment training if needed.

4. The case manager is responsible for co-ordinating the total rehabilitative plan, collaborating with and coordinating the services provided by all members of the healthcare team, including the home healthcare nurse who will be responsible for directing the client's care after discharge from the rehabilitation unit.

Content – Management of Care: **Category of Health Alteration** *– Musculoskeletal:* **Integrated Processes** *– Nursing Process: Implementation:* **Client Needs** *– Safe and Effective Care Environment: Management of Care:* **Cognitive Level** *– Comprehension*

MAKING NURSING DECISIONS: The test taker must be knowledgeable of the role of all members of the multidisciplinary healthcare team as well as HIPAA rules and regulations. These will be tested on the NCLEX-RN® exam.

38. 1. **The rehabilitation nurse must recognize and address sexual issues in order to promote feelings of self-worth that are essential to total rehabilitation. The age of the client should not matter, but this client is young; therefore, this is priority.**
2. This is not a psychosocial intervention, and the social worker or occupational therapist usually addresses the home situation.
3. This is not necessarily a psychosocial intervention, but it should be addressed so the client can be independent. The social worker usually addresses transportation.
4. The client may or may not need psychological counseling, but the priority psychosocial intervention of the rehabilitation nurse is to discuss the client's sexuality needs.

Content – Medical/Surgical: **Category of Health Alteration** *– Musculoskeletal:* **Integrated Processes** *– Nursing Process: Implementation:* **Client Needs** *– Psychosocial Integrity: Therapeutic Communication:* **Cognitive Level** *– Application*

MAKING NURSING DECISIONS: The NCLEX-RN® blueprint includes Therapeutic Communication as a subcategory of Psychosocial Integrity. The nurse should allow clients and family to ventilate feelings and address psychosocial concerns.

39. 1. The nurse could apologize for the UAP's comments, but this is not the first intervention.
2. This is a violation of HIPAA and the nurse should tell this to the UAP, but it is not the first intervention.
3. The nurse should not allow the conversation to continue. The UAP is violating confidentiality and is gossiping about another client.
4. **The nurse should stop the conversation immediately, and asking the UAP to go to**

the nurse's station does not embarrass the UAP. Gossiping about another client is a violation of his or her privacy, and a breach of protected health information under HIPAA.

Content – Legal: **Category of Health Alteration** *– Musculoskeletal:* **Integrated Processes** *– Nursing Process: Implementation:* **Client Needs** *– Safe and Effective Care Environment: Management of Care:* **Cognitive Level** *– Application*

MAKING NURSING DECISIONS: There will be management questions on the NCLEX-RN®. In many instances, there is no test-taking strategy. The nurse must be knowledgeable of management issues. The Health Insurance Portability and Accountability Act (HIPAA) was passed into law in 1996 to standardize the exchange of information between healthcare providers, and to ensure patient record confidentiality.

40. 1. After two verbal warnings, the clinical manager should document the behavior and start formal proceedings to correct the staff nurse's behavior.
2. The human resources department would not need to be notified until the clinical manager has decided to terminate the staff nurse's employment.
3. **Every hospital has a procedure for termination if the employee is not performing as expected. After two verbal warnings, the clinical manager should document the employee's actions in writing and implement the hospital policy for possible termination.**
4. The clinical manager cannot allow the nurse to go home because this will affect the care of the clients during the shift. It would cause a hardship on the other staff members.

Content – Management: **Category of Health Alteration** *– Musculoskeletal:* **Integrated Processes** *– Nursing Process: Implementation:* **Client Needs** *– Safe and Effective Care Environment: Management of Care:* **Cognitive Level** *– Application*

MAKING NURSING DECISIONS: There will be management questions on the NCLEX-RN®. In many instances, there is no test-taking strategy. The nurse must be knowledgeable of management issues.

41. 1. **The LPN's scope of practice allows the LPN to take telephone orders.**
2. The LPN's scope of practice does not include assessment.
3. The registered dietician would be the most appropriate team member to teach about diets.

ANSWERS

4. The unlicensed assistive personnel (UAP) could obtain the intake and output; therefore, this is not an appropriate assignment for an LPN.
    Content – Medical/Surgical: **Category of Health Alteration** *– Musculoskeletal:* **Integrated Processes** *– Nursing Process: Planning:* **Client Needs** *– Safe and Effective Care Environment: Management of Care:* **Cognitive Level** *– Comprehension*

MAKING NURSING DECISIONS: The nurse cannot assign assessment, teaching, evaluation, or an unstable client to a LPN. The LPN can transcribe HCP orders and can call HCPs on the phone to obtain orders for a client.

42. 1. The client with COPD would be expected to have low oxygen and high CO_2 levels in the arterial blood; therefore, this laboratory result would not warrant intervention from the charge nurse.
    2. This WBC level is within normal limits; therefore, this client does not warrant immediate intervention from the charge nurse.
    3. **Antibiotic therapy can result in a superinfection that destroys the normal bacterial flora of the intestines and produces diarrhea. Diarrhea, in turn, causes an increased excretion of potassium, resulting in hypokalemia. This K+ level is below normal, and the charge nurse should notify the healthcare provider.**
    4. This glucose level is slightly elevated, and TPN is high in glucose; therefore, this laboratory result does not require immediate intervention.
    Content – Medical/Surgical: **Category of Health Alteration** *– Musculoskeletal:* **Integrated Processes** *– Nursing Process: Assessment:* **Client Needs** *– Physiological Integrity: Reduction of Risk Potential:* **Cognitive Level** *– Analysis*

MAKING NURSING DECISIONS: The nurse must be knowledgeable of normal laboratory values. These values must be memorized and the nurse must be able to determine if the laboratory value is normal for the client's disease process or medications the client is taking.

43. 1. The nurse is an employee of the hospital and cannot witness documents for clients.
    2. **This is the correct action to take; the nurse is an employee of the hospital directly involved in providing care and cannot witness documents for clients.**
    3. This is incorrect information; the document should be witnessed by individuals who are not family members or employees of the hospital providing direct care.

4. The living will must be witnessed by two individuals when the client is signing it, but it does not have to be notarized.
    Content – Legal: **Category of Health Alteration** *– Musculoskeletal:* **Integrated Processes** *– Nursing Process: Implementation:* **Client Needs** *– Safe and Effective Care Environment: Management of Care:* **Cognitive Level** *– Comprehension*

MAKING NURSING DECISIONS: The NCLEX-RN® blueprint includes nursing care that is ruled by legal requirements. The nurse must be knowledgeable of these issues.

44. 1. The nurse should ensure the client has appropriate shoes when ambulating, but the priority is safety of the client, which means using a gait belt.
    2. **The nurse's priority is to ensure the safety of the client, and placing a safety gait belt around the client's waist before ambulating the client helps to ensure safety. The gait belt provides a handle to hold onto the client securely during ambulation.**
    3. The nurse should explain the procedure to the client, but it is not priority over ensuring safety for the client while walking in the hall.
    4. The nurse should make sure there is a clear path to walk, but the priority intervention is to protect the client if he or she falls, and that can be prevented by placing a gait belt around the client's waist.
    Content – Medical/Surgical: **Category of Health Alteration** *– Integumentary:* **Integrated Processes** *– Nursing Process: Implementation:* **Client Needs** *– Physiological Integrity: Reduction of Risk Potential: Cognitive Level* *– Application*

MAKING NURSING DECISIONS: The NCLEX-RN® blueprint includes adhering to safety standards when caring for clients.

45. 1. Being a client advocate means the nurse will support the client's wishes, but in some situations the nurse must adhere to the medical regimen. Telling the client he or she does not have to attend therapy is detrimental to the client's recovery and is not being a client advocate.
    2. Being a client advocate means the nurse will support the client's wishes, but in some situations the nurse must adhere to the medical regimen. Talking to the physical therapist will not help the client's recovery.
    3. **Finding ways for the client to perform the exercises by the physical therapist is supporting the medical regimen. This action supports client advocacy. PTs cannot prescribe.**

4. Discussing the client concerns does not help the client's recovery; therefore, this statement does not support client advocacy.
*Content – Management of Care: **Category of Health Alteration** – Musculoskeletal: **Integrated Processes** – Nursing Process: Implementation: **Client Needs** – Physiological Integrity: Physiological Adaptation: **Cognitive Level** – Application*

MAKING NURSING DECISIONS: There will be management questions on the NCLEX-RN® addressing client advocacy. A client advocate acts as a liaison between clients and healthcare providers to help improve or maintain a high quality of healthcare.

46. 1. As long as the client gives permission, the nurse can discuss the client's condition with anyone.
2. The nurse can answer questions over the phone with the client's permission. It may be difficult for the client's wife to come to the rehabilitation unit.
3. The client and wife are allowed and encouraged to come to the multidisciplinary team meeting, but the nurse should talk to the wife on the phone.
4. **The nurse can talk to anyone the client requests. This is not a violation of HIPAA as long as the client gives permission for the nurse to share information.**
*Content – Legal: **Category of Health Alteration** – Musculoskeletal: **Integrated Processes** – Nursing Process: Implementation: **Client Needs** – Health Promotion and Maintenance: **Cognitive Level** – Application*

MAKING NURSING DECISIONS: There will be management questions on the NCLEX-RN®. In many instances, there is no test-taking strategy. The nurse must be knowledgeable of management issues. The Health Insurance Portability and Accountability Act (HIPAA) was passed into law in 1996 to standardize the exchange of information between healthcare providers, and to ensure patient record confidentiality.

47. 1, 2, and 3 are correct.
1. **An antibiotic ointment, such as Polysporin, should be applied thinly four times daily. Polysporin can be purchased without a prescription.**
2. **Children should be kept home from school until the lesions crust over.**
3. **Use separate towels for the client. The client's towels, pillowcases, and sheets should be changed after the first day of treatment. The clothing should be changed and laundered daily for the first 2 days.**

4. Crusts should be removed before the ointment is applied. Soak a soft, clean cloth in a mixture of one-half cup of white vinegar and a quart of lukewarm water. Press a cloth on the crusts for 10 to 15 minutes three or four times daily. Then gently wipe off the crusts and apply a little antibiotic ointment.
5. The child does not have to wear sterile gloves.
*Content – Medical/Surgical: **Category of Health Alteration** – Integumentary: **Integrated Processes** – Nursing Process: Implementation: **Client Needs** – Safe and Effective Care Environment: Safety and Infection Control: **Cognitive Level** – Application*

MAKING NURSING DECISIONS: This is an alternate type of question included in the NCLEX-RN®. The nurse must be able to select all the options that answer the question correctly. There are no partially correct answers.

48. 1. The nurse's scope of practice includes teaching the client how to use equipment.
2. **This is a violation of HIPAA. The client's right to confidentiality is being compromised because anyone could read the client's record on the computer. The charge nurse should intervene.**
3. The nurse can discuss a client situation with the HCP; therefore, this action does not require intervention.
4. The nurse should refer a client with a spiritual need to the chaplain. It is not necessary to know what the need is only that the chaplain needs to see the client.
*Content – Management of Care: **Category of Health Alteration** – Integumentary: **Integrated Processes** – Nursing Process: Implementation: **Client Needs** – Safe and Effective Care Environment, Management of Care: **Cognitive Level** – Planning*

MAKING NURSING DECISIONS: There will be management questions on the NCLEX-RN®. In many instances, there is no test-taking strategy; the nurse must be knowledgeable of management issues. The Health Insurance Portability and Accountability Act (HIPAA) was passed into law in 1996 to standardize the exchange of information between healthcare providers, and to ensure patient record confidentiality.

49. 1. Vitiligo is a common skin disorder in which white spots appear on the skin, usually occurring on both sides of the body in the same location. The client would not need an immediate appointment.
2. **Allergic contact dermatitis occurs when skin comes in contact with an allergen the client is sensitive or allergic to. Symptoms include redness, swelling, blistering,**

itching, and weeping. This client has an acute dermatological condition and should be seen immediately.

3. Angiomas are not dangerous or contagious. Angiomas do not need to be treated unless they bleed or bother the client. This client does not need an immediate appointment.

4. The client may have shingles but it cannot be determined at this time. The rash of shingles begins as red patches that soon develop blisters, often on one side of the body. It is treated with Acyclovir (Zovirax) but at this time the nurse would not need to make an appointment immediately.

Content – Medical/Surgical: Category of Health Alteration – Integumentary: Integrated Processes – Nursing Process: Assessment: Client Needs – Physiological Integrity: Reduction of Risk Potential: Cognitive Level – Analysis

MAKING NURSING DECISIONS: The test taker must determine which sign/symptom is not expected for the disease process. If the sign/symptom is not expected, then the nurse should assess the client first. This type of question is determining if the nurse is knowledgeable of signs/symptoms of a variety of disease processes.

50. 1. An MRI is not the diagnostic test used to confirm the diagnosis of basal cell carcinoma.
2. A washing is not used to confirm the diagnosis of basal cell carcinoma.
3. **The only way to tell for sure if a skin growth is cancerous is to biopsy it.**
4. A biopsy will definitively diagnosis the skin cancer.

Content – Medical/Surgical: Category of Health Alteration – Integumentary: Integrated Processes – Nursing Process: Analysis: Client Needs – Physiological Integrity, Physiological Adaptation: Cognitive Level – Analysis

MAKING NURSING DECISIONS: The nurse must be knowledgeable of normal diagnostic tests pre- and post-procedure. These interventions must be memorized, and to ensure the client is safe, the nurse must be able to determine if the client is able to have the diagnostic procedure and post-procedure care.

51. Correct Answer: 5, 3, 1, 2, 4
These are the best practices for helping a client use a cane when ambulating.
5. **The gait belt is applied to ensure safety of the patient and the person assisting the client to ambulate.**
3. **The client should use the strong hand to control the assistive device.**

1. **The client should move the cane forward to provide a stable support for the weaker leg when it is moved.**
2. **The client should move the weaker leg even with the supportive cane while maintaining the stronger leg in place.**
4. **Finally, the stronger leg can move to a position even with the weak leg and cane.**

Content – Medical/Surgical: Category of Health Alteration – Musculoskeletal: Integrated Processes – Nursing Process: Implementation: Client Needs – Physiological Integrity: Reduction of Risk Potential: Cognitive Level – Application

MAKING NURSING DECISIONS: The NCLEX-RN® has alternate types of questions including putting interventions in rank order. The test taker must put the interventions in the correct order to get the answer correct.

52. 1. Adequate skin care is an appropriate intervention to help prevent pressure ulcers, but it is not the priority intervention.
2. **The priority intervention to prevent skin impairment is frequent position changes along with skin care and nutritional support.**
3. Sufficient nutritional intake will help prevent pressure ulcers but it is not the priority intervention.
4. The use of any mechanical device does not eliminate the need for turning and repositioning the client to help prevent pressure ulcers.

Content – Medical/Surgical: Category of Health Alteration – Integumentary: Integrated Processes – Nursing Process: Implementation: Client Needs – Physiological Integrity: Reduction of Risk Potential: Cognitive Level – Application

MAKING NURSING DECISIONS: Test questions asking the test taker to select the priority intervention means all the options may be plausible. The test taker has to determine the most important.

53. 1. Assessing the client's breath sounds is an appropriate intervention, but if the client is in distress the nurse should intervene to help the client's body.
2. The client should be encouraged to cough and deep breathe but it will not help oxygenate the client, which is the priority for the client with a fat embolism.
3. **Oxygen must be administered to treat hypoxia, which occurs after a fat embolism; therefore, this is the nurse's first intervention.**
4. The HCP may or may not administer heparin therapy, but it would not be the first intervention the nurse would implement.

*Content – Medical/Surgical: **Category of Health Alteration** – Musculoskeletal: **Integrated Processes** – Nursing Process: Implementation: **Client Needs** – Physiological Integrity: Reduction of Risk Potential: **Cognitive Level** – Application*

MAKING NURSING DECISIONS: The nurse should use the nursing process when answering questions asking which intervention the nurse should implement first. If the client is in distress, do not assess; the nurse needs to address the client's physiological needs. The nurse should use Maslow's Hierarchy of Needs, which states that oxygenation needs are priority.

54. 1. The wounds need to be kept sterile to decrease chance of infection, but the priority for electrical burn wounds is to monitor for cardiac problems.
    2. All clients need to have vital signs assessed, but the priority for electrical burn wounds is to monitor for cardiac problems.
    3. The client's oxygenation level should be monitored, but the priority for electrical burns is cardiac problems.
    4. **The electrical current in the body bounces off bone and goes through muscle. The heart is a muscle; therefore, the priority intervention is for the nurse to apply cardiac monitors to assess for lethal dysrhythmias that may occur.**

*Content – Medical/Surgical: **Category of Health Alteration** – Integumentary: **Integrated Processes** – Nursing Process: Implementation: **Client Needs** – Physiological Integrity: Reduction of Risk Potential: **Cognitive Level** – Application*

MAKING NURSING DECISIONS: The test taker should try to determine what is different about the client's disease process/disorder. All clients need to have vital signs assessed and oxygenation levels monitored—what is different for the client with an electrical burn?

55. 1. The nurse should have another staff member to assist with the lift, but it is not priority over safety of the client in the equipment.
    2. **This is priority because the safety of the client must be ensured. If the client is not placed correctly in the lift sleeve, the client could fall. Electric lifts are powered either through a standard electrical outlet or by a rechargeable battery. The lifting is completely controlled through a hand control, eliminating any physical exertion by the caregiver.**
    3. The nurse should lift the client slowly but it is not priority.
    4. The stretcher should be locked and ready for the transfer but the client is priority.

*Content – Medical/Surgical: **Category of Health Alteration** – Musculoskeletal: **Integrated Processes** – Nursing Process: Implementation: **Client Needs** – Safe and Effective Care Environment: Safety and Infection Control: **Cognitive Level** – Application*

MAKING NURSING DECISIONS: If the test taker is trying to determine the correct answer between option 2 and 4, the test taker should select the client's body over any type of equipment. All these options are plausible for a nurse to implement, but safety of the client is priority.

56. 1. Grade A indicates the client is independent in feeding, bathing, and toileting.
    2. Grade C indicates the client has some functioning areas of ADLs.
    3. Grade E indicates the client will need more assistance with ADLs.
    4. **Grade G indicates the client is dependent in all six functions including bathing, feeding, toileting, continence, dressing, and transferring. This client would require the nurse to delegate activities of daily living to the UAP.**

*Content – Management of Care: **Category of Health Alteration** – Musculoskeletal: **Integrated Processes** – Nursing Process: Planning: **Client Needs** – Physiological Integrity: Physiological Adaptation: **Cognitive Level** – Comprehension*

MAKING NURSING DECISIONS: This is a knowledge-based question but pertinent to rehabilitation nursing. The test taker must realize either a grade A or G would be the answer since in most scales, but not all, the higher the number, the more severe the condition.

57. 1. The arm should be elevated to decrease edema, not placed in the dependent position, which is lower than the heart.
    2. **Moist heat, immobilization, elevation, and systemic antibiotics are the treatments for cellulitis, which is an inflammation of subcutaneous tissue.**
    3. Antistaphylococcal soap (Hibiclen, Lever 2000, Dial) is prescribed for staph infection.
    4. The affected area should be left open to air, not wrapped by ACE bandage.

*Content – Medical/Surgical: **Category of Health Alteration** – Integumentary: **Integrated Processes** – Nursing Process: Implementation: **Client Needs** – Health Promotion and Maintenance: **Cognitive Level** – Application*

MAKING NURSING DECISIONS: The nurse must know the expected medical treatment for the client. This is a knowledge-based question.

58. Correct Answer: 2, 5, 3, 4, 1
    This is the procedure in correct order when transferring a client from the bed to a wheelchair.

ANSWERS

2. **The wheelchair should be ready for the client to transfer to and is the first step.**

5. **The brakes should be locked so the chair will not move during the transfer.**

3. **The client should support him- or herself when moving with the stronger side.**

4. **The client next shifts the weight forward so he/she can pivot into the chair.**

1. **The client should not attempt until he/she feels the chair on the back of the legs so the client knows where the chair is.**

Content – Management of Care: **Category of Health Alteration** *– Musculoskeletal:* **Integrated Processes** *– Nursing Process: Implementation:* **Client Needs** *– Safe and Effective Care Environment: Management of Care:* **Cognitive Level** *– Application*

MAKING NURSING DECISIONS: The NCLEX-RN® has alternate types of questions including ranking interventions in priority order. The test taker must put the interventions in the correct order to get the answer correct.

59. 1. **The residual limb of an AKA should be elevated after 48 hours to help prevent contractures. Since the client is in the rehabilitation unit, it is past 48 hours.**

2. The LPN could give the HS snacks to the clients but the UAP could also do this; therefore, it is not appropriate for the LPN to do this task.

3. The UAP cannot perform sterile procedures, so this cannot be delegated to a UAP.

4. The nurse cannot assign assessment to the LPN.

Content – Medical/Surgical: **Category of Health Alteration** *– Integumentary:* **Integrated Processes** *– Nursing Process: Planning:* **Client Needs** *– Safe and Effective Care Environment: Management of Care:* **Cognitive Level** *– Synthesis*

MAKING NURSING DECISIONS: The nurse cannot delegate assessment, teaching, evaluation, medications, or an unstable client to the UAP. The nurse cannot assign assessment, teaching, evaluation, or an unstable client to the LPN.

60. 1. The nurse cannot delegate assessment to the UAP.

2. **The UAP can clean the client's dentures, so this task should be delegated.**

3. The UAP should not perform passive range-of-motion exercises because it could lead to harm if not done correctly. The nurse should perform passive ROM.

4. The client's right leg should be elevated to decrease edema, not in a dependent position, which is hanging off the bed.

Content – Medical/Surgical: **Category of Health Alteration** *– Integumentary:* **Integrated Processes** *– Nursing Process: Planning:* **Client Needs** *– Safe and Effective Care Environment: Management of Care:* **Cognitive Level** *– Synthesis*

MAKING NURSING DECISIONS: The nurse cannot delegate assessment, teaching, evaluation, medication, or an unstable client to a UAP. The nurse must be knowledgeable about interventions that cannot be delegated, and in some cases, the intervention should not be implemented at all—such as option 1.

61. 1. A sterile environment should be maintained, but the priority is fluid volume because the client is at risk for hypovolemia.

2. **The priority intervention in the first 24 hours for the client with a third degree burn is maintaining intravascular volume so the client will not die from hypovolemic shock.**

3. Preventing infection is important but initially maintaining fluid volume is priority.

4. The nurse should assess the client's pain, but for a client with third degree burns over both the legs the priority is maintaining fluid volume.

Content – Medical/Surgical: **Category of Health Alteration** *– Integumentary:* **Integrated Processes** *– Nursing Process: Implementation:* **Client Needs** *– Physiological Integrity: Reduction of Risk Potential:* **Cognitive Level** *– Analysis*

MAKING NURSING DECISIONS: The nurse must know the expected medical treatment for the client. This is a knowledge-based question.

62. 1. **Orthostatic hypotension is a side effect of administering the beta-blocker medication atenolol; therefore, this medication should be questioned.**

2. Rocephin is an antibiotic and these signs/symptoms would not warrant questioning this medication.

3. Bisacodyl is a laxative and light-headedness would not warrant questioning this medication.

4. Light-headedness is a side effect of beta blockers and should not be administered until further assessment and notification of the healthcare provider.

Content – Medical/Surgical: **Category of Health Alteration** *– Drug Administration:* **Integrated Processes** *– Nursing Process: Assessment:* **Client Needs** *– Physiological Integrity: Pharmacological and Parenteral Therapies:* **Cognitive Level** *– Analysis*

MAKING NURSING DECISIONS: The NCLEX-RN® has alternate types of questions such as this one.

It is an application-style question and the test taker needs to be able to read a medication administration record (MAR) as well as know the side effects of medications.

63. **1, 2, and 4 are correct.**
    1. **Acupuncture is traditional Chinese medicine, which involves the use of sharp, thin needles that are inserted in the body at very specific points and is believed to adjust and alter the body's energy flow into healthier patterns.**
    2. **Guided imagery is the use of relaxation and mental visualization to improve mood and/or physical well-being.**
    3. A compression sequential device is a pneumatic device used to prevent DVT from the legs and arms. This is medically approved and is not a CAM.
    4. **Music therapy is a technique of complementary alternative medicine that uses music prescribed in a skilled manner by trained therapists. Programs are designed to help patients overcome physical, emotional, intellectual, and social challenges.**
    5. Muscle-strengthening exercises are not a CAM. It is performed as physical therapy and is a medical treatment.
    *Content – Management of Care: **Category of Health Alteration** – Complementary Alternative Medication: **Integrated Processes** – Nursing Process: Planning: **Client Needs** – Physiological Integrity: Pharmacological and Parenteral Therapies: **Cognitive Level** – Synthesis*

MAKING NURSING DECISIONS: This is an alternate type of question in which the test taker must select all options to get the question correct. The NCLEX-RN® tests complementary alternate medicine according to the test blueprint.

64. 1. **This is the reason for referring a client to a vocational counselor.**
    2. This describes the physiatrist who is a physician specializing in rehabilitative care.
    3. This is the reason for referring a client to an occupational therapist.
    4. This is the reason for referring a client to the recreational therapist.
    *Content – Management of Care: **Category of Health Alteration** – Musculoskeletal: **Integrated Processes** – Nursing Process: Implementation: **Client Needs** – Physiological Integrity: Physiological Adaptation: **Cognitive Level** – Comprehension*

MAKING NURSING DECISIONS: The nurse must know the role of the client's multidisciplinary team in rehabilitation. The nurse must be able to refer to the appropriate team member to help with rehabilitation for the client.

65. 1. This question may be asked but it is not assessing daily schedules and habits.
    2. **Assessment of daily schedules and habits includes questions concerning hygiene practices, eating, elimination, sexual activity, sleep, work, exercise, and recreational activities.**
    3. Asking about insurance does not help the nurse assess the client's daily schedules and habits.
    4. This question can be asked but it does not address daily schedules and habits.
    *Content – Management of Care: **Category of Health Alteration** – Integumentary: **Integrated Processes** – Nursing Process: Planning: **Client Needs** – Physiological Integrity: Basic Care and Comfort: **Cognitive Level** – Synthesis*

MAKING NURSING DECISIONS: The nurse must be able to ask appropriate questions when completing assessments, especially in rehabilitation nursing.

66. 1. **The vancomycin needs to have a peak and trough drawn every third or fourth dose depending on the HCP's order.**
    2. Protonix does not have a required laboratory test on a routine basis.
    3. Silvadene does not have a required laboratory test on a routine basis.
    4. Morphine does not have a required laboratory test on a routine basis.
    *Content – Medical/Surgical: **Category of Health Alteration** – Integumentary: **Integrated Processes** – Drug Administration: **Client Needs** – Physiological Integrity: Pharmacological and Parenteral Therapies: **Cognitive Level** – Comprehension*

MAKING NURSING DECISIONS: This is an alternate type of question included in the NCLEX-RN® blueprint. The test taker must be able to read a medication administration record (MAR), be knowledgeable of medications, and be able to make an appropriate decision as to the nurse's most appropriate intervention.

67. **Answer: 1 tablet**
    The medication comes in 40 mg tablets. On M/W/F the patient should receive 1/2 tablet, on Su/T/Th/Sa the patient should receive 1 whole tablet.
    *Content – Medical/Surgical: **Category of Health Alteration** – Drug Administration: **Integrated Processes** – Nursing Process: Implementation: **Client Needs** – Physiological Integrity; Pharmacological and Parenteral Therapies: **Cognitive Level** – Application*

MAKING NURSING DECISIONS: The NCLEX-RN® blueprint includes dosage calculations under Pharmacological and Parenteral Therapies.

ANSWERS

This category is included under Physiological Integrity, which promotes physical health and wellness by providing care and comfort, reducing client risk potential, and managing health alterations.

68. 1, 2, and 3 are correct.
   1. The HHA is capable of weighing a client and documenting the finding.
   2. An HHA can offer the SO time away from the home to do personal business.
   3. This is within the HHA's capabilities.
   4. Taking the patient to perform personal business in the HHA's vehicle is crossing boundaries, particularly when the business involves finances.
   5. The HHA is not capable of performing assessments and making nursing judgments based on the findings.

   Content – *Management of Care:* **Category of Health Alteration** – *Neurosensory:* **Integrated Processes** – *Nursing Process: Planning:* **Client Needs** – *Safe and Effective Care Environment: Management of Care:* **Cognitive Level** – *Synthesis*

MAKING NURSING DECISIONS: This is an alternate type of question included in the NCLEX-RN®. The nurse must be able to select all the options that answer the question correctly. There are no partially correct answers.

69. 1. The emergency services need to come to the mall immediately. This woman is having an allergic reaction to something and this is a potentially life-threatening emergency.
   2. **The nurse should determine if the woman has medication available that will save her life. If she doesn't, the nurse will have to wait for the ambulance.**
   3. The client with allergies should wear a medical alert bracelet to let anyone know what she is allergic to, but the first intervention is to try and save the woman's life by giving epinephrine to the client.
   4. The nurse should protect the client's head but it is not the priority intervention.

Content – *Medical/Surgical:* **Category of Health Alteration** – *Integumentary:* **Integrated Processes** – *Nursing Process: Implementation:* **Client Needs** – *Physiological Integrity: Reduction of Risk Potential:* **Cognitive Level** – *Application*

MAKING NURSING DECISIONS: When the question asks which intervention should be implemented first, it means all the options are something a nurse could implement but only one should be implemented first. The nurse should use the nursing process to determine the appropriate intervention: If the client is in distress, do not assess; if the client is not in distress, then the nurse should assess.

70. Correct Answer: 3, 1, 5, 2, 4
   3. This patient has a change in normal sputum production. Frequently, patients diagnosed with obstructive pulmonary diseases are placed on steroid therapy. Steroid therapy can mask an infection. The only symptom of an infection may be a change in the color of the sputum.
   1. This patient has a deep wound that needs to be assessed.
   5. This test can be performed by the nurse with a portable machine. The HCP may need to adjust the patient's medication based on the results.
   2. This is a medication to increase the patient's WBC production.
   4. This is expected behavior for a client with Alzheimer's disease.

   Content – *Medical/Surgical:* **Category of Health Alteration** – *Respiratory:* **Integrated Processes** – *Nursing Process: Assessment:* **Client Needs** – *Physiological Integrity: Reduction of Risk Potential:* **Cognitive Level** – *Analysis*

MAKING NURSING DECISIONS: This is an alternate type of question that requires the nurse to assess clients in order of priority. This requires the nurse to evaluate each client's situation and determine which situations are life threatening, which situations are expected for the client's situation, or which client has a psychosocial problem.

CLINICAL SCENARIO ANSWERS AND RATIONALES

The correct answer number and rationale for why it is the correct answer are given in **boldface type.** Rationales for why the other possible answer options are incorrect also are given, but they are not in boldface type.

1. 1. Sunburn is an example of this depth of burn; a superficial partial-thickness burn affects the epidermis and the skin is reddened and blanches with pressure.
   2. **Deep partial-thickness burns are scalds and flash burns that injure the epidermis, upper dermis, and portions of the deeper dermis. This causes pain, blistered and mottled red skin, and edema.**
   3. Full-thickness burns are caused by flame, electric current, or chemicals, and include the epidermis, entire dermis, and sometimes subcutaneous tissue, and may also involve connective tissue, muscle, and bone.
   4. First degree burn is another name for a superficial partial-thickness burn.

2. 1. **After airway, the most urgent need is preventing irreversible shock by replacing fluids and electrolytes.**
   2. This is important, but it is not priority over fluid volume balance. Curling's ulcer is an acute peptic ulcer of the duodenum resulting as a complication from severe burns when reduced plasma volume leads to sloughing of the gastric mucosa.
   3. Prevention of infection is priority but not prior to maintaining fluid and electrolyte balance for the first 48 to 72 hours. The client will die if fluid and electrolyte balance is not maintained.
   4. An escharotomy, an incision that releases the scar tissue, prevents the body from being able to expand and enables chest excursion in circumferential chest burns. The client has not had time to develop eschar.

3. 1. This is a pertinent problem because the body's protective barrier, the skin, has been compromised and there is an impaired immune response, but it is not priority over pain.
   2. **Pain is the client's priority problem. The client has a full-thickness burn, which has no pain but the deep partial-thickness burns are very painful.**
   3. Burn wound edema, pain, and potential joint contractures can cause mobility deficits, but the first priority is preventing infection so wound healing can occur.

4. After the initial 48 to 72 hours, fluid and electrolyte imbalance is no longer priority. This client is 4 days post–initial burn.

4. 1, 2, and 5 are correct.
   1. **Hand washing is the number one intervention used to prevent infection, which is priority for the client with a burn.**
   2. **The client is at risk for infection and visitors with infections should not be allowed to visit the client.**
   3. The client must have a high-protein diet to help with tissue growth.
   4. Invasive lines and tubing should be changed daily.
   5. **Prophylactic antibiotics are administered to help prevent infection.**

5. 1. **The UAP can put the pulse oximeter on the client's finger and record the number. Ms. Kathy must evaluate the reading to determine if it is within normal limits.**
   2. The dressing change is a sterile procedure; therefore, this cannot be delegated to the UAP.
   3. This is a medication and the nurse cannot delegate medication administration to a UAP.
   4. Kathy cannot delegate assessment to the UAP.

6. 1. Severe pain would be expected in a client with these types of burns; therefore, it would not warrant notifying the healthcare provider.
   2. **A pulse oximeter reading greater than 93% is WNL. Therefore, a 90% reading indicates the client is in respiratory distress and requires Mr. Rob to notify the healthcare provider.**
   3. The client's vital signs show an elevated temperature, pulse, and respiration, along with a low blood pressure, but these vital signs would not be unusual for a client with severe burns.
   4. Fluid and electrolyte balance must be evaluated to ensure the output is at least 30 mL an hour. This output is within normal limits; therefore, the data do not warrant notifying a HCP.

7. 1. Ice should never be applied to a burn because this will worsen the tissue damage by causing vasoconstriction.
   2. **Cool water gives immediate and striking relief from pain and limits local tissue edema and damage.**
   3. Burn ointment should not be applied until the burning has stopped. The client should first put the hand in cool water.

4. The client should be told to go to the emergency department, not the doctor's office, for burn care.

8. 1. The skin should be kept dry. The skin should be patted completely dry after each bath.
   2. The client should be pre-medicated, but is not the responsibility of the UAPs to ensure this intervention is implemented.
   3. Clients should be turned at least every 1 to 2 hours to prevent pressure areas on the skin. Prevention of pressure areas is priority to a client with a burn.
   4. All employees in any healthcare facility are responsible for providing care within their scope of services. UAPs can turn clients to help prevent pressure ulcers.

9. 1. The UAP cannot touch TPN; it is administered via a subclavian line and should be considered a medication. The nurse cannot delegate assessment, teaching, evaluation, medications, or an unstable client.
   2. The UAP can care for a client receiving a continuous tube feeding and should elevate the HOB to prevent aspiration pneumonia.
   3. The UAP can assist a client with a meal.
   4. The UAP can add Thick-It to water prior to giving it to a client; it will help prevent the client from choking.

10. 1. The client with full- and partial-thickness burns is expected to have pain and it should be assessed but not prior to a client having difficulty breathing.
    2. The client does not have 30 mL urine output an hour (this should be 240 mL/8 hours) and the client should be assessed but not prior to a client with airway problems.
    3. When determining which client to see first, Ms. Glada should use Maslow's Hierarchy of Needs and assess the client with airway problems first.
    4. No palpable pulse indicates neurovascular compromise but it is not priority over airway problems.

Hematological and Immunological Management

All the kindness which a man puts out into the world works on the heart and thoughts of mankind.

—Albert Schweitzer

QUESTIONS

1. The client diagnosed with breast cancer who is positive for the *BRCA* gene is requesting advice from the nurse about treatment options. Which statement is the nurse's best response?
   1. "If it were me in this situation, I would consider having a bilateral mastectomy."
   2. "What treatment options has your healthcare provider (HCP) discussed with you?"
   3. "You should discuss your treatment options with your HCP."
   4. "Have you talked with your significant other (SO) about the treatment options available to you?"

2. The staff nurse answers the telephone on a medical unit and the caller tells the nurse that he has planted a bomb in the facility. Which actions should the nurse implement? **Select all that apply.**
   1. Do not touch any suspicious object.
   2. Call 911, the emergency response system.
   3. Try to get the caller to provide additional information.
   4. Immediately pull the red emergency wall lever.
   5. Write down exactly what the caller says.

3. The new graduate working on a medical unit night shift is concerned that the charge nurse is drinking alcohol on duty. On more than one occasion, the new graduate has smelled alcohol when the charge nurse returns from a break. Which action should the new graduate nurse implement first?
   1. Confront the charge nurse with the suspicions.
   2. Talk with the night supervisor about the concerns.
   3. Ignore the situation unless the nurse cannot do her job.
   4. Ask to speak to the nurse educator about the problem.

4. The nurse is completing a head-to-toe assessment on a client diagnosed with breast cancer and notes a systolic murmur that the nurse was not informed of during report. Which action should the nurse implement first?
   1. Notify the HCP about the new cardiac complication.
   2. Document the finding in the client's chart and tell the charge nurse.
   3. Check the chart to determine whether this is the first time a murmur has been identified.
   4. Ask the client whether she has ever been told she has an abnormal heartbeat.

5. The client diagnosed with lung cancer has a hemoglobin and hematocrit (H&H) of 13.4 mg/dL and 40.1, a WBC count of 7800, and a neutrophil count of 62%. Which action should the nurse implement?
   1. Place the client in reverse isolation.
   2. Notify the HCP.
   3. Make sure no flowers are taken into the room.
   4. Continue to monitor the client.

6. The charge nurse observes two unlicensed assistive personnel (UAPs) arguing in the hallway. Which action should the nurse implement first in this situation?
   1. Tell the manager to check on the UAPs.
   2. Instruct the UAPs to stop arguing in the hallway.
   3. Have the UAPs go to a private room to talk.
   4. Mediate the dispute between the UAPs.

7. The graduate nurse is working with an unlicensed assistive personnel (UAP) who has been an employee of the hospital for 12 years. However, tasks delegated to the UAP by the graduate nurse are frequently not completed. Which action should the graduate nurse take first?
   1. Tell the charge nurse the UAP will not do tasks as delegated by the nurse.
   2. Write up a counseling record with objective data and give it to the manager.
   3. Complete the delegated tasks and do nothing about the insubordination.
   4. Address the UAP to discuss why the tasks are not being done as requested.

8. The client is diagnosed with laryngeal cancer and is scheduled for a laryngectomy next week. Which intervention would be priority for the clinic nurse?
   1. Assess the client's ability to swallow.
   2. Refer the client to a speech therapist.
   3. Order the client's preoperative lab work.
   4. Discuss the client's operative permit.

9. The charge nurse is making assignments for the surgical unit. Which client should be assigned to the new graduate nurse?
   1. The 84-year-old client who has a chest tube that is draining bright red blood.
   2. The 38-year-old client who is 1 day postoperative with a temperature of 101.2°F.
   3. The 42-year-old client who has just returned to the unit after a breast biopsy.
   4. The 55-year-old client who is complaining of unrelenting abdominal pain.

10. Which task is most appropriate for the surgical nurse to assign to the licensed practical nurse (LPN)?
    1. Tell the LPN to administer the aminoglycoside antibiotic to the client.
    2. Request the LPN to empty the client's indwelling urinary catheter.
    3. Instruct the LPN to assess the client who was just transferred from PACU.
    4. Ask the LPN to determine if the client understands the discharge teaching.

11. The primary nurse informs the shift manager that one of the unlicensed assistive personnel (UAPs) is falsifying vital signs. Which action should the shift manager implement first?
    1. Notify the unit manager of the potential situation of falsifying vital signs.
    2. Take the assigned client's vital signs and compare them with the UAP's results.
    3. Talk to the UAP about the primary nurse's allegation.
    4. Complete a counseling record and place in the UAP's file.

12. The client tells the nurse, "I am not sure my surgeon is telling me the truth about my prognosis." The nurse knows the client has terminal cancer but the healthcare provider is not telling the client per the family's request. Which statement is the nurse's best response?
    1. "I think you should know you have terminal cancer."
    2. "You do have a right to a second opinion."
    3. "You are concerned your surgeon is not telling you the truth."
    4. "I think you should talk to your surgeon about your concerns."

13. The nurse hung the wrong intravenous antibiotic for the postoperative client. Which intervention should the nurse implement first?
1. Assess the client for any adverse reactions.
2. Complete the incident or adverse occurrence report.
3. Administer the correct intravenous antibiotic medication.
4. Notify the client's healthcare provider.

14. The 24-year-old male client diagnosed with testicular cancer is scheduled for a unilateral orchiectomy. Which priority intervention should the clinic nurse implement?
1. Teach the client to turn, cough, and deep breathe.
2. Discuss the importance of sperm banking.
3. Explain about the testicular prosthesis.
4. Refer the client to the American Cancer Society (ACS).

15. The female client in the preoperative holding area tells the nurse that she had a reaction to a latex diaphragm. Which intervention should the nurse perform first?
1. Notify the operating room personnel.
2. Label the client's chart with the allergy.
3. Place a red allergy band on the client.
4. Inform the client to tell all HCPs of the allergy.

16. The nurse, a licensed practical nurse (LPN), and the unlicensed assistive personnel (UAP) are caring for clients in a critical care unit. Which task would be most appropriate for the nurse to assign/delegate?
1. Instruct the UAP to obtain the client's serum glucose level.
2. Request the LPN to change the central line dressing.
3. Ask the LPN to bathe the client and change the bed linens.
4. Tell the UAP to obtain urine output for the 12-hour shift.

17. Which task should the critical care nurse delegate to the unlicensed assistive personnel (UAP)?
1. Check the pulse oximeter reading for the client on a ventilator.
2. Take the client's sterile urine specimen to the laboratory.
3. Obtain the vital signs for the client in an Addisonian crisis.
4. Assist the HCP with performing a paracentesis at the bedside.

18. The critical care charge nurse is making client assignments. Which client should the charge nurse assign to the nurse who is pregnant?
1. The client with intracavity radiation for cervical cancer who developed ARDS.
2. The client who is HIV positive and admitted for chest pain R/O myocardial infarction.
3. The client who is immunosuppressed and diagnosed with cytomegalovirus (CMV).
4. The client receiving I131 iodine for hyperthyroidism who had a motor vehicle accident (MVA).

19. The intensive care nurse is caring for a client and notes blood oozing out from under the Tegaderm dressing over the peripheral intravenous site, bleeding gums, and blood in the indwelling urinary catheter bag. Which intervention should the nurse implement first?
1. Check the client's hemoglobin/hematocrit (H&H) level.
2. Monitor the client's pulse oximeter reading.
3. Apply pressure to the intravenous site.
4. Notify the client's healthcare provider.

20. A client diagnosed with AIDS dementia is angry and yells at everyone entering the room. None of the critical care staff want to be assigned to this client. Which intervention would be most appropriate for the nurse manager to use in resolving this situation?
1. Explain that this attitude is a violation of the client's rights.
2. Request the HCP to transfer the client to the medical unit.
3. Discuss some possible options with the nursing staff.
4. Try to find a nurse who does not mind being assigned to the client.

21. Which situation would prompt the healthcare team to utilize the client's advance directive when needing to make decisions for the client?
    1. The client with a head injury who is exhibiting decerebrate posturing.
    2. The client with a C-6 SCI who is on a ventilator.
    3. The client in ESRD who is being placed on dialysis.
    4. The client diagnosed with terminal cancer who is mentally retarded.

22. Which staff nurse should the charge nurse in the intensive care unit (ICU) send to the medical unit?
    1. The nurse who has worked in the unit for 18 months.
    2. The nurse who is orienting to the critical care unit.
    3. The nurse who has been working at the hospital for 2 months.
    4. The nurse who has 12 years' experience in this ICU unit.

23. The confused client in the critical care unit is attempting to pull out the IV line and the indwelling urinary catheter. Which action should the nurse implement first?
    1. Ask a family member to stay with the client.
    2. Request the UAP to stay with the client.
    3. Place the client in a chest restraint.
    4. Notify the HCP to obtain a restraint order.

24. Which tasks should the long-term care nurse delegate to the unlicensed assistive personnel (UAP)? **Select all that apply.**
    1. Instruct the UAP to perform the a.m. care for the clients.
    2. Tell the UAP to wash the hair of the female clients.
    3. Ask the UAP to cut the toenails of the clients.
    4. Request the UAP to turn the clients every shift.
    5. Instruct the UAP to empty the clients' wastebaskets.

25. The nurse notes the unlicensed assistive personnel (UAP) tied a sheet around the client in the chair so the client will not fall out. Which action should the nurse implement first?
    1. Praise the UAP for being concerned about the safety of the client.
    2. Remove the sheet from the client immediately.
    3. Explain to the UAP the sheet is a form of restraint and cannot be tied around the client.
    4. Assess the client's need for restraints and notify the healthcare provider for an order.

26. The charge nurse in the long-term care center is making assignments for licensed practical nurses (LPNs) and unlicensed assistive personnel (UAPs) on the day shift. Which task is most appropriate to assign to the LPN?
    1. Instruct the LPN to place anti-thrombolism hose on the client.
    2. Ask the LPN to escort the client outside to smoke a cigarette.
    3. Tell the LPN to administer the tube feeding to the client.
    4. Request the LPN to change the client's colostomy bag.

27. The nurse is caring for clients on a skilled nursing unit. Which task should not be delegated to the unlicensed nursing personnel (UAP)?
    1. Instruct the UAP to apply sequential compression devices to the client on strict bed rest.
    2. Ask the UAP to assist the radiology tech to perform a STAT portable chest x-ray.
    3. Request the UAP to prepare the client for a wound debridement at the bedside.
    4. Tell the UAP to obtain the intakes and outputs for all the clients on the unit.

28. The older adult client receiving chemotherapy complains that food just does not taste like it used to. Which intervention should the medical unit nurse implement first?
    1. Ask the dietician to consult with the client on food preferences.
    2. Medicate the client before meals with an antiemetic medication.
    3. Ask the HCP to suggest an over-the-counter nutritional supplement.
    4. Check the client's current weight with the client's usual weight.

29. The nurse is assigned to a quality improvement committee to decide on a quality improvement project for the unit. Which issue should the nurse discuss at the committee meetings?
    1. Systems that make it difficult for the nurses to do their job.
    2. How unhappy the nurses are with their current pay scale.
    3. Collective bargaining activity at a nearby hospital.
    4. The number of medication errors committed by another nurse.

30. The female nurse is discussing an upcoming surgical procedure with a 76-year-old male client diagnosed with cancer. Which action is an example of the ethical principle of fidelity?
    1. The nurse makes sure the client understands the procedure before signing the permit.
    2. The nurse refuses to disclose the client's personal information to the CNO.
    3. The nurse tells the client his diagnosis when the family did not want him to know.
    4. The nurse tells the client that she does not know the client's diagnosis.

31. Which client laboratory data should the nurse report to the HCP immediately?
    1. The elevated amylase report on a client diagnosed with acute pancreatitis.
    2. The elevated WBC count on a client diagnosed with a septic leg wound.
    3. The urinalysis report showing many bacteria in a client receiving chemotherapy.
    4. The serum glucose level of 235 mg/dL on a client diagnosed with type 1 diabetes.

32. The charge nurse in a long-term care facility is reviewing the male resident's laboratory data and notes the following: H&H, 13/39; WBC count, 5.25 (10^3); and platelets, 39 (10^3). Which instructions should the nurse give to the unlicensed assistive personnel (UAP) caring for the client?
    1. Place the client in reverse isolation immediately.
    2. Administer oxygen during strenuous activities.
    3. Do not shave the resident with a safety razor.
    4. Check the resident's temperature every 4 hours.

33. The clinic RN manager is discussing osteoporosis with the clinic staff. Which activity is an example of a secondary nursing intervention when discussing osteoporosis?
    1. Obtain a bone density evaluation test on a female client older than 50.
    2. Perform a spinal screening examination on all female clients.
    3. Encourage the client to walk 30 minutes daily on a hard surface.
    4. Discuss risk factors for developing osteoporosis.

34. A client had an allergic reaction to penicillin, an antibiotic, and was admitted to the hospital 2 weeks ago. The client is being seen at the clinic for a follow-up visit. Which priority intervention should the nurse implement?
    1. Recommend the client wear a medical alert bracelet.
    2. Encourage the client to tell the pharmacy about the allergy.
    3. Tell the client not to be around any person taking penicillin.
    4. Allow the client to ventilate feelings about the hospitalization.

35. Which action would be most appropriate for the clinic nurse who suspects another staff nurse of stealing narcotics from the clinic?
    1. Confront the staff nurse with the suspicion.
    2. Call the state board of nurse examiners.
    3. Notify the director of nurses immediately.
    4. Report the suspicion to the clinic's HCP.

36. The clinic nurse administered 200,000 units of intramuscular penicillin to a client. Which priority intervention should the nurse implement?
    1. Place a bandage over the intramuscular injection site.
    2. Tell the client to put a warm compress over the injection site.
    3. Document the medication injection in the client's chart.
    4. Inform the client to stay in the waiting room for 30 minutes.

37. The female home health (HH) aide calls the office and reports pain after feeling a pulling sensation in her back when she was transferring the client from the bed to the wheelchair. Which priority action should the HH nurse tell the HH aide?
    1. Explain how to perform isometric exercises.
    2. Instruct her to go to the local emergency room.
    3. Tell her to complete an occurrence report.
    4. Recommend that she apply an ice pack to the back.

38. The female client with osteoarthritis is 6 weeks postoperative for open reduction and internal fixation of the right hip. The home health (HH) aide tells the HH nurse the client will not get in the shower in the morning because she "hurts all over." Which action would be most appropriate by the HH nurse?
    1. Tell the HH aide to allow the client to stay in bed until the pain goes away.
    2. Instruct the HH aide to get the client up to a chair and give her a bath.
    3. Explain to the HH aide that the client should get up and take a warm shower.
    4. Arrange an appointment for the client to visit her healthcare provider.

39. The home health (HH) nurse is discussing the care of a client with an HH aide. Which task can the HH nurse delegate to the HH aide?
    1. Instruct the HH aide to assist the client with a shower.
    2. Ask the HH aide to prepare the breakfast meal for the client.
    3. Request that the HH aide take the client to an HCP's appointment.
    4. Tell her to show the client how to use a glucometer.

40. The home health (HH) care agency director is teaching a class to the HH aides concerning safety in HH nursing. Which statement by the HH aide indicates the director needs to re-teach safety information?
    1. "It is all right to call the agency if I am afraid of going into the home."
    2. "I should wear my uniform and name tag when I go into the home."
    3. "I must take my cellular phone when visiting the client's home."
    4. "It is all right if I don't wear gloves when touching bodily fluids."

41. The home healthcare (HH) agency director is making assignments. Which client should be assigned to the most experienced HH nurse?
    1. The client who is recovering from Guillain-Barré syndrome who reports being tired all the time.
    2. The client who has multiple Stage 3 and 4 pressure ulcers on the sacral area.
    3. The client who is 2 weeks postoperative for laryngectomy secondary to laryngeal cancer.
    4. The client who is being discharged from service within the next week.

42. The home health (HH) nurse is visiting a female client diagnosed with colon cancer who has had a sigmoid colostomy. The client is crying and tells the nurse that she was told the cancer has spread and she will die very soon. Which intervention should the nurse implement?
    1. Discuss the possibility of being placed on hospice services.
    2. Contact the client's oncologist to discuss the client's prognosis.
    3. Ask the client whether she has planned her funeral services.
    4. Recommend the client get a second opinion concerning her prognosis.

43. The client tells the home health (HH) nurse, "My oncologist told me they can't do anything else for my cancer. I do not want my children to know, but I had to tell someone. You won't tell them, will you?" Which statement is the nurse's best response?
    1. "Since you told me about the prognosis, I must talk to your children."
    2. "I don't think it is a good idea not to tell your children; they should know."
    3. "I will not say anything to your children, but I will contact the HH doctor."
    4. "You are concerned I might talk to your children about your prognosis."

44. The home health (HH) hospice nurse is making rounds. Which client should the nurse assess first?
1. The client with end-stage heart failure who has increasing difficulty breathing.
2. The client whose family has planned to surprise her with an early birthday party.
3. The client who is complaining of being tired and irritable all the time.
4. The client with chronic lung disease who has not eaten for 3 days.

45. A client diagnosed with cancer and receiving chemotherapy is brought to the emergency department (ED) after vomiting bright red blood. Which intervention should the nurse implement first?
1. Check to see which antineoplastic medications the client has received.
2. Start an IV of normal saline with an 18-gauge intravenous catheter.
3. Investigate to see whether the client has a do not resuscitate (DNR) order written.
4. Call the oncologist to determine what lab work to order.

46. The nurse is called to the room of a male client diagnosed with lung cancer by the client's wife because the client is not breathing. The client has discussed having a DNR order written but has not made a decision. Which interventions should the nurse implement first?
1. Ask the spouse whether she wants the client to be resuscitated.
2. Tell the spouse to leave the room and then perform a slow code.
3. Assess the client's breathing and call a code from the room.
4. Notify the oncologist the client has arrested.

47. The female client who is dying asks to see her son, but the son refuses to come to the hospital. Which action should the nurse implement first?
1. Call the son and tell him he must come to see his mother before it is too late.
2. Ask the social worker to call the son and see whether the son will come to the hospital.
3. Check with the family to see whether they can discuss the issue with the son.
4. Do nothing because to intervene in a private matter would be boundary crossing.

48. The nurse is caring for clients on an oncology unit. Which client should the nurse assess first?
1. The client diagnosed with leukemia who is afebrile and has a white blood cell (WBC) count of 100,000 mm³.
2. The client who has undergone four rounds of chemotherapy and is nauseated.
3. The client diagnosed with lung cancer who has absent breath sounds in the lower lobes.
4. The client diagnosed with rule out (R/O) breast cancer who had a negative biopsy this a.m.

49. The nurse caring for clients on an oncology unit is administering medications. Which medication should the nurse administer first?
1. The antinausea medication to the male client who thinks he may get sick.
2. The pain medication to the female client who has pain she rates a 2.
3. The loop diuretic to the female client who had an output greater than the intake.
4. The nitroglycerin paste to the male client who is diagnosed with angina pectoris.

50. The staff nurse is caring for a client who was diagnosed with pancreatic cancer during an exploratory laparotomy. Which client problem is priority for postoperative day 1?
1. Ineffective coping.
2. Fluid and electrolyte imbalance.
3. Risk for infection.
4. Potential for suicidal thoughts.

QUESTIONS

51. The male client who was just told he has 6 months to live tells the nurse, "This can't be happening. I am too young to die." Which statement is the nurse's best response?
1. "I can contact the chaplain to come talk to you."
2. "I will leave you alone and come back in a little while."
3. "Is there anyone I can call to come be with you?"
4. "If it is all right with you I am going to sit here with you."

52. The nurse administered pain medication 30 minutes ago to a client diagnosed with terminal cancer. Thirty minutes after the medication, the client tells the nurse "I don't think you gave me anything. My pain is even worse than before." Which intervention(s) should the nurse implement? **Select all that apply.**
1. Attempt to determine whether the client is experiencing spiritual distress.
2. Ask the client to rate the current pain on the numeric pain scale.
3. Reposition the client to relieve pressure on the pain site.
4. Call the HCP to request an increase in pain medication.
5. Explain to the client he or she should relax and let the medication take effect.

53. Which member of the healthcare team should be assigned to a dying client who is having frequent symptoms of distress?
1. The unlicensed assistive personnel (UAP) who can be spared to sit with the client.
2. The licensed practical nurse (LPN) who has grown attached to the family.
3. The registered nurse (RN) who has experience as a hospice nurse.
4. The registered nurse (RN) who graduated 2 months ago.

54. During the morning assessment, the client diagnosed with cancer complains of nausea most of the time. Based on the client's medication administration record (MAR), which intervention should the day nurse implement first?

Client's Name: Mr. B		Admit Number: 543216		Allergies: NKDA
Height: 67 inches		Weight: 74.2 kg 163 pounds		Diagnosis: Cancer of the Pancreas
Date:	Medication	0701–1500	1501–2300	2301–0700
	Morphine sulfate 2 mg q2 hours PRN IVP			
	Promethazine (Phenergan) 12.5 mg IVP q4 hours PRN			
	Prochlorperazine (Compazine) 5 mg PO tid PRN			
	Hydrocodone (Vicodin) PO q4–6 hours PRN 5 mg			
Signature/Initials		Day Nurse RD/DN	Night Nurse RN/NN	

1. Administer the prescribed antiemetic promethazine (Phenergan) PRN.
2. Administer the prescribed antiemetic prochlorperazine (Compazine) ac.
3. Discuss changing the order for Compazine to routine with the HCP.
4. Assess the client to see whether pain is the cause of the nausea.

55. The infection control nurse notices a rise in nosocomial infection rates on the surgical unit. Which action should the infection control nurse implement first?
1. Hold an in-service for the staff on the proper method of hand washing.
2. Tell the unit manager to decide on a corrective measure.
3. Arrange to observe the staff at work for several shifts.
4. Form a hospital-wide quality improvement project.

56. The unlicensed assistive personnel (UAP) is preparing to provide postmortem care to a client with a questionable diagnosis of anthrax. Which instruction is priority for the nurse to provide to the UAP?
    1. The UAP is not at risk for contracting an illness.
    2. The UAP should wear a mask, gown, and gloves.
    3. The UAP may skip performing postmortem care.
    4. Ask whether the UAP is pregnant before she enters the client's room.

57. The client on a medical unit died of a communicable disease. Which information should the nurse provide to the mortuary workers?
    1. No information can be released to the mortuary service.
    2. The nurse should tell the funeral home the client's diagnosis.
    3. Ask the family for permission to talk with the mortician.
    4. Refer the funeral home to the HCP for information.

58. The nurse and unlicensed assistive personnel (UAP) are caring for a group of clients on a medical unit. Which action by the UAP requires immediate intervention by the nurse?
    1. The UAP dons unsterile gloves before emptying a urinary catheter bag.
    2. The UAP places clean linen in all of the clients' rooms for the day.
    3. The UAP uses a different plastic bag for every client when getting ice.
    4. The UAP massages the client's trochanter when turning the client.

59. The charge nurse is making assignments on a surgical unit. Which client should be assigned to the least experienced nurse?
    1. The client who had a vaginal hysterectomy and still has an indwelling catheter.
    2. The client who had an open cholecystectomy and has gray drainage in the tube.
    3. The client who had a hip replacement and states something popped while walking.
    4. The client who had a Whipple procedure and reports being thirsty all the time.

60. The unit manager on an oncology unit receives a complaint about the care a client received from the night shift nurse. Which action should the unit manager implement first?
    1. Ask the night charge nurse to make sure the nurse does the work.
    2. Request the nurse come in to discuss the care provided.
    3. Discuss the situation with the client making the complaint.
    4. Document this occurrence and place in the nurse's employee file.

61. The female client was admitted to the orthopedic unit for injuries received during a domestic argument. The client tells the nurse, "I am afraid my husband will kill me if I leave him. It was my fault anyway." Which statement is the nurse's best response?
    1. "What did you do to set him off like that?"
    2. "Do you have a plan for safety if you go back?"
    3. "Why do you think it was your fault?"
    4. "You should leave him before it is too late."

62. The husband of a client on the surgical unit comes to the desk and asks the nurse, "What is my wife's biopsy report?" Which intervention is the nurse's best action?
    1. Check the chart to see whether the client has allowed the spouse to have information.
    2. Obtain the pathology report and tell the husband the results of the biopsy.
    3. Call the HCP and arrange a time for the husband to meet with the HCP.
    4. Inform the client and husband of the biopsy results at the same time.

63. A new graduate nurse is assigned to work with an unlicensed assistive personnel (UAP) to provide care for a group of clients. Which action by the graduate nurse is the best method to evaluate whether delegated care is being provided?
    1. Check with the clients to see whether they are satisfied.
    2. Ask the charge nurse whether the UAP is qualified.
    3. Make rounds to see that the clients are being turned.
    4. Watch the UAP perform all the delegated tasks.

64. The charge nurse is making assignments on a pediatric unit. Which client should be assigned to the licensed practical nurse (LPN)?
1. The 6-year-old client diagnosed with sickle cell crisis.
2. The 8-year-old client diagnosed with biliary atresia.
3. The 10-year-old client diagnosed with anaphylaxis.
4. The 11-year-old client diagnosed with pneumonia.

65. The nurse administered erythropoietin alpha (Epogen), a biological response modifier, to a client diagnosed with anemia. Which of the following data indicates the client may be experiencing an adverse reaction?
1. BP 200/124.
2. Apical pulse 54.
3. Hematocrit 38%.
4. Long bone pain.

66. The client diagnosed with sickle cell disease complains of joint pain rated 10 on a pain scale of 1 to 10. Which intervention should the nurse implement first?
1. Administer a narcotic analgesic to the client.
2. Check the ID prior to administering the medication.
3. Assess the client to rule out (R/O) complications.
4. Obtain the medication from the narcotics box.

67. The nurse is caring for a client diagnosed with acquired immunodeficiency syndrome (AIDS). Which client problem is priority?
1. Body image disturbance.
2. Impaired coping.
3. Risk for infection.
4. Self-care deficit.

68. The nurse and licensed practical nurse (LPN) are caring for clients on an oncology unit. Which client should be assigned to the LPN?
1. The client diagnosed with acute leukemia who is on a continuous infusion of antineoplastic medications.
2. The client newly diagnosed with cancer of the lung who is being admitted for placement of an implanted port.
3. The client diagnosed with an ovarian tumor weighing 22 pounds who is being prepared for surgery in the morning.
4. The client diagnosed with pancreatic cancer who complains of frequent, unrelenting abdominal pain.

69. The nurse has received the morning shift report on an oncology unit. Which client should the nurse assess first?
1. The client diagnosed with leukemia who has a white blood cell (WBC) count of 1.2 (10^3).
2. The client diagnosed with a brain tumor who has a headache rated as a 2 on a pain scale of 1 to 10.
3. The client diagnosed with breast cancer who is upset and crying.
4. The client diagnosed with lung cancer who is dyspneic on exertion.

70. The nurse is caring for a female client diagnosed with systemic lupus erythematosus (SLE). Which of the following client-reported data has priority?
1. The client reports that she has trouble finding makeup to cover the rash across her nose.
2. The client tells the unlicensed assistive personnel (UAP) to close the drapes because sunlight is bad for her.
3. The client notices a bright red color in the bedside commode.
4. The client complains of joint stiffness and requests a pain medication.

71. The nurse caring for a client newly diagnosed with protein calorie malnutrition secondary to acquired immune deficiency syndrome (AIDS) writes a nursing problem of "altered nutrition: less than body requirements." Which nursing interventions should the nurse implement? **Select all that apply.**
1. Place the client on daily weights.
2. Have the client identify preferred foods.
3. Refer to the dietician.
4. Monitor bedside glucose levels four times a day.
5. Perform central line dressing changes every 72 hours.

72. The client diagnosed with congestive heart failure and iron deficiency anemia is prescribed a unit of packed red blood cells (PRBC). Rank the interventions in order of performance.
1. Administer furosemide (Lasix), a loop diuretic, between units.
2. Check the client's hemoglobin and hematocrit.
3. Assess the client's lung sounds and periphery.
4. Have the client sign a permit to receive blood.
5. Return the empty blood bags to the laboratory.

73. The nurse working in a rheumatology clinic is teaching a 34-year old female client with rheumatoid arthritis (RA) about the disease-modifying antirheumatic drug methotrexate. Which information has the highest priority?
1. Teach the client to take measures to ensure she does not become pregnant.
2. Inform the client to keep the follow-up appointments with the clinic.
3. Have the client see a dietician if she loses her appetite.
4. Tell the client to keep a diary of her symptoms to bring to appointments with her.

74. The 28-year-old female client in the outpatient clinic has been told that her test for the human immune deficiency virus (HIV) is positive. Which interventions should the nurse implement? **Select all that apply.**
1. Discuss having regular gynecological examinations.
2. Assist the client to make her funeral arrangements.
3. Refer the client to a social worker.
4. Encourage the client to take the highly active antiretroviral therapy (HAART).
5. Teach the client to follow a healthy life style.

HEMATOLOGICAL AND IMMUNOLOGICAL CLINICAL SCENARIO

Ms. Cindy is the charge nurse on an inpatient oncology unit. She is working with two RNs, Ms. Mary and Ms. Kathy, along with an LPN, Ms. Brenda, and two UAPs, Ms. Teresa and Ms. Paula. They are working on Saturday from 0700 to 1900. There are 10 clients on the 15-bed unit.

1. Ms. Mary and Ms. Brenda are caring for clients. Which client should be assigned to the LPN, Ms. Brenda?
   1. The client newly diagnosed with chronic lymphocytic leukemia.
   2. The client who is 4 hours post-procedure bone marrow biopsy.
   3. The client who is receiving PRBCs with hemoglobin of 6.
   4. The client who is receiving antineoplastic medications.

2. Which client should Ms. Cindy assign to the medical-surgical nurse who is being pulled to work on the oncology unit for this shift?
   1. The client diagnosed with non-Hodgkin's lymphoma who is having complications from daily radiation treatments.
   2. The client diagnosed with Hodgkin's disease who is being prepared for a bone marrow transplant.
   3. The client diagnosed with leukemia who has petechiae covering both anterior and posterior body surfaces.
   4. The client diagnosed with ovarian cancer who is 1 day postoperative total abdominal hysterectomy.

3. Ms. Kathy, an RN, and Ms. Teresa, the UAP, are caring for a group of clients. Which information provided by Ms. Teresa warrants immediate intervention by Ms. Kathy?
   1. The client diagnosed with bladder cancer who has bright red blood in the urinal.
   2. The client receiving chemotherapy who is complaining of pain in the mouth.
   3. The client with a biological response modifier who has a T 99.2°F, P 68, R 24, and BP of 198/102.
   4. The client receiving a steroid who is complaining of having a rounded swollen face.

4. Ms. Kathy is caring for a client that is 1 day postoperative sigmoid resection and notes bright red bleeding on the midline abdominal incision. Which intervention should Ms. Kathy implement first?
   1. Assess the client's vital signs.
   2. Reinforce the abdominal dressing.
   3. Notify the healthcare provider.
   4. Place the client in the Trendelenburg position.

5. Which nursing task should Ms. Kathy, the RN, delegate to Ms. Paula, the UAP?
   1. Discontinue the client's subclavian intravenous catheter.
   2. Empty the Jackson Pratt drainage tube and record amount.
   3. Determine if the client's pain medication has been effective.
   4. Perform irrigation for the client who is 2 days post-op abdominoperineal resection.

6. The client is 2 days post-ureterosigmoidostomy for cancer of the bladder. Which assessment data warrants Ms. Mary notifying the HCP?
   1. The client has excreted urine from the rectum.
   2. The client's abdominal incision is slightly reddened.
   3. The client has an apical rate of 98 and B/P 114/80.
   4. The client has a low-grade fever and a hard, rigid abdomen.

7. Ms. Mary identifies a problem of "anticipatory grieving" for a client diagnosed with Stage 4 ovarian cancer. Which nursing intervention is priority for this client?
   1. Request the client is referred to hospice.
   2. Encourage the client to make plans for her funeral.
   3. Allow the client to verbalize feelings about having cancer.
   4. Discuss an advance directive and a power of attorney for healthcare.

8. The client diagnosed with ovarian cancer has had five courses of chemotherapy. Which laboratory data warrant immediate intervention by Ms. Mary?
   1. Absolute neutrophil count (ANC) of 681 mm/dL.
   2. Platelet count of 175,000.
   3. Red blood cell count of 5.0×10^6.
   4. Hemoglobin of 11.2 and hematocrit 37%.

9. Ms. Mary is performing a head-to-toe assessment on a Hispanic client diagnosed with prostate cancer. The nurse notes an irregular-shaped lesion with some scabbed-over areas surrounding the lesion. Which intervention should Ms. Mary implement first?
   1. Take no action since this is a common lesion found on Hispanic skin.
   2. Assess the lesion by completing the ABCDs of skin cancer.
   3. Document the findings in the client's nurse's notes.
   4. Instruct the client to make sure the HCP checks the lesion.

10. The female client diagnosed with pancreatic cancer has an advance directive (AD) stipulating no cardiopulmonary resuscitation. Which intervention should Ms. Kathy implement first?
    1. Notify the client's healthcare provider about the AD.
    2. Determine if the client has discussed the AD with significant others.
    3. Place a copy of the advance directive in the client's chart.
    4. Give the original advance directive to the client.

CLINICAL SCENARIO

ANSWERS AND RATIONALES

The correct answer number and rationale for why it is the correct answer are given in **boldface type.** Rationales for why the other possible answer options are incorrect also are given, but they are not in boldface type.

1. 1. This is boundary crossing because the nurse does not have breast cancer. The nurse should assess what information the client is really seeking and then explain the treatment or refer the client, as appropriate.
   2. **The nurse must assess what information the client actually needs. To do this, the nurse must know what treatment options have been suggested to the client. Assessment is the first step in the nursing process.**
   3. This may be needed after the nurse further assesses the situation, but this is not the first intervention.
   4. The client needs information about treatment options from a designated HCP; the significant other would not have such information/suggestions.
   Content – Medical/Surgical: ***Category of Health Alteration –*** *Oncology:* ***Integrated Processes –*** *Nursing Process: Assessment:* ***Client Needs –*** *Health Promotion and Maintenance:* ***Cognitive Level –*** *Analysis*

2. 1, 3, and 5 are correct.
   1. **The nurse should begin a systematic search of the unit after activating the bomb scare emergency plan, and if any suspicious objects are found the nurse should not touch them, and should notify the bomb squad.**
   2. The nurse should notify the house supervisor and administration because they are responsible for notifying the police department.
   3. **The nurse should stay calm and try to keep the caller on the telephone. The nurse should attempt to get as much information from the caller as possible. The nurse can jot a note to someone nearby to initiate the bomb scare procedure.**
   4. The red emergency levers in hospitals are to notify the fire departments of a fire, not a bomb scare.
   5. **The nurse should try to transcribe exactly what the caller says; this may help identify who is calling and where a bomb might be placed.**
   Content – Management: ***Category of Health Alteration –*** *Oncology:* ***Integrated Processes –*** *Nursing Process: Implementation:* ***Client Needs –*** *Safe and Effective Care Environment: Safety and Infection Control:* ***Cognitive Level –*** *Comprehension*

MAKING NURSING DECISIONS: The nurse must be knowledgeable of hospital emergency preparedness. Students as well as new employees receive this information in hospital orientations and are responsible for implementing procedures correctly. The NCLEX-RN® blueprint includes questions on the Safe and Effective Care Environment.

3. 1. The new graduate must work under this charge nurse; confronting the nurse would not resolve the issue because the nurse can choose to ignore the new graduate. Someone in authority over the charge nurse must address this situation with the nurse.
   2. **The night supervisor or the unit manager has the authority to require the charge nurse to submit to drug screening. In this case, the supervisor on duty should handle the situation.**
   3. The new graduate is bound by the nursing practice acts to report potentially unsafe behavior regardless of the position the nurse holds.
   4. The nurse educator would not be in a position of authority over the charge nurse.
   Content – Management: ***Category of Health Alteration –*** *Oncology:* ***Integrated Processes –*** *Nursing Process: Implementation:* ***Client Needs –*** *Safe and Effective Care Environment: Management of Care:* ***Cognitive Level –*** *Application*

MAKING NURSING DECISIONS: When the nurse is deciding on a course of action involving other staff members, a rule of thumb is this: If the individual the nurse is concerned about is superior in job title to the nurse, then the nurse should go through the chain of command to the next level of superior. If the individual is subordinate in job title to the nurse, then the nurse should confront the individual.

4. 1. This should be done if the murmur is a new finding; however, the nurse should investigate the finding further before notifying the HCP.
   2. This should be done, but assessing the client's situation is the nurse's priority.
   3. **Although the client was not admitted for a cardiac problem, she may have had a murmur for a while, and the previous nurse did not pick it up or did not mention it in the report because it was a long-standing physiological finding in this client. The nurse should research the chart for a current history and physical to determine whether the HCP is aware of the condition.**

4. The nurse should not ask the client because this could scare or alarm the client needlessly.
   Content – Medical/Surgical: **Category of Health Alteration** *– Oncology:* **Integrated Processes** *– Nursing Process: Assessment:* **Client Needs** *– Physiological Integrity: Reduction of Risk Potential:* **Cognitive Level** *– Analysis*

5. 1. The client's lab work does not indicate an increased risk for infection. The client does not need to be placed in reverse isolation.
   2. The lab work is within normal limits. The nurse does not need to notify the HCP.
   3. The client is not at an increased risk for infection; therefore, the client may have flowers in the room.
   4. **This client's lab work is within normal limits. The nurse should continue to monitor the client.**
   Content – Medical/Surgical: **Category of Health Alteration** *– Hematology:* **Integrated Processes** *– Nursing Process: Implementation:* **Client Needs** *– Physiological Integrity: Reduction of Risk Potential:* **Cognitive Level** *– Analysis*

6. 1. The nurse should stop the behavior occurring in a public place. The charge nurse can discuss the issue with the UAPs and determine whether the manager should be notified.
   2. **The first action is to stop the argument from occurring in a public place. The charge nurse should not discuss the UAPs' behavior in public.**
   3. The second action is to have the UAPs go to a private area before resuming the conversation.
   4. The charge nurse may need to mediate the disagreement; this would be the third step.
   Content – Management: **Category of Health Alteration** *– Hematology:* **Integrated Processes** *– Communication and Documentation:* **Client Needs** *– Safe and Effective Care Environment: Management of Care:* **Cognitive Level** *– Comprehension*

7. 1. The graduate nurse should handle the situation directly with the UAP first before notifying the charge nurse.
   2. This may need to be completed, but not prior to directly discussing the behavior with the UAP.
   3. The graduate nurse must address the insubordination with the UAP, not just complete the tasks that are the responsibility of the UAP.
   4. **The graduate nurse must discuss the insubordination directly with the UAP first. The nurse must give objective data as to when and where the UAP did not follow through with the completion of assigned tasks.**
   Content – Management: **Category of Health Alteration** *– Oncology:* **Integrated Processes** *– Communication and Documentation:* **Client Needs** *– Safe and Effective Care Environment: Management of Care:* **Cognitive Level** *– Application*

8. 1. The client's ability to swallow is not impaired prior to the surgical procedure.
   2. **The client will not be able to speak after the removal of the larynx; therefore, referral to a speech therapist who will be able to discuss an alternate means of communication is priority.**
   3. The HCP, not the nurse, is responsible for ordering the preoperative laboratory work.
   4. The HCP, not the nurse, is responsible for discussing the operative permit.
   Content – Oncology: **Category of Health Alteration** *– Oncology:* **Integrated Processes** *– Nursing Process: Planning:* **Client Needs** *– Physiological Integrity: Physiological Adaptation:* **Cognitive Level** *– Synthesis*

MAKING NURSING DECISIONS: The test taker must be aware of the setting that ultimately dictates the appropriate intervention. The adjectives will clue the test taker to the setting. In this question, the words "clinic nurse" clue the test taker to the setting. The test taker must also remember the nurse's scope of practice and realize that options 3 and 4 are outside the nurse's scope of practice.

9. 1. This client is not stable and requires a more experienced nurse.
   2. An elevated temperature indicates a potential complication of surgery; therefore, this client requires a more experienced nurse.
   3. **Of the four clients, the one who is most stable is the client who has just undergone a breast biopsy; therefore, this client would be the most appropriate to assign to a new graduate nurse.**
   4. Unrelenting pain requires further assessment; therefore, the client should be assigned to a more experienced nurse.
   Content – Medical/Surgical: **Category of Health Alteration** *– Oncology:* **Integrated Processes** *– Nursing Process: Planning:* **Client Needs** *– Safe and Effective Care Environment: Management of Care:* **Cognitive Level** *– Synthesis*

MAKING NURSING DECISIONS: When the test taker is deciding which client should be assigned to a new graduate, the most stable client should be assigned to the least experienced nurse.

10. 1. **The LPN can administer intravenous antibiotic medication according to the LPN scope of practice.**
    2. The UAP should be instructed to empty the indwelling urinary catheter, not the LPN.
    3. The LPN should not be assigned to assess a client.

4. The LPN should not be assigned to evaluate the client's understanding of the discharge teaching.

Content – Medical/Surgical: **Category of Health Alteration** *– Oncology:* **Integrated Processes** *– Nursing Process: Planning:* **Client Needs** *– Safe and Effective Care Environment: Management of Care:* **Cognitive Level** *– Synthesis*

MAKING NURSING DECISIONS: The nurse cannot assign assessment, teaching, evaluation, or an unstable client to an LPN.

11. 1. This should not be implemented until verification of the allegation is complete, and the shift manager has discussed the situation with the UAP.

2. **The shift manager should have objective data about the allegation of falsifying vital signs prior to confronting the UAP; therefore, the shift manager should take the client's vital signs and compare them with the UAP's results before taking any other action.**

3. The shift manager should not confront the UAP until objective data are obtained to support the allegation.

4. Written documentation should be the last action when resolving staff issues.

Content – Management: **Category of Health Alteration** *– Oncology:* **Integrated Processes** *– Nursing Process: Implementation:* **Client Needs** *– Safe and Effective Care Environment: Management of Care:* **Cognitive Level** *– Application*

12. 1. If the nurse tells the client the truth at this time, the client may ask, "What happens now? How long do I have to live?" In this situation, the nurse should not tell the client the truth.

2. The client does have a right to a second opinion but in this situation the nurse should encourage the client to talk to the surgeon.

3. This is a therapeutic response that encourages the client to ventilate his or her feelings, but the client needs answers. This is not the best response by the nurse.

4. **Since the nurse knows the client is terminal, it would be best for the nurse to encourage the client to talk to the surgeon. The client needs the truth and the surgeon is the person who should tell it to the client.**

Content – Medical/Surgical: **Category of Health Alteration** *– Oncology:* **Integrated Processes** *– Nursing Process: Implementation:* **Client Needs** *– Psychosocial Integrity:* **Cognitive Level** *– Analysis*

MAKING NURSING DECISIONS: The nurse needs to be able to guide clients to the correct person when they have questions about their healthcare.

13. 1. **The nurse should first assess the client prior to taking any other action to determine if the client is experiencing any untoward reaction.**

2. An incident report must be completed by the nurse, but not prior to taking care of the client.

3. The nurse should administer the correct medication, but not prior to assessing the client.

4. The client's HCP must be notified but the nurse should be able to provide the HCP with pertinent client information, so this is not the first intervention.

Content – Medical/Surgical: **Category of Health Alteration** *– Oncology:* **Integrated Processes** *– Nursing Process: Implementation:* **Client Needs** *– Physiological Integrity: Pharmacological and Parenteral Therapies:* **Cognitive Level** *– Analysis*

MAKING NURSING DECISIONS: Whenever something happens to the client, the nurse should first assess the client prior to taking any other action.

14. 1. The client must be taught postoperative care, but this is not the priority intervention of the clinic nurse.

2. **Sperm banking will allow the client's sperm to be kept until the time the client wants to conceive a child. This is priority because it must be done between the clinic visit and admission to the hospital for the procedure. The unilateral orchiectomy will not result in sterility, but the subsequent treatments may cause sterility.**

3. The nurse can discuss the testicular prosthesis, but this is not priority over sperm banking because the prosthesis may or may not be inserted at the time of surgery.

4. A referral to the ACS is appropriate, but is not the most important information a 24-year-old male client needs at this time.

Content – Oncology: **Category of Health Alteration** *– Oncology:* **Integrated Processes** *– Nursing Process: Planning:* **Client Needs** *– Physiological Integrity: Physiological Adaptation:* **Cognitive Level** *– Synthesis*

15. 1. **Because the client is in the preoperative holding area, the immediate safety need for the client is to inform the operating room personnel so that no latex gloves or equipment will come into contact with the client. Person-to-person communication for a safety issue ensures that the information is not overlooked.**

2. The nurse should label the chart with the allergy, but because the client is in the preoperative holding area, this is not the first intervention.

3. The nurse should place a red allergy band on the client, but because the client is in the preoperative holding area, this is not the first intervention.
4. The nurse should always teach the client, but at this time the first intervention is the client's safety, which is why the OR team should be notified.

Content – Medical/Surgical: **Category of Health Alteration** *– Oncology:* **Integrated Processes** *– Communication and Documentation:* **Client Needs** *– Physiological Integrity: Reduction of Risk Potential:* **Cognitive Level** *– Application*

16. 1. The serum blood glucose level requires a venipuncture, which is not within the scope of the UAP's expertise. The laboratory technician would be responsible for obtaining a venipuncture.
2. This is a sterile dressing change and requires assessing the insertion site for infection; therefore, this would not be the most appropriate task to assign to the LPN.
3. The nurse should ask the UAP to bathe the client and change bed linens because this is a task the UAP can perform. The LPN could be assigned higher-level tasks.
4. **The UAP can add up the urine output for the 12-hour shift; however, the nurse is responsible for evaluating whether the urine output is what is expected for the client.**

Content – Management of Care: **Category of Health Alteration** *– Oncology:* **Integrated Processes** *– Nursing Process: Planning:* **Client Needs** *– Safe and Effective Care Environment: Management of Care:* **Cognitive Level** *– Synthesis*

MAKING NURSING DECISIONS: When the test taker is deciding which option is the most appropriate task to delegate/assign, the test taker should choose the task that allows each member of the staff to function at his or her full scope of practice. Do not assign a task to a staff member that requires a higher level of expertise than the staff member has, and do not assign a task to a staff member when another staff member with a lower level of expertise can do it.

17. 1. The client on the ventilator is unstable; therefore, the nurse should not delegate any tasks to the UAP.
2. **The UAP can take specimens to the laboratory; it is not medications and not vital to the client.**
3. The client in an Addisonian crisis is unstable; therefore, the nurse should not delegate any tasks to the UAP.
4. The UAP cannot assist the HCP with an invasive procedure at the bedside.

Content – Medical/Surgical: **Category of Health Alteration** *– Oncology:* **Integrated Processes** *– Nursing Process: Planning:* **Client Needs** *– Safe and Effective Care Environment: Management of Care:* **Cognitive Level** *– Synthesis*

MAKING NURSING DECISIONS: The nurse cannot delegate assessment, teaching, evaluation, medication, or an unstable client to a UAP.

18. 1. The client with intracavity radiation could cause problems with the pregnant nurse's fetus, so she should not be assigned to this client.
2. **The pregnant nurse can be assigned to a client who is HIV positive. The nurse must adhere to Standard Precautions.**
3. The cytomegalovirus could harm the nurse's fetus, so the pregnant nurse should not be assigned to this client.
4. The I131 is radioactive iodine and a pregnant nurse should not be near radiation.

Content – Medical/Surgical: **Category of Health Alteration** *– Hematology:* **Integrated Processes** *– Nursing Process: Planning:* **Client Needs** *– Safe and Effective Care Environment: Management of Care:* **Cognitive Level** *– Synthesis*

MAKING NURSING DECISIONS: The NCLEX-RN® has questions asking the test taker to address making assignments on units. Nurses who are pregnant should not care for clients whose condition can harm the fetus.

19. 1. The nurse will need to check the client's H&H but not prior to notifying the HCP. The client has disseminated intravascular coagulation (DIC).
2. Monitoring the client's pulse oximeter reading would be an intervention the nurse could implement but it is not the first intervention for a client with DIC.
3. Applying pressure to the IV site will not help stop the bleeding since the client's coagulation factors have been exhausted. The client must receive heparin therapy.
4. **The client is exhibiting signs of DIC, which requires intravenous therapy. This is a life-threatening complication that requires immediate medical intervention, so the nurse must notify the HCP first.**

Content – Medical/Surgical: **Category of Health Alteration** *– Hematology:* **Integrated Processes** *– Nursing Process: Implementation:* **Client Needs** *– Physiological Integrity: Reduction of Risk Potential:* **Cognitive Level** *– Analysis*

MAKING NURSING DECISIONS: When the stem of the question provides all the data needed to determine whether the client is in life-threatening distress, the nurse must contact the client's healthcare provider.

ANSWERS

20. 1. The feelings of the staff are not a violation of the client's rights. Refusing to care for the client is a violation of the client's rights.
2. Transferring the client to the medical unit solves the problem for the critical care unit, but the client's behavior should be addressed by the healthcare team. This is not the most appropriate intervention for the nurse manager.
3. **This would be the most appropriate intervention because it allows the staff to have input into resolving the problem. When staff have input into resolving the situation, then there is ownership of the problem.**
4. One nurse cannot be on duty 24 hours a day. The nurse manager should try to allow the staff to identify options to address the client's behavior.
Content – *Management of Care:* **Category of Health Alteration** – *Hematology:* **Integrated Processes** – *Nursing Process: Planning:* **Client Needs** – *Safe and Effective Care Environment: Management of Care:* **Cognitive Level** – *Application*

21. 1. **The client must have lost decision-making capacity because of a condition that is not reversible, or must be in a condition that is specified under state law, such as a terminal, persistent vegetative state, irreversible coma, or as specified in the advance directive. A client who is exhibiting decerebrate posturing is unconscious and unable to make decisions.**
2. The client on a ventilator has not lost the ability to make healthcare decisions. The nurse can communicate by asking the client to blink his or her eyes to yes/no questions.
3. The client receiving dialysis is alert and does not lose the ability to make decisions; therefore, the advance directive should not be consulted to make decisions for the client.
4. Mental retardation does not mean the client cannot make decisions for him- or herself unless the client has a legal guardian who has a durable power of attorney for healthcare. If the client has a legal guardian, then the client cannot complete an advance directive.
Content – *Medical/Surgical:* **Category of Health Alteration** – *Oncology:* **Integrated Processes** – *Nursing Process: Assessment:* **Client Needs** – *Physiological Integrity: Basic Care and Comfort:* **Cognitive Level** – *Analysis*

22. 1. **This nurse should be sent to the medical unit because, with 18 months' experience, the nurse is familiar with the hospital routine and would be helpful to the medical unit but is not the most experienced ICU nurse on duty.**

2. The nurse who is still orienting to the unit should not be sent to the medical unit. The nurse in orientation should be kept with the nurse preceptor.
3. The nurse who is new to the hospital should not be sent to a new unit with which he or she is unfamiliar.
4. The nurse with 12 years' experience should be kept on in the ICU because his or her expertise would be more helpful for client care than a nurse with 18 months' experience.
Content – *Management:* **Category of Health Alteration** – *Oncology:* **Integrated Processes** – *Nursing Process: Planning:* **Client Needs** – *Safe and Effective Care Environment: Management of Care:* **Cognitive Level** – *Synthesis*

23. 1. The family may or may not be able to control the client's behavior but the nurse should not ask a family member first. The CCU usually has mandated visiting hours.
2. **The nurse should first ensure the client's safety by having someone stay at the bedside with the client, and then call the HCP, and finally apply mitt restraints.**
3. This is a form of restraint and is against the law unless the nurse has a healthcare provider's order. This is the least restrictive form of restraint but would not be helpful if the client is pulling at tubes.
4. The nurse must notify the healthcare provider before putting the client in restraints; restraints must be used only in an emergency situation, for a limited time, and for the protection of the client.
Content – *Medical/Surgical:* **Category of Health Alteration** – *Hematology:* **Integrated Processes** – *Nursing Process: Implementation:* **Client Needs** – *Safe and Effective Care Environment: Safety and Infection Control:* **Cognitive Level** – *Application*

24. 1 and 2 are correct.
1. **The UAP can perform a.m. care; therefore, this can be delegated to the UAP.**
2. **Washing the hair of female clients can be delegated to the UAP.**
3. The UAP should not cut the toenails of clients; this should be referred to a podiatrist.
4. The clients should be turned every 2 hours, not every shift.
5. The housekeeping department should empty the wastebaskets, not the UAP.
Content – *Medical/Surgical:* **Category of Health Alteration** – *Hematology:* **Integrated Processes** – *Nursing Process: Planning:* **Client Needs** – *Safe and Effective Care Environment: Management of Care:* **Cognitive Level** – *Synthesis*

MAKING NURSING DECISIONS: The nurse cannot delegate assessment, teaching, evaluation, medications, and an unstable client to the UAP.

25. 1. The nurse can praise the UAP for safety concerns but first the sheet must be removed because it is a form of restraint and is illegal.
    2. **The nurse must remove the sheet since it is a restraint. There must be an HCP's order prior to restraining a client.**
    3. The nurse should discuss the restraint policy with the UAP but not prior to removing the restraint.
    4. The nurse should determine if the client needs restraints for safety and then call and obtain the order, but not prior to removing the sheet. A chest restraint could be used to secure the client to the chair if needed.
       Content – Medical/Surgical: **Category of Health Alteration** – Hematology: **Integrated Processes** – Nursing Process: Implementation: **Client Needs** – Safe and Effective Care Environment: Safety and Infection Control: **Cognitive Level** – Application

MAKING NURSING DECISIONS: The nurse must ensure the UAP provides legal and ethical nursing care to the clients in the long-term care facility.

26. 1. The UAP could place anti-thrombolism hose on the client.
    2. The UAP should not escort the client outside to smoke a cigarette, the UAP will be off the unit and this encourages poor health habits.
    3. **The LPN should administer a tube feeding, not the UAP.**
    4. The UAP can change a colostomy bag on a client who has had it for an extended period of time, which is implied since the client is in a long-term care center.
       Content – Medical/Surgical: **Category of Health Alteration** – Hematology: **Integrated Processes** – Nursing Process: Planning: **Client Needs** – Safe and Effective Care Environment: Management of Care: **Cognitive Level** – Synthesis

MAKING NURSING DECISIONS: The charge nurse should not assign a task to the LPN that a UAP could implement.

27. 1. The UAP can apply sequential compression devices to the client on strict bed rest.
    2. The UAP can assist with a portable STAT chest x-ray as long as it is not a female UAP who is pregnant.
    3. **The client will need to be pre-medicated for a wound debridement; therefore, this task cannot be delegated to the UAP.**
    4. The UAP can obtain intake and outputs for clients.
       Content – Medical/Surgical: **Category of Health Alteration** – Hematology: **Integrated Processes** – Nursing Process: Planning: **Client Needs** – Safe and

Effective Care Environment: Management of Care: **Cognitive Level** – *Synthesis*

MAKING NURSING DECISIONS: The nurse cannot delegate assessment, teaching, evaluation, medications, and an unstable client to the UAP. The nurse cannot delegate premedicating the client.

28. 1. Asking the dietitian to consult with the client is a good intervention, but the nurse should assess the impact of the change in taste on the client.
    2. The client did not complain of nausea. Antiemetic medication is used to prevent nausea associated with food odors and attempting to eat.
    3. The nurse can recommend an over-the-counter supplement to increase nutrition, but the nurse should first assess the impact of the problem. Over-the-counter supplements are expensive, and the nurse should suggest the client try malts, milkshakes, and fortified soups. Then, if the client does not like or gets tired of the taste, a family member can consume the food and it is not wasted.
    4. **Checking the client's weight change over a period of time is the first step in assessing the client's nutritional status and the impact of the taste changes on the client.**
       Content – Medical/Surgical: **Category of Health Alteration** – Oncology: **Integrated Processes** – Nursing Process: Assessment: **Client Needs** – Physiological Integrity: Reduction of Risk Potential: **Cognitive Level** – Analysis

MAKING NURSING DECISIONS: The test taker should employ a systematic approach to problem-solving. The nursing process is a systematic approach, and assessment is the first step of the nursing process.

29. 1. **A quality improvement project looks at the way tasks are performed and attempts to see whether the system can be improved. A medication delivery system in which it takes a long time for the nurse to receive a STAT or "now" medication is an example of a system that needs improvement and should be addressed by a quality improvement committee.**
    2. Financial reimbursement of the staff is a management issue, not a quality improvement issue.
    3. Collective bargaining is an administrative issue, not a quality improvement issue.
    4. The number of medication errors committed by a nurse is a management-to-nurse issue and does not involve a systems issue, unless several nurses have committed the same

error because the system is not functioning appropriately.

Content – Management: **Category of Health Alteration –** *Hematology:* **Integrated Processes –** *Nursing Process: Implementation:* **Client Needs** *– Safe and Effective Care Environment: Safety and Infection Control:* **Cognitive Level** *– Application*

30. 1. This is an example of autonomy. The client needs all pertinent information prior to making an informed choice.
    2. **This is an example of fidelity. Fidelity is the duty to be faithful to commitments and involves keeping information confidential and maintaining privacy and trust.**
    3. This is an example of veracity, the duty to tell the truth.
    4. This is an example of nonmalfeasance, the duty to do no harm. This avoids telling a client facing surgery that he has cancer.

Content – Nursing Ethics: **Category of Health Alteration –** *Oncology:* **Integrated Processes –** *Nursing Process: Implementation:* **Client Needs** *– Psychosocial Integrity:* **Cognitive Level** *– Comprehension*

31. 1. An elevated amylase would be expected in a client diagnosed with acute pancreatitis. The nurse would not need to call the HCP immediately.
    2. An elevated WBC would be expected in a client diagnosed with a septic (infected) leg wound. The nurse would not need to call the HCP immediately.
    3. **The urinalysis report showing many bacteria is indicative of an infection. Clients receiving chemotherapy are at high risk of developing an infection. The nurse should notify the HCP immediately.**
    4. This blood glucose level is above normal range but would not be particularly abnormal for a client diagnosed with type 1 diabetes. The nurse would not need to call the HCP immediately.

Content – Medical/Surgical: **Category of Health Alteration –** *Oncology:* **Integrated Processes –** *Nursing Process: Assessment:* **Client Needs** *– Physiological Integrity: Reduction of Risk Potential:* **Cognitive Level** *– Analysis*

32. 1. The resident's WBC count is within normal limits and indicates an ability to resist infection. The nurse should not place this resident in reverse isolation.
    2. The resident's H&H is slightly lower than normal but not low enough to cause dyspnea during activity. The resident does not need oxygen.
    3. **The resident's platelet count is very low and could cause the resident to bleed.**

The nurse should initiate bleeding precautions that include not using sharp blades to shave the resident and using soft-bristle toothbrushes.
    4. The client is not at risk for developing an infection. The client does not need his temperature checked every 4 hours.

Content – Medical/Surgical: **Category of Health Alteration –** *Hematology* **Integrated Processes –** *Nursing Process: Implementation:* **Client Needs** *– Physiological Integrity: Reduction of Risk Potential:* **Cognitive Level** *– Analysis*

33. 1. **A secondary nursing intervention includes screening for early detection. The bone density evaluation will determine the density of the bone and is diagnostic for osteoporosis.**
    2. Spinal screening examinations are performed on adolescents to detect scoliosis. This is a secondary nursing intervention, but not to detect osteoporosis.
    3. Teaching the client is a primary nursing intervention. This is an appropriate intervention to help prevent osteoporosis, but it is not a secondary intervention.
    4. Discussing risk factors is an appropriate intervention, but it is not a secondary nursing intervention.

Content – Medical/Surgical: **Category of Health Alteration –** *Hematological:* **Integrated Processes –** *Nursing Process: Analysis:* **Client Needs** *– Health Promotion and Maintenance:* **Cognitive Level** *– Comprehension*

34. 1. **This is the nurse's priority intervention because any emergency personnel who may come into contact with the client should be aware of the client's allergy. A penicillin allergy can kill the client.**
    2. The client's pharmacy can be made aware of the allergy, but this is helpful only when the client is having prescriptions filled.
    3. Unless the client has an allergy to penicillin dust, which is rare, coming into contact with another person taking penicillin will not cause the client to have an allergic reaction.
    4. Therapeutic communication allows the client to ventilate feelings, which is an appropriate intervention, but it is not priority over teaching the client how to prevent a potentially life-threatening reaction.

Content – Medical/Surgical: **Category of Health Alteration –** *Hematological:* **Integrated Processes –** *Nursing Process: Implementation:* **Client Needs** *– Physiological Integrity: Physiological Adaptation:* **Cognitive Level** *– Analysis*

35. 1. The clinic nurse should not confront the staff nurse without objective data that support the allegation.
2. The state board of nurse examiners cannot do anything to the nurse until the nurse has been convicted of the crime. Many states have programs to help addicted nurses, and some states may revoke the nurse's license to practice nursing.
3. **The clinic nurse should report the suspicions so that appropriate actions can be taken, such as a urine drug screen for the nurse, watching the nurse for the behavior, and possibly notifying the police department.**
4. The nurse should follow the chain of command, which does not include the HCP.
*Content – Legal: **Category of Health Alteration –** Hematological: **Integrated Processes –** Communication and Documentation: **Client Needs –** Safe and Effective Care Environment: Management of Care: **Cognitive Level –** Application*

36. 1. The nurse can or cannot place a bandage over the injection site. This is not a priority intervention.
2. Warm compresses will help increase the absorption of the medication, but this is not the priority nursing intervention.
3. The medication injection must be documented in the client's chart in a clinic, just as it must be in an acute care area, but documentation is not priority over a possible life threatening allergic reaction.
4. **The client is at risk for having an allergic reaction to the penicillin, which is a life-threatening complication. Therefore, the client must stay in the waiting room for at least 30 minutes so the nurse can determine whether an allergic reaction is occurring.**
*Content – Medical/Surgical: **Category of Health Alteration –** Hematological: **Integrated Processes –** Nursing Process: Evaluation: **Client Needs –** Physiological Integrity: Pharmacological and Parenteral Therapies: **Cognitive Level –** Application*

37. 1. Isometric exercises such as weight lifting increase muscle mass. The HH nurse should not instruct the HH aide to do this type of exercises.
2. The HH aide may go to the emergency department, but the HH nurse should address the aide's back pain. Many times, the person with back pain does not need to be seen in the emergency room.
3. An occurrence report explaining the situation is important documentation and should be completed. It provides the staff member

with the required documentation to begin a workers' compensation case for payment of medical bills. However, the HH nurse on the phone should help decrease the HH aide's pain, not worry about paperwork.
4. **The HH aide is in pain, and applying ice to the back will help decrease pain and inflammation. The HH nurse should be concerned about a co-worker's pain. Remember: Ice for acute pain and heat for chronic pain.**
*Content – Medical/Surgical: **Category of Health Alteration –** Musculoskeletal: **Integrated Processes –** Nursing Process: Implementation: **Client Needs –** Safe and Effective Care Environment: Safety and Infection Control: **Cognitive Level –** Application*

38. 1. Allowing the client to stay in bed is inappropriate because a client with osteoarthritis should be encouraged to move, which will decrease the pain.
2. A bath at the bedside does not require as much movement from the client as getting up and walking to the shower. This is not an appropriate action for a client with osteoarthritis.
3. **Movement and warm or hot water will help decrease the pain; the worst thing the client can do is not to move. The HH aide should encourage the client to get up and take a warm shower or bath.**
4. Osteoarthritis is a chronic condition, and the HCP could not do anything to keep the client from "hurting all over."
*Content – Medical/Surgical: **Category of Health Alteration –** Musculoskeletal: **Integrated Processes –** Nursing Process: Implementation: **Client Needs –** Physiological Integrity: Reduction of Risk Potential: **Cognitive Level –** Comprehension*

39. 1. **The HH aide's responsibility is to care for the client's personal needs, which include assisting with a.m. care.**
2. The HH aide is not responsible for cooking the client's meals.
3. The HH aide is not responsible for taking the client to appointments. This also presents an insurance problem, since the client is in the HH aide's car.
4. Even in the home, the HH nurse should not delegate teaching.
*Content – Management of Care: **Category of Health Alteration –** Hematological: **Integrated Processes –** Nursing Process: Planning: **Client Needs –** Safe and Effective Care Environment: Management of Care: **Cognitive Level –** Synthesis*

MAKING NURSING DECISIONS: The nurse cannot delegate assessment, evaluation, teaching, medications, or care of an unstable client to a UAP, including an HH aide.

40. 1. If the HH aide is fearful for any reason, the HH aide should not go into the home and should notify the agency. The employee's safety is important. This statement does not require re-teaching.
    2. For safety purposes, the HH aide should be clearly identified when entering the client's neighborhood and home. This statement does not require re-teaching.
    3. The HH aide should be able to contact the HH nurse or agency about any potential or actual concerns. This is for the safety of the client as well as the employee. This statement does not require re-teaching.
    4. **Standard precautions apply in the home as in the hospital. If the HH aide has the potential to touch the client's bodily fluids, then the aide should wear gloves and wash his or her hands. The statement indicates the HH aide needs re-teaching.**
    Content – Medical/Surgical: **Category of Health Alteration** *– Musculoskeletal* **Integrated Processes** *– Teaching/Learning:* **Client Needs** *– Safe and Effective Care Environment: Safety and Infection Control:* **Cognitive Level** *– Analysis*

MAKING NURSING DECISIONS: According to the NCLEX-RN® test blueprint, staff education is a component of the management of care.

41. 1. The client diagnosed with Guillain-Barré syndrome would have been on bed rest for days to weeks and would be in a debilitated state; therefore, reports of being tired all the time would be expected. This client would not require the most experienced nurse.
    2. **The client with pressure ulcers requires meticulous nursing care and a nurse who has experience with wounds. The most experienced nurse should be assigned this client.**
    3. The client with a laryngectomy has received teaching prior to and after the procedure and would not require extensive teaching or nursing care; therefore, this client would not require the most experienced nurse.
    4. Discharge teaching starts on admission into the home healthcare agency; therefore, most of the teaching would have been completed, and this client would not need the most experienced nurse.
    Content – Medical/Surgical: **Category of Health Alteration** *– Integumentary:* **Integrated Processes** *– Nursing Process: Planning:* **Client Needs** *– Safe and Effective Care Environment: Management of Care:* **Cognitive Level** *– Synthesis*

42. 1. **Hospice is a service for clients who have less than 6 months to live. If the client has been told she will die "very soon,"** then this is probably less than 6 months. If the client does not die within the 6 months, she will not automatically be discharged from hospice. Each client is assessed individually for the need to remain in hospice care. If the client does not want any heroic measures and wants to die at home, then hospice will provide these services. This intervention would be appropriate for the HH nurse.
    2. The HH nurse is not responsible for discussing the client's prognosis. The oncologist would have to write a letter stating the client had less than 6 months to live to be placed on hospice services. The client should discuss this with the oncologist, not the HH nurse.
    3. Because the client is crying and upset, it would be more appropriate for the nurse to discuss a plan for living and hospice services than to discuss what is going to happen after she dies. At some point this should be done, but this is not an appropriate time.
    4. The client does have a right to a second opinion, but the nurse should not tell the client this unless the client is questioning the diagnosis.
    Content – Management of Care: **Category of Health Alteration** *– Oncology:* **Integrated Processes** *– Nursing Process: Planning:* **Client Needs** *– Psychosocial Integrity:* **Cognitive Level** *– Synthesis*

43. 1. The client is an adult and the nurse must respect the client's confidentiality. The nurse does not have to tell the children.
    2. This is giving advice and is not the nurse's role.
    3. **The nurse not telling the children respects the client's wishes and confidentiality but the healthcare providers should be told of new client circumstances, as the information applies to the client's care.**
    4. This is a therapeutic response but the client did not indicate that she or he thought the nurse would talk about the client's status to the children. The client just wanted to tell someone.
    Content – End-of-Life: **Category of Health Alteration** *– Oncology:* **Integrated Processes** *– Nursing Process: Assessment:* **Client Needs** *– Psychological Integrity: End-of-Life Care:* **Cognitive Level** *– Analysis*

MAKING NURSING DECISIONS: When the test taker is deciding on a therapeutic response, then the test taker must determine whether there is a response that directly addresses the problem or whether a therapeutic conversation is indicated.

44. 1. **This client may need oxygen or an intervention to keep the client comfortable. This client should be seen first.**

2. This client does not have priority over difficulty breathing.

3. This client does not have priority over difficulty breathing.

4. This client does not have priority over difficulty breathing.

Content – Medical/Surgical: **Category of Health Alteration** *– Cardiovascular:* **Integrated Processes** *– Nursing Process: Assessment:* **Client Needs** *– Physiological Integrity: Reduction of Risk Potential:* **Cognitive Level** *– Analysis*

MAKING NURSING DECISIONS: The test taker should apply some systematic approach when answering priority questions. Maslow's Hierarchy of Needs should be used when determining which client to assess first. The test taker should start at the bottom of the pyramid, where physiological needs are priority.

45. 1. The medications are not important at this time. The client is bleeding.

 2. **The client is at risk for shock. The nurse should take steps to prevent vascular collapse. Starting the IV is the priority.**

 3. This is not important in the emergency department.

 4. Prevention of circulatory collapse is the priority. The nurse could anticipate an order for a complete blood count (CBC) and a type and crossmatch.

Content – Medical/Surgical: **Category of Health Alteration** *– Oncology:* **Integrated Processes** *– Nursing Process: Implementation:* **Client Needs** *– Physiological Integrity: Reduction of Risk Potential:* **Cognitive Level** *– Application*

MAKING NURSING DECISIONS: The test taker must be aware of the setting, which dictates the appropriate intervention. The adjectives will cue the test taker to the setting, in this case, the emergency department. The test taker must also remember the nurse's scope of practice. Starting an IV with normal saline is within a nurse's scope of practice.

46. 1. It is too late to ask this question. This decision must be made prior to an arrest situation.

 2. The nurse should not hesitate to call a code, and a full code must be performed, not a slow code.

 3. **These are the first steps of a code.**

 4. This should be done by someone at the desk, not by the nurse responding to the emergency.

Content – Medical/Surgical: **Category of Health Alteration** *– Respiratory:* **Integrated Processes** *– Nursing Process: Implementation:* **Client Needs** *– Physiological Integrity: Reduction of Risk Potential:* **Cognitive Level** *– Application*

MAKING NURSING DECISIONS: The nurse must react immediately in an emergency situation and should not hesitate. The nurse should immediately begin cardiopulmonary resuscitation (CPR) and follow the hospital's protocol.

47. 1. The son has a right to refuse to come to the hospital regardless of what the nurse thinks the son should do. The nurse is unaware of the family dynamics that led to this dilemma.

 2. This is only placing another healthcare professional in the picture and would not be the best option.

 3. **Other family members are more likely to understand the family dynamics and would be the best ones to intervene in the situation.**

 4. The nurse should attempt to assist in reconciliation between the client and her son if possible.

Content – End-of-Life: **Category of Health Alteration** *– Oncology:* **Integrated Processes** *– Caring:* **Client Needs** *– Psychosocial Integrity:* **Cognitive Level** *– Application*

48. 1. This is an expected lab value for a client diagnosed with leukemia. The client's bone marrow is overproducing immature white blood cells and clogging the bloodstream.

 2. **This client is complaining of nausea, which is an uncomfortable experience. The nurse should attempt to intervene and treat the nausea. This client should be seen first.**

 3. Absent breath sounds are expected in a client diagnosed with lung cancer.

 4. A negative biopsy is a good result. This client does not need to be seen first.

Content – Oncology: **Category of Health Alteration** *– Oncology:* **Integrated Processes** *– Nursing Process: Analysis:* **Client Needs** *– Safe and Effective Care Environment: Management of Care:* **Cognitive Level** *– Analysis*

MAKING NURSING DECISIONS: When deciding which client to assess first, the test taker should determine whether the signs/symptoms the client is exhibiting are normal or expected for the client situation. After eliminating the expected options, the test taker should determine which situation is unexpected or causing the client distress.

49. 1. **Anticipatory nausea is a very real problem for clients diagnosed with cancer and undergoing treatment. If this problem is not rectified quickly and progresses to vomiting, the client may not get relief. This medication should be administered first.**

2. This is considered mild pain and can be treated after the anticipatory nausea.

3. This is expected and indicates the medication is working. This medication does not have priority.

4. This is a routine medication and can be administered after the nausea and pain medications. Sublingual nitroglycerin is administered for acute chest pain, angina.

Content – Medical/Surgical; **Category of Health Alteration** *– Oncology:* **Integrated Processes** *– Nursing Process: Assessment:* **Client Needs** *– Physiological Integrity: Reduction of Risk Potential:* **Cognitive Level** *– Analysis*

50. 1. Ineffective coping is a psychological problem that would not have priority on the first day after major abdominal surgery.

2. **After major trauma, the body undergoes a fluid shift. The possibility of fluid and electrolyte imbalance is the top priority problem for 1 day after major abdominal surgery.**

3. This could be a priority, but a potential or risk is not priority over an actual problem.

4. A potential psychological problem would not have priority on the first day after major abdominal surgery.

Content – Medical/Surgical: **Category of Health Alteration** *– Oncology:* **Integrated Processes** *– Nursing Process: Planning:* **Client Needs** *– Physiological Integrity: Reduction of Risk Potential:* **Cognitive Level** *– Synthesis*

MAKING NURSING DECISIONS: When the test taker is deciding which client problem is priority, physiological problems usually are priority, and an actual problem is priority over a potential problem.

51. 1. The nurse should address the client's spiritual faith but at this time this is not the nurse's best response.

2. The nurse should not leave the client alone after receiving this type of news.

3. The nurse should ensure someone is with the client but it is not the nurse's best response.

4. **The nurse's best response is to stay with the client and allow the client to ventilate his feelings of denial, fear, and hopelessness.**

Content – End-of-Life: **Category of Health Alteration** *– Oncology:* **Integrated Processes** *– Nursing Process: Implementation:* **Client Needs** *– Psychosocial Integrity:* **Cognitive Level** *– Application*

MAKING NURSING DECISIONS: The nurse needs to be able to address the client's psychosocial needs and allowing the client to ventilate feelings is an appropriate intervention. A nurse who is a good listener is a very special nurse.

52. **1, 3, and 4 are correct.**
1. **Spiritual distress can greatly affect the perception of pain. If the client is not receiving relief from pain medication, the nurse should explore other variables that could affect the perception of pain.**

2. Clients experiencing chronic pain may or may not be able to rate their pain on a pain scale. The client has provided all the information about the pain that is currently needed. The pain is greater than it was before the medication.

3. **This is an alternative to medication that may provide some minimal relief while other interventions are being attempted.**

4. **The nurse should notify the HCP that the current pain regimen is not effective.**

5. This is a condescending statement and would tend to agitate the client more than help.

Content – End-of-Life: **Category of Health Alteration** *– Drug Administration:* **Integrated Processes** *– Nursing Process: Assessment:* **Client Needs** *– Physiological Integrity: Basic Care and Comfort:* **Cognitive Level** *– Analysis*

53. 1. The charge nurse should not assign a UAP to care for a client in spiritual distress. This is outside of the UAP's functions.

2. The charge nurse should not delegate or assign care based on a personal relationship of the nurse with the family. The nurse most qualified to care for the client's needs should be assigned to the client.

3. **A hospice nurse has experience in managing symptoms associated with the dying process. This is the best nurse to care for this client.**

4. A new graduate would not have the experience or knowledge to manage the symptoms as effectively as an experienced hospice nurse.

Content – End-of-Life: **Category of Health Alteration** *– Oncology:* **Integrated Processes** *– Nursing Process: Planning:* **Client Needs** *– Safe and Effective Care Environment: Management of Care:* **Cognitive Level** *– Synthesis*

MAKING NURSING DECISIONS: When the test taker is deciding which option is the most appropriate task to delegate/assign, the test taker should choose the task that allows each member of the staff to function within his or her full scope of abilities.

54. 1. The nurse could administer the Phenergan as a one-time medication administration or whenever the client asks for it, but this is not a proactive intervention.

2. **Administering the PRN Compazine prophylactically before meals is a proactive stance and assists the client in maintaining**

his or her nutrition. **This is the best action. If the client responds well to the regimen, the nurse should discuss changing the order to become a routine medication.**

3. If the client responds well to the PRN Compazine, the nurse should discuss changing the order to become a routine medication instead of just PRN.

4. The client did not complain of pain. Nausea can be caused by pain, but it can also be caused by any number of other reasons. The nurse should be concerned with controlling the symptom.

*Content – Medical/Surgical: **Category of Health Alteration** – Oncology: **Integrated Processes** – Nursing Process: Assessment: **Client Needs** – Physiological Integrity: Pharmacological and Parenteral Therapies: **Cognitive Level** – Analysis*

55. 1. The infection control nurse should evaluate the problem fully before deciding on a course of action.

2. The infection control nurse should assess the staff member's delivery of care and use standard nursing practice before deciding on a course of action with the unit manager.

3. **This is an action that will allow the infection control nurse to observe compliance with standard nursing practices such as hand washing. Once the nurse has attempted to determine a cause, then a corrective action can be implemented.**

4. The entire hospital has not shown an increased infection rate; only one unit has shown an increase.

*Content – Medical/Surgical: **Category of Health Alteration** – Oncology: **Integrated Processes** – Nursing Process: Planning: **Client Needs** – Safe and Effective Care Environment: Safety and Infection Control: **Cognitive Level** – Synthesis*

56. 1. The UAP may be at risk of contacting the illness.

2. **The UAP should wear appropriate personal proactive equipment when providing any type of care.**

3. The UAP should not be told to skip performing assigned tasks.

4. The fetus is not affected by anthrax so a pregnant nurse could care for the client, taking the same precautions as a nurse who is not pregnant.

*Content – Medical/Surgical: **Category of Health Alteration** – Respiratory: **Integrated Processes** – Nursing Process: Implementation: **Client Needs** – Safe and Effective Care Environment: Safety and Infection Control: **Cognitive Level** – Application*

57. 1. The mortuary service is considered part of the healthcare team in this case. The personnel in the funeral home should be made aware of the client's diagnosis.

2. **The mortuary service is considered part of the healthcare team. In this case, the personnel in the funeral home should be made aware of the client's diagnosis.**

3. The nurse does not need to ask the family for permission to protect the funeral home workers.

4. The nurse, not the HCP, releases the body to the funeral home.

*Content – End-of-Life: **Category of Health Alteration** – Hematological: **Integrated Processes** – Nursing Process: Implementation: **Client Needs** – Safe and Effective Care Environment: Safety and Infection Control: **Cognitive Level** – Comprehension*

58. 1. This is the correct procedure when coming into contact with blood and body fluids. The nurse does not need to intervene.

2. This may be wasteful if the linens are not used because the client is discharged, but it does not warrant immediate intervention by the nurse until the unit has a problem with linen overusage. This action saves the UAP time.

3. This is the correct procedure for getting ice. The nurse does not need to intervene.

4. **Massaging pressure points increases tissue damage and increases the risk of skin breakdown. The nurse should intervene and stop this action by the UAP.**

*Content – Medical/Surgical: **Category of Health Alteration** – Integumentary: **Integrated Processes** – Nursing Process: Analysis: **Client Needs** – Safe and Effective Care Environment: Management of Care: **Cognitive Level** – Application*

59. 1. **This client has had a common surgical procedure and is not experiencing a complication. The least experienced nurse could care for this client.**

2. Green bile in a T-tube is expected, but a gray tint to the drainage indicates an infection. An experienced nurse should be assigned to this client.

3. A popping feeling when ambulating indicates the hip joint may have dislocated. An experienced nurse should be assigned to this client.

4. A Whipple procedure involves removing most of the pancreas. The symptoms indicate the client is not metabolizing glucose (symptom of diabetes mellitus). An experienced nurse should be assigned to this client.

*Content – Medical/Surgical: **Category of Health Alteration** – Genitourinary: **Integrated Processes** – Nursing Process: Planning: **Client Needs** – Safe and*

ANSWERS

Effective Care Environment: Management of Care: ***Cognitive Level*** *– Synthesis*

60. 1. The unit manager should talk to the client first, not ask the night charge nurse to watch the nurse. This step may be needed if a doubt does surface about the nurse's performance.
2. This is the second step in this process if the manager determines the complaint is valid.
3. **The first step is to discuss the complaint with the client. This step lets the client know that the client is being heard, and the manager is able to ask any questions to clarify the complaint.**
4. The occurrence may need to be documented and placed in the employee's file, but this is not the unit manager's first intervention.
Content *– Management:* ***Category of Health Alteration*** *– Oncology:* ***Integrated Processes*** *– Communication and Documentation:* ***Client Needs*** *– Safe and Effective Care Environment: Management of Care:* ***Cognitive Level*** *– Application*

61. 1. This is blaming the client. No one has the right to abuse the client.
2. **The nurse must assess the client's safety and provide a referral to a women's center. This is the nurse's best response.**
3. The client does not owe the nurse an explanation of her feelings. This is not a good response to the client.
4. The nurse is advising. The decision whether to leave the abuser or not must be the client's decision.
Content *– Management of Care:* ***Category of Health Alteration*** *– Musculoskeletal:* ***Integrated Processes*** *– Caring:* ***Client Needs*** *– Psychosocial Integrity:* ***Cognitive Level*** *– Synthesis*

62. 1. **Even though the spouse of the client is making the request, the nurse should still check to make sure that the client has listed the husband as being allowed to receive information. The Health Insurance Portability and Accountability Act (HIPAA) regulations do not allow for release of information to anyone not specifically designated by the client.**
2. The nurse cannot do this unless the client has designated that her husband is allowed to receive information.
3. The HCP as well as the nurse must abide by HIPAA.
4. The HCP is responsible for divulging biopsy results. If the spouse is present when the HCP enters the room and the client allows the spouse to stay, then consent for receiving information is implied.

Content *– Legal:* ***Category of Health Alteration*** *– Oncology:* ***Integrated Processes*** *– Communication and Documentation:* ***Client Needs*** *– Safe and Effective Care Environment: Management of Care:* ***Cognitive Level*** *– Comprehension*

63. 1. The clients would not understand the importance of the specific tasks. Clients will tell the nurse whether the UAP is pleasant when in the room but not whether the delegated tasks have been completed.
2. The nurse retains responsibility for the delegated tasks. The charge nurse may be able to tell the nurse that the UAP has been checked off as being competent to perform the care, but would not know whether the care was actually provided.
3. **The nurse retains responsibility for the care. Making rounds to see that the care has been provided is the best method to evaluate the care.**
4. The nurse would not have time to complete his or her own work if the nurse watched the UAP perform all of the UAP's work.
Content *– Management:* ***Category of Health Alteration*** *– Oncology:* ***Integrated Processes*** *– Communication and Documentation:* ***Client Needs*** *– Safe and Effective Care Environment: Management of Care:* ***Cognitive Level*** *– Synthesis*

64. 1. A client in a crisis should be assigned to a registered nurse (RN).
2. Biliary atresia involves liver failure and multiple body systems. This client should be assigned to an RN.
3. Anaphylaxis is an emergency situation. The client should be assigned to an RN.
4. **The LPN can administer routine medications and care for clients who have no life-threatening conditions.**
Content *– Medical/Surgical:* ***Category of Health Alteration*** *– Respiratory:* ***Integrated Processes*** *– Nursing Process: Planning:* ***Client Needs*** *– Safe and Effective Care Environment: Management of Care:* ***Cognitive Level*** *– Synthesis*

65. 1. **Erythropoietin stimulates the bone marrow to produce red blood cells. An adverse reaction to Epogen is hypertension, which this client has, with a BP of 200/124. Hypertension can cause the dose of erythropoietin to be decreased or discontinued.**
2. Epogen does not affect the pulse.
3. A hematocrit of 38% would indicate the medication is effective.
4. A side effect of the medication is long bone pain. This can be treated with a non-narcotic analgesic. This is not an adverse reaction.

*Content – Medical/Surgical: **Category of Health Alteration – Hematological: Integrated Processes –** Nursing Process: Evaluation: **Client Needs –** Physiological Integrity: Pharmacological and Parenteral Therapies: **Cognitive Level –** Analysis*

66. 1. The nurse should assess the client for complications before administering the medication.
    2. This should occur, but not before assessing the client for complications.
    3. **The first step in administering a PRN pain medication is to assess the client for a complication that may require the nurse to notify the HCP or implement an independent nursing intervention.**
    4. This is not the first intervention.
    *Content – Medical/Surgical: **Category of Health Alteration – Hematological: Integrated Processes –** Nursing Process: Assessment: **Client Needs –** Physiological Integrity: Pharmacological and Parenteral Therapies: **Cognitive Level –** Analysis*

67. 1. Clients diagnosed with acquired immunodeficiency syndrome (AIDS) may have body image disturbance issues related to weight loss and Kaposi's sarcoma lesions, but these are psychological problems, and physiological problems have priority.
    2. Impaired coping is a psychological problem, and physiological problems are priority.
    3. **The basic problem with a client diagnosed with AIDS is that the immune system is not functioning normally. This increases the risk for infection. This is the priority client problem.**
    4. Self-care deficit is a psychosocial problem, not a physiological problem.
    *Content – Management of Care: **Category of Health Alteration – Hematological: Integrated Processes –** Nursing Process: Planning: **Client Needs –** Physiological Integrity: Reduction of Risk Potential: **Cognitive Level –** Synthesis*

68. 1. The infusion of antineoplastic medications is limited to chemotherapy- and biotherapy-competent registered nurses. A qualified registered nurse should be assigned to this client.
    2. This client should be assigned to a registered nurse who can answer the client's questions about the cancer and cancer treatments.
    3. **This client is pre-op, and the LPN can prepare a client for surgery. A 22-pound tumor indicates a benign ovarian cyst.**
    4. An experienced registered nurse should be assigned to this client because the client is unstable, with unrelenting pain.
    *Content – Medical/Surgical: **Category of Health Alteration – Oncology: Integrated Processes –** Nursing Process: Planning: **Client Needs –** Safe and Effective*

*Care Environment: Management of Care: **Cognitive Level –** Synthesis*

69. 1. A low WBC count is expected in a client diagnosed with leukemia. This client does not need to be assessed first.
    2. A client diagnosed with a brain tumor would be expected to have a mild headache. This client does not need to be assessed first.
    3. **The client is upset and crying. When all the information in the options is expected and not life threatening, then psychological issues have priority. This client should be seen first.**
    4. Dyspnea on exertion is expected in a client diagnosed with lung cancer. This client does not need to be assessed first.
    *Content – Medical/Surgical: **Category of Health Alteration – Oncology: Integrated Processes –** Nursing Process: Assessment: **Client Needs –** Physiological Integrity: Reduction of Risk Potential: **Cognitive Level –** Analysis*

70. 1. A butterfly rash is one of the clinical manifestations of SLE; this statement does not alert the nurse to a new finding.
    2. Photosensitivity is a clinical manifestation of SLE and does not alert the nurse to a new problem.
    3. **Bright red in the bedside commode indicates blood, alerting the nurse to possible renal involvement. The healthcare provider must be notified so that diagnostic test can be ordered and steps taken to limit the damage to the kidneys.**
    4. Joint stiffness is related to the SLE and is a clinical manifestation. The nurse will medicate the client for pain but the priority is to limit damage to the kidneys.
    *Content – Medical/Surgical: **Category of Health Alteration – Altered Immune Response: Integrated Processes –** Nursing Process: Assessment: **Client Needs –** Health Promotion and Maintenance: **Cognitive Level –** Analysis*

MAKING NURSING DECISIONS: When deciding on the priority, the test taker must decide between clinical signs/symptoms that are normally found in clients who have the diagnosis and are not life threatening and those that can be life threatening or life altering.

71. **1, 2, and 3 are correct.**
    1. **The client's daily weights will provide information as to fluid balance and nutrition deficits.**
    2. **The client's preferred foods can be used to help increase the client's appetite and should be provided whenever possible on the meal trays.**

3. The dietician can be the nurse's best ally when caring for a client with nutritional problems.

4. Glucose levels are monitored when a client is on total parenteral nutrition (TPN), not for a client newly diagnosed with a nutritional problem.

5. This would be appropriate for a client on TPN.

*Content – Medical/Surgical: **Category of Health Alteration** – Altered Immune Response: **Integrated Processes** – Nursing Process: Assessment: **Client Needs** – Health Promotion and Maintenance: **Cognitive Level** – Analysis*

MAKING NURSING DECISIONS: The test taker must note words that give a hint as to the extent of a problem, such as "newly," in the stem of the question. This eliminates options 4 and 5. Words matter. "Left" or "right," "only," "all"—words such as these can eliminate or define the option.

72. **Correct Answer: 2, 4, 3, 1, 5**

2. Of the steps listed, the nurse should check the client's hemoglobin and hematocrit. Most healthcare facilities have a procedure to administer PRBCs only when the H/H are less than 8 and 24. Blood is a scarce commodity, and unless the client is scheduled for surgery there are other means of providing care of the client without the administration of blood products.

4. The client must consent to receiving blood and blood products. If the client will not allow the blood to be administered, then the procedure stops here.

3. The nurse must determine the client's physical status prior to picking up the blood in case the nurse assesses a client situation that requires the nurse to get in touch with the healthcare provider.

1. If ordered, a diuretic is usually administered between the units of blood to prevent fluid volume overload.

5. The blood bags can be returned to the laboratory after the blood has infused.

*Content – Medical/Surgical: **Category of Health Alteration** – Hematology: **Integrated Processes** – Nursing Process: Implementation: **Client Needs** – Health Promotion and Maintenance: **Cognitive Level** – Analysis*

MAKING NURSING DECISIONS: Rank order questions can be answered by the test taker placing himself/herself at the client's bedside and asking, "What would I really do first?"

73. 1. Methotrexate can cause fetal abnormalities or loss of the fetus. The client should be placed on birth control for the duration of administration of this medication and for 2 years post.

2. This is a standard instruction for many disease processes but it is not priority over prevention of pregnancy.

3. This medication can produce nausea and nutritional intake is important, but not over preventing a pregnancy and possible complications.

4. Keeping a diary of symptoms and questions is a good idea but the priority is to prevent an unplanned pregnancy.

*Content – Medical/Surgical: **Category of Health Alteration** – Altered Immune Response: **Integrated Processes** – Nursing Process: Implementation: **Client Needs** – Health Promotion and Maintenance: **Cognitive Level** – Analysis*

MAKING NURSING DECISIONS: If the stem of the question gives an age, then it is usually an important indication of what the question is actually asking. In this question an age and a gender, female, are both given. Any time the client is a female of childbearing age, the test taker must consider there may be another potential client, the fetus.

74. **1, 4 and 5 are correct.**

1. Females who are HIV positive are at risk for multiple gynecological problems.

2. This is not in the scope of practice of a nurse, and clients newly diagnosed are living 20 years or longer with the virus.

3. Nothing in the stem indicated a need for this referral.

4. HAART regimens are responsible for the improved prognosis of HIV+ clients.

5. A healthy life style will improve the client's ability to maintain her health.

*Content – Medical/Surgical: **Category of Health Alteration** – Altered Immune Response: **Integrated Processes** – Nursing Process: Implementation: **Client Needs** – Health Promotion and Maintenance: **Cognitive Level** – Analysis*

MAKING NURSING DECISIONS: When answering select all questions, each option is answered as a true/false question. One option cannot rule out another.

CLINICAL SCENARIO ANSWERS AND RATIONALES

The correct answer number and rationale for why it is the correct answer are given in **boldface type**. Rationales for why the other possible answer options are incorrect also are given, but they are not in boldface type.

1. 1. The newly diagnosed client will need to be taught about the disease and about treatment options. The registered nurse cannot delegate teaching to an LPN.
   2. **This is post-procedure care for a stable client; therefore, Ms. Mary could assign Ms. Brenda, the LPN, to care for this client. Ms. Mary cannot assign assessment, teaching, evaluation, or an unstable client to Ms. Brenda.**
   3. This client has hemoglobin of 6, which is extremely low; this client is not stable, and should not be assigned to Ms. Brenda, the LPN.
   4. The LPN cannot administer antineoplastic (chemotherapy) medications to the client. The chemotherapy nurse must be an RN with additional education in chemotherapy medication.

2. 1. This client is receiving treatments that can have life-threatening side effects; the nurse is not experienced with this type of client.
   2. Bone marrow transplants are very specific to oncology clients; therefore, this client would not be appropriate to assign to a float nurse.
   3. This is expected in a client with leukemia, but it indicates a severely low platelet count; a nurse with more experience should care for this client.
   4. **A medical-surgical nurse should be able to care for a client who is 1 day postoperative abdominal surgery; therefore, this client can be assigned to a floating nurse.**

3. 1. This is expected from this client and does not warrant immediate attention.
   2. This is stomatitis and is expected with a client receiving chemotherapy.
   3. **Biological response modifiers that stimulate the bone marrow can increase the client's blood pressure to dangerous levels. This BP is very high and warrants immediate attention.**
   4. This client is experiencing steroid toxicity, which is called "moon" face and is expected; therefore, this client does not warrant immediate intervention.

4. 1. **Ms. Kathy should assess the client's vital signs to determine if the client is hemorrhaging. Hypotension and tachycardia indicate hemorrhaging, potentially a life-threatening emergency.**
   2. The nurse may need to reinforce the dressing if the dressing becomes too saturated, but this would be after a thorough assessment is completed.
   3. The nurse should assess the situation before notifying the HCP.
   4. The client may be put in the Trendelenburg position.

5. 1. Ms. Paula cannot discontinue a subclavian line; this is a higher level nursing intervention.
   2. **Ms. Paula can empty the JP and reapply negative pressure. Ms. Kathy cannot delegate assessment, teaching, evaluation, medications, or an unstable client.**
   3. Evaluation of the effectiveness of a PRN medication must be done by the nurse.
   4. The UAP should not do the initial colostomy irrigation, but the client would not have fecal output 2 days postoperative surgery.

6. 1. A ureterosigmoidostomy is a surgical procedure wherein the ureters, which carry urine from the kidneys, are diverted into the sigmoid colon. It is done as a treatment for bladder cancer, where the urinary bladder had to be removed. This is expected; therefore, it does not warrant notifying the HCP.
   2. This may indicate the client has an incisional infection, but the HCP can be notified of this on rounds since this is not life threatening.
   3. The AP and B/P are within normal range; therefore, this does not warrant notifying the healthcare provider.
   4. **This client is exhibiting signs/symptoms of peritonitis, which is a life-threatening complication secondary to abdominal surgery; therefore, the nurse should notify the healthcare provider.**

7. 1. Referral to hospice is an appropriate intervention for this client but it does not apply to the identified problem of anticipatory grieving.
   2. At this time the client should consider funeral arrangements but the priority intervention is to assist the client to deal with the loss of her life. That is accomplished by therapeutic communication.

3. Therapeutic communication is the priority intervention for a client diagnosed with Stage 4 cancer and an identified problem of anticipatory grieving. Allowing the client to work through the steps of grieving is accomplished by encouraging the client to express feelings.

4. An advance directive and a durable power of attorney for healthcare are appropriate interventions for a client diagnosed with Stage 4 cancer but this does not address the problem of anticipatory grieving.

8. 1. An absolute neutrophil count of 681 indicates the client does not have sufficient mature white blood cells or granulocytes to act as a defense against infections. This client needs to be placed in reverse isolation and receive Neulasta, a biological response modifier.

2. A platelet count of 175,000 is within normal range. Thrombocytopenia is less than 100,000; therefore, Ms. Mary does not need to intervene.

3. A red blood cell count of 5,000,000 is within normal limits. $(5.0 \times 10^6 [1,000,000] = 5,000,000)$.

4. This H&H is a little low but it is not life threatening; therefore, this does not warrant intervention.

9. 1. The nurse should complete an assessment of the lesion. This is not a common lesion found on Hispanic clients.

2. This is part of assessing the lesion and should be completed. The ABCDs of skin cancer detection include the following: (1) Asymmetry—Is the lesion balanced on both sides with an even surface? (2) Borders—Are the borders rounded and smooth or notched and indistinct? (3) Color—Is the color a uniform light brown or is it variegated and darker or reddish purple? (4) Diameter—A diameter exceeding 4–6 mm is considered suspicious.

3. Ms. Mary should document the findings in the chart but it is not Ms. Mary's first nursing intervention.

4. Instructing the client to also notify the HCP to assess the lesion should be done, but does not have priority.

10. 1. The HCP should be made aware of the AD so a do not resuscitate (DNR) order can be written. Only the HCP can write this order. Ms. Kathy should notify the HCP to get the DNR written immediately. The order must be written before an arrest occurs or CPR will be initiated.

2. The AD should be discussed between the client and the significant others but the AD is still valid even if the significant others do not agree and the HCP can write the DNR order based on the client's wishes.

3. A copy is placed in the client's chart to notify all healthcare team members of the client's decisions, but this is not the priority intervention.

4. Giving the client a copy of the AD is good but it is not the priority intervention.

Women's Health Management

Science may have found a cure for most evils, but it has found no remedy for the worst of them all—the apathy of human beings.

—Helen Keller

QUESTIONS

1. Which client should the postpartum nurse assess first after receiving the a.m. shift report?
   1. The client who is complaining of perineal pain when urinating.
   2. The client who saturated multiple peri-pads during the night.
   3. The client who is refusing to have the newborn in the room.
   4. The client who is crying because the baby will not nurse.

2. Which newborn infant would warrant immediate intervention by the nursery nurse?
   1. The 1-hour-old newborn who has abundant lanugo.
   2. The 6-hour-old newborn whose respirations are 52.
   3. The 12-hour-old newborn who is turning red and crying.
   4. The 24-hour-old newborn who has not passed meconium.

3. The client in labor is showing late decelerations on the fetal monitor. Which intervention should the nurse implement first?
   1. Notify the healthcare provider (HCP) immediately.
   2. Instruct the client to take slow, deep breaths.
   3. Place the client in the left lateral position.
   4. Prepare for an immediate delivery of the fetus.

4. The nurse walks into the client's room to check on the mother and her newborn. The client states another nurse just took her baby back to the nursery. Which intervention should the nurse implement first?
   1. Initiate an emergency Code Pink, indicating an infant abduction.
   2. Ask the mother to describe the nurse who took the baby.
   3. Determine whether the infant was returned to the nursery.
   4. Ask the mother whether the nurse asked for the code word.

5. The nurse in the labor and delivery department is caring for a client whose abdomen remains hard and rigid between contractions and the fetal heart rate is 100. Which client problem is priority?
   1. Alteration in comfort.
   2. Ineffective breathing pattern.
   3. Risk for fetal demise.
   4. Fluid and electrolyte imbalance.

6. The nurse working in a women's health clinic is returning telephone calls. Which client should the nurse contact first?
   1. The 16-year-old client who is complaining of severe lower abdominal cramping.
   2. The 27-year-old primigravida client who is complaining of blurred vision.
   3. The 48-year-old perimenopausal client who is expelling dark-red blood clots.
   4. The 68-year-old client who thinks her uterus is falling out of her vagina.

7. The charge nurse has received laboratory results for clients on the postpartum unit. Which client would warrant intervention by the nurse?
   1. The client whose white blood cell count is 18,000 mm³.
   2. The client whose serum creatinine level is 0.8 mg/dL.
   3. The client whose platelet count is 410,000 mm³.
   4. The client whose serum glucose level is 280 mg/dL.

8. The nurse on the postpartum unit is administering a.m. medications. Which medication should the nurse administer first?
   1. The sliding scale insulin to the client diagnosed with type 1 diabetes.
   2. The stool softener to the client complaining of severe constipation.
   3. The non-narcotic analgesic to the client complaining of headache, rated as a 3 on a pain scale of 1 to 10.
   4. The rectal suppository for the client complaining of hemorrhoidal pain.

9. The labor and delivery nurse is performing a vaginal examination and assesses a prolapsed cord. Which intervention should the nurse implement first?
   1. Place the client in the Trendelenburg position.
   2. Ask the father to leave the delivery room.
   3. Request the client not to push during contractions.
   4. Prepare the client for an emergency C-section.

10. Which newborn infant would the nursery nurse assess first?
    1. The 3-hour-old newborn who weighs 6 pounds and 2 ounces.
    2. The 4-hour-old newborn delivered at 42 weeks' gestation.
    3. The 6-hour-old newborn who is 22 inches long.
    4. The 8-hour-old newborn who was born at 40 weeks' gestation.

11. Which antepartum client should the charge nurse assign to the most experienced nurse?
    1. The 34-week gestation client who is receiving brethine and is on strict bed rest.
    2. The 36-week gestation client in active labor whose fetus has a Biophysical Profile of 10.
    3. The 38-week gestation client who is 10 cm dilated and 100% effaced.
    4. The 42-week gestation client who has been pushing for 4 hours and has yellow amniotic fluid.

12. A nurse has been floated from the medical unit to the postpartum unit. Which client should be assigned to this nurse?
    1. The 4-hour postpartum client whose fundus is not midline.
    2. The 8-hour postpartum client who has saturated 3 peri-pads in 1 hour.
    3. The 14-hour postpartum client who experienced eclampsia during delivery.
    4. The 23-hour postpartum client who is being discharged home this morning.

13. Which priority intervention should the nurse implement for the 38-week gestation client who is receiving epidural anesthesia?
    1. Place the client in the fetal position.
    2. Assess the client's respiratory rate.
    3. Pre-hydrate the client with intravenous fluid.
    4. Ensure the client has been NPO for 4 hours.

14. The 28-year-old female client is being scheduled for an emergency appendectomy. Which priority question should the emergency department nurse ask the client?
1. "Are you currently breastfeeding?"
2. "Have you ever had general anesthesia?"
3. "Do you have any medication allergies?"
4. "Is there any chance you are pregnant?"

15. Which client should the labor and delivery charge nurse assign to the most experienced nurse?
1. The client who has a fetal heart rate of 130 bpm.
2. The client who has non-reassuring fetal heart rate patterns.
3. The client who is scheduled for a cesarean section.
4. The client having a vaginal birth who has been pushing for 1 hour.

16. The female unlicensed assistive personnel (UAP) informs the nurse she has helped the 1-day postpartum client change her peri-pad three times in the last 4 hours. Which action should the nurse implement?
1. Ask the UAP why the nurse was not notified earlier.
2. Go to the room and check the client immediately.
3. Instruct the UAP to massage the client's uterus.
4. Document the finding in the client's chart.

17. The unlicensed assistive personnel (UAP) is assisting the nurse in the newborn nursery. Which action by the UAP would warrant intervention?
1. The UAP swaddles the infant securely in a blanket.
2. The UAP uses gloves when changing the infant.
3. The UAP is bathing the newborn with a bar of soap.
4. The UAP wipes down the crib with a disinfectant.

18. The charge nurse is making assignments in the labor and delivery department. Which client should be assigned to the most experienced nurse?
1. The 26-week gestational client who is having Braxton Hicks contractions.
2. The 32-week gestational client who is having triplets and is on bed rest.
3. The 38-week gestational client whose contractions are 3 minutes apart.
4. The 39-week gestational client who has late decelerations on the fetal monitor.

19. Which task should the nurse on the postpartum unit delegate to the unlicensed assistive personnel (UAP)?
1. Instruct the UAP to prepare a sitz bath for the client.
2. Ask the UAP to call the laboratory for a stat complete blood cell (CBC) count.
3. Tell the UAP to show the mother how to breastfeed.
4. Have the UAP check the client's fundus.

20. A nurse from the medical-surgical unit is assigned to the postpartum unit. Which client should the charge nurse assign to the medical-surgical nurse?
1. The client who has developed mastitis and is trying to breastfeed.
2. The client who had a vaginal hysterectomy and oophorectomy.
3. The client who is having difficulty bonding with her infant.
4. The unmarried client who is giving her child up for adoption.

21. The unlicensed assistive personnel (UAP) responds to a code in the newborn nursery. Which task should the house supervisor delegate to the UAP?
1. Tell the UAP to sit with the family in the waiting room.
2. Give medication to the nurse from the crash cart.
3. Assist the nurse anesthetist with intubation.
4. Instruct the UAP to obtain supplies for the code.

22. Which action by the nursery nurse would warrant immediate intervention by the charge nurse?
    1. The nurse allows an experienced volunteer to rock an infant.
    2. The nurse puts a gloved finger into the newborn's mouth.
    3. The nurse performs the Ortoloni maneuver on the newborn.
    4. The nurse requests the LPN to bathe the newborn infant.

23. The RN and unlicensed assistive personnel (UAP) are caring for clients on a postpartum unit. Which task would be most appropriate for the RN to assign to the UAP?
    1. Perform an in-and-out catheterization.
    2. Complete the client's discharge instructions.
    3. Escort the client to the car and check for a car seat.
    4. Spray anesthetic foam on the client's episiotomy.

24. The charge nurse is making assignments on the postpartum unit. Which client should be assigned to the licensed practical nurse (LPN)?
    1. The client who has delivered her sixth baby and has just returned to her room.
    2. The client who had a C-section yesterday and is running a low-grade fever.
    3. The client who had a vaginal delivery this morning and has foul-smelling lochia.
    4. The client who is 1 day post–vaginal delivery who is ambulating in the hall.

25. The nurse and unlicensed assistive personnel (UAP) are caring for babies in the newborn nursery. Which action by the UAP would warrant immediate intervention?
    1. The UAP does not check the mother's identification (ID) band with the infant's ID band.
    2. The UAP brings the mother a full package of newborn diapers.
    3. The UAP applies baby lotion to the newborn while the mother is watching.
    4. The UAP tells the father to support the newborn's head.

26. Which task should the postpartum nurse not delegate to the unlicensed assistive personnel (UAP)?
    1. Tell the UAP to assess the vital signs of the client 4 hours post–vaginal delivery.
    2. Request the UAP to pass out the breakfast trays to the clients.
    3. Instruct the UAP to administer Rhogam to the client who is Rh-negative.
    4. Ask the UAP to remove the client's indwelling urinary catheter.

27. Which behavior by the unlicensed assistive personnel (UAP) warrants immediate intervention by the postpartum nurse?
    1. The UAP helped the client with an episiotomy apply an ice pack to the perineal area.
    2. The UAP pushes the PCA button for the 8-hour post-op C-section client.
    3. The UAP uses non-sterile gloves to remove the client's peri-pad.
    4. The UAP encourages the client to eat all of the food on the breakfast tray.

28. The charge nurse is making assignments on a postpartum unit that has two registered nurses (RNs), two licensed practical nurses (LPNs), and two unlicensed assistive personnel (UAPs). Which task/assignment is most appropriate?
    1. Instruct the UAP to evaluate how the mother and infant are bonding.
    2. Tell the RN to change the sharps container in the medication room.
    3. Ask the LPN to administer ibuprofen to the client experiencing afterbirth pains.
    4. Request the LPN to care for the client who is 6 hours postpartum who had eclampsia.

29. The nurse instructed the unlicensed assistive personnel (UAP) to provide a sitz bath to the postpartum client with hemorrhoids. Which priority intervention should the nurse implement?
    1. Document the sitz bath in the client's nurse's notes.
    2. Follow-up to ensure the UAP gave the sitz bath.
    3. Assess the client's hemorrhoids every 4 hours.
    4. Discuss the importance of not getting constipated.

30. Which newborn should the charge nurse in the nursery assign to the licensed practical nurse (LPN)?
    1. The 4-hour newborn who was born at 42 weeks.
    2. The 8-hour newborn who is jittery and irritable.
    3. The 18-hour newborn whose mother was addicted to heroin.
    4. The 22-hour newborn who was born vaginally after 2 hours of pushing.

31. The client being seen in the obstetric (OB) clinic tells the nurse, "I don't think it is right that the judge is making me get a contraceptive implant just because they don't think I am a good mother." Which ethical principle does the requirement violate?
    1. Autonomy.
    2. Justice.
    3. Fidelity.
    4. Beneficence.

32. The client in labor is diagnosed with pregnancy-induced hypertension and has preeclampsia. Which interventions should the nurse implement? **Select all that apply.**
    1. Monitor the intravenous (IV) magnesium sulfate.
    2. Check the client's telemetry monitor.
    3. Assess the client's deep tendon reflexes.
    4. Administer furosemide (Lasix) intravenous push (IVP).
    5. Notify the nursery when delivery is imminent or has occurred.

33. The father of a newborn infant tells the nurse excitedly, "Someone just took our baby and they didn't know the code word." Which action should the nurse implement first?
    1. Tell the father to remain calm and go back to his wife.
    2. Assign staff members to block all exits from the unit.
    3. Page a Code Pink, indicating an infant abduction.
    4. Question the father about what exactly happened in the room.

34. The client who delivered twins 3 days ago calls the women's health clinic and tells the nurse, "I am having hip pain that makes it difficult for me to walk." Which statement is the nurse's best response?
    1. "I am going to make you an appointment to see the HCP today."
    2. "This often occurs a few days after delivery and will go away with time."
    3. "Are you performing the Kegel exercises 10 to 20 times a day?"
    4. "The pain may decrease if you empty your bladder every 2 hours."

35. The 36-week gestational client has just delivered a stillborn infant. Which intervention should the nurse implement?
    1. Call the sudden infant death syndrome (SIDS) support group.
    2. Refer the client to the maternal child case manager.
    3. Notify the hospital chaplain of the fetal demise.
    4. Contact Child Protective Services.

36. The client who is 20 weeks' gestation comes to the women's health clinic, and the nurse notices bruises on her abdomen and back. Which response is most appropriate for the nurse?
    1. "Please tell me who is abusing you."
    2. "This could cause you to lose your baby."
    3. "How did you get these bruises?"
    4. "Do you feel safe in your home?"

37. The boyfriend comes to the postpartum unit and demands his girlfriend's room number. The nurse can smell alcohol on the man's breath, and he is acting erratically. Which action should the nurse implement?
    1. Explain to the client her boyfriend is causing problems.
    2. Give the boyfriend the client's room number.
    3. Contact hospital security to come to the unit.
    4. Tell the boyfriend that he can't be here if he is drunk.

38. The nurse is caring for a postpartum client who is a Jehovah's Witness and needs a RhoGAM injection. Which question should the nurse ask the client?
    1. "Rhogam is a blood product. Do you want the injection?"
    2. "Do you know what type blood your husband has?"
    3. "Did you know that you have Rh-negative blood?"
    4. "Do you know whether your insurance will pay for the shot?"

39. The nurse is administering medications to clients on a postpartum floor. Which medication should the nurse question administering?
    1. The rubella vaccine to the postpartum client who has a negative titer.
    2. The yearly flu vaccine to a client who reports an allergy to eggs.
    3. The PPD to a client who suspects she was exposed to tuberculosis.
    4. The hepatitis B vaccine to a client who is breastfeeding.

40. Which client would the newborn nursery nurse assess first after receiving shift report?
    1. The newborn who has chignon.
    2. The newborn with caput succedaneum.
    3. The newborn who has a cephalohematoma.
    4. The newborn who has a port-wine stain.

41. Which statement indicates to the postpartum nurse the discharge teaching to the first-time mother is effective?
    1. "I should contact my baby's doctor if she refuses two or more feedings."
    2. "My baby will have green liquid stools for at least 1 month after I take her home."
    3. "I must administer AquaMephyton elixir once a day with formula to my daughter."
    4. "If my daughter has thick, yellow-colored stool I will call her doctor."

42. Which primigravida client should the clinic nurse report to the certified nurse midwife?
    1. The 12-week gestation client complaining of nausea and vomiting.
    2. The 24-week gestation client complaining of ankle edema.
    3. The 32-week gestation client reporting of facial edema.
    4. The 38-week gestation client reporting urinary frequency.

43. The nurse is caring for a postpartum client in the "taking in" phase. Which intervention is most appropriate for the nurse to implement?
    1. Ask the client to demonstrate how to change the infant's diaper.
    2. Determine if the client's blood is Rh-negative or Rh-positive.
    3. Allow the client to ventilate feelings about the birth of her infant.
    4. Discuss the advantages of breastfeeding over bottle feeding.

44. Which data should the nurse assess on the 2-hour postpartum client who delivered vaginally? **Select all that apply.**
    1. Palpate the client's breasts.
    2. Check the client's vaginal discharge.
    3. Assess the client's pedal pulses.
    4. Inspect the client's surgical incision.
    5. Check the client's pupillary response.

45. Which action by the nurse warrants intervention by the charge nurse on the postpartum unit?
    1. The nurse offers the Muslim client a ham sandwich and salad for lunch.
    2. The nurse asks the Seventh Day Adventist client if she needs anything for her Sabbath on Saturday.
    3. The nurse offers the Asian client who is febrile hot water instead of cold water.
    4. The nurse explains to the Jehovah's Witness client who is Rh-negative that Rhogam is a blood product.

46. The nurse volunteering in a free clinic has been caring for a female client for several weeks. The client states, "My husband and I been trying to have a baby for 6 years. What can we do?" Which statement is the nurse's best response?
    1. "You should discuss your concerns with the doctor when he comes in."
    2. "Infertility treatments are very expensive and you would have to pay for it."
    3. "You are concerned because you have not been able to get pregnant."
    4. "Have you tried the rhythm method to try and conceive a child?"

47. Which client should the labor and delivery nurse assess first after receiving report?
    1. The client who is 10 cm dilated and 100% effaced.
    2. The client who is exhibiting early decelerations on the fetal monitor.
    3. The client who is vacillating about whether or not to have an epidural.
    4. The client who is upset because her obstetrician is on vacation.

48. The nurse is caring for clients in a women's health clinic. Which client warrants intervention by the nurse?
    1. The pregnant client who has hematocrit and hemoglobin levels of 11/33.
    2. The pregnant client who has a fasting blood glucose level of 110 mg/dL.
    3. The pregnant client who has 3+ proteins in her urine.
    4. The pregnant client who has a white blood cell count of 11,500 mm^3.

49. The client is 1 day postpartum, and the nurse notes the fundus is displaced laterally to the right. Which nursing intervention should be implemented first?
    1. Prepare to perform an in-and-out catheterization.
    2. Assess the bladder using the bladder scanner.
    3. Massage the client's fundus for 2 minutes.
    4. Assist the client to the bathroom to urinate.

50. While making rounds, the charge nurse notices the client's chart has been left on the bedside table. Which action should the charge nurse implement first?
    1. Ask the client's nurse who left the chart at the bedside.
    2. Leave the chart at the bedside until talking to the nurse.
    3. Tell the nurse this could be a violation of HIPAA.
    4. Take the client's chart back to the nurse's station.

51. The 27-year-old female client is being scheduled for a chest x-ray. Which question should the nurse ask the client?
    1. "Have you ever had a chest x-ray before?"
    2. "Is there any chance you may be pregnant?"
    3. "When was the date of your last period?"
    4. "Do you have any allergies to shellfish?"

52. The clinical manager is reviewing hospital occurrence reports and notes that the nurse on the postpartum unit has documented three medication errors in the last 2 months. Which action should the clinical manager implement first?
    1. Initiate the formal counseling procedure for multiple medication errors.
    2. Continue to monitor the nurse for any further medication errors.
    3. Discuss the errors with the nurse to determine whether there is a medication system problem.
    4. Arrange for the nurse to attend a medication administration review course.

53. The nursery nurse is assessing newborns. Which newborn would require immediate intervention by the nurse?
    1. The newborn who remains in the fetal position when lying supine.
    2. The newborn whose toes flare out when the lateral heel is stroked.
    3. The newborn whose head turns toward the cheek being stroked.
    4. The newborn who extends the arms when hearing a loud noise.

54. The client on the postpartum unit tells the nurse, "My husband thinks he is the father of my baby but he is not. What should I tell him?" Which response supports the ethical principal of no maleficence?
1. "You should tell him the truth before he becomes attached to the infant."
2. "How do you think your husband will feel if he knows he is not the father?"
3. "I know my husband would want to know if my child was his or not."
4. "Do you know what the real father is planning on doing about the baby?"

55. The chief nursing officer of the hospital instructed the clinical manager of the post-partum unit to research a change in the system of delivery of care. Which statement best describes modular nursing?
1. Nurses are designated the primary responsible persons for client care.
2. A nurse and UAP are assigned a group of postpartum clients.
3. Nursing staff members are divided into groups responsible for client care.
4. Nurses are assigned specific tasks rather than specific clients.

56. Which action by the postpartum clinical manager would be most effective in producing a smooth transition to the new medication delivery system?
1. Counsel any nurses who cannot adapt to the change.
2. Ask the staff to vote on accepting the new system.
3. Have an open-door policy to discuss the change.
4. Send written documentation of the change by hospital e-mail.

57. During an interview, the pregnant client at the women's health clinic hesitantly tells the nurse, "I think I should let someone know that I can't stop eating dirt. I crave it all the time." Which action should the nurse implement first?
1. Explain that the behavior is normal.
2. Ask whether the client is taking the prenatal vitamins.
3. Check the client's hemoglobin and hematocrit (H&H).
4. Determine whether there is a history of pica in the family.

58. The client who is 16 weeks pregnant calls and tells the office nurse, "My husband's insurance has changed and they say I can't use you anymore." Which statement is the nurse's best response?
1. "If we continue to see you it will cost you a lot more money."
2. "Because you are already pregnant your insurance company must pay."
3. "You are concerned you don't want to change doctors at this time."
4. "Can your husband get a supplemental policy to cover this pregnancy?"

59. The 16-year-old mother of a 1-day-old infant wants her son circumcised. Which intervention should the nurse implement?
1. Request the client's mother sign the permit.
2. Determine whether the insurance will pay for the procedure.
3. Refer the client to the social worker to apply for Medicaid.
4. Have the 16-year-old client sign for informed consent.

60. The clinical manager is presenting a lecture on collective bargaining. One of the nurse participants asks, "What happens if nurses decide to go on strike?" Which statement is the clinical nurse manager's best response?
1. "The UAPs and managers will have to take care of the clients."
2. "If nurses go on strike it is considered abandonment of the clients."
3. "The clients will get better care once the nurses' demands are met."
4. "The nurses must give a 10-day notice before a strike takes place."

61. Which client should the newborn nurse refer to the hospital ethics committee?
1. The newborn who is anencephalic whose parents want everything done.
2. The newborn whose 16-year-old mother wants to place the infant up for adoption.
3. The newborn whose mother is a known cocaine user and is HIV positive.
4. The newborn who needs a unit of blood and the parents are refusing consent.

62. The client has delivered a 37-week gestation infant whose cord was wrapped around the neck. The infant died in utero. Which interventions should the nurse implement? **Select all that apply.**
   1. Allow the mother to hold and cuddle the infant.
   2. Have the mother transferred to the medical unit.
   3. Encourage the father to talk about his child to the nurse.
   4. Recommend to the parents that the child be cremated.
   5. Discourage the client from giving the infant a name.

63. Which action would be most important for the clinical manager to take regarding a primary nurse who has received numerous compliments from the clients and their families about the excellent care she provides?
   1. Ask the nurse what she does that makes her care so special.
   2. Document the comments on the nurse's performance evaluation.
   3. Acknowledge the comments with a celebration on the station.
   4. Take no action because excellent care is expected by all nurses.

64. The client asks the nurse in the women's health clinic, "I am so miserable during my premenstrual syndrome I can't even go to work. Please help me." Which interventions should the nurse implement? **Select all that apply.**
   1. Increase the amount of colas and coffee daily.
   2. Avoid simple sugars such as cakes and candy.
   3. Drink at least two glasses of red wine nightly.
   4. Decrease the intake of foods high in salt.
   5. Adhere to a regular schedule for sleep.

65. The nurse is completing the admission assessment on a 12-weeks-pregnant client who is visiting the women's health clinic. The client tells the nurse, "I am a vegan and will not drink any milk or eat any meat." Which intervention should the nurse implement?
   1. Recommend the client eat grains, legumes, and nuts daily.
   2. Suggest that the client eat at least two eggs every day.
   3. Discuss not adhering to the vegan diet during pregnancy.
   4. Explain that a vegan diet does not require iron supplements.

66. The charge nurse of the postpartum unit is making assignments. Which patients should be assigned to the medical-surgical nurse who has been assigned to the unit for the day? **Select all that apply.**
   1. The patient who delivered 4 hours ago and is complaining of pain.
   2. The patient who is being discharged and needs discharge teaching about breastfeeding.
   3. The patient who is being treated for HELLP syndrome.
   4. The patient who is 30 weeks' gestation on a fetal monitor.
   5. The patient who is gravida 8 and on a Pitocin drip.

67. The labor and delivery nurse is preparing to assist the anesthetist to insert an epidural catheter in a patient close to delivery. Which picture indicates the correct position to assist the patient to assume?

1.

2.

3.

4.

68. The 34-week pregnant patient in the labor and delivery unit is on a magnesium sulfate, an anticonvulsant, intravenous drip for eclampsia. The labor and delivery nurse assesses the patient's reflexes as absent with repeated stimulation. Which nursing intervention should the nurse implement first?

Deep Tendon Reflex Scale

0 = absent despite reinforcement
1 = present only with reinforcement
2 = normal
3 = increased but normal
4 = markedly hyperactive, with clonus

1. Notify the obstetrician.
2. Document the finding as absent.
3. Have another nurse assess the reflexes.
4. Turn off the magnesium drip.

69. The public health nurse is working at a sexually transmitted disease (STD) clinic. The female client has been diagnosed with gonorrhea. Which nursing interventions should the nurse implement? Rank in order of performance.
1. Notify the client's sexual partners of potential exposure to an STD.
2. Complete the report to the Centers for Disease Control and Prevention.
3. Teach the client safe sex procedures.
4. Administer the prescribed antibiotic to the client.
5. Ask the client to provide a list of sexual partners.

70. The emergency department nurse observed a motor vehicle accident (MVA) on her way home from work. The driver of one of the vehicles is obviously several months pregnant. Which nursing intervention should the nurse implement first?
1. Determine the length of gestation.
2. Assess the driver for signs of trauma.
3. Check to see if the patient was wearing a seat belt.
4. Monitor for fetal heart tones.

71. The nurse is caring for a 34-year-old female client who tells the nurse, "I have been diagnosed with a human papillomavirus (HPV) infection in my mouth. I don't understand. I get cervical smears for that." Which is the nurse's best response?
1. "You must have had oral sex to get the HPV infection in your mouth."
2. "You should have a smear made of your mouth every 6 months from now on."
3. "I would have the test repeated; it is not possible to have an HPV infection in the mouth."
4. "This infection is on the rise from oral contact with a person who has the infection."

72. The nurse is teaching a health class for 14- to 18-year-old females. Which information regarding sexually transmitted diseases (STDs) should the nurse include in the discussion?
1. The acquired immunodeficiency syndrome (AIDS) virus is only transmitted through multiple exposures.
2. The use of a condom during intercourse ensures that a sexually transmitted disease is not passed from one partner to the other.
3. The more sexual contacts an individual has both for oral sex and intercourse, the greater the probability that individual has of contracting an STD.
4. Syphilis and gonorrhea are easily treatable and no lasting effects will be experienced with either of these infections.

MATERNAL-CHILD CLINICAL SCENARIO

Ms. Helen is the charge nurse on the maternal child unit for the 7a–7p shift. She has four RNs, Ms. Kathy, Ms. Judy, Ms. Glada, and Ms. Patricia, a new graduate who has just completed a 3-month orientation. There are three unlicensed assistive personnel (UAP) working on the unit, Ms. Monica, Ms. Janice, and Ms. Gail.

1. Which postpartum client should Ms. Helen assign to the most inexperienced nurse, Ms. Patricia?
   1. The client who has hemorrhoids and is complaining of pain.
   2. The client who saturated multiple peri-pads during the night.
   3. The client who is refusing to have the newborn in the room.
   4. The client who is crying because the baby will not nurse.

2. Which newborn infant would warrant immediate intervention by Ms. Kathy, the nursery nurse?
   1. The 1-hour-old newborn who has tiny, white, hard spots on the nose.
   2. The 6-hour-old newborn who has a respiratory rate of 24.
   3. The 12-hour-old newborn who is turning red and crying.
   4. The 18-hour-old newborn who has a viscous, sticky tar, odorless stool.

3. The laboring client is showing late decelerations on the fetal monitor. After placing the client in the left lateral position, which intervention should Ms. Glada implement first?
   1. Notify the client's obstetrician immediately.
   2. Encourage the client to pant when the contraction occurs.
   3. Administer oxytocin (Pitocin) intravenously.
   4. Prepare for an immediate delivery of the fetus.

4. Ms. Helen is monitoring laboratory results for clients on the postpartum unit. Which client would warrant intervention by Ms. Helen?
   1. The client who had a vaginal delivery and who has a white blood cell count of 15,000 mm^3.
   2. The client who had a C-section who has a serum potassium level of 4.8 mEq/L.
   3. The client with preeclampsia who has a platelet count of 90,000 mm^3.
   4. The client with gestational diabetes who has a serum glucose level of 140 mg/dL.

5. Ms. Helen is making assignments in the labor and delivery department. Which client should be assigned to Ms. Judy, the most experienced nurse?
   1. The 26-week gestational client who is having Braxton Hicks contractions.
   2. The 32-week gestational client who is having twins and is on bed rest.
   3. The 38-week gestational client who is 100% effaced and 10 cm dilated.
   4. The 39-week gestational client who has early decelerations on the fetal monitor.

6. Which task should Ms. Glada, postpartum nurse, delegate to the unlicensed assistive personnel (UAP)?
   1. Instruct the UAP to take the client whose fundus is not midline to the bathroom.
   2. Ask the UAP to take the vital signs for the client diagnosed with HELLP syndrome.
   3. Tell the UAP to assist the mother with breastfeeding her newborn daughter.
   4. Request the UAP to administer Rhogam to the mother who is Rh-negative.

7. A float nurse from the medical-surgical unit is assigned to the postpartum unit. Which client should Ms. Helen assign to the float nurse?
   1. The client who had a fetal demise at 34 weeks' gestation.
   2. The client who has a boggy fundus that massaging has not helped.
   3. The client who has had six saturated peri-pads in the last shift.
   4. The unmarried client who is giving her child up for adoption.

8. Ms. Judy is administering medications to clients on a postpartum floor. Which medication should Ms. Judy question administering?
   1. The yearly flu vaccine to a client who reports an allergy to tomatoes.
   2. The hepatitis B vaccine to a client who is breastfeeding.
   3. The Rhogam to the mother who is Rh-negative and whose infant is Rh-positive.
   4. The rubella vaccine to the postpartum client who has a positive titer.

9. Which client should Ms. Kathy, the newborn nursery nurse, assess first after receiving shift report?
   1. The Asian newborn who has purple-colored splotches on the lower back.
   2. The Caucasian newborn with a purple-colored area on the right side of the face.
   3. The Hispanic newborn who has a red rash, "flea bites," on the chest.
   4. The African American newborn who has edema between suture lines.

10. Ms. Kathy, the nursery nurse, is assessing newborns. Which newborn would require further assessment by Ms. Kathy?
    1. The newborn who remains in the fetal position when lying supine.
    2. The newborn whose toes flare out when the lateral heel is stroked.
    3. The newborn who acts like he is walking when his feet are placed on a hard surface.
    4. The newborn who grasps the finger when it is placed in his hand.

CLINICAL SCENARIO

ANSWERS AND RATIONALES

The correct answer number and rationale for why it is the correct answer are given in **boldface type.** Rationales for why the other possible answer options are incorrect also are given, but they are not in boldface type.

1. 1. This pain may be related to an episiotomy or perineal tear, but this client is not priority over a client who may be hemorrhaging.
   2. **Saturating multiple peri-pads indicates heavy bleeding, which may indicate hemorrhaging. The nurse should assess this client first.**
   3. The nurse needs to assess this client for possible maternal/infant bonding problems, but this is a psychosocial issue that should be addressed after a physiological issue, such as possible hemorrhaging.
   4. This client is going to require some time to be taught, but this is not priority over a client who is hemorrhaging.
   Content – Women's Health: ***Category of Health Alteration*** *– Women's Health:* ***Integrated Processes –*** *Nursing Process: Assessment:* ***Client Needs*** *– Physiological Integrity: Reduction of Risk Potential:* ***Cognitive Level –*** *Analysis*

MAKING NURSING DECISIONS: The test taker should apply some systematic approach when answering a priority question. Maslow's Hierarchy of Needs should be used when determining which client to assess first. The test taker should start at the bottom of the pyramid, and physiological needs are priority.

2. 1. The newborn with lanugo is normal and would not warrant immediate intervention by the nurse.
   2. The normal respiratory rate for a newborn is 30 to 60; therefore, this would not warrant immediate intervention.
   3. The newborn who is turning red when crying is not in distress; therefore, this would not warrant immediate intervention.
   4. **The newborn who has not passed meconium 24 hours after birth must be evaluated for intestinal obstruction or a congenital abnormality. This could be caused by an imperforate anus, Hirschsprung's disease, cystic fibrosis, or several other possibilities. This newborn warrants immediate intervention.**
   Content – Newborn: ***Category of Health Alteration –*** *Women's Health:* ***Integrated Processes –*** *Nursing Process: Assessment:* ***Client Needs*** *– Physiological Integrity, Reduction of Risk Potential:* ***Cognitive Level –*** *Synthesis*

MAKING NURSING DECISIONS: When deciding which client to assess first, the test taker should determine whether the signs/symptoms the client is exhibiting are normal or expected for the client situation. After eliminating the expected options, the test taker should determine which situation is more life threatening.

3. 1. The nurse should first intervene to increase blood supply to the fetus; therefore, notifying the HCP is not the nurse's first intervention.
   2. Slow, deep breaths may help decrease the mother's anxiety, but the nurse's first intervention is to increase blood supply to the fetus.
   3. **The left lateral position will improve placental blood flow and oxygen supply to the fetus. This should be the nurse's first intervention.**
   4. The nurse should prepare for an emergency C-section, but this is not the nurse's first intervention.
   Content – Women's Health: ***Category of Health Alteration*** *– Women's Health:* ***Integrated Processes –*** *Nursing Process: Implementation:* ***Client Needs –*** *Physiological Integrity: Reduction of Risk Potential:* ***Cognitive Level –*** *Application*

MAKING NURSING DECISIONS: When the test taker is deciding when to notify an HCP, the test taker should look at the other three options and determine whether one of the options should be implemented prior to notifying the HCP. Another option may, for example, provide information the HCP will need in order to make a decision.

4. 1. Once the nurse definitely determines the infant is not in the nursery, then a Code Pink should be initiated. This notifies all hospital personnel of a possible infant abduction.
   2. This will be done if the infant was not returned to the nursery, but this is not the first intervention.
   3. **The nurse should first determine whether another staff member returned the infant to the nursery. The nurse should not call a false alarm.**
   4. There are many safety precautions to prevent infant abductions, and most facilities have a code word that is changed daily. The mother must ask anyone who wants to take the infant out of the mother's room for the code word. This is not the nurse's first intervention.

Content – Newborn: Category of Health Alteration – Obstetrics: Integrated Processes – Nursing Process: Implementation: Client Needs – Safe and Effective Care Environment: Management of Care: Cognitive Level – Application

5. 1. Pain for the mother is a priority, but it is not priority over potential death of the fetus.
   2. The client is not having trouble breathing; therefore, this would not be a priority problem. Altered gas exchange would be an appropriate problem for the fetus.
   3. **The client is exhibiting signs of abruptio placentae, and a decreased heart rate indicates a compromised fetus. This problem will lead quickly to the death of the fetus. Therefore, it is the priority problem.**
   4. All pregnant women experience an increase in fluid volume status and some resulting electrolyte imbalance; therefore, this is not a priority problem.

Content – Women's Health: Category of Health Alteration – Women's Health: Integrated Processes – Nursing Process: Planning: Client Needs – Physiological Integrity: Reduction of Risk Potential: Cognitive Level – Synthesis

6. 1. The client with severe lower abdominal cramping should be called to determine whether she is currently menstruating, but this is not priority over a pregnant client with symptoms of preeclampsia.
   2. **Blurred vision is a symptom of preeclampsia, and this is the client's first pregnancy. This client should be contacted first and told to come into the clinic for further evaluation.**
   3. The expulsion of dark-red blood clots indicates the client is going through menopause. This is not a life-threatening situation because dark-red blood does not indicate frank bleeding.
   4. This is uncomfortable for the client and indicates the need for a hysterectomy or instructions in the insertion and use of a pessary device to hold the uterus in place, but it is not life threatening.

Content – Women's Health Category of Health Alteration – Women's Health: Integrated Processes – Nursing Process: Assessment: Client Needs – Physiological Integrity: Reduction of Risk Potential: Cognitive Level – Analysis

MAKING NURSING DECISIONS: When deciding which client to assess first, the test taker should determine whether the signs/symptoms the client is exhibiting are normal or expected for the client situation. After eliminating the expected options, the test taker should determine which situation is more life threatening.

7. 1. The white blood cell count rises normally during labor and postpartum—up to 25,000; therefore, this does not warrant intervention.
   2. The serum creatinine level is within normal limits; therefore, this client does not warrant immediate intervention.
   3. Platelets show marked increase 3 to 5 days after birth, but the client who is 1 to 2 days postpartum would have a slightly increased platelet count. Normal platelet count is 150,000 to 450,000, so this client's count is within normal limits.
   4. **This glucose level is elevated, and the nurse should investigate further as to why the glucose level is abnormal. The normal glucose level is 70 to 120 mg/dL.**

Content – Women's Health Category of Health Alteration – Women's Health: Integrated Processes – Nursing Process: Evaluation: Client Needs – Physiological Integrity: Reduction of Risk Potential: Cognitive Level – Synthesis

8. 1. **The client with type 1 diabetes must receive insulin prior to eating; therefore, this must be administered first.**
   2. The stool softener will take several days to soften the stool; therefore, this medication does not need to be administered first.
   3. The client with a headache is not priority over a type 1 diabetic patient who needs sliding scale coverage. This client should receive medication after the insulin-dependent diabetic receives insulin.
   4. The rectal suppository is administered to shrink the hemorrhoids and has a local anesthetic effect, but it would not be priority over the sliding scale insulin.

Content – Women's Health: Category of Health Alteration – Drug Administration: Integrated Processes – Nursing Process: Implementation: Client Needs – Physiological Adaptation: Pharmacological and Parenteral Therapies: Cognitive Level – Application

9. 1. **A prolapsed cord is an emergency situation because the prolapsed cord could compromise the fetus's blood supply. Placing the client in the Trendelenburg position will cause the fetus to reverse back into the uterus, which will take the pressure off the umbilical cord. The safety of the fetus is priority.**
   2. In emergency situations, the nurse may need to request visitors to leave the delivery room, depending on how visitors are acting during the crisis, but this is not the first intervention.
   3. This is an appropriate intervention, but the nurse's priority is getting pressure off the umbilical cord.

ANSWERS

4. The fetus is in distress and the nurse must prepare for an emergency C-section, but it is not the nurse's first intervention.
   Content – Women's Health: **Category of Health Alteration** *– Women's Health:* **Integrated Processes** *– Nursing Process: Implementation:* **Client Needs** *– Physiological Integrity: Reduction of Risk Potential:* **Cognitive Level** *– Application*

10. 1. The newborn who weighs 6 pounds and 2 ounces is within normal weight for a newborn; therefore, the nurse would not need to assess this baby first.
    2. **The newborn delivered at 42 weeks is postmature and is at risk for hypoglycemia and hypothermia because the placenta begins to deteriorate after 40 weeks and subcutaneous fat is utilized to support the infant's life. The nurse should assess this baby first just because of the 42-week gestation.**
    3. The newborn who is 22 inches long is longer than most infants, but this infant would not need to be assessed first.
    4. The newborn delivered at 40 weeks' gestation is within normal gestation time; therefore, the nurse would not need to assess this baby first.
    Content – Newborn: **Category of Health Alteration** *– Women's Health:* **Integrated Processes** *– Nursing Process: Assessment:* **Client Needs** *– Health Promotion and Maintenance:* **Cognitive Level** *– Analysis*

MAKING NURSING DECISIONS: When deciding which client to assess first, the test taker should determine whether the signs/symptoms the client is exhibiting are normal for the client situation. After eliminating the expected options, the test taker should determine which situation is more life threatening.

11. 1. This client is preterm but is stable according to the data in the option. Brethine is a uterine relaxant and the client should be on strict bed rest.
    2. A Biophysical Profile is used to determine if the fetus is ready to make the trip down the vaginal canal. Two points are given to fetal breathing movements, gross body movements, fetal tone (flexion), amniotic fluid volume, and reactive (or not) non-stress test, with a score of 10 being the best.
    3. This client is ready to deliver the fetus; therefore, the most experienced nurse would not need to be assigned to this client.
    4. **This client is postmature and the fetus is at risk for meconium; therefore, this client should be assigned to the most experienced nurse.**

Content – Women's Health: **Category of Health Alteration** *– Women's Health:* **Integrated Processes** *– Nursing Process: Planning:* **Client Needs** *– Safe and Effective Care Environment: Management of Care:* **Cognitive Level** *– Synthesis*

MAKING NURSING DECISIONS: The test taker must determine which client is least stable and assign this client to the most experienced nurse.

12. 1. This client needs to urinate since the number one reason for a displaced fundus is a full bladder. Since a medical nurse may not know how to palpate a fundus, this client should be assigned to a more experienced nurse.
    2. This client may be hemorrhaging and should be assigned to a more experienced nurse.
    3. **This client is still at risk for a seizure but a medical nurse should be able to care for a client who has a seizure. This client should be assigned to the medical nurse.**
    4. This nurse must evaluate the mother's ability to care for the new infant or complete discharge teaching; therefore, a more experienced nurse should be assigned to this client.
    Content – Women's Health: **Category of Health Alteration** *– Women's Health:* **Integrated Processes** *– Nursing Process: Planning:* **Client Needs** *– Safe and Effective Care Environment: Management of Care:* **Cognitive Level** *– Synthesis*

MAKING NURSING DECISIONS: The test taker must determine which client is most stable or which client may be at risk for a complication a medical nurse could care for safely.

13. 1. The client should be in the fetal position but the possibility of anesthesia ascending the spinal cord is priority.
    2. **If the anesthesia ascends the spinal cord the client will quit breathing; therefore, this is the priority intervention.**
    3. The client should be pre-hydrated but it is not a priority over airway.
    4. Clients are made NPO to prevent aspiration pneumonia secondary to vomiting if the client is undergoing general anesthesia, not epidural anesthesia.
    Content – Women's Health: **Category of Health Alteration** *– Women's Health:* **Integrated Processes** *– Nursing Process: Implementation:* **Client Needs** *– Physiological Integrity: Reduction of Risk Potential:* **Cognitive Level** *– Comprehension*

MAKING NURSING DECISIONS: The test taker should apply Maslow's Hierarchy of Needs. Airway is priority. Remember that priority intervention means all the options are something the RN can implement, but there is only one correct option.

14. 1. There is nothing in the stem of the question that suggests the client has an infant. It is a question the nurse could ask the female client but it is not a priority.
2. This is a question the nurse could ask the client, but since the question states the client is a 28-year-old female, age and gender are pertinent to which option the test taker should select.
3. This is a question all clients should be asked, but the adjectives describing the client as "a 28-year-old" and "female" should identify the fourth option as the most priority question.
4. **Since the client will have to have anesthesia for the surgery and the client is within childbearing age, the nurse should determine whether the client is pregnant.**

*Content – Medical/Surgical: **Category of Health Alteration** – Gastrointestinal: **Integrated Processes** – Nursing Process: Assessment: **Client Needs** – Physiological Integrity: Reduction of Risk Potential: **Cognitive Level** – Analysis*

MAKING NURSING DECISIONS: The test taker must acknowledge adjectives in questions when determining the correct answer. When the stem gives the client a gender and an age, it is pertinent to the correct answer.

15. 1. Normal fetal heart rate is 110 to 160 beats a minute so this client is stable.
2. **Non-reassuring fetal heart rate patterns indicate the fetus is in danger, which requires a more experienced nurse.**
3. A scheduled C-section is a stable client, so a less experienced nurse could care for this client.
4. Pushing for 1 hour prior to a vaginal birth is normal; therefore, a less experienced nurse could care for this client.

*Content – Women's Health: **Category of Health Alteration** – Women's Health: **Integrated Processes** – Nursing Process: Planning: **Client Needs** – Safe and Effective Care Environment: Management of Care: **Cognitive Level** – Synthesis*

MAKING NURSING DECISIONS: The most experienced nurse should be assigned to the most critical client. Non-reassuring fetal heart patterns indicate the infant is in distress.

16. 1. The nurse should first assess the client to determine whether the UAP was negligent in reporting before talking to the UAP.
2. **This client may or may not be experiencing excessive bleeding, but the nurse's first intervention is to assess the client.**
3. Excessive bleeding could indicate the uterus is boggy, which would require the nurse to massage the uterus. This assessment and intervention cannot be delegated to a UAP.
4. The nurse should not document any information before verifying the client situation.

*Content – Women's Health: **Category of Health Alteration** – Women's Health: **Integrated Process:** Nursing Process: Assessment: **Client Needs** – Safe and Effective Care Environment: Management of Care: **Cognitive Level** – Analysis*

MAKING NURSING DECISIONS: Any time the nurse receives information from another staff member about a client who may be experiencing a complication, the nurse must assess the client. The nurse should not make decisions about client's needs based on another staff member's information.

17. 1. The infant should be securely swaddled in a blanket to maintain body heat.
2. The UAP should wear nonsterile gloves when being exposed to blood or body fluids.
3. **When bathing a newborn, soap is not necessary. Soap can be very drying to the skin; therefore, this action warrants intervention by the nurse.**
4. The UAP should wipe the crib with disinfectant to decrease the potential for contamination.

*Content – Newborn: **Category of Health Alteration** – Obstetrics: Integrated Process: Nursing Process: Assessment: **Client Needs** – Health Promotion and Maintenance: **Cognitive Level** – Analysis*

18. 1. Braxton Hicks contractions are irregular contractions of the uterus throughout the pregnancy and are not true labor. This client would not need to be assigned to the most experienced nurse.
2. The client having triplets on bed rest is not in imminent danger; therefore, this client would not need the most experienced nurse.
3. This client is progressing normally and would not require the most experienced nurse.
4. **Late decelerations on the fetal monitor indicate fetal distress; this is a life-threatening situation, and an emergency C-section may be necessary. The charge nurse should assign the most experienced nurse to this client.**

*Content – Women's Health: **Category of Health Alteration** – Women's Health: Integrated Process: Nursing Process: Planning: **Client Needs** – Safe and Effective Care Environment: Management of Care: **Cognitive Level** – Synthesis*

MAKING NURSING DECISIONS: The test taker must determine which client is the most unstable and assign this client to the most experienced nurse.

19. 1. **The UAP can provide hygiene care to the client. A sitz bath requires the UAP to check the temperature of the water and does not require nursing judgment.**
 2. The UAP's primary responsibility is direct client care. The unit secretary, not the UAP, should call the laboratory.
 3. The nurse cannot delegate teaching to the UAP.
 4. The nurse cannot delegate assessment; therefore, the UAP cannot check the client's fundus.

 Content – Women's Health: ***Category of Health Alteration*** *– Women's Health: Integrated Process: Nursing Process: Planning* ***Client Needs*** *– Safe and Effective Care Environment: Management of Care:* ***Cognitive Level*** *– Synthesis*

MAKING NURSING DECISIONS: The nurse cannot delegate assessment, evaluation, teaching, administration of medications, or care of an unstable client to a UAP.

20. 1. A client with mastitis who is trying to breastfeed requires a nurse experienced in the postpartum unit who can teach the client about breastfeeding and assess for complications.
 2. **This is a routine surgical procedure that would not require the nurse to have any specialized postpartum experience. This client would be most appropriate to assign the float nurse who has experience on the medical-surgical unit.**
 3. A client who is having difficulty bonding would require a nurse with experience in the postpartum unit to care for the client as well as document pertinent information if bonding does not occur.
 4. There are many legal issues surrounding an adoption as well as caring for the mother who is giving up her child; this client should be assigned a nurse more experienced in postpartum care.

 Content – Women's Health: ***Category of Health Alteration*** *– Women's Health: Integrated Process: Nursing Process: Planning:* ***Client Needs*** *– Safe and Effective Care Environment: Management of Care:* ***Cognitive Level*** *– Synthesis*

MAKING NURSING DECISIONS: The test taker must determine which client requires the least amount of specialized knowledge and assign the float nurse to that client. Remember, legal issues, teaching, and psychosocial concepts require the more experienced nurse.

21. 1. An experienced nurse, a chaplain, or social worker should be assigned to sit with the family during this crisis.

 2. Even though the UAP is not administering the medication, the UAP should not be handing the nurse medication in a crisis situation.
 3. The UAP cannot assist with intubation; this must be assigned to a nurse or respiratory therapist.
 4. **The UAP can stand by and be ready to obtain any supplies needed for the code. This would be a most appropriate task to delegate in an emergency situation.**

 Content – Newborn: ***Category of Health Alteration*** *– Women's Health:* ***Integrated Process*** *– Nursing Process: Planning:* ***Client Needs*** *– Safe and Effective Care Environment: Management of Care:* ***Cognitive Level*** *– Synthesis*

22. 1. Volunteers are often asked to rock irritable infants so that the nurse can have more time to perform higher-level nursing care for the infants. This action would not warrant immediate intervention by the charge nurse.
 2. The nurse is using palpation to determine whether the newborn has a cleft palate. This assessment is within the scope of the newborn nursery nurse.
 3. **The Ortoloni maneuver is performed to assess developmental hip dysplasia. A pediatrician or a nurse practitioner only should perform this maneuver because it can cause further damage if it is done incorrectly.**
 4. The LPN can bathe a newborn infant; therefore, this would not warrant immediate intervention by the charge nurse.

 Content – Newborn: ***Category of Health Alteration*** *– Musculoskeletal:* ***Integrated Process*** *– Nursing Process: Implementation:* ***Client Needs*** *– Safe and Effective Care Environment: Management of Care:* ***Cognitive Level*** *– Application*

23. 1. This client is unable to urinate, which may or may not be a complication of the delivery/anesthesia. Catheterization is a sterile procedure, and many facilities do not allow the UAP to perform sterile procedures. The nurse should not delegate this task.
 2. This is teaching, and the nurse cannot delegate teaching to the UAP.
 3. **The infant must be transported in a car safety seat. Many facilities will lend or give the client a car seat if one is not available. The UAP can determine whether there is a car seat and take the appropriate action if there is not one.**
 4. Anesthetic foam is topical medication, and the nurse cannot delegate medication administration to the UAP.

*Content – Women's Health: **Category of Health Alteration** – Women's Health: **Integrated Processes** – Nursing Process: Planning: **Client Needs** – Safe and Effective Care Environment: Management of Care: **Cognitive Level** – Synthesis*

MAKING NURSING DECISIONS: The nurse cannot delegate assessment, evaluation, teaching, medications, or an unstable client to a UAP.

24. 1. The more pregnancies the client has had, the more likely it will be that the uterus will not contract to prevent bleeding. The RN should be assigned to this client.
    2. A client with a fever and a surgical incision may be experiencing a complication and should be assigned to an RN.
    3. Foul-smelling lochia indicates the client has an infection; therefore, this client should not be assigned to the LPN.
    4. **The client who is ambulating is stable and not exhibiting any complications; therefore, this client should be assigned to the LPN.**

*Content – Women's Health: **Category of Health Alteration** – Women's Health: Integrated Process: Nursing Process: Planning: **Client Needs** – Safe and Effective Care Environment: Management of Care: **Cognitive Level** – Synthesis*

MAKING NURSING DECISIONS: The test taker must determine which client is the most stable, which makes this an "except" question. Three clients are either unstable or have potentially life-threatening conditions.

25. 1. **The Joint Commission and safety standards mandate that all hospital personnel must check the parent's ID band with the infant's ID band before releasing the infant to the care of the mother or father.**
    2. The UAP can bring diapers to the mother; therefore, this would not warrant immediate intervention.
    3. The UAP can put lotion on the infant while the mother is watching because this is not teaching.
    4. This may be teaching, but the UAP is making sure the newborn is safe; therefore, this action would not warrant immediate intervention.

*Content – Women's Health: **Category of Health Alteration** – Women's Health: Integrated Process: Nursing Process: Evaluation: **Client Needs** – Safe and Effective Care Environment: Management of Care: **Cognitive Level** – Synthesis*

26. 1. The UAP can take vital signs on a stable client.
    2. The UAP can pass out breakfast trays.

3. Rhogam is a medication that cannot be delegated to the UAP.
4. The UAP can remove an indwelling urinary catheter. It is not a medication.

*Content – Women's Health: **Category of Health Alteration** – Drug Administration: **Integrated Process** – Nursing Process: Planning: **Client Needs** – Safe and Effective Care Environment: Management of Care: **Cognitive Level** – Synthesis*

MAKING NURSING DECISIONS: The nurse cannot delegate assessment, teaching, evaluation, medication, or an unstable client to a UAP.

27. 1. Ice packs are applied to acute injuries, so this intervention is appropriate for the UAP.
    2. **Only the client pushes the PCA pump; therefore, this action requires immediate intervention by the nurse.**
    3. Using non-sterile gloves is appropriate when handling blood and body fluids, so this is an appropriate intervention for the UAP.
    4. The UAP can encourage a client to eat the food on the breakfast tray; therefore, this behavior does not warrant immediate intervention.

*Content – Women's Health: **Category of Health Alteration** – Women's Health: **Integrated Process** – Nursing Process: Evaluation: **Client Needs** – Safe and Effective Care Environment: Management of Care: **Cognitive Level** – Synthesis*

MAKING NURSING DECISIONS: The phrase "warrants immediate intervention" means one of the options is inappropriate for the UAP to perform.

28. 1. The UAP cannot assess, teach, evaluate, administer medications, or care for an unstable client.
    2. The sharps container can be changed by a housekeeper, UAP, or an LPN, so this is not an appropriate task to assign to the RN.
    3. **The LPN can administer medications, and ibuprofen has an antiprostaglandin effect that is appropriate for a client experiencing afterbirth pains.**
    4. The charge nurse should not assign a LPN an unstable client. This client may have another seizure and should be monitored closely for at least 24 to 48 hours post-delivery.

*Content – Women's Health: **Category of Health Alteration** – Women's Health: **Integrated Processes** – Nursing Process: Planning: **Client Needs** – Safe and Effective Care Environment: Management of Care: **Cognitive Level** – Synthesis*

MAKING NURSING DECISIONS: The nurse must know what can be delegated and assigned to the UAP and LPN. There will be numerous

ANSWERS

questions on NCLEX-RN® concerning delegation and assignment. Remember that the nurse may not delegate the following to the UAP: assessment, teaching, evaluation, administering medications, or the care of an unstable client. The nurse cannot assign assessment, teaching, evaluation, or an unstable client to the LPN.

29. 1. The nurse should document the sitz bath but it is not priority over making sure the UAP gave the sitz bath.
    2. **The most important intervention for the nurse to do when delegating a task is to follow up to ensure it was done.**
    3. The nurse should assess the client, but the priority intervention is to ensure the UAP completed the assigned task.
    4. The nurse should ensure the client does not get constipated, but the test taker must read the stem of the question to determine how to answer it correctly.
    Content – Women's Health: *Category of Health Alteration* – Women's Health: *Integrated Process* – Nursing Process: Implementation: *Client Needs* – Physiological Integrity: Basic Care and Comfort: *Cognitive Level* – Application

MAKING NURSING DECISIONS: When the question asks which option is the priority intervention, it means one or more of the options are something a nurse can implement. The test taker must determine what the question is asking in order to select the right answer. There is always something in the stem of the question that will help the test taker determine the correct option.

30. 1. This newborn is postmature and may have complications, so she should be assigned to an RN.
    2. The newborn is experiencing hypoglycemia and should be assigned to an RN.
    3. The newborn is a risk for going through heroin withdrawals and should be assigned to an RN.
    4. **The newborn born vaginally after 2 hours' labor is stable and should be assigned to the LPN.**
    Content – Newborn: *Category of Health Alteration* – Women's Health: *Integrated Process* – Nursing Process: Planning: *Client Needs* – Safe and Effective Care Environment: Management of Care: *Cognitive Level* – Synthesis

MAKING NURSING DECISIONS: The test taker must decide which newborn should be assigned to the LPN: the most stable, or a more critical newborn. Once the test taker makes this decision, the newborn who is most stable should be selected to be assigned to the LPN.

31. 1. This requirement is violating the client's autonomy, which is a client's right to self-determination without outside control. This approach has been used as a condition of probation, to allow women accused of child abuse/neglect to get out of a jail term.
    2. Justice is the duty to treat all clients fairly, without regard to age, socioeconomic status, and other variables.
    3. Fidelity is the duty to be faithful to commitments.
    4. Beneficence is the duty to do good actively for the clients.
    Content – Women's Health: *Category of Health Alteration* – Women's Health: *Integrated Process* – Nursing Process: Evaluation: *Client Needs* – Psychosocial Integrity: *Cognitive Level* – Synthesis

MAKING NURSING DECISIONS: The nurse must be cognizant of ethical principles that guide nursing and healthcare practices. The judge is acting under legal guidelines that can supersede the client's rights.

32. 1, 3, and 5 are correct.
    1. **Magnesium sulfate, a uterine relaxant, is the drug of choice to help prevent seizures. The medication relaxes smooth muscles and reduces vasoconstriction, thus promoting circulation to the vital organs of the mother and increasing placental circulation to the fetus.**
    2. The mother is not placed on telemetry, but continuous electronic fetal monitoring is required to identify fetal heart rate patterns that suggest fetal compromise.
    3. **The deep tendon reflexes are monitored to determine the effectiveness of the magnesium sulfate.**
    4. After delivery, the mother will excrete large volumes of fluid, a sign of recovery from preeclampsia. However, the loop diuretic Lasix would not be given before delivery because it may lead to hypovolemia.
    5. **The nursery should be notified of the delivery so it will be prepared for the neonate. Because the client is in labor, the baby will be born within a reasonable time frame.**
    Content – Women's Health: *Category of Health Alteration* – Women's Health: *Integrated Process* – Nursing Process: Implementation: *Client Needs* – Physiological Integrity: Reduction of Risk Potential: *Cognitive Level* – Application

33. 1. The nurse should encourage the father to remain calm for his wife in this crisis situation, but this is not the first intervention.

2. Assigning staff members is part of the Code Pink protocol, but it is not the nurse's first intervention.
3. **The nurse's first intervention is to call a Code Pink. Then, the nurse should institute all other nursing interventions. The infant's safety is priority.**
4. The nurse should question the father for exact details, but the nurse should first call the Code Pink so that the person who took the infant can be found.

*Content – Women's Health: **Category of Health Alteration** – Women's Health: **Integrated Process** – Nursing Process: Implementation: **Client Needs** – Safe and Effective Care Environment: Safety and Infection Control: **Cognitive Level** – Application*

MAKING NURSING DECISIONS: The nurse is responsible for knowing and complying with hospital protocols as well as the local, state, and federal standards of care.

34. 1. This pain is normal and does not require seeing the HCP today.
2. **During the first few days after delivery, levels of the hormone relax and gradually subside, and the ligaments and cartilage of the pelvis return to their pre-pregnancy position. These changes cause hip and joint pain that interfere with ambulation. The mother should understand that the pain is temporary and does not indicate a problem.**
3. Kegel exercises tone up the client's peritoneal muscles after a pregnancy. These exercises would not help hip and joint pain.
4. Emptying the bladder will not help the client's joint and hip pain.

*Content – Women's Health: **Category of Health Alteration** – Women's Health: **Integrated Process** – Nursing Process: Evaluation: **Client Needs** – Physiological Integrity, Physiological Adaptation: **Cognitive Level** – Synthesis*

35. 1. SIDS occurs to infants who are living, not to infants in utero.
2. The case manager is responsible for coordinating care between disciplines for clients with chronic illnesses. This client has lost a baby and would not need a referral to a case manager.
3. **According to the NCLEX-RN® test blueprint, management of care includes appropriate use of referrals. The chaplain is responsible for intervening in a case where there is spiritual distress. A loss of a child is devastating.**
4. Child Protective Services (CPS) are notified only if the child is being abused. This baby

died in utero; therefore, CPS would not be notified, except in states where the mother is a drug abuser or has chronic alcoholism.

*Content – Women's Health: **Category of Health Alteration** – Women's Health: **Integrated Processes** – Nursing Process: Implementation: **Client Needs** – Psychosocial Integrity: **Cognitive Level** – Application*

36. 1. This statement is making the assumption the client is being abused—which is probably true—but the nurse should not put words in the client's mouth. Because this is a legal issue, the nurse cannot suggest in any manner, verbally or physically, to the client that abuse is occurring. If the client is being abused and decides to file charges, then the accused can use the defense that indeed he or she was not abusing the client and the client decided to consider his or her actions as abuse only after the nurse suggested it.
2. This is a true statement, but it is judgmental and would not encourage a therapeutic relationship with the client.
3. Research indicates that abusive situations escalate during pregnancy, particularly with the woman being hit in the abdominal area; therefore, this question is not necessary. These bruises indicate that abuse is occurring.
4. **The nurse's best intervention is to assess the safety of the client and infant and provide information to the client about a safe haven.**

*Content – Women's Health: **Category of Health Alteration** – Women's Health: **Integrated Processes** – Nursing Process: Assessment: **Client Needs** – Safe and Effective Care Environment, Safety and Infection Control: **Cognitive Level** – Analysis*

MAKING NURSING DECISIONS: The nurse is responsible for knowing and complying with local, state, and federal standards of care.

37. 1. The nurse should not upset the client by telling her that her boyfriend is creating problems.
2. The nurse should not allow a person displaying this behavior to remain on the unit.
3. **The nurse should first contact hospital security to intervene and escort the boyfriend off the unit.**
4. Confronting a drunken individual could escalate the situation. The nurse should contact security to take care of this situation.

*Content – Women's Health: **Category of Health Alteration** – Obstetrics: **Integrated Processes** – Nursing Process: Implementation: **Client Needs** – Safe and Effective Care Environment: Safety and Infection Control: **Cognitive Level** – Application*

ANSWERS

38. 1. **Jehovah's Witnesses do not believe in accepting blood products, but it is the individual's choice. The nurse is a client advocate and should make sure the client is aware that without the injection her next pregnancy could result in erythroblastosis fetalis. However, with the injection her religious belief may be compromised because Rhogam is a blood product.**
2. The father of the baby must be Rh-positive; otherwise, the baby would not be Rh-positive and the mother would not require the Rhogam injection. The baby's blood type determines whether the mother needs the Rhogam injection.
3. When administering Rhogam to the client, this question is not pertinent. Rhogam is prescribed only for Rh-negative mothers who have Rh-positive babies, or within 72 hours of a miscarriage.
4. The client's insurance status is not pertinent information for the nurse caring for the client.

Content – Women's Health: ***Category of Health Alteration** – Drug Administration:* ***Integrated Processes** – Nursing Process: Implementation:* ***Client Needs** – Psychosocial Integrity:* ***Cognitive Level** – Application*

MAKING NURSING DECISIONS: Any time there is a cultural or religious factor in the question, the test taker should be aware that this will affect the correct answer.

39. 1. The nurse would not question administering this medication because a negative titer means the client is not immune to rubella (German measles). This vaccine prevents rubella infection and possible severe congenital defects in a fetus in a subsequent pregnancy.
2. **The flu vaccine is made using duck eggs; therefore, the nurse should question the administration of this vaccine to a client who is allergic to eggs.**
3. A positive PPD test determines whether the client was exposed to tuberculosis.
4. The nurse would not question administering the hepatitis B vaccine to a mother who is breastfeeding because 1-day-old infants receive the vaccine.

Content – Women's Health: ***Category of Health Alteration** – Drug Administration:* ***Integrated Processes** – Nursing Process: Assessment:* ***Client Needs** – Health Promotion and Maintenance:* ***Cognitive Level** – Analysis*

40. 1. A chignon is newborn scalp edema created by vacuum extraction and will resolve within a few days of delivery. This infant would not need to be assessed first.
2. Caput succedaneum appears over the vertex of the newborn's head as a result of pressure against the mother's cervix during labor. The edematous area crosses suture lines, is soft, and varies in size. It resolves quickly and disappears within 12 hours to several days after birth. This newborn would not need to be seen first.
3. **A cephalohematoma results when there is bleeding between the periosteum and the skull from pressure during birth. The firm swelling is not present at birth but develops within the first 24 to 48 hours. Any time a client is bleeding, it warrants intervention by the nurse.**
4. A port-wine stain, nevus flammeus, is a permanent, flat, reddish purple mark that varies in size and location and does not blanch with pressure. This would not require immediate intervention from the nurse.

Content – Newborn: ***Category of Health Alteration** – Women's Health:* ***Integrated Processes** – Nursing Process: Assessment:* ***Client Needs** – Physiological Integrity: Reduction of Risk Potential:* ***Cognitive Level** – Analysis*

41. 1. **Refusal of two or more feedings indicates the infant has a problem that requires the mother notify the healthcare provider. This indicates the mother understands the discharge teaching.**
2. Green liquid stools indicate a problem and require the mother notify the healthcare provider.
3. AquaMephyton (vitamin K) is administered intramuscularly to the infant in the newborn nursery to prevent the infant from bleeding because the gastrointestinal tract is sterile when the infant is born and requires bacteria to synthesize vitamin K from the food eaten by the infant.
4. The infant will have meconium stool for a few weeks after being born, so the mother should not notify the healthcare provider.

Content – Women's Health: ***Category of Health Alteration** – Women's Health:* ***Integrated Processes** – Nursing Process: Evaluation:* ***Client Needs** – Health Promotion and Maintenance:* ***Cognitive Level** – Synthesis*

MAKING NURSING DECISIONS: When the question asks, "Which statement indicates the teaching is effective?" the test taker must select the option with correct information.

42. 1. Nausea and vomiting is normal for a 12-week gestation client.
2. Ankle edema is expected in a 24-week gestation client.
3. **Facial edema is a sign of pregnancy-induced hypertension, which requires the clinic nurse to contact the certified nurse midwife.**
4. The increasing size of the uterus compresses on the bladder, leading to increased frequency of urination so this is an expected finding.

Content – Women's Health: **Category of Health Alteration** – Women's Health: **Integrated Processes –** Nursing Process: Assessment: **Client Needs –** Physiological Integrity: Reduction of Risk Potential: **Cognitive Level** – Analysis

MAKING NURSING DECISIONS: The test taker should ask "Is it normal for . . . ?" For example, "Is it normal for the 12-week gestation client to have nausea and vomiting?" If this is normal, then the nurse would not need to notify anyone of this finding.

43. 1. The "taking in" phase is the first phase the mother goes through after the delivery. The mother is not ready to learn or be taught anything in this phase.
2. This is a nursing intervention but is not part of the "taking in" phase.
3. **The client during the "taking in" phase is self-absorbed and needs to be cared for, so allowing the client to talk about her own experience is the most appropriate intervention.**
4. The client in the "taking in" phase is not ready to learn or be taught anything.

Content – Women's Health: **Category of Health Alteration** – Women's Health: **Integrated Processes –** Nursing Process: Implementation: **Client Needs –** Psychosocial Integrity: **Cognitive Level** – Comprehension

MAKING NURSING DECISIONS: The test taker must not only know what the "taking in" phase is, but must be able to apply it. Remembering information is not the same as being able to apply the information.

44. 1 and 2 are correct.
1. **The breasts should be palpated to assess for fullness or engorgement.**
2. **The nurse should check for the amount, color, and consistency of vaginal discharge.**
3. The nurse should assess for deep vein thrombosis (DVT) but this does not include assessing pedal pulses.
4. The client with a vaginal delivery will not have a surgical incision.

5. The nurse does not need to check pupillary response for a postpartum client; this would be appropriate for a client with a neurological disorder.

Content – Women's Health: **Category of Health Alteration** – Women's Health: **Integrated Processes –** Nursing Process: Assessment: **Client Needs –** Physiological Integrity: Reduction of Risk Potential: **Cognitive Level** – Analysis

MAKING NURSING DECISIONS: The test taker must select one or more options when asked to answer "select all that apply" questions. The key to the assessment data is a postpartum client. The test taker does not get partial credit for the answer—all appropriate options must be selected to get the question correct.

45. 1. **The Muslim religion does not allow the consumption of pork products, so this warrants intervention by the charge nurse.**
2. The Sabbath day for Seventh Day Adventist is Saturday so this does not warrant intervention.
3. Asians who believe in the hot-cold theory of disease will often not drink cold fluids or eat cold foods during the postpartum period, so this does not warrant immediate intervention.
4. Jehovah's Witnesses do not take blood products so this action does not warrant intervention.

Content – Women's Health: **Category of Health Alteration** – Women's Health: **Integrated Processes –** Nursing Process: Assessment: **Client Needs –** Physiological Integrity: Reduction of Risk Potential: **Cognitive Level** – Analysis

MAKING NURSING DECISIONS: The nurse must attempt to support a client's cultural beliefs. This is a knowledge-based question but the nurse must be knowledgeable of cultural beliefs.

46. 1. The HCP in a free clinic would not be able to refer this client to an infertility clinic because of cost. The nurse can discuss this with the client.
2. **If the couple has not been able to conceive in 6 years, then a referral to an infertility clinic would be appropriate, but the tests and treatment for infertility are very expensive. The client is being seen in a free clinic, which indicates a lack of funds. The nurse has a relationship with this client over the time period "several weeks." The nurse should answer the client's question.**

ANSWERS

3. This is a therapeutic response, which does not answer the client's question, "What can we do?"
4. If the client has not conceived in 6 years, this is not a probable solution to the client's concern.

*Content – Women's Health: **Category of Health Alteration** – Women's Health: **Integrated Processes** – Nursing Process: Implementation: **Client Needs** – Psychosocial Integrity: **Cognitive Level** – Application*

47. 1. **The client who is 10 cm dilated and 100% effaced is ready to deliver the fetus; therefore, the nurse should assess this client first.**
2. Early decelerations are not associated with fetal compromise and require no added interventions; therefore, this client would not need to be assessed first.
3. This client does not have an immediate need; therefore, the nurse should not assess this client first.
4. This is causing distress to the mother, but there is nothing the nurse can do about this situation. The on-call obstetrician will have to deliver the fetus.

*Content – Women's Health: **Category of Health Alteration** – Women's Health: **Integrated Processes** – Nursing Process: Assessment: **Client Needs** – Safe and Effective Care Environment: Management of Care: **Cognitive Level** – Analysis*

48. 1. The pregnant client has an increased circulating blood volume, which results in a slight decrease of the hemoglobin and hematocrit; therefore, this client would not warrant intervention.
2. The normal fasting blood glucose level is 70 to 120 mg/dL; therefore, this client does not warrant intervention by the nurse.
3. **Protein in the urine indicates the client is at risk for pregnancy-induced hypertension; therefore, this client warrants intervention and further assessment by the nurse.**
4. The white blood cell count increases during pregnancy; the normal range is 5,000 to 12,000 and rises during labor. This client does not warrant intervention.

*Content – Women's Health: **Category of Health Alteration** – Women's Health: **Integrated Processes** – Nursing Process: Assessment: **Client Needs** – Physiological Integrity: Reduction of Risk Potential: **Cognitive Level** – Analysis*

49. 1. If the client is unable to urinate, then the nurse will have to perform an in-and-out catheterization to empty the bladder. However, the nurse should implement the least invasive intervention.

2. The nurse could use a bladder scanner to determine whether the bladder was full, but the first intervention is to ask the client to urinate.
3. Massaging the fundus will not put the fundus in a midline position until the bladder is empty.
4. **The number one reason for a displaced fundus is a full bladder. The nurse should always do the least invasive procedure, which is to ask the client to attempt to void. The emptying of the bladder should allow the fundus to return to the midline position.**

*Content – Women's Health: **Category of Health Alteration** – Women's Health: **Integrated Processes** – Nursing Process: Implementation: **Client Needs** – Physiological Integrity: Reduction of Risk Potential: **Cognitive Level** – Application*

50. 1. Anyone could have left the client's chart at the bedside, such as the HCP or the radiology technician. The charge nurse should first determine the facts before taking further action.
2. The charge nurse should take the client's chart back to the nurse's station.
3. This could be a violation of HIPAA because anyone entering the client's room could read the client's chart, but this is not the charge nurse's first intervention.
4. **The charge nurse should first take the client's chart back to the nurse's station and then determine who left it at the client's bedside, and why.**

*Content – Legal: **Category of Health Alteration** – Women's Health: **Integrated Processes** – Nursing Process: Implementation: **Client Needs** – Safe and Effective Care Environment: Management of Care: **Cognitive Level** – Application*

51. 1. The nurse really does not need to know when the client had her last chest x-ray when scheduling this chest x-ray.
2. **The nurse should ask whether the client may be pregnant because if there is a chance of pregnancy, the client should not have an x-ray. Any time a female client is of childbearing age and is having any type of x-ray, this question should be asked.**
3. The date of the client's last period would not affect the client's having a chest x-ray.
4. This question would be asked if the client was receiving some type of contrast or dye.

*Content – Women's Health: **Category of Health Alteration** – Women's Health: **Integrated Processes** – Nursing Process: Assessment: **Client Needs** – Physiological Integrity: Reduction of Risk Potential: **Cognitive Level** – Comprehension*

52. 1. The clinical manager should first talk to the nurse to determine what is causing the medication error.
2. Three medication errors in a short period of time require the clinical manager to investigate the cause.
3. **This should be the clinical manager's first intervention, to assess whether the system is responsible for the medication errors or whether it is a nursing error problem. For example, a system error problem would be that the medication is not available at the prescribed time.**
4. This may be needed, but it is not the nurse's first intervention. If the clinical manager determines the nurse is at fault, then this could be a possible action.

*Content – Management: **Category of Health Alteration –** Women's Health: **Integrated Processes –** Nursing Process: Implementation: **Client Needs –** Safe and Effective Care Environment: Safety and Infection Control: **Cognitive Level –** Application*

53. 1. **When the infant is placed in the supine position, the infant should extend the arm and leg on the side to which the head is turned and then flex the extremities on the other. This is known as the tonic-neck reflex or fencing reflex, which is normal for the newborn. The newborn remaining in a fetal position when supine warrants further intervention to assess for neurological problems.**
2. The Babinski reflex is elicited by stroking the lateral sole of the foot from the heel forward. Normal reflex is that the toes flare outward and the big toe dorsiflexes. This is a normal response for an infant but is abnormal in an adult, indicating neurological deficit in the adult. Therefore, this does not warrant immediate intervention.
3. This is the rooting reflex, which is normal for a newborn. This would not warrant immediate intervention.
4. The Moro reflex or the startle reflex is a sharp extension and abduction of arm with thumbs and forefingers in a C-position followed by flexion and adduction to embrace position. This response occurs with loud noise or when the newborn is startled. This would not warrant immediate intervention.

*Content – Women's Health: **Category of Health Alteration –** Women's Health: **Integrated Processes –** Nursing Process: Assessment: **Client Needs –** Physiological Integrity: Physiological Adaptation: **Cognitive Level –** Analysis*

54. 1. This is the ethical principle of veracity, which is truth telling.

2. **No maleficence is the duty to do no harm. Many ethicists think that the principle of no maleficence has priority over other ethical principles except for autonomy. No maleficence allows the nurse to answer a question or make a decision that does not create further complications for the client.**
3. This is paternalism, which is giving advice and telling the client what is best for her.
4. This is an assessment question that could guide the nurse in helping the client make a decision, but it does not demonstrate the ethical principle of no maleficence.

*Content – Nursing Ethics: **Category of Health Alteration –** Women's Health: **Integrated Processes –** Nursing Process: Implementation: **Client Needs –** Psychosocial Integrity: **Cognitive Level –** Application*

55. 1. This statement describes primary care, which is a type of nursing care delivery.
2. **Modular nursing is frequently called care pairs, in which nurses are paired with other less well-trained caregivers to provide nursing care to group clients.**
3. This statement describes team nursing, which is a type of nursing care delivery.
4. This statement describes functional nursing, in which there is a charge nurse, a medication nurse, and a treatment nurse.

*Content – Nursing Trends: **Category of Health Alteration –** Women's Health: **Integrated Processes –** Nursing Process: Implementation: **Client Needs –** Safe and Effective Care Environment: Management of Care: **Cognitive Level –** Comprehension*

56. 1. Threatening and attempting to manipulate the staff will create distrust and anger, which will not facilitate a smooth transition for the medication delivery system.
2. This action is not fair because the new system is being implemented whether the staff members vote for it or not. There are situations, resulting from financial or other constraints, which require the clinical manager to implement a change without the input of the staff.
3. **To be an effective change agent, the manager needs to develop a sense of trust, establish common goals, and facilitate effective communication.**
4. Sending the documentation by hospital e-mail is pertinent to ensure all staff members receive the information, but it is not effective in producing a smooth transition and reduction of resistance to the change.

*Content – Management: **Category of Health Alteration –** Women's Health: **Integrated Processes –** Nursing Process: Implementation: **Client Needs –** Safe and Effective Care Environment: Management of Care: **Cognitive Level –** Application*

57. 1. This behavior may be normal for some individuals and may not be detrimental to the infant or mother, but the nurse must investigate the situation first before making this statement.

2. Clay and dirt in the gut may decrease the absorption of nutrients such as iron. Therefore, asking this question is appropriate, but the first intervention should be to determine whether there are complications related to pica.

3. **Pica, ingesting substances not normally considered food, may decrease the intake of food and therefore essential nutrients. Iron deficiency was once thought to be a cause of pica but is now considered a result. The nurse must first assess to determine whether the behavior is detrimental to the mother or infant before further action is taken.**

4. Pica may be related to cultural beliefs about materials that will ensure a healthy mother and infant. This should not be the nurse's first intervention. The safety of mother and fetus is priority. If the H&H is within normal limits, the nurse should support the cultural belief.

Content – Women's Health: **Category of Health Alteration** *– Women's Health:* **Integrated Processes** *– Diagnosis:* **Client Needs** *– Physiological Integrity: Reduction of Risk Potential:* **Cognitive Level** *– Analysis*

58. 1. **Insurance companies contract with certain providers to provide care to the client at a reduced rate. Using this doctor, who is not a preferred provider of care, will result in a greater out-of-pocket expense for the client.**

2. This is not a true statement, and the nurse should not give the client false information, especially about money.

3. This therapeutic response is to encourage the client to ventilate feelings. This client needs factual information.

4. Most insurance companies will not cover a preexisting condition for 1 year after the policy is initiated; therefore, this pregnancy may not be covered.

Content – Women's Health: **Category of Health Alteration** *– Women's Health:* **Integrated Processes** *– Nursing Process: Implementation:* **Client Needs** *– Health Promotion and Maintenance:* **Cognitive Level** *– Comprehension*

59. 1. The 16-year-old client must sign for her child's care. The grandmother does not have the authority to sign informed consent for the procedure.

2. The cost of the procedure should not be a factor for the nurse when discussing a medical procedure with the client.

3. The client is not requesting assistance to pay the medical bills; therefore, this intervention is not appropriate.

4. **A 16-year-old mother has the right to make decisions for her child; therefore, the mother must sign the informed consent for the procedure.**

Content – Legal: **Category of Health Alteration** *– Women's Health:* **Integrated Processes** *– Nursing Process: Implementation:* **Client Needs** *– Safe and Effective Care Environment: Management of Care:* **Cognitive Level** *– Application*

60. 1. The UAPs may or may not cross the picket line, and the managers will not be able to provide care to all the clients. This is not the best response.

2. Abandonment is leaving the shift without notifying the supervisor after accepting the assignment. Going on strike with a 10-day notice is not abandonment.

3. This may or may not be a true statement; therefore, it is not the best response.

4. **Federal law requires that there must be a 10-day notice before going on a strike. This gives the hospital a chance to prepare for the strike and make changes to ensure client safety.**

Content – Management: **Category of Health Alteration** *– Women's Health:* **Integrated Processes** *– Nursing Process: Implementation:* **Client Needs** *– Safe and Effective Care Environment: Management of Care:* **Cognitive Level** *– Application*

61. 1. **Anencephaly is a congenital abnormality that entails an absence of all or a major part of the brain. The infant has no chance of life outside of a healthcare institution. The healthcare team refers situations to the ethics committee to help resolve dilemmas when caring for clients.**

2. This is not an ethical dilemma because the 16-year-old client has a right to place her infant up for adoption. This would not need to be referred to an ethics committee.

3. If the nurse wants to take the child away from the mother, then this must be reported to Child Protective Services. Therefore, this is not an ethical dilemma. The nurse has a law that directs the decision. This would not need to be referred to an ethics committee.

4. This is a legal issue, not an ethical issue. The healthcare team can request the hospital attorney to take these parents to court and

request a court order to administer blood. The parents do not have the right to refuse life-sustaining treatment for their child.

Content – Nursing Ethics: **Category of Health Alteration** *– Women's Health:* **Integrated Processes** *– Communication and Documentation:* **Client Needs** *– Safe and Effective Care Environment: Management of Care:* **Cognitive Level** *– Analysis*

62. **1, 2, and 3 are correct.**
   1. **The mother should be encouraged to hold and cuddle the infant to help with the grieving process.**
   2. **The mother should not be required to stay on a unit where she can hear crying infants and happy families. This is a very cruel action to take. The nurse should transfer the client to another unit.**
   3. **The nurse should remember the father has lost the baby, too. Acknowledging and encouraging the father to talk about his loss will help with his grieving process.**
   4. The nurse should not impose his or her beliefs about funerals on the client. This is a boundary crossing violation.
   5. Grief support groups recommend giving the infant a name because it acknowledges the infant's existence.

   Content – Newborn: **Category of Health Alteration** *– Women's Health:* **Integrated Processes** *– Nursing Process: Implementation:* **Client Needs** *– Psychosocial Integrity:* **Cognitive Level** *– Application*

63. 1. The clinical manager could ask the primary nurse why she provides such excellent care, but it is not the most important action. Excellence in care should be documented in writing in nurse's personnel file to support merit raises, transfers, and promotions.
   2. **The clinical manager should recognize the comments of clients/families during the performance evaluation. Excellence in care should be documented in writing in nurse's personnel file to support merit raises, transfers, and promotions. Many healthcare facilities have employee recognition programs.**
   3. This is a possible action, but this could single out the nurse and cause dissension among the other staff. Parties on the unit should celebrate the unit's accomplishments, not a single individual.
   4. Excellent care is the expectation of all clinical managers, but when the multiple clients/families recognize the nurse's care, then there should be documentation in the nurse's personnel file.

Content – Management: **Category of Health Alteration** *– Women's Health:* **Integrated Processes** *– Nursing Process: Implementation:* **Client Needs** *– Safe and Effective Care Environment: Management of Care:* **Cognitive Level** *– Application*

64. **2, 4, and 5 are correct.**
   1. The client should decrease the amount of caffeine, which includes coffee, teas, cola, and chocolate, because caffeine increases irritability, insomnia, anxiety, and nervousness.
   2. **Avoiding simple sugars will prevent rebound hypoglycemia, which will exacerbate the signs/symptoms of PMS.**
   3. Alcohol is a central nervous system depressant and aggravates the depression associated with PMS. This is not an appropriate intervention.
   4. **Decreasing the intake of salt will decrease fluid retention, thereby decreasing edema.**
   5. **Insomnia is a symptom of PMS, and a regular schedule for sleep will help decrease the severity of the PMS.**

   Content – Women's Health: **Category of Health Alteration** *– Women's Health:* **Integrated Processes** *– Nursing Process: Implementation:* **Client Needs** *– Physiological Integrity: Physiological Adaptation:* **Cognitive Level** *– Application*

65. 1. **Vegans are individuals who avoid animal proteins, which are complete proteins that contain all the essential amino acids the body cannot synthesize from other sources. Vegetable proteins lack one or more of the essential amino acids, so the vegan must combine different plant proteins, grains, legumes, and nuts, to allow for intake of all essential amino acids. Vegans avoid all animal products and have difficulty meeting adequate nutritional protein needs.**
   2. Vegans avoid animal products, and if she does not drink milk she will not eat eggs.
   3. The nurse should assist the client in adhering to cultural, spiritual, or personal beliefs, not try to talk the client into changing her beliefs unless it is a danger to the fetus or the mother.
   4. A vegan diet requires extra iron supplements; iron in the vegetarian diet is poorly absorbed because of the lack of heme iron that comes from meat.

   Content – Women's Health: **Category of Health Alteration** *– Women's Health:* **Integrated Processes** *– Nursing Process: Implementation:* **Client Needs** *– Health Promotion and Maintenance:* **Cognitive Level** *– Application*

ANSWERS

66. 1 and 4 are correct.
1. **This patient has delivered her infant and has pain. The medical-surgical nurse can care for this patient.**
2. This patient requires teaching, a knowledge base the medical-surgical nurse could not be assumed to have encountered on a medical-surgical unit.
3. HELLP syndrome stands for H—hemolysis (the breakdown of red blood cells), EL—elevated liver enzymes, LP—low platelet count. HELLP syndrome is a group of symptoms that occur in pregnant women who have preeclampsia or eclampsia. Symptoms include fatigue or feeling unwell, fluid retention and excess weight gain, headache, nausea and vomiting that continues to get worse, pain in the upper right part of the abdomen, blurry vision, nosebleed or other bleeding that won't stop easily (rare), and seizures or convulsions (rare). A medical-surgical nurse does not have the expertise required to care for this patient.
4. **This is a preterm patient who is on a monitor. The medical-surgical nurse can care for this patient. If something occurs on the monitor or the patient goes into labor, the nurse can get help.**
5. Pitocin is a medication that stimulates uterine contraction; it is used to induce labor or postpartum to help a boggy uterus to contract. It must be administered by a nurse familiar with the medication and its potential adverse effects.
Content – Women's Health: **Category of Health Alteration** *– Women's Health:* **Integrated Processes** *– Nursing Process: Planning:* **Client Needs** *– Safe and Effective Care Environment: Management of Care:* **Cognitive Level** *– Synthesis*

MAKING NURSING DECISIONS: The test taker must decide on each option individually. Would the medical-surgical nurse have the knowledge and skill to care for the patient or should the patient be cared for by a nurse more familiar with the specialized area of ante partum and postpartum care?

67. 1. This is a semi-Fowler's position, useful for increasing ease of breathing, etc., but it does not provide access to the epidural space.
2. This is the Sims position used for administering an enema.
3. **This position allows for a space to be created between the vertebrae and allow the anesthetist to insert the catheter into the epidural space.**

4. The laboring patient would not be able to lie on the stomach.
Content – Women's Health: **Category of Health Alteration** *– Women's Health:* **Integrated Processes** *– Nursing Process: Implementation:* **Client Needs** *– Physiological Integrity: Reduction of Risk Potential:* **Cognitive Level** *– Comprehension*

MAKING NURSING DECISIONS: The test taker should assess which position would allow access to the anatomical area needed to insert the catheter, remembering that the epidural space is part of the central nervous system.

68. 1. The nurse should notify the healthcare practitioner (HCP) after making sure no more magnesium is administered to the patient
2. Documenting the data is important but does not come before safety of the patient or notifying the HCP.
3. It is not necessary for the nurse to have his/her finding verified prior to acting to protect the patient.
4. **The adverse effects of parenterally administered magnesium sulfate usually are the result of magnesium intoxication. These include flushing, sweating, hypotension, depressed reflexes, flaccid paralysis, hypothermia, circulatory collapse, and cardiac and central nervous system depression proceeding to respiratory paralysis. This patient is demonstrating magnesium toxicity. The nurse should immediately discontinue the magnesium.**
Content – Women's Health: **Category of Health Alteration** *– Drug Administration:* **Integrated Processes** *– Nursing Process: Implementation:* **Client Needs** *– Physiological Integrity: Pharmacological and Parenteral Therapies:* **Cognitive Level** *– Application*

MAKING NURSING DECISIONS: The test taker should read all graphs, charts, or legends very carefully when choosing an option. Absent reflexes should indicate a need for an action on the part of the nurse. Documentation, while important, is not directly taking care of the patient and should only be chosen first when the data supplied is normal.

69. Correct Answer: 4, 5, 3, 1, 2
4. **The client came to the clinic for treatment and it should be the first intervention.**
5. **All sexual partners of the client should be notified of possible exposure to an STD. This is the responsibility of the public health nurse.**

3. The nurse's only opportunity to teach the client about safe sex practices may be this clinic visit.

1. The nurse should attempt to notify the sexual partners of client to prevent spread of the disease to other unsuspecting individuals.

2. The report is filed monthly or quarterly.

Content – Women's Health: **Category of Health Alteration** *– Women's Health:* **Integrated Processes** *– Nursing Process: Implementation:* **Client Needs** *– Safe and Effective Care Environment: Safety and Infection Control:* **Cognitive Level** *– Comprehension*

MAKING NURSING DECISIONS: The test taker must logically deduce the steps for the nurse to implement. Care of the client is first. Next the nurse must consider other clients who may be affected and get the names and contact information of the sexual partners; this must be done prior to being able to contacting the individual. Reports and documentation are last.

70. 1. At the scene of an accident, it is not important how far along the driver is.

2. **The driver must be assessed for signs of trauma before anything else can be done. If the patient dies, then the fetus will die too.**

3. Whether or not the driver was wearing a seat belt is a legal matter, and possible assessment data for the labor and delivery nurse to determine potential trauma to the fetus, but not at the scene of the accident.

4. This might be done if the nurse has a stethoscope, but the mother's status is first since the fetus's life depends on her.

Content – Women's Health: **Category of Health Alteration** *– Women's Health:* **Integrated Processes** *– Nursing Process: Implementation:* **Client Needs** *– Physiological Integrity: Reduction of Risk Potential:* **Cognitive Level** *– Application*

MAKING NURSING DECISIONS: The nurse has two patients in this scenario, the mother and the fetus, but one life definitely depends on the status of the other. All the options in this question have words that can be used to indicate assessment, so the test taker must choose the first assessment that must be made.

71. 1. The infection can come from kissing someone who has the infection in the mouth as well as oral sex. This is not the best statement.

2. Smear of oral tissue is not done routinely.

3. Due to oral sex and frequent partner changes transferring the organism from mucous membranes to mucous membranes via oral sex or kissing, the infection is the fastest rising incidence of causation for head and neck cancers

4. **Human papillomavirus (HPV) infections are increasing exponentially and many younger persons are developing mouth infections and cancers from HPV.**

Content – Women's Health: **Category of Health Alteration** *– Women's Health:* **Integrated Processes** *– Nursing Process: Implementation:* **Client Needs** *– Physiological Integrity: Reduction of Risk Potential:* **Cognitive Level** *– Application*

MAKING NURSING DECISIONS: The nurse must keep up to date with health issues. This is an issue that occurs in particular among the young adult population.

72. 1. The AIDS virus can be transmitted during the first exposure to it. The class should be taught no exposure is safe.

2. The use of condoms is somewhat protective but it does not guarantee protection from transmitting a sexually transmitted disease.

3. **The more exposure there is to blood or body fluids from another individual (more partners), the greater the chance there is of developing an STD.**

4. Both syphilis and gonorrhea are usually treatable but lasting problems can occur. For example, pelvic inflammatory disease can scar the fallopian tube and cause fertility issues.

Content – Women's Health: **Category of Health Alteration** *– Women's Health:* **Integrated Processes** *– Nursing Process: Implementation:* **Client Needs** *– Physiological Integrity: Reduction of Risk Potential:* **Cognitive Level** *– Application*

MAKING NURSING DECISIONS: The test taker could eliminate option 2 because of the word "ensure"; there are no guarantees in medicine. The test taker can also eliminate option 4 because of the word "no," as this is an absolute word. The test taker must read carefully because the words in the stem and in the options can give clues as to the correct answer.

CLINICAL SCENARIO ANSWERS AND RATIONALES

The correct answer number and rationale for why it is the correct answer are given in boldface type. Rationales for why the other possible answer options are incorrect also are given, but they are not in boldface type.

1. 1. **This pain needs to be assessed and pain medication administered. A new graduate would be able to care for this client safely.**
   2. Saturating multiple peri-pads indicates heavy bleeding, which may indicate hemorrhaging. A more experienced nurse should be assigned to this client.
   3. The nurse needs to assess this client for possible maternal/infant bonding problems and would require a nurse who has experience with psychosocial problems. This client should be assigned to a more experienced nurse.
   4. This client requires a nurse who is knowledgeable and experienced in breastfeeding; therefore, a more experienced nurse should be assigned to this client.

2. 1. These are called milia and look like pimples; they will fade within a few days and do not warrant immediate intervention.
   2. **The normal respiratory rate for a newborn is 30 to 60; therefore, this information warrants immediate intervention.**
   3. The newborn who is turning red when crying is not in distress; therefore, this would not warrant immediate intervention.
   4. The newborn should pass meconium within 24 hours of birth and it is viscous and sticky like tar, and has no odor. This would not warrant intervention by Ms. Kathy.

3. 1. **The fetus is in distress and after increasing blood supply by placing the client in the left lateral position, Ms. Glada needs to contact the obstetrician for immediate C-section.**
   2. Panting during contractions will help prevent the client from pushing but it is not the first intervention. This client needs immediate evaluation by an obstetrician.
   3. Oxytocin is a uterine stimulant and this fetus is in distress and does not need uterine contractions. This is an inappropriate intervention.
   4. The nurse needs to prepare for immediate delivery of the fetus but not prior to contacting the obstetrician. The nurse cannot perform a C-section.

4. 1. The white blood cell count rises normally during labor and postpartum—up to 25,000 mm³; therefore, this does not warrant intervention.
   2. The serum potassium level is within normal limits, 3.5 to 5.5 mEq/L so this client does not warrant immediate intervention by Ms. Helen.
   3. **HELLP syndrome is a group of symptoms that occur in pregnant women who have hemolysis (H), elevated liver enzymes (EL), and low platelet count (LP), which occurs in women who are severely preeclamptic and eclamptic. Normal platelet count is 150,000 to 450,000, so this client's platelet count requires immediate intervention.**
   4. This glucose level is elevated, but since the client had gestational diabetes this blood glucose level does not require immediate intervention.

5. 1. Braxton Hicks contractions are irregular contractions of the uterus throughout the pregnancy and are not true labor. This client would not need to be assigned to Ms. Judy.
   2. The client having twins on bed rest is not in imminent danger; therefore, this client would not to be assigned to Ms. Judy.
   3. **This client is ready to deliver; therefore Ms. Judy should be assigned to this client since the other three clients are not experiencing any life-threatening complications.**
   4. Early decelerations on the fetal monitor do not indicate fetal distress; therefore, this client does not need to be assigned to Ms. Judy.

6. 1. **The UAP can assist the client to the bathroom to urinate. The UAP cannot assess the client's fundus. The number one reason for a non-midline fundus is a full bladder. Ms. Glada cannot delegate assessment, teaching, evaluation, medication administration, or an unstable client to the UAP.**
   2. The client with a HELLP syndrome is unstable; therefore, Ms. Glada, should not delegate these vital signs to the UAP.
   3. Ms. Glada cannot delegate teaching to the UAP.
   4. Ms. Glada cannot delegate medication administration to the UAP.

7. 1. **The float nurse should be able to address the psychosocial concerns of the mother and family. The client has no physiological problems so the float nurse could care**

for this client. Often, the mother with a fetal demise is transferred to a medical-surgical unit so she does not have to hear babies crying.

2. A boggy uterus indicates a potentially life-threatening situation and requires an experienced postpartum nurse to care for this client.

3. This client is potentially hemorrhaging and requires a more experienced nurse to care for her.

4. There are many legal issues surrounding an adoption as well as caring for the mother who is giving up her child; this client should be assigned a nurse more experienced in postpartum care.

8. 1. The flu vaccine is made using duck eggs; therefore, Ms. Judy should question the administration of this vaccine to a client who is allergic to eggs, not tomatoes.

2. The nurse would not question administering the hepatitis B vaccine to a mother who is breastfeeding because 1-day-old infants receive the vaccine.

3. Rhogam should be administered to the client since the baby is Rh-positive. This will help prevent erthroblastosis fetalasis in the woman's next pregnancy.

4. **The nurse would question administering this medication because a positive titer means the client is immune to rubella (German measles).**

9. 1. Mongolian spots are blue- or purple-colored splotches on the baby's lower back and buttocks. The spots are caused by a concentration of pigmented cells that usually disappear in the first 4 years of life. This newborn does not need to be assessed first.

2. A port-wine stain is a flat pink-, red-, or purple-colored birthmark. These are caused by a concentration of dilated tiny blood vessels called capillaries. The most effective way of treating port-wine stains is with a special type of laser done when the baby is older. This newborn does not need to be assessed first.

3. Erythema toxicum is a red rash on newborns that is often described as "flea bites." The rash is common on the chest and back, but may be found all over. It does not require any treatment and disappears by itself in a few days; therefore, Ms. Kathy does not need to assess this newborn first.

4. **A cephalohematoma results when there is bleeding between the periosteum and the skull from pressure during birth. The firm swelling, edema, is not present at birth but develops within the first 24 to 48 hours. Any time a client is bleeding, it warrants intervention by the nurse.**

10. 1. **When the infant is placed in the supine position, the infant should extend the arm and leg on the side to which the head is turned and then flex the extremities on the other. This is known as the tonic-neck reflex or fencing reflex, which is normal for the newborn. The newborn remaining in a fetal position when supine warrants further intervention to assess for neurological problems.**

2. The Babinski reflex is elicited by stroking the lateral sole of the foot from the heel forward. Normal reflex is that the toes flare outward and the big toe dorsiflexes. This is a normal response for an infant but is abnormal in an adult, indicating neurological deficit in the adult. Therefore, this does not warrant immediate intervention.

3. The stepping reflex is intact when the nurse places the baby on a flat surface. The baby will "walk" by placing one foot in front of the other. This is expected and does not warrant intervention by Ms. Judy.

4. The grasp reflex is elicited by placing a finger on the infant's open palm. The hand will close around the finger. Newborn infants have strong grasps and can almost be lifted from the examination table if both hands are used. This would not warrant intervention.

Pediatric Health Management

People are like stained-glass windows. They sparkle and shine when the sun is out but when the darkness sets in, their true beauty is revealed only if there is light from within.

—Elisabeth Kübler-Ross

QUESTIONS

1. The nurse is working in the emergency department (ED) of a children's medical center. Which client should the nurse assess first?
   1. The 1-month-old infant who has developed colic and is crying.
   2. The 2-year-old toddler who was bitten by another child at the day-care center.
   3. The 6-year-old school-age child who was hit by a car while riding a bicycle.
   4. The 14-year-old adolescent whose mother suspects her child is sexually active.

2. The 8-year-old client diagnosed with a vaso-occlusive sickle cell crisis is complaining of a severe headache. Which intervention should the nurse implement first?
   1. Administer 6 L of oxygen via nasal cannula.
   2. Assess the client's neurological status.
   3. Administer a narcotic analgesic by intravenous push (IVP).
   4. Increase the client's intravenous (IV) rate.

3. The 6-year-old client who has undergone abdominal surgery is attempting to make a pinwheel spin by blowing on it with the nurse's assistance. The child starts crying because the pinwheel won't spin. Which action should the nurse implement first?
   1. Praise the child for the attempt to make the pinwheel spin.
   2. Notify the respiratory therapist to implement incentive spirometry.
   3. Encourage the child to turn from side to side and cough.
   4. Demonstrate how to make the pinwheel spin by blowing on it.

4. The nurse is caring for clients on the pediatric medical unit. Which client should the nurse assess first?
   1. The child diagnosed with type 1 diabetes who has a blood glucose level of 180 mg/dL.
   2. The child diagnosed with pneumonia who is coughing and has a temperature of 100°F.
   3. The child diagnosed with gastroenteritis who has a potassium (K+) level of 3.9 mEq/L.
   4. The child diagnosed with cystic fibrosis who has a pulse oximeter reading of 90%.

5. The nurse has received the a.m. shift report for clients on a pediatric unit. Which medication should the nurse administer first?
1. The third dose of the aminoglycoside antibiotic to the child diagnosed with methicillin-resistant *Staphylococcus aureus* (MRSA).
2. The IVP steroid methylprednisolone (Solu-Medrol) to the child diagnosed with asthma.
3. The sliding scale insulin to the child diagnosed with type 1 diabetes mellitus.
4. The stimulant methylphenidate (Ritalin) to a child diagnosed with attention deficit-hyperactivity disorder (ADHD).

6. The nurse enters the client's room and realizes the 9-month-old infant is not breathing. Which interventions should the nurse implement? Prioritize the nurse's actions from first (1) to last (5).
1. Perform cardiac compression 30:2.
2. Check the infant's brachial pulse.
3. Administer two puffs to the infant.
4. Determine unresponsiveness.
5. Open the infant's airway.

7. The 3-year-old client has been admitted to the pediatric unit. Which task should the nurse instruct the unlicensed assistive personnel (UAP) to perform first?
1. Orient the parents and child to the room.
2. Obtain an admission kit for the child.
3. Post the child's height and weight at the HOB.
4. Provide the child with a meal tray.

8. The clinic nurse is preparing to administer an intramuscular (IM) injection to the 2-year-old toddler. Which intervention should the nurse implement first?
1. Immobilize the child's leg.
2. Explain the procedure to the child.
3. Cleanse the area with an alcohol swab.
4. Administer the medication in the thigh.

9. The nurse is writing a care plan for the 5-year-old child diagnosed with gastroenteritis. Which client problem is priority?
1. Imbalanced nutrition.
2. Fluid volume deficit.
3. Knowledge deficit.
4. Risk for infection.

10. Which data would warrant immediate intervention from the pediatric nurse?
1. Proteinuria for the child diagnosed with nephrotic syndrome.
2. Petechiae for the child diagnosed with leukemia.
3. Drooling for a child diagnosed with acute epiglottitis.
4. Elevated temperature in a child diagnosed with otitis media.

11. Which client should the pediatric nurse assess first after receiving the a.m. shift report?
1. The 6-month old child diagnosed with bacterial meningitis who is irritable and crying.
2. The 9-month old child diagnosed with tetralogy of Fallot (TOF) who has edema of the face.
3. The 11-month old child diagnosed with Reye syndrome who is lethargic and vomiting.
4. The 13-month-old child diagnosed with diarrhea who has sunken eyeballs and decreased urine output.

12. The pediatric clinic nurse is triaging telephone calls. Which client's parent should the nurse call first?
1. The 4-month-old child who had immunizations yesterday and the parent is reporting a high-pitched cry and a 103°F fever.
2. The 8-month-old whose parent is reporting the child is pulling on the right ear and has a fever.
3. The 2-year-old child who has patent ductus arteriosis whose parent reports running out of digoxin.
4. The 3-year-old child whose mother called and reported her daughter may have chickenpox.

13. The parent of a 12-year-old male child with a left below-the-knee cast calls the pediatric clinic nurse and tells the nurse, "My son's foot is cold and he told me it feels like his foot is asleep." Which action should the nurse implement first?
1. Prepare to bifurcate the left below-the-knee cast.
2. Tell the parent to bring the child to the office.
3. Instruct the parent to elevate the left leg on two pillows.
4. Notify the child's orthopedist of the situation.

14. Which child requires the nurse to notify the healthcare provider?
1. The 1-year-old child with iron deficiency anemia who has dark-colored stool.
2. The 3-year-old child with phenylketonuria (PKU) whose parent does not feed the child any meat or milk products.
3. The 5-year-old child with rheumatic heart fever who is having difficulty breathing.
4. The 7-year-old child diagnosed with acute glomerulonephritis who has dark "tea"-colored urine.

15. The pediatric nurse on the surgical unit has just received a.m. shift report. Which client should the nurse assess first?
1. The 3-week-old child 1 day postoperative with surgical repair of a myelomeningocele who has bulging fontanels.
2. The 3-month-old child 2 days postoperative temporary colostomy secondary to Hirschsprung's disease who has a moist, pink stoma.
3. The 9-month-old child with a cleft palate repair who is spitting up formula and refusing to eat.
4. The 4-year-old child 1 day postoperative for repair of hypospadias who has clear amber urine draining from indwelling catheter.

16. The charge nurse has assigned a staff nurse to care for an 8-year-old client diagnosed with cerebral palsy. Which nursing action by the staff nurse would warrant immediate intervention by the charge nurse?
1. The staff nurse performs gentle range-of-motion (ROM) exercises to extremities.
2. The staff nurse puts the client's bed in the lowest position possible.
3. The staff nurse takes the client in a wheelchair to the activity room.
4. The staff nurse places the child in semi-Fowler's position to eat lunch.

17. The nurse and the unlicensed assistive personnel (UAP) are caring for clients on the pediatric unit. Which action by the nurse indicates appropriate delegation?
1. The nurse requests the UAP to check the circulation on the child with a cast.
2. The nurse asks the UAP to feed an infant who has just had a cleft palate repair.
3. The nurse has the UAP demonstrate a catheterization for a child with a neurogenic bladder.
4. The nurse checks to make sure the UAP's delegated tasks have been completed.

18. The nurse on a pediatric unit has received the a.m. shift report and tells the unlicensed assistive personnel (UAP) to keep the 2-year-old child NPO for a procedure. At 0830, the nurse observes the mother feeding the child. Which action should the nurse implement first?
1. Determine what the UAP did not understand about the instruction.
2. Tell the HCP the UAP did not follow the nurse's direction.
3. Ask the mother why she was feeding her child if the child was NPO.
4. Notify the dietary department to hold the child's meal trays.

19. The charge nurse on the six-bed pediatric burn unit is making shift assignments and has one registered nurse (RN), one scrub technician, one unlicensed assistive personnel (UAP), and a unit secretary. Which client care assignment indicates the best use of the hospital personnel?
1. The RN performs daily whirlpool dressing changes.
2. The unit secretary transcribes the HCP's orders.
3. The scrub technician medicates the client prior to dressing changes.
4. The UAP places the current laboratory results on the chart.

20. The RN and the UAP are caring for clients on a pediatric surgical unit. Which tasks would be most appropriate to delegate to the UAP? **Select all that apply.**
1. Pass dietary trays to the clients.
2. Obtain routine vital signs on the clients.
3. Complete the preoperative checklist.
4. Change linens on the clients' beds.
5. Document the clients' intake and output.

21. Which client should the charge nurse on the pediatric unit assign to the most experienced nurse?
1. The 4-year-old child diagnosed with hemophilia receiving factor VIII.
2. The 8-year-old child with headaches who is scheduled for a CT scan.
3. The 6-year-old child recovering from a sickle cell crisis.
4. The 11-year-old child newly diagnosed with rheumatoid arthritis.

22. The charge nurse is making shift assignments on a pediatric oncology unit. Which delegation/assignment would be most appropriate?
1. Delegate the unlicensed assistive personnel (UAP) to obtain routine blood work from the central line.
2. Instruct the licensed practical nurse (LPN) to contact the leukemia support group.
3. Assign the chemotherapy-certified RN to administer chemotherapeutic medication.
4. Have the dietitian check the meal trays for the amount eaten.

23. The nurse observes the unlicensed assistive personnel (UAP) bringing a cartoon video to a 6-year-old female child on bed rest so that she can watch it on the television. Which action should the nurse take?
1. Tell the UAP that the child should not be watching videos.
2. Explain that this is the responsibility of the child life therapist.
3. Praise the UAP for providing the child with an appropriate activity.
4. Notify the charge nurse that the UAP gave the child videos to watch.

24. Which newborn should the nurse in the neonatal intensive care unit (NICU) assign to a new graduate who has just completed an NICU internship?
1. The 1-day-old infant diagnosed with a myelomeningocele.
2. The 2-week-old infant who was born 6 weeks premature.
3. The 3-hour-old infant who is being evaluated for esophageal atresia.
4. The 1-week-old infant diagnosed with tetralogy of Fallot.

25. The newly hired nurse is working on a pediatric unit and needs the unlicensed assistive personnel (UAP) to obtain a urine specimen on an 11-month-old infant. Which statement made to the UAP indicates the nurse understands the delegation process?
    1. "Be sure to weigh the diaper when obtaining the urine specimen."
    2. "Do you know how to apply the urine collection bag?"
    3. "Use a small indwelling catheter when obtaining the urine specimen."
    4. "I need for you to get a urine specimen on the infant."

26. Which task is most appropriate for the pediatric nurse to delegate to the unlicensed assistive personnel (UAP)?
    1. Ask the UAP to orient the parents and child to the room.
    2. Tell the UAP to prepare the child for an endoscopy.
    3. Request the UAP to log roll the client who had a spinal surgery.
    4. Instruct the UAP to assess the child's developmental level.

27. Which behavior by the unlicensed assistive personnel (UAP) warrants intervention by the nurse?
    1. The UAP weighs the child's diaper on a scale and records the urine output on the intake & output (I&O) sheet.
    2. The UAP sits with the child while the parent goes down to the cafeteria to get something to eat.
    3. The UAP bathes the child with congenital dislocated hip with the Pavlik harness on the child.
    4. The UAP applies wrist restraints on the 7-month-old who is 1 day postoperative cleft palate repair.

28. The nurse is caring for pediatric clients. Which tasks are most appropriate to assign to an unlicensed assistive personnel (UAP) and/or a licensed vocational nurse (LPN)? **Select all that apply.**
    1. Instruct the LPN to teach the parent of a child new diagnosed with type 1 diabetes.
    2. Tell the UAP to apply an ice collar to the child who is 1 day postoperative tonsillectomy.
    3. Ask the UAP to place ointment on a child's diaper rash around the anal area.
    4. Request the LPN to double-check the medication dose for the child receiving an antibiotic.
    5. Tell the LPN to transcribe the healthcare provider's orders for the child with cystic fibrosis.

29. The nurse is discharging a 4-month-old child with a temporary colostomy. Which intervention should the nurse implement?
    1. Request the UAP to complete the discharge written documentation.
    2. Tell the LPN to show the parent how to irrigate the colostomy.
    3. Ask the UAP to remove the child's intravenous catheter.
    4. Request the UAP to escort the parent and child to the car.

30. The unlicensed assistive personnel (UAP) tells the nurse the child with Down syndrome who is 2 days postoperative appendectomy is having pain. Which intervention should the nurse implement first?
    1. Tell the UAP to check the child's vital signs.
    2. Assess the child's abdominal dressing and pain immediately.
    3. Notify the healthcare provider.
    4. Check the MAR for last time pain medication was administered.

31. The 8-year-old male child in the pediatric unit is refusing to ambulate postoperatively. Which intervention would be most appropriate?
   1. Give the child the option to ambulate now or after lunch.
   2. Ask the parents to insist the child ambulate in the hall.
   3. Refer the child to the child developmental therapist.
   4. Tell the child he can watch a video game if he cooperates.

32. The clinic nurse overhears a mother in the waiting room tell her 6-year-old son, "If you don't sit down and be quiet, I am going to get the nurse to give you a shot." Which action should the nurse implement?
   1. Do not take any action because the mother is attempting to discipline her son.
   2. Tell the child the nurse would not give him a shot because the mother said to.
   3. Report this verbally abusive behavior to Child Protective Services.
   4. Tell the mother this behavior will cause her son to be afraid of the nurses.

33. The parents of an infant born with Down syndrome are holding their infant and crying. The father asks, "I have heard children like this are hard to take care of at home." Which referral would be most appropriate for the parents?
   1. The Web site for the National Association for Down Syndrome.
   2. The hospital chaplain.
   3. A Down syndrome support group.
   4. A geneticist.

34. The charge nurse on the pediatric unit hears the overhead announcement of Code Pink (infant abduction), newborn nursery. Which action should the charge nurse implement?
   1. Send a staff member to the newborn nursery.
   2. Explain the situation to the clients and visitors.
   3. Continue with the charge nurse's responsibilities.
   4. Station a staff member at all the unit exits.

35. The mother of a 4-year-old child diagnosed with Duchenne's muscular dystrophy is overwhelmed and asks the nurse, "I have been told a case manager will come and talk to me. What will they do for me?" Which statement indicates the nurse understands the role of the case manager?
   1. "You will have a case manager so that the hospital can save money."
   2. "She will make sure your child gets the right medication for muscular dystrophy."
   3. "She will help you find the resources you need to care for your child."
   4. "The case manager helps your child to have a normal life expectancy."

36. The nurse is assigned to the pediatric unit performance improvement committee. The unit is concerned with IV infection rates. Which action should the nurse implement first when investigating the problem?
   1. Contact central supply for samples of IV start kits.
   2. Obtain research to determine the best length for IV dwell time.
   3. Identify how many IV infections have occurred in the last year.
   4. Audit the charts to determine if hospital policy is being followed.

37. The clinic nurse is discussing a tubal ligation with a 17-year-old adolescent with Down syndrome. The adolescent does not want the surgery, but her parents (who are also in the room) are telling her she must have it. Which statement by the nurse would be an example of the ethical principle of justice?
   1. "I think this requires further discussion before scheduling this procedure."
   2. "You will not be able to have children after you have this procedure."
   3. "You should have this procedure because you could not care for a child."
   4. "You can refuse this procedure and your parents can't make you have it."

38. The school nurse has referred an 8-year-old student for further evaluation of vision. The single mother has told the school nurse she does not have the money for the evaluation or glasses. Which action by the nurse would be an example of client advocacy?
   1. Tell the mother the child cannot read the board.
   2. Refer the mother to a local service organization.
   3. Ask the mother if the family is on Medicaid.
   4. Loan the mother money for the examination.

39. The emergency department (ED) nurse is scheduling the 16-year-old client for an emergency appendectomy. Which intervention should the nurse implement when obtaining permission for the surgery?
   1. Withhold the narcotic pain medication until the client signs the permit.
   2. Have the client's parent or legal guardian sign the operative permit.
   3. Explain the procedure to the client and the parents in simple terms.
   4. Get a visitor from the ED waiting area to witness the parent's signature.

40. The unit manager has been notified by central supply that many client items are missing from stock and have not been charged to the client. Which action should the nurse manager implement regarding the lost charges?
   1. Send out a memo telling the staff to follow the charge procedures.
   2. Form a performance improvement committee to study the problem.
   3. Determine whether the items in question are being restocked daily.
   4. Schedule a staff meeting to discuss how to prevent further lost charges.

41. Which child's behavior warrants notifying the child developmental specialist?
   1. The 1-year-old child who cries when the parent leaves the room.
   2. The 2-year-old child who can talk in two- or three-word sentences.
   3. The 3-year-old child who is toilet trained for bowel and bladder.
   4. The 4-year-old child who throws frequent temper tantrums.

42. Which child should the nurse assign to the new graduate who has just completed orientation to the pediatric unit?
   1. The 5-year-old child admitted in a sickle cell crisis whose patient-controlled analgesia (PCA) pump is not controlling the child's pain.
   2. The 6-year-old child in Russell's traction for a fractured femur who has insertion pin sites that are inflamed and infected.
   3. The 12-year-old child who is newly diagnosed with type 1 diabetes who needs medication teaching.
   4. The 16-year-old female diagnosed with scoliosis who is being admitted for insertion of a spinal rod in the morning.

43. Which action by the emergency department (ED) nurse warrants intervention by the charge nurse?
   1. The nurse is elevating the right arm of a child who appears to have fractured the wrist.
   2. The nurse is notifying Child Protective Services for a child who is suspected of being sexually abused.
   3. The nurse is assessing the tonsils on a 4-year-old child who has a sore throat and is drooling.
   4. The nurse is obtaining a midstream urine specimen for the child who is complaining of burning upon urination.

44. The day shift nurse is preparing to administer 0730 medications to the 12-year-old child diagnosed with type 1 diabetes. The child's 0730 blood glucose level is 252. Which insulin coverage should the nurse administer?

Client's Name:		Account Number: 13456	Allergies: NKA	
Date	Medication	2301–0700	0701–1500	1501–2300
	Sliding scale regular insulin ac & hs <150 no insulin 151–200 4 units 201–250 6 units 251–300 8 units 301 notify HCP			
	10 units regular insulin 20 units NPH insulin	0730		
Signature/Initials		Day Nurse RN/DN	Night Nurse RN/NN	

1. Regular insulin 6 units.
2. Regular insulin 18 units and NPH 20 units.
3. Regular insulin 10 units and NPH 20 units.
4. Regular insulin 8 units.

45. Which interventions should the nurse implement to help establish a nurse/parent relationship? **Select all that apply.**
1. Include the parents when developing the plan of care for their child.
2. Encourage the parents to hold their child as much as possible.
3. Allow the parents to verbalize their feelings of fear and anxiety.
4. Tell the parents to never leave while the child is hospitalized.
5. Request the parents to bring toys from home the child will enjoy.

46. The nurse is caring for clients on the pediatric unit. Which child would warrant a referral to the early childhood development specialist?
1. The 9-month-old child who says only "mama" or "dada."
2. The 11-month-old child who walks hanging onto furniture.
3. The 8-month-old child who sits by leaning forward on both hands.
4. The 4-month-old infant who turns from the abdomen to the back.

47. The 10-year-old child diagnosed with leukemia is scheduled for a bone marrow aspiration. Which intervention is most important when obtaining informed consent for the procedure?
1. Obtain assent from the child.
2. Have the parent sign the permit.
3. Refer any questions to the HCP.
4. Witness the signature on the permit.

48. The 13-year-old client has just delivered a 4-pound baby boy. The stepfather of the client becomes verbally abusive to the nurse when he is asked to leave the room. The client is withdrawn and silent. Which legal action should the nurse implement?
1. Call hospital security to come to the room.
2. Contact Child Protective Services.
3. Refer the child to the social worker.
4. Ask the client whether she feels safe at home.

49. The fire alarm on the pediatric unit has just started sounding. Which action should the charge nurse implement first?
1. Call the hospital operator to find out the location of the fire.
2. Ensure that all visitors and clients are in the room with the door closed.
3. Prepare to evacuate the clients and visitors down the stairs.
4. Make a list of which clients are not currently on the unit.

50. A nurse overhears two other nurses talking about a client in the hospital dining room. Which action should the nurse implement first?
1. Notify the HIPAA officer about the breach of confidentiality.
2. Immediately report the two nurses to their clinical manager.
3. Document the situation in writing and submit to the Chief Nursing Officer (CNO).
4. Tell the two nurses they are violating the client's confidentiality.

51. The nurse is caring for newborns in the nursery. Which newborn warrants immediate intervention by the nurse?
1. The 8-hour-old newborn who has not passed meconium.
2. The 15-hour-old newborn who is slightly jaundiced.
3. The 4-hour-old newborn who is jittery and irritable.
4. The 10-hour-old newborn who will not stop crying.

52. At 1300, the nurse is assessing a 12-year-old child who is complaining of abdominal pain and rating it as a 5 on a scale of 1 to 10. Which intervention should the nurse implement?

Client's Name:		Account Number: 123456	Allergies: NKDA	
Height: 60 inches		**Weight:** 98 pounds		
Date	**Medication**	**2301–0700**	**0701–1500**	**1501–2300**
	Maalox 30 mL q1 hour PRN			
	Acetominophen (Tylenol) 650 mg PO q6 hours PRN			
	Hydrocodone (Vicodin) 5 mg PO PRN pain q4–6 hours	0600 NN		
	Morphine 2 mg IVP PRN pain q4 hours			
Signature/Initials		**Day Nurse RN/DN**	**Night Nurse RN/NN**	

1. Administer 30 mL of Maalox PO.
2. Administer 650 mg of Tylenol PO.
3. Administer 5 mg of hydrocodone PO.
4. Administer 2 mg of morphine IVP.

53. The nurse who has never worked on the maternity ward has been pulled from the surgical unit to work in the newborn nursery. Which assignment would be most appropriate for the nurse to accept?
1. Perform an assessment on the newborn.
2. Assist the pediatrician with a circumcision.
3. Gavage feed a newborn who is 8 hours old.
4. Transport newborns to the mothers' room.

54. The nurse is instructing the unlicensed assistive personnel (UAP) on gross motor skill activity that is appropriate for a developmentally delayed 9-month-old infant. Which activity should the nurse delegate to the UAP?
   1. Help the child to sit without support.
   2. Teach the child to catch the beach ball.
   3. Reward the child with food for sitting up.
   4. Teach the child to blow a kiss.

55. Which incident should the primary nurse report to the clinical manager concerning a violation of information technology guidelines?
   1. The nurse keeps the computer screen turned away from public view.
   2. The nurse researches medications using the online formulary.
   3. The nurse shares the computer access code with another nurse.
   4. The nurse logs off the computer when leaving the terminal.

56. The nurse is caring for clients in a pediatric emergency department (ED). Which client should the nurse assess first?
   1. The child with a dog bite on the left hand who is bleeding.
   2. The child who has a laceration on the right side of the forehead.
   3. The child with a fractured tibia who will not move the foot.
   4. The child who has ingested a bottle of prenatal vitamins.

57. The nurse is caring for a client in a children's medical center. Which behavior indicates the nurse understands the pediatric client's rights?
   1. The nurse administers an injection without talking to the child.
   2. The nurse covers the 5-year-old child's genitalia during a code.
   3. The nurse discusses the child's condition with the grandparents.
   4. The nurse leaves an uncapped needle at the client's bedside.

58. The home health nurse is planning the care of a 14-year-old client diagnosed with leukemia who is receiving chemotherapy. Which psychosocial problem is priority for this client?
   1. Diversional activity deficit.
   2. High risk for infection.
   3. Social isolation.
   4. Hopelessness.

59. The nurse is administering IV fluids to a 3-year-old client. Which action by the nurse would warrant intervention by the charge nurse?
   1. The nurse places the IV on an infusion pump.
   2. The nurse does not use a volume-controlled chamber.
   3. The nurse checks the child's IV site every hour.
   4. The nurse labels the IV tubing with date and time.

60. The nurse is caring for clients on a psychiatric pediatric unit. Which action by the nurse is reportable to the state board of nursing?
   1. The nurse leaves for lunch and does not return to complete the shift.
   2. The nurse fails to check the ID band when administering medications.
   3. The nurse has had three documented medication errors in the last 3 months.
   4. The nurse has admitted to having an affair with another staff member.

61. The nurse is working in a free healthcare clinic. Which client situation warrants further investigation?
   1. The child diagnosed with rheumatoid arthritis who is wearing a copper bracelet.
   2. The mother of a child with a sunburn who is using juice from an aloe vera plant on the burn.
   3. The grandmother who reports rubbing Vick's Vapo-Rub on the child's chest for a cold.
   4. The father who tells the nurse that the child receives a variety of herbs every day.

62. The unlicensed assistive personnel (UAP) tells the primary nurse that the 4-year-old child is alone in the room because the mother went to the cafeteria to get something to eat. Which action should the nurse implement first?
    1. Arrange for the mother to have a tray sent to the room.
    2. Go to the cafeteria and ask the mother to return to the room.
    3. Tell the UAP to stay with the child until the mother returns.
    4. Notify social services that the mother left the child alone.

63. The nurse is evaluating an 18-month-old child in the pediatric clinic. Which data would indicate to the nurse that the child is not meeting tasks according to Erikson's Stages of Psychosocial Development?
    1. The child stamps his or her foot and says "no" frequently.
    2. The child does not interact with the mother.
    3. The child cries when the mother leaves the room.
    4. The child responds when called by name.

64. Which statement by the female charge nurse indicates she has an autocratic leadership style?
    1. "You must complete all the a.m. care before you take your morning break."
    2. "I don't care how the work is done as long as it is completed on time."
    3. "I would like to talk to you about your ideas on a new staffing mix."
    4. "I think we should have a pot luck lunch tomorrow because it is Saturday."

65. The nurse is evaluating the care of a 5-year-old client with a cyanotic congenital heart defect. Which client outcome would support that discharge teaching has been effective?
    1. The mother makes the child get up when squatting.
    2. The child is playing in the dayroom without oxygen.
    3. The father buys the child a baseball and a bat.
    4. The nurse finds unopened packs of salt on the meal tray.

66. The nurse is administering morning medications on a pediatric unit. Which action should the nurse take first when preparing to administer medication to the client T.R.?

Client Name: T.R.		Account Number: 5948726	Allergies: milk and dairy products	
Height: 21 inches		Weight in pounds: 15 Weight in kg: 6.82	Date of Birth: 2 weeks ago	
Date: Today	Medication	2301–0700	0701–1500	1501–2300
	Digoxin 0.125 mg/5 mL q day PO		0900	
	250 mL 0.33% DextroseIV @ 10 mL/hour	0215 NN via buretrol setup and IV pump		
Signature/Initials		Night Nurse RN/NN	Day Nurse RN/DN	

1. Check the client's apical pulse rate.
2. Ask the parent for the baby's date of birth.
3. Look to see if a digoxin level has been drawn.
4. Call the healthcare provider to discuss the digoxin.

67. The nurse working in a pediatrician's office is preparing to administer the initial HIB vaccination to a 2-month-old infant. Which is the preferred site for the injection?

1. A
2. B
3. C
4. D

68. The nurse is preparing to administer an intravenous piggyback to an 8-year-old child. The child has an IV running at 45 mL per hour. The medication comes prepared in 50 mL of NS. At which rate should the nurse set the IV pump? _____

69. The unconscious 4-year-old child is brought to the emergency department by paramedics; the child has bruises covering the torso in varying stages of healing. The nurse notes small burn marks on the child's genitalia. Which actions should the nurse implement? **Select all that apply.**
1. Notify Child Protective Services.
2. Ask the parent how the child was injured.
3. Perform a thorough examination for more injuries.
4. Tell the parents that the police have been called.
5. Prepare the child for skull x-rays and a CT scan.

70. The 24-month-old toddler is admitted to the pediatric unit with vomiting and diarrhea. Which interventions should the nurse implement? Rank in order of performance.
1. Teach the parent about weighing diapers to determine output status.
2. Show the parent the call light and explain safety regimens.
3. Assess the toddler's tissue turgor.
4. Place the appropriate size diapers in the room.
5. Take the toddler's vital signs.

PEDIATRIC CLINICAL SCENARIO

Ms. Laura is the charge nurse in a pediatric emergency department (ED). She has three registered nurses working, Ms. Polly, Mr. Aaron, and Ms. Ruth. There are two unlicensed assistive personnel (UAP), Ms. Michelle and Ms. Diane.

1. Which child should Ms. Laura assess first?
   1. The 1-month-old infant who crying, is inconsolable, and has inspiratory retractions.
   2. The 4-year-old toddler with cystic fibrosis who has a pulse oximeter reading of 93%.
   3. The 6-year-old child with gastroenteritis who has a potassium level of 3.6 mEq/L.
   4. The 14-year-old child with type 2 diabetes with a blood glucose level of 210 mg/dL.

2. Which task should Ms. Laura delegate to Ms. Michelle, the UAP?
   1. Take the vital signs of a child who is having a sickle cell crisis.
   2. Place oxygen via nasal cannula on a child diagnosed with cystic fibrosis.
   3. Obtain the weight of the child who is diagnosed with nephrotic syndrome.
   4. Escort the child diagnosed with traumatic brain injury (TBI) to the intensive care unit (ICU).

3. Ms. Laura is observing Mr. Aaron administer an intramuscular (IM) injection to a 2-year-old toddler. Which action by Mr. Aaron warrants intervention by Ms. Laura?
   1. He immobilizes the child's leg.
   2. He explains the procedure to the child.
   3. He places the syringe in the sharps container.
   4. He recaps the needle after administering the medication.

4. Which task should Ms. Ruth not delegate to the Ms. Diane, the UAP?
   1. Document the intake and output (I&O) on the child diagnosed with congestive heart failure (CHF).
   2. Feed the child who is experiencing an acute exacerbation of inflammatory bowel disease (IBD).
   3. Elevate the child's leg who just had a cast applied for a fractured right ankle.
   4. Take the child's catheterized urine specimen to the laboratory.

5. Which client should Ms. Laura assign to Ms. Polly, the most experienced pediatric emergency department nurse?
   1. The 1-year-old child who is tugging at the right ear and has a temperature of 100.4°F.
   2. The 6-year-old child who is wheezing and complaining of chest tightness.
   3. The 8-year-old female child who is complaining of burning when she urinates.
   4. The 11-year-old child with bilateral crackles and a productive cough.

6. The 13-year-old child is admitted to the emergency department with nucal rigidity, a positive Kernig's sign, a positive Brudzinki's sign, and an elevated temperature. Which intervention should Ms. Laura implement first?
   1. Administer acetaminophen (Tylenol) PO with water.
   2. Place the child in droplet isolation.
   3. Prepare the child for a lumbar puncture.
   4. Notify the hospital infection control nurse.

7. Mr. Aaron answers the phone and a distraught woman says, "My daughter just drank a bottle of cleaning solution." Which intervention should Mr. Aaron implement first?
   1. Tell the mother to bring the child to the emergency department immediately.
   2. Ask the mother how old the child is and how much the child weighs.
   3. Ask the mother if she has syrup of ipecac that could be given to the child.
   4. Tell Ms. Laura to call poison control immediately.

8. The 8-year-old child is brought to the emergency department by his parents with a pencil penetrating the right eye. Which intervention should Ms. Laura implement first?
   1. Remove the object with a lightly moistened gauze pad.
   2. Ask the parents about child medical history and any known allergies.
   3. Stabilize the pencil in place and patch the left eye.
   4. Assess the child's vital signs and pulse oximeter reading.

9. Mr. Aaron is caring for a 7-year-old child who was hit in the head with a baseball. One hour ago the child had a 15 on the Glasgow Coma Scale and now has a 12. Which intervention should Mr. Aaron implement first?
   1. Notify the hospital neurologist immediately.
   2. Document the findings in the chart.
   3. Complete a Glasgow Coma Scale in 2 hours.
   4. Place the child in the high-Fowler's position.

10. Which client should Ms. Laura assign to Mr. Aaron, the least experienced nurse in the emergency department?
    1. The child whose parent reports the child had a sore throat and is now drooling.
    2. The child who has a distended abdomen and absent bowel sounds.
    3. The child who has an edematous and contused right ankle.
    4. The child whose parent reports the child has blood in his urine.

11. Which nursing task should Ms. Ruth delegate to Ms. Michelle, the UAP?
    1. Escort the child who is being discharged via wheelchair out to the parent's car.
    2. Determine if a child's growth and developmental level is on target.
    3. Explain how to care for the below-the-knee cast to the parents.
    4. Assist the healthcare provider to suture a child's leg laceration.

ANSWERS AND RATIONALES

The correct answer number and rationale for why it is the correct answer are given in **boldface type**. Rationales for why the other possible answer options are incorrect also are given, but they are not in boldface type.

1. 1. The main sign of colic is intense crying; therefore, this is expected and would not warrant the nurse's assessing the child first.
   2. A human bite is dangerous, but it is not life threatening.
   3. **The child hit by a car should be assessed first because he or she may have life-threatening injuries that must be assessed and treated promptly.**
   4. This client is not priority over a client with a physiological problem.

   Content – Pediatrics: **Category of Health Alteration –** *Gastrointestinal:* **Integrated Processes –** *Nursing Process: Assessment:* **Client Needs –** *Health Promotion and Maintenance:* **Cognitive Level –** *Analysis*

2. 1. Administering oxygen may help decrease the sickling of the cells, but this should not be the first intervention to address the client's headache.
   2. **Because the client is complaining of a headache, the nurse should first rule out cerebrovascular accident (CVA) by assessing the client's neurological status and then determine whether it is a headache that can be treated with medication.**
   3. Prior to administering any pain medication to a client, the nurse must first assess the client to determine whether the pain is what is expected with the disease process or whether it is a complication that requires further nursing intervention.
   4. Only after CVA has been ruled out should the nurse medicate the client. Adequate hydration will help decrease sickling of the cells, but this is not the first intervention to address the client's pain.

   Content – Pediatrics: **Category of Health Alteration –** *Hematology:* **Integrated Processes –** *Nursing Process:* **Implementation:** *Client Needs – Health Promotion and* **Maintenance:** *Cognitive Level – Application*

3. 1. **The nurse should always praise the child for attempts at cooperation even if the child did not accomplish what the nurse asked.**
   2. This action can be taken by the nurse after praising the child for the attempt.

   3. This action is appropriate and should be implemented, but not before the nurse praises the child for the attempt.
   4. The nurse can demonstrate the correct technique for the child, but not before praising the child for the attempt.

   Content – Pediatrics: **Category of Health Alteration –** *Gastrointestinal:* **Integrated Processes –** *Nursing Process:* **Implementation:** *Client Needs – Health Promotion and* **Maintenance:** *Cognitive Level – Application*

4. 1. A 180 mg/dL glucose level for a child with type 1 diabetes is not life threatening, and the nurse would not assess this child first.
   2. The nurse would expect the child with pneumonia to have these signs/symptoms; therefore, the nurse would not assess this child first.
   3. This is a normal potassium level; therefore, the nurse would not assess this child first.
   4. **A pulse oximeter reading of less than 93% is significant and indicates hypoxia, which is life threatening; therefore, this child should be assessed first.**

   Content – Pediatrics: **Category of Health Alteration –** *Respiratory:* **Integrated Processes –** *Nursing Process:* **Assessment:** *Client Needs – Physiological Integrity:* **Reduction of Risk Potential:** *Cognitive Level – Analysis*

MAKING NURSING DECISIONS: When deciding which client to assess first, the test taker should determine whether the signs/symptoms the client is exhibiting are normal or expected for the client situation. After eliminating the expected options, the test taker should determine which situation is more life threatening.

5. 1. The third dose of an antibiotic would not be priority over sliding scale insulin because insulin must be administered prior to the breakfast meal.
   2. Routine medications have a 1-hour leeway before and after the scheduled time; therefore, this medication does not have to be administered first.
   3. **Sliding scale insulin is ordered ac, which is before meals; therefore, this medication must be administered first after receiving the a.m. shift report.**
   4. Routine medications have a 1-hour leeway before and after the scheduled time; therefore, this medication does not have to be administered first.

   Content – Pediatric: **Category of Health Alteration –** *Drug Administration:* **Integrated Processes –** *Nursing*

*Process: Implementation: **Client Needs** – Physiological Integrity: Pharmacological and Parenteral Therapies: **Cognitive Level** – Application*

6. **Correct Answer: 4, 5, 3, 2, 1**

4. **The nurse must first determine the infant's responsiveness by thumping the baby's feet.**

5. **The nurse should then open the child's airway using the head-tilt chin-lift technique, with care taken not to hyperextend the neck. Then the nurse should look, listen, and feel for respirations.**

3. **The nurse then administers quick puffs of air while covering the child's mouth and nose, preferably with a rescue mask.**

2. **The nurse should determine whether the infant has a pulse by checking the brachial artery.**

1. **If the infant has no pulse, the nurse should begin chest compressions using two fingers at a rate of 30:2.**

*Content – Pediatrics: **Category of Health Alteration** – Respiratory: **Integrated Processes** – Nursing Process: Implementation: **Client Needs** – Physiological Integrity: Reduction of Risk Potential: **Cognitive Level** – Synthesis*

7. 1. **The first intervention after the child is admitted to the unit is to orient the parents and child to the room, the call system, and the hospital rules, such as not leaving the child alone in the room.**

2. This task is within the scope of the UAP, but it is not priority over orienting the child/parents to the room.

3. The height/weight should be posted in case the client codes, but this can be done after the child/parents are oriented to the room.

4. The child should receive a meal tray, but not before orientation to the room.

*Content – Pediatrics: **Category of Health Alteration** – Safety: **Integrated Processes** – Nursing Process: Planning: **Client Needs** – Safe and Effective Care Environment: Management of Care: **Cognitive Level** – Synthesis*

8. 1. The nurse should immobilize the child's leg, but it is not the first intervention.

2. **The nurse must explain any procedure in words the child can understand. It does not matter how old the child is.**

3. This is an appropriate intervention, but it is not the first intervention.

4. This is an appropriate intervention, but it is not the first intervention.

*Content – Pediatrics: **Category of Health Alteration** – Drug Administration: **Integrated Processes** – Nursing Process: Implementation: **Client Needs** – Physiological Integrity: Pharmacological and Parenteral Therapies: **Cognitive Level** – Application*

9. 1. This is not the priority problem because lack of fluids is more life threatening to a child than lack of food.

2. **The child diagnosed with gastroenteritis is at high risk for hypovolemic shock resulting from vomiting and diarrhea; therefore, maintaining fluid and electrolyte homeostasis is priority.**

3. Knowledge deficit is a psychosocial diagnosis, and although it is important to teach the parents and child, it is not priority over a physiological problem.

4. The child already has an infection; thus there is no risk.

*Content – Pediatrics: **Category of Health Alteration** – Gastrointestinal: **Integrated Processes** – Nursing Process: Planning: **Client Needs** – Safe and Effective Care Environment: Management of Care: **Cognitive Level** – Synthesis*

MAKING NURSING DECISIONS: The test taker should use Maslow's Hierarchy of Needs to determine the client's priority problem. Physiological problems are priority.

10. 1. The child diagnosed with nephrotic syndrome would be expected to have proteinuria.

2. The child diagnosed with leukemia would be expected to have petechaie.

3. **Drooling indicates the child is having trouble swallowing, and the epiglottis is at risk of completely occluding the airway. This warrants immediate intervention. The nurse should notify the HCP and obtain an emergency tracheostomy tray for the bedside.**

4. A child with an ear infection would be expected to have an elevated temperature.

*Content – Pediatrics: **Category of Health Alteration** – Respiratory: **Integrated Processes** – Nursing Process: Assessment: **Client Needs** – Physiological Integrity: Reduction of Risk Potential: **Cognitive Level** – Analysis*

MAKING NURSING DECISIONS: When deciding which client to assess first, the test taker should determine whether the signs/symptoms the client is exhibiting are normal or expected for the client situation. After eliminating the expected options, the test taker should determine which situation is more life threatening.

11. 1. Irritability and crying are expected signs/symptoms for a child with bacterial meningitis; therefore, this child does not need to be assessed first.

2. The child with TOF would be expected to have signs of congestive heart failure so this child would not be assessed first.

3. The child with Reye syndrome would present with lethargy and vomiting so this child would not be assessed first.

4. **Sunken eyeballs and decreased urine output are signs of dehydration, which is a life-threatening complication of diarrhea; therefore, this child should be assessed first.**

*Content – Pediatrics: **Category of Health Alteration** – Endocrine: **Integrated Processes** – Nursing Process: Assessment: **Client Needs** – Safe and Effective Care Environment: Management of Care: **Cognitive Level** – Analysis*

MAKING NURSING DECISIONS: The test taker must determine if the signs/symptoms are normal for the disease process; if the signs/symptoms are normal, then the nurse should not assess the child first. If two or more are not expected, then the nurse must determine which is more life threatening, needs further assessment, or needs notification of the healthcare provider.

12. 1. **A high fever and high-pitched crying may indicate a reaction to the immunizations; therefore, this parent needs to be called first to bring the child to the clinic.**

2. This child probably has an ear infection, which needs to be seen but is not priority over a reaction to immunizations.

3. The nurse needs to call in a prescription for the digoxin but not prior to calling the parent whose child is having a reaction to an immunization.

4. The child may need to be seen but primarily kept in isolation so this parent does not need to be called first.

*Content – Pediatrics: **Category of Health Alteration** – Drug Administration: **Integrated Processes** – Nursing Process: Assessment: **Client Needs** – Physiological Integrity: Reduction of Risk Potential: **Cognitive Level** – Analysis*

MAKING NURSING DECISIONS: The test taker must determine if the signs/symptoms are normal for the disease process; if the signs/symptoms are not normal, then the nurse should call this parent first.

13. 1. These are signs/symptoms of neurovascular compromise and the cast may need to be cut (bifurcated) but it is not the first intervention.

2. The child should be brought to the office but the parent should first attempt to decrease edema by elevating the extremity.

3. **The nurse should first take care of the client's body by having the parent elevate the left leg.**

4. The orthopedist should be notified but it is not the first intervention.

*Content – Pediatrics: **Category of Health Alteration** – Musculoskeletal: **Integrated Processes** – Nursing Process: Implementation: **Client Needs** – Physiological Integrity: Reduction of Risk Potential: **Cognitive Level** – Application*

MAKING NURSING DECISIONS: When the question asks the nurse which intervention should be implemented first, it means all the interventions are possible. The nurse should implement an action that will help the client's situation first.

14. 1. The child with iron-deficiency anemia would be taking an iron elixir, which causes the stool to be black.

2. The child with PKU should not eat any meats, milk, dairy, and eggs since the child lacks the enzyme that breaks down phenylalanine.

3. **A complication of rheumatic heart disease is valvular disorders that may be manifested by respiratory problems; therefore, the nurse should notify the child's healthcare provider.**

4. The child with acute glomerulonephritis would be expected to have dark urine.

*Content – Pediatrics: **Category of Health Alteration** – Cardiovascular: **Integrated Processes** – Nursing Process: Assessment: **Client Needs** – Health Promotion and Maintenance: **Cognitive Level** – Analysis*

MAKING NURSING DECISIONS: The nurse should notify the healthcare provider of any signs/symptoms that are not expected with the disease process or are signs of a complication.

15. 1. **Bulging fontanels is a sign of increased intracranial pressure, which is a complication of neurological surgery; therefore, this child should be assessed first.**

2. A moist, pink stoma is normal; therefore, this child does not need to be assessed first.

3. This child needs to be assessed but is not priority over a child with a surgical, possibly life-threatening, complication.

4. The child will have an indwelling urinary catheter and clear amber urine is normal so this child does not need to be assessed first.

*Content – Pediatrics: **Category of Health Alteration** – Neurological: **Integrated Processes** – Nursing Process: Assessment: **Client Needs** – Physiological Integrity: Reduction of Risk Potential: **Cognitive Level** – Analysis*

MAKING NURSING DECISIONS: The test taker must determine if the signs/symptoms are expected for the surgical procedure. If the signs/symptoms are not expected, this child should be assessed first. If two are not expected,

then the child with a life-threatening complication should be assessed first.

16. 1. It is appropriate for the nurse to perform ROM exercises to help prevent contractures, specifically scissoring of the legs. This action would not require intervention.
    2. Safety issues should always be addressed, and keeping the bed in the lowest position may prevent injury to the child.
    3. Taking the child to the activity room is being a client advocate and would not warrant intervention.
    4. **The child should be positioned upright to prevent aspiration during meals; therefore, this action would require the charge nurse to intervene.**
    Content – *Pediatrics:* ***Category of Health Alteration*** – *Neurological:* ***Integrated Processes*** – *Nursing Process: Assessment:* ***Client Needs*** – *Safe and Effective Care Environment: Management of Care:* ***Cognitive Level*** – *Analysis*

17. 1. The UAP cannot assess a client; therefore, this is an inappropriate delegation.
    2. The child with a cleft palate repair is at risk for choking or damaging the incision site; therefore, this task should not be delegated to a UAP.
    3. Demonstrating is teaching, and the UAP cannot teach a client.
    4. **The last step of delegating to a UAP is for the nurse to evaluate and determine whether the delegated tasks have been completed and performed correctly. This indicates the nurse has delegated appropriately.**
    Content – *Pediatrics:* ***Category of Health Alteration*** – *Management of Care:* ***Integrated Processes*** – *Nursing Process: Planning:* ***Client Needs*** – *Safe and Effective Care Environment: Management of Care:* ***Cognitive Level*** – *Synthesis*

MAKING NURSING DECISIONS: When delegating to a UAP, the nurse must follow the four rights of clinical delegation: the right task, to the right person, using the right communication, and providing the right feedback. The right feedback includes determining whether the delegated tasks were performed correctly.

18. 1. **Communication to the UAP must be clear, concise, correct, and complete. The nurse must determine why there was a lack of communication, which resulted in the child receiving food; therefore, this action should be implemented first.**
    2. The nurse retains ultimate accountability for any delegated tasks and cannot blame the UAP for the child's being fed by the mother. The HCP needs to be notified to cancel the procedure.
    3. The nurse should talk to the mother about why the child was being fed, but the nurse must first determine whether the UAP told the mother not to feed the child and that the child was to be given nothing by mouth.
    4. This action is too late to take care of the situation.
    Content – *Management:* ***Category of Health Alteration*** – *Management of Care:* ***Integrated Processes*** – *Nursing Process: Implementation:* ***Client Needs*** – *Safe and Effective Care Environment: Safety and Infection Control:* ***Cognitive Level*** – *Application*

19. 1. The scrub technician is assigned to perform daily whirlpool dressing changes, which is a lengthy procedure. Therefore, assigning the one RN to this task would be inappropriate because he or she cannot be unavailable for an extended period of time.
    2. **One of the responsibilities of the unit secretary is to transcribe the HCP's orders, but the licensed nurse retains total responsibility for the correctness and accuracy of the transcribed orders.**
    3. The scrub technician cannot administer medications.
    4. The unit secretary and laboratory personnel are responsible for posting laboratory data into the client's charts. The UAP should be on the unit taking care of the clients.
    Content – *Pediatrics:* ***Category of Health Alteration*** – *Integumentary:* ***Integrated Processes*** – *Nursing Process: Planning:* ***Client Needs*** – *Safe and Effective Care Environment: Management of Care:* ***Cognitive Level*** – *Synthesis*

20. **1, 2, 4, and 5 are correct.**
    1. **The UAP can pass the dietary trays to the clients because it does not require judgment.**
    2. **One of the responsibilities of the UAP is taking routine vital signs on clients.**
    3. The nurse must complete the preoperative checklist because it requires nursing judgment to determine whether the client is ready for surgery.
    4. **One of the responsibilities of the UAP is changing bed linens.**
    5. **The UAP can document the client's intake and output, but the UAP cannot evaluate the numbers.**
    Content – *Pediatrics:* ***Category of Health Alteration*** – *Management of Care:* ***Integrated Processes*** – *Nursing Process: Planning:* ***Client Needs*** – *Safe and Effective Care Environment: Management of Care:* ***Cognitive Level*** – *Application*

21. 1. The administration of blood products does not require the most experienced nurse.
    2. Preparing a child for a routine procedure does not require the most experienced nurse.
    3. The child recovering from a sickle cell crisis would not require the most experienced nurse.
    4. **The child newly diagnosed with a chronic disease, which will have acute exacerbations, requires extensive teaching; therefore, the most experienced nurse should be assigned to this child and family.**
    *Content – Pediatrics: **Category of Health Alteration –** Management of Care: **Integrated Processes –** Nursing Process: Planning: **Client Needs –** Safe and Effective Care Environment: Management of Care: **Cognitive Level –** Synthesis*

22. 1. Only a nurse can withdraw blood from a central line.
    2. The social worker or case manager is responsible for referring clients to support groups. This is not an expected responsibility of a floor nurse/LPN.
    3. **Only chemotherapy-certified RNs can administer antineoplastic, chemotherapeutic medications. This is a national minimal standard of care according to the Oncology Nursing Society.**
    4. The dietician is responsible for ensuring that the proper food is provided along with evaluating the child's nutritional intake, not checking the amount of food eaten—this is the responsibility of the nursing staff.
    *Content – Pediatrics: **Category of Health Alteration –** Oncology: **Integrated Processes –** Nursing Process: Planning:**Client Needs –** Safe and Effective Care Environment: Management of Care: **Cognitive Level –** Synthesis*

23. 1. A 6-year-old child on bed rest needs an appropriate activity to help with distraction; a cartoon video would be an age-appropriate activity.
    2. The child life therapist is responsible for recreational and developmental activity for the hospitalized child, but any staff member should address the child's psychosocial needs.
    3. **Part of the delegation process is to evaluate the UAP's performance of duties, and the nurse should praise any initiative on the part of the UAP in being a client advocate.**
    4. Videos are one of the few age-appropriate activities to occupy a 6-year-old on bed rest; therefore, there is no reason to notify the charge nurse.
    *Content – Management: **Category of Health Alteration –** Management of Care: **Integrated Processes –** Nursing Process: Implementation: **Client***

*Needs – Safe and Effective Care Environment: Management of Care: **Cognitive Level –** Application*

24. 1. The newborn with the myelomeningocele has a portion of the spinal cord and membranes protruding through the back and is at risk for hydrocephalus and meningitis; this client should be assigned to a more experienced nurse.
    2. **The new graduate who has completed the NICU internship should be able to care for a premature infant because care is primarily supportive.**
    3. Esophageal atresia, a congenital anomaly in which the esophagus does not completely develop, is a clinical and surgical emergency. It puts the newborn at risk for aspiration because the upper esophagus ends in a blind pouch with the lower part of the esophagus connected to the trachea. This newborn should be assigned to a more experienced nurse.
    4. Tetralogy of Fallot is a cyanotic, congenital anomaly. It includes a combination of four defects of the heart, all of which result in unoxygenated blood being pumped into the systemic circulation. This newborn must be assigned to an experienced nurse.
    *Content – Pediatrics: **Category of Health Alteration –** Cardiac: **Integrated Processes –** Nursing Process: Planning: **Client Needs –** Safe and Effective Care Environment: Management of Care: **Cognitive Level –** Synthesis*

MAKING NURSING DECISIONS: The test taker must determine which client is the most stable, which makes this an "except" question. Three clients are either unstable or have potentially life-threatening conditions.

25. 1. Weighing the diaper is the procedure for determining the infant's urinary output and is not part of the procedure for obtaining a urine specimen.
    2. **The NCSBN position paper in 1995 defined delegation as transferring to a competent individual the authority to perform a selected nursing task in a selected situation. The nurse retains the accountability for the delegation. The nurse must determine whether the UAP has the ability and knowledge to perform a task. This question clarifies whether the UAP has the ability to obtain a urine specimen.**
    3. Obtaining a urine specimen with an indwelling catheter on an 11-month-old infant would require more expertise than a UAP would have on the pediatric unit.

ANSWERS

Furthermore, it does not determine whether the UAP understands how to do the procedure.

4. This statement does not determine whether the UAP understands how to perform the procedure of obtaining a urine specimen from an 11-month-old infant.

*Content – Management: **Category of Health Alteration** – Management of Care: **Integrated Processes** – Nursing Process: Assessment: **Client Needs** – Safe and Effective Care Environment: Management of Care: **Cognitive Level** – Analysis*

26. 1. **The UAP can orient the parents and child to the room, and demonstrate how to use the call light, how the bed works, or how the television works.**
2. The UAP cannot prepare a child for endoscopy; this requires assessment and evaluation to determine if the child is ready for the procedure.
3. There must be at least two people to log roll a child, and the UAP cannot do this procedure alone.
4. The nurse cannot delegate assessment to the UAP.

*Content – Pediatrics: **Category of Health Alteration** – Management of Care: **Integrated Processes** – Nursing Process: Planning: **Client Needs** – Safe and Effective Care Environment: Management of Care: **Cognitive Level** – Synthesis*

MAKING NURSING DECISIONS: The nurse cannot delegate assessment, teaching, evaluation, medications, or an unstable client to a UAP.

27. 1. The UAP can weigh the diapers and obtain urine output. The nurse must evaluate the output.
2. A child under 12 years of age cannot be left alone in the room, and the UAP could stay with the child while the parent gets something to eat.
3. The Pavlik harness should not be removed, so bathing the child in the harness is appropriate and does not warrant intervention.
4. **The 7-month-old should have elbow restraints, not wrist restraints. Elbow restraints prevent the child from putting fingers into the mouth, but allow the child to move the arms.**

*Content – Pediatrics: **Category of Health Alteration** – Management of Care: **Integrated Processes** – Nursing Process: Assessment: **Client Needs** – Safe and Effective Care Environment: Management of Care: **Cognitive Level** – Analysis*

MAKING NURSING DECISIONS: The nurse is responsible for supervising and evaluating the care

the UAP provides to any clients. The nurse must intervene and correct the UAP's behavior.

28. **2, 3, 4, and 5 are correct.**
1. The nurse cannot assign teaching to the LPN.
2. **The UAP can apply an ice collar since the client is stable.**
3. **The UAP can apply ointment to a diaper rash—it is a medication but it can be applied by the UAP.**
4. **The LPN can double-check a dose of medication. The nurse can assign medication administration to an LPN.**
5. **The LPN can transcribe a healthcare provider's orders.**

*Content – Pediatrics: **Category of Health Alteration** – Management of Care: **Integrated Processes** – Nursing Process: Planning: **Client Needs** – Safe and Effective Care Environment: Management of Care: **Cognitive Level** – Synthesis*

MAKING NURSING DECISIONS: The nurse cannot delegate assessment, teaching, evaluation, medications, or an unstable client to a UAP. The nurse cannot assign assessment, teaching, evaluation, or an unstable client to an LPN.

29. 1. The nurse cannot delegate teaching to the UAP.
2. The LPN could teach a client how to irrigate a colostomy, but a 4-month-old is incontinent of stool; therefore, irrigating the colostomy is not done.
3. The LPN or nurse should remove the IV catheter of a 4-month-old child, not the UAP.
4. **The UAP can escort the child and parents to the car.**

*Content – Pediatrics: **Category of Health Alteration** – Gastrointestinal: **Integrated Processes** – Nursing Process: Implementation: **Client Needs** – Health Promotion and Maintenance: **Cognitive Level** – Application*

MAKING NURSING DECISIONS: The nurse cannot delegate assessment, teaching, evaluation, medications, or an unstable client to a UAP. The nurse cannot assign assessment, teaching, evaluation, or an unstable client to an LPN. Many questions on the NCLEX-RN® are evaluating the test taker's knowledge of the disease process or surgical procedure, as well as delegation/assignments.

30. 1. The UAP can take vital signs but the nurse should assess the child to determine whether this is routine postoperative pain (expected), or whether a complication is occurring.
2. A rule of thumb—if anyone else gives the nurse information about a client, the

nurse should first assess the client before taking any further action.

3. The nurse may need to notify the HCP, but not before assessing the child.

4. The nurse may need to administer pain medication but not prior to assessing the child.

Content – Pediatrics: **Category of Health Alteration –** *Gastrointestinal:* **Integrated Processes –** *Nursing Process: Implementation:* **Client Needs –** *Physiological Integrity: Reduction of Risk Potential:* **Cognitive Level –** *Application*

MAKING NURSING DECISIONS: When the question asks, "Which intervention should the nurse implement first?" it means all or at least more than one option is plausible. Remember: If another person, a machine, or laboratory datum provides information about the client, the nurse should assess the client first.

31. 1. **The nurse should offer the child choices that ensure cooperation with the therapeutic regimen. The choices are when the child will ambulate, not whether the child will ambulate.**

2. The nurse could ask the parents for help in making sure the client ambulates, but this may cause a rift in the nurse/parent/child relationship. This is not the most appropriate intervention.

3. The child development therapist could assist with activities that would encourage the client to ambulate, but the nurse should take control of the situation and ensure the client ambulates. This is not the most appropriate intervention.

4. This is bribery, and the nurse should not use this technique to ensure cooperation with the therapeutic regimen.

Content – Pediatric: **Category of Health Alteration –** *Management of Care:* **Integrated Processes –** *Caring:* **Client Needs –** *Safe and Effective Care Environment:* **Management of Care: Cognitive Level –**

32. 1. The nurse must take action or the child will be afraid of the nurse.

2. The nurse should discuss the inappropriate comment with the mother, not with the child.

3. If every nurse who overheard this type of comment reported it to Child Protective Services, it would only unnecessarily increase the workload in an already overloaded system. Furthermore, reporting perceived potential abuse to Child Protective Services is a very serious accusation.

4. **The nurse should explain to the mother that threatening the child with a shot will cause the child to be frightened of**

healthcare professionals. This type of comment is inappropriate and should not be used to discipline a child.

Content – Pediatrics: **Category of Health Alteration –** *Management of Care:* **Integrated Processes –** *Nursing Process: Implementation:* **Client Needs –** *Psychosocial Integrity:* **Cognitive Level –** *Application*

33. 1. There is a Web site to obtain information about Down syndrome, but this type of referral would not be the most appropriate for parents who need to deal with emotional aspects of having a child with special needs.

2. The hospital chaplain is an important part of the multidisciplinary healthcare team but would not have specialized knowledge regarding caring for a special needs child.

3. **According to the NCLEX-RN® test plan, referrals are included in management of care. The most appropriate referral would be to a support group where other parents who have special needs children can share their feelings and provide advice on how to care for their child in the home.**

4. Although Down syndrome results from a trisomy chromosome 21, it is primarily associated with maternal age over 35 years. Furthermore, a geneticist would not have specialized knowledge regarding caring for a special needs child.

Content – Pediatrics: **Category of Health Alteration –** *Management of Care:* **Integrated Processes –** *Diagnosis:* **Client Needs –** *Safe and Effective Care Environment:* **Management of Care: Cognitive Level –** *Knowledge*

34. 1. The newborn nursery does not need any more people in the area. Personnel are needed to monitor any and all exits.

2. The purpose of using code names to alert hospital personnel of emergency situations is to avoid panic among the clients and visitors; therefore, the nurse should not explain the situation to the clients and visitors.

3. Any time there is an overhead emergency announcement, the charge nurse is responsible for following the hospital emergency plan.

4. **Code Pink means an infant has been abducted from the newborn nursery. The priority intervention is to prevent the abductor from taking the child from the hospital, which can be prevented by placing a staff member at all of the unit exits.**

Content – Pediatrics: **Category of Health Alteration –** *Management of Care:* **Integrated Processes –** *Nursing Process: Implementation:* **Client Needs –** *Safe and Effective Care Environment: Safety and Infection Control:* **Cognitive Level –** *Application*

MAKING NURSING DECISIONS: The nurse must be knowledgeable of hospital emergency preparedness. Students as well as new employees receive this information in hospital orientations and are responsible for implementing procedures correctly. The NCLEX-RN® blueprint includes questions on the safe and effective care environment.

35. 1. Even though case management is a strategy to ensure coordination of care while reducing costs, the nurse should not share this with the mother.
    2. The case manager is not responsible for ensuring that the client receives the correct medication; it is the responsibility of the HCP.
    3. **According to the NCLEX-RN® test blueprint, questions on case management are included. The case manager will coordinate the care for a client with a chronic illness with other members of the multidisciplinary healthcare team. This attempts to prevent duplication of services and allows the mother to have a specific individual to coordinate services to meet the child's needs.**
    4. The life expectancy of a child with Duchenne's muscular dystrophy is approximately 25 years. The case manager is not responsible for helping the child have a normal life expectancy.
    Content – Management of Care: **Category of Health Alteration** *– Management of Care:* **Integrated Processes** *– Nursing Process: Implementation:* **Client Needs** *– Safe and Effective Care Environment: Management of Care:* **Cognitive Level** *– Comprehension*

36. 1. Although this would not be the first step in investigating a problem, this action may be initiated if it is determined to be the cause for the increase in infection rates.
    2. The nurse should utilize evidenced-based practice research when proposing changes because it is part of the performance improvement process, but it is not the first intervention when investigating the problem.
    3. **The first intervention is to determine the extent of the problem and who owns the problem. The NCLEX-RN® test blueprint includes performance improvement (quality improvement) in the management of care content.**
    4. This action may need to be implemented once it is determined whether there is a problem with IV infection rates. However, this would be the second step in the process.
    Content – Management: **Category of Health Alteration** *– Management of Care:* **Integrated Processes** *– Nursing Process: Implementation:* **Client Needs** *– Safe*

and Effective Care Environment: Safety and Infection Control: **Cognitive Level** *– Comprehension*

37. 1. **The ethical principle of justice is to treat all clients fairly, without regard to age, socioeconomic status, or any other variable, including clients with special needs. This statement supports the adolescent's right to her opinion even though she has Down syndrome.**
    2. If the adolescent needs clarification of the procedure, this would be an appropriate response, which is an example of the ethical principle of veracity or truth telling.
    3. This statement is an example of the ethical principle of paternalism, in which the nurse knows what is best for the client.
    4. This is an example of autonomy, in which the client has the right to self-determination. The Nuremburg Code of ethics specifically supports the rights of individuals with special needs against being forced to participate in procedures they do not want.
    Content – Pediatrics: **Category of Health Alteration –** *Reproductive:* **Integrated Processes** *– Nursing Process: Evaluation:* **Client Needs** *– Psychosocial Integrity:* **Cognitive Level** *– Synthesis*

38. 1. Although this may be the case, this is not client advocacy, and doing so may make the mother feel guilty about not being able to afford glasses for her child.
    2. **This is an example of client advocacy because many local service organizations, such as the Lions Club or the Rotary Club, will subsidize the cost of the vision test and glasses.**
    3. Medicaid does not pay for glasses, and it is not the school nurse's business whether the family is on Medicaid.
    4. The nurse should not loan the mother money because this crosses professional boundaries.
    Content – Pediatrics: **Category of Health Alteration –** *Neurosensory:* **Integrated Processes** *– Nursing Process: Implementation:* **Client Needs** *– Health Promotion and Maintenance* **Cognitive Level** *– Application*

39. 1. The 16-year-old client is not old enough to sign the permit; therefore, pain medication would not be withheld.
    2. **Legally, a child under the age of 18 must have a parent or legal guardian sign for informed consent. The nurse should determine whether the child is aware of the situation and assents to the procedure.**
    3. The surgeon is responsible for explaining the procedure; the nurse is responsible for witnessing the signature on the operative permit.

4. The nurse is responsible for witnessing the signature. Having a visitor sign the operative permit is a violation of HIPAA.

Content – Pediatrics: **Category of Health Alteration –** *Gastrointestinal:* **Integrated Processes –** *Nursing Process:* **Implementation: Client Needs –** *Safe and Effective Care Environment: Management of Care:* **Cognitive Level –** *Application*

40. 1. A written memo does not allow the staff to have input into how to correct the problem. This memo might lead to blaming and arguments among the staff.

2. The performance improvement committee is designed to improve client care, not to address management issues.

3. This is implying that the unit manager does not believe the central supply lost charges. If the unit manager has this concern, it should be addressed directly with the central supply supervisor.

4. **Because the staff is responsible for following the hospital procedure for charging for items used in client care, the unit manager should discuss this with staff to determine what should be done to correct the problem.**

Content – Management: **Category of Health Alteration –** *Management of Care:* **Integrated Processes –** *Nursing Process:* **Implementation: Client Needs –** *Safe and Effective Care Environment: Management of Care:* **Cognitive Level –** *Application*

41. 1. A 1-year-old child who cries when the parent leaves the room is developmentally on target.

2. The 2-year-old who can speak in two- or three-word sentences is developmentally on target.

3. The 3-year-old should be toilet trained by this age.

4. **The toddler (age 1–3) is expected to throw temper tantrums, but a 4-year-old child should not be doing this; therefore, the child is not developmentally on target and the child developmental specialist should be notified.**

Content – Pediatrics: **Category of Health Alteration –** *Growth and Development:* **Integrated Processes –** *Nursing Process:* **Evaluation: Client Needs –** *Psychosocial Integrity:* **Cognitive Level –** *Synthesis*

MAKING NURSING DECISIONS: The pediatric nurse must be knowledgeable of the normal developmental tasks for each age. The Joint Commission mandates all children in a pediatric unit must have a developmental assessment and intervention if the child is not on task.

42. 1. The child with uncontrolled pain would require a more experienced nurse.

2. Infected skeletal pin sites can lead to osteomyelitis, which would require a more experienced nurse.

3. This child and parents require extensive teaching and should be assigned to a more experienced nurse.

4. **The new graduate should be able to complete preoperative teaching and prepare the young client for surgery. This client is stable.**

Content – Pediatrics: **Category of Health Alteration –** *Management of Care:* **Integrated Processes –** *Nursing Process:* **Planning: Client Needs –** *Safe and Effective Care Environment: Management of Care:* **Cognitive Level –** *Synthesis*

MAKING NURSING DECISIONS: An inexperienced nurse should be assigned the most stable client.

43. 1. Elevating the arm to help decrease edema is an appropriate intervention and does not warrant intervention.

2. The nurse is legally obligated to notify CPS for any suspected child abuse.

3. **A child who is drooling may have epiglottitis and opening the mouth may lead to respiratory distress. This action warrants intervention by the charge nurse.**

4. The nurse needs to confirm a urinary tract infection by obtaining a urine specimen.

Content – Pediatrics: **Category of Health Alteration –** *Immunoinflammatory:* **Integrated Processes –** *Nursing Process:* **Assessment: Client Needs –** *Safe and Effective Care Environment: Management of Care:* **Cognitive Level –** *Analysis*

MAKING NURSING DECISIONS: The test taker must be able to apply assessment data and interventions to determine if the action is appropriate. This is an NCLEX-RN® style application question.

44. 1. The nurse must administer the scheduled insulin dose along with the sliding scale coverage; therefore, this is the incorrect dose.

2. **The nurse must administer the scheduled dose along with an additional 8 units, so the total dose is 18 units regular insulin and NPH 20 units. The nurse should not administer two injections to the child.**

3. This is the scheduled dose and does not include the sliding scale coverage.

4. This covers the sliding scale coverage but not the scheduled dose.

Content – Pediatrics: **Category of Health Alteration –** *Drug Administration:* **Integrated Processes –** *Nursing Process:* **Implementation: Client Needs –** *Physiological Integrity: Pharmacological and Parenteral Therapies:* **Cognitive Level –** *Analysis*

MAKING NURSING DECISIONS: This is a knowledge-based question concerning managing a child's disease. There are no test-taking hints for this type of question.

45. 1 and 3 are correct.
    1. **Including the parents in developing the plan of care will help establish a positive relationship.**
    2. Holding their child will help with the child/parent relationship, but not with the nurse/parent relationship.
    3. **Allowing the parents to vent their feelings will help form a positive nurse/parent relationship.**
    4. The nurse must not make the parents feel guilty if they have to work while the child is hospitalized. A relative can stay with the child if parents have to work.
    5. This will help the child/parent relationship not the nurse/parent relationship.

    Content – Pediatrics: *Category of Health Alteration – Management of Care:* **Integrated Processes** *– Nursing Process: Implementation:* **Client Needs** *– Psychosocial Integrity:* **Cognitive Level** *– Application*

MAKING NURSING DECISIONS: "Select all that apply" questions require the test taker to select more than one option as a correct answer. There are no partial points given for partially correct answers.

46. 1. The 9-month-old infant's language and cognitive skills include imitating sounds, saying single syllables, and beginning to put syllables together. Using "mama" and "dada" indicates this child is developmentally on target.
    2. The 10- to 12-month-old infant can walk with one hand held or cruise the furniture, but will usually crawl to get places more rapidly. This behavior indicates the child is developmentally on target.
    3. **The 8-month-old infant should be able to sit steadily unsupported; therefore, this child is developmentally delayed and warrants a referral to the early childhood development specialist. Leaning forward on both hands to sit is normal for a 6-month-old.**
    4. The 4-month-old infant should be able to turn from the abdomen to back; therefore, this child is developmentally on target.

    Content – Pediatrics: *Category of Health Alteration – Growth and Development:* **Integrated Processes** *– Nursing Process: Assessment:* **Client Needs** *– Health Promotion and Maintenance:* **Cognitive Level** *– Analysis*

47. 1. **The most important intervention for this child is to make sure the child has some control and input into the decision making. It is customary to obtain assent from children 7 years of age and older. Assent means the child has been fully informed about the procedure and concurs with those giving the informed consent.**
    2. The parents must sign the permit because the child is under age 18, but the most important intervention is to make sure the child is included and aware of decisions being made about his or her body.
    3. The nurse may be able to clarify some of the child's or parent's questions and does not need to refer all questions to the HCP.
    4. Witnessing the signature on the permit is required prior to the child's having surgery, but it is not the most important intervention.

    Content – Pediatrics: *Category of Health Alteration – Hematology:* **Integrated Processes** *– Nursing Process: Implementation:* **Client Needs** *– Psychosocial Integrity:* **Cognitive Level** *– Comprehension*

48. 1. The nurse should call hospital security when a client or visitor is being abusive, but this is not a legal action.
    2. **Legally, the nurse is required to report any suspected child abuse. A 13-year-old child who is having a baby and is withdrawn and silent along with a potential abuser who is trying to control access to the child should make the nurse suspect child abuse.**
    3. Referring the client to a social worker is not a legal action.
    4. Asking the client whether she feels safe at home is an appropriate assessment question, but it is not a legal action.

    Content – Pediatrics: *Category of Health Alteration – Obstetrics:* **Integrated Processes** *– Nursing Process: Implementation:* **Client Needs** *– Safe and Effective Care Environment, Safety and Infection Control:* **Cognitive Level** *– Application*

49. 1. The charge nurse must first make sure that clients and visitors are safe. Someone will notify the charge nurse about the location of the fire.
    2. **Safety of the clients and visitors is priority; therefore, ensuring that they are in a room with the door closed is the first intervention.**
    3. The charge nurse may need to prepare for evacuation, but it is not the first intervention.
    4. Although making a list of clients not currently on the unit is an appropriate intervention, the charge nurse must first ensure the

safety of the clients and visitors who are on the pediatric unit.

*Content – Pediatrics: **Category of Health Alteration –** Management of Care: **Integrated Processes** – Nursing Process: Implementation: **Client Needs** – Safe and Effective Care Environment: Safety and Infection Control: **Cognitive Level** – Comprehension*

50. 1. The HIPAA officer can be notified of the breach of confidentiality, but the nurse must first confront the two nurses and correct the behavior.
    2. The nurses can be reported to their clinical manager, but the nurse must first confront the two nurses and correct the behavior.
    3. The situation can be documented in writing and turned into the HIPAA officer (not the CNO), but the nurse must first confront the two nurses and correct the behavior.
    4. **This is a violation of HIPAA; therefore, the nurse must first confront the two nurses and correct the behavior.**

    *Content – Pediatrics: **Category of Health Alteration –** Management of Care: **Integrated Processes** Nursing Process: Implementation: **Client Needs** – Safe and Effective Care Environment: Management of Care: **Cognitive Level** – Application*

51. 1. The nurse would not be concerned about not passing meconium until at least 24 hours after delivery.
    2. The nurse would not be concerned about a newborn who is slightly jaundiced until after 24 hours after delivery, at which point the HCP would investigate to determine whether the jaundice is pathological.
    3. **A newborn who is jittery and irritable needs to be assessed first for possible hypoglycemia. The nurse could feed the newborn glucose water or provide more frequent, regular feedings.**
    4. Although the nurse should determine why the newborn will not stop crying, the newborn who is showing signs of hypoglycemia warrants immediate intervention.

    *Content – Pediatrics: **Category of Health Alteration –** Endocrine: **Integrated Processes** – Nursing Process: Evaluation: **Client Needs** – Physiological Integrity: Reduction of Risk Potential: **Cognitive Level** – Synthesis*

52. 1. An antacid is administered to neutralize gastric acidity and help with heartburn, not abdominal pain.
    2. A non-narcotic analgesic is used to treat mild pain, a 2 to 4 on a pain scale.
    3. **A narcotic analgesic is used for moderate-to-severe pain; a 5 is considered moderate pain. The child received a dose at 0600, which relieved the pain for**

7 hours; therefore, this would be the most appropriate medication.
    4. An IVP narcotic analgesic should be administered for severe pain, that is, pain greater than 7 on a pain scale of 1 to 10.

    *Content – Pediatrics: **Category of Health Alteration –** Drug Administration: **Integrated Processes** – Nursing Process: Implementation: **Client Needs** – Physiological Integrity: Pharmacological and Parenteral Therapies: **Cognitive Level** – Application*

53. 1. The nurse should not accept any assignment for which he or she is unqualified. A newborn assessment requires specialized knowledge and skills to detect potential complications.
    2. The nurse who is not familiar with the procedure or the unit should not be assigned to assist a pediatrician to perform a procedure.
    3. This is a dangerous procedure because the nurse must insert a tube into the newborn's stomach. A nurse who is not familiar with this procedure should refuse the assignment.
    4. **Any nurse can take an infant to the mother's room and check the bands to ensure the right infant is with the right mother. This is an appropriate task for a nurse who has never worked in the nursery.**

    *Content – Pediatrics: **Category of Health Alteration –** Management of Care: **Integrated Processes** – Nursing Process: Planning: **Client Needs** – Safe and Effective Care Environment: Management of Care: **Cognitive Level** – Synthesis*

54. 1. **The 9-month-old infant should be able to sit without support. Therefore, the nurse should instruct the UAP to perform the developmental task of helping the child sit without support.**
    2. Teaching a child to catch a beach ball would be appropriate for a 15- to 18-month-old child, so the nurse should not instruct the UAP to perform this task.
    3. The UAP should not use food as a reward or comfort measure because it may lead to childhood obesity.
    4. Teaching a child how to blow a kiss is a language/cognitive activity and will not help the child's gross motor development.

    *Content – Pediatrics: **Category of Health Alteration –** Neurological: **Integrated Processes** – Nursing Process: Planning: **Client Needs** – Safe and Effective Care Environment: Management of Care: **Cognitive Level** – Synthesis*

55. 1. Making sure no one can view the screen is an appropriate information technology guideline.

ANSWERS

2. Researching medication online is ensuring safe and effective nursing care and shows that the nurse is keeping abreast of new medications.

3. **According to the NCLEX-RN® test blueprint, the nurse must be knowledgeable of information technology. Giving another nurse his or her access code is a very serious violation of information technology guidelines and should be reported.**

4. Logging off the computer is an appropriate information technology guideline.

Content – Legal: *Category of Health Alteration* – *Management of Care:* ***Integrated Processes*** – *Nursing Process: Implementation:* ***Client Needs*** – *Safe and Effective Care Environment: Management of Care:* ***Cognitive Level*** – *Application*

56. 1. A dog bite is an emergency, but it is not life threatening; therefore, this child would not be assessed first.
2. The child with a head laceration must be assessed, but not before a child who might die of medication poisoning.
3. The child with a fractured tibia would not be expected to move the foot.
4. **A child who ingested a bottle of prenatal vitamins presents a medication poisoning that is a potentially life-threatening situation. This child must be assessed first to determine how many vitamins were taken, how long ago they were taken, and whether or not the vitamins contained iron. The child's neurological status must also be assessed.**

Content – Pediatrics: *Category of Health Alteration* – *Drug Administration:* ***Integrated Processes*** – *Nursing Process: Assessment:* ***Client Needs*** – *Physiological Integrity: Reduction of Risk Potential:* ***Cognitive Level*** – *Analysis*

57. 1. The pediatric client has the right to an explanation of procedures being done to his or her body.
2. **The pediatric client has a right to be treated with dignity and respect. Just because the child is being coded does not mean the nurse should allow the child's body to be exposed to everyone in the room.**
3. The pediatric client has a right to confidentiality, and the parents/legal guardians are the only individuals who have a right to the child's health information. Talking to the grandparents is a violation of HIPAA unless the parents have approved.
4. The nurse is responsible and accountable to protect the health, safety, and rights of the pediatric client. Leaving an uncapped needle

at the bedside could cause serious harm to the child.

Content – Pediatrics: *Category of Health Alteration* – *Management of Care:* ***Integrated Processes*** – *Nursing Process: Evaluation:* ***Client Needs*** – *Safe and Effective Care Environment: Management of Care:* ***Cognitive Level*** – *Synthesis*

58. 1. Diversional activity deficit would be appropriate if the client did not have sufficient activities to keep him or her occupied. Most children of this age will watch television, play video games, or read books.
2. The client has leukemia and is receiving chemotherapy, which leads to an increased risk of infection; however, this is a physiological problem, not a psychosocial problem.
3. **The client will be isolated from peers and schools because of the high risk of infection resulting from the immunosuppression secondary to chemotherapy and the disease process. At this stage, the child needs to be developing peer relationships and independence from parents. Therefore, social isolation is the priority psychosocial problem for this client.**
4. The nurse should not identify hopelessness because childhood leukemia has a good prognosis.

Content – Pediatrics: *Category of Health Alteration* – *Oncology:* ***Integrated Processes*** – *Nursing Process: Planning:* ***Client Needs*** – *Psychosocial Integrity:* ***Cognitive Level*** – *Synthesis*

59. 1. Placing the IV line on an infusion pump helps to make sure the client does not receive an overload of IV fluid. Most facilities require an IV pump and volume-controlled chamber when administering fluids in a pediatric clinic.
2. **A volume-controlled chamber (Buretrol) is a device that is used with children when administering IV fluids. The chamber is filled with 1 hour's amount of fluid so that the child will not inadvertently receive an overload of fluid. Fluid volume overload is a potentially life-threatening situation in children.**
3. The site should be checked frequently to ensure that the IV does not infiltrate; therefore, this does not warrant intervention.
4. The IV tubing should not be used longer than 72 hours; therefore, labeling the tubing with the date and time would not warrant intervention.

Content – Pediatrics: *Category of Health Alteration* – *Drug Administration:* ***Integrated Processes*** – *Nursing Process: Evaluation:* ***Client Needs*** – *Physiological Integrity: Pharmacological and Parenteral Therapies:* ***Cognitive Level*** – *Synthesis*

60. 1. **Abandonment is a reportable offense to the state board of nursing in every state. Reportable offenses could result in stipulations made to the nurse's license.**
2. This is failure to follow the five rights of medication administration, but it is not a reportable offense.
3. Multiple medication errors are a management issue, not a reportable offense.
4. Having an affair with a fellow employee is not a reportable offense.
Content – Pediatric: **Category of Health Alteration –** *Mental Health:* **Integrated Processes** *– Nursing Process: Evaluation:* **Client Needs** *– Safe and Effective Care Environment: Management of Care:* **Cognitive Level** *– Synthesis*

61. 1. A copper bracelet may or may not help the child with rheumatoid arthritis, but because it will not hurt the child, it does not warrant further investigation.
2. Aloe vera is used in many topical burn preparations; therefore, this practice would not warrant further investigation.
3. Vick's VapoRub may or may not help the child's cold, but, because it will not hurt the child, it does not warrant further investigation.
4. **Herbal products are not regulated by the Food and Drug Administration, and there is very little (if any) research on herbal use with children. The nurse should at least investigate which herbs the child is receiving before taking further action.**
Content – Pediatric: **Category of Health Alteration –** *Drug Administration:* **Integrated Processes** *– Nursing Process: Evaluation:* **Client Needs** *– Safe and Effective Care Environment: Management of Care:* **Cognitive Level** *– Synthesis*

62. 1. This is an appropriate nursing intervention so that the mother will not have to leave her child, but it is not the first intervention. The child's safety is priority.
2. The nurse could go to the cafeteria and tell the mother to return to the room, but during this time the UAP should stay with the child.
3. **The child's safety is priority; therefore, the nurse should have the UAP stay with the child until the mother returns.**
4. Social services would not need to be notified at this time. If the mother continually leaves the child alone, then this would be an appropriate action.
Content – Pediatric: **Category of Health Alteration –** *Safety:* **Integrated Processes** *– Nursing Process: Implementation:* **Client Needs** *– Safe and Effective Care Environment: Safety and Infection Control:* **Cognitive Level** *– Comprehension*

63. 1. An 18-month-old child should be throwing temper tantrums. This indicates the child is developing a sense of autonomy.
2. **An 18-month-old child should cling to the mother and interact continuously with the primary caregiver. A child not interacting with the mother is not meeting the task of developing a sense of autonomy.**
3. The child has met the task of trust when he or she cries if the mother leaves the room.
4. When a child responds to his or her name, it indicates a sense of identity; therefore, the task is met.
Content – Pediatric: **Category of Health Alteration –** *Neurological:* **Integrated Processes** *– Nursing Process: Assessment:* **Client Needs** *– Psychosocial Integrity:* **Cognitive Level** *– Analysis*

64. 1. **An autocratic manager uses an authoritarian approach to direct the activities of others. This individual makes most of the decisions alone without input from other staff members.**
2. A laissez-faire manager maintains a permissive climate with little direction or control.
3. A democratic manager is people oriented and emphasizes efficient group functioning. The environment is open, and communication flows both ways.
4. A democratic manager is people oriented and emphasizes efficient group functioning.
Content – Management: **Category of Health Alteration –** *Management of Care:* **Integrated Processes** *– Nursing Process: Implementation:* **Client Needs** *– Safe and Effective Care Environment: Management of Care:* **Cognitive Level** *– Comprehension*

65. 1. Squatting relieves the hypoxic episodes, and the child should be able to remain in the squatting position.
2. The child with a cyanotic, congenital heart defect should have oxygen when being active.
3. This indicates the father does not understand that the child will not be able to participate in active sports because of the stress that is placed on the heart.
4. **This behavior indicates the child understands the importance of salt restriction because of potential congestive heart failure.**
Content – Pediatric: **Category of Health Alteration –** *Cardiovascular:* **Integrated Processes** *– Nursing Process: Evaluation:* **Client Needs** *– Health Promotion and Maintenance:* **Cognitive Level** *– Synthesis*

66. 1. This is appropriate once the dose has been adjusted for a neonate.
2. This is appropriate once the dose has been adjusted for a neonate.

3. At 2 weeks old there probably will not be a level yet.

4. **Digoxin can be administered to neonates but this is an adult dose: the neonate maintenance dose is 4–8 mcg/kg; 0.125 mg equals 125 mcg. The dose for a 6.82 kg infant would be 27–54 mcg per day.**

Content – Pediatric: ***Category of Health Alteration –*** *Drug Administration:* ***Integrated Processes –*** *Nursing Process: Implementation:* ***Client Needs –*** *Physiological Integrity: Pharmacological and Parenteral Therapies:* ***Cognitive Level –*** *Application*

67. 1. The infant's arm does not have enough tissue for an injection.

2. The infant has a poorly developed dorso gluteal muscle and the sciatic nerve is in this area of the body. Injecting a needle into the nerve could cause permanent damage.

3. Vaccines are not administered into the abdomen.

4. **The anterior lateral thigh muscle (vastus lateralus) is the preferred site for an infant to receive an injection. It is the largest muscle the infant has and is far away from nerves.**

Content – Pediatric: ***Category of Health Alteration –*** *Drug Administration:* ***Integrated Processes –*** *Nursing Process: Implementation:* ***Client Needs –*** *Physiological Integrity: Pharmacological and Parenteral Therapies:* ***Cognitive Level –*** *Comprehension*

68. **Answer: 45 mL per hour.**
The IV pump is set at an hourly rate. Pediatric clients receive medications at the rate per hour prescribed by the healthcare provider. Increasing the rate to a higher rate is not within the realm of nursing judgment. The medication should be administered at the rate determined by the healthcare provider to be a safe volume.

Content – Pediatric: ***Category of Health Alteration –*** *Drug Administration:* ***Integrated Processes –*** *Nursing Process: Implementation:* ***Client Needs –*** *Physiological Integrity: Pharmacological and Parenteral Therapies:* ***Cognitive Level –*** *Application*

69. **1, 3, and 5 are correct.**
1. **This child has injuries consistent with child abuse. Child Protective Services and the police should be notified.**

2. This could result in not being able to prosecute the perpetrator if the nurse is not trained in forensic medicine.

3. **The nurse should determine the full extent of the child's injuries.**

4. The nurse should not notify the parent of the potential involvement. The police are fully capable of doing this for themselves. The nurse could instigate an inflammatory situation with this action.

5. **The child needs x-ray studies to determine the extent of internal injuries.**

Content – Pediatric: ***Category of Health Alteration –*** *Integumentary:* ***Integrated Processes –*** *Nursing Process: Implementation:* ***Client Needs –*** *Safe and Effective Care Environment: Safety and Infection Control:* ***Cognitive Level –*** *Application*

70. **Correct Answer: 5, 3, 2, 4, 1**
5. **Taking the vital signs is part of the assessment and a beginning point for the nurse.**

3. **Since the child has been losing fluids, the nurse should assess tissue turgor to try and determine whether fluid replacement by the parents has been effective.**

2. **The nurse should make sure that the parents do not leave the child alone in the room and make sure the parents are aware of any safety measures used to protect the toddler from abduction and how to call the nurse in case of need.**

4. **The parents will need to change diapers so the child will not develop skin irritation problems.**

1. **When the nurse provides diapers it is a good opportunity to teach the parents about weighing the diapers before and after the child soils them.**

Content – Pediatric: ***Category of Health Alteration –*** *Gastrointestinal:* ***Integrated Processes –*** *Nursing Process: Implementation:* ***Client Needs –*** *Physiological Integrity: Reduction of Risk Potential:* ***Cognitive Level –*** *Analysis*

CLINICAL SCENARIO ANSWERS AND RATIONALES

The correct answer number and rationale for why it is the correct answer are given in boldface type. Rationales for why the other possible answer options are incorrect also are given, but they are not in boldface type.

1. 1. **The child who is having respiratory difficulty, inspiratory retractions, should be assessed first. Remember Maslow's Hierarchy of Needs.**
   2. A pulse oximeter reading of 93% is within normal limits (93%–100%). It is on the low side because CF is chronic hypoxia and a low arterial oxygen level is expected.
   3. This is a normal potassium level; therefore, the nurse would not assess this child first.
   4. A 210 mg/dL glucose level for a child with type 2 diabetes is not life threatening, and the nurse would not assess this child first.

2. 1. The child in a sickle cell crisis is not stable; therefore, Ms. Laura should not delegate this task to a UAP.
   2. Oxygen is considered a medication and Ms. Laura cannot delegate medication administration to a UAP.
   3. **The child with nephrotic syndrome experiences weight gain secondary to edema, which is expected with this disease process. This child is stable, and the UAP can obtain weights; therefore, Ms. Laura can delegate this task to the UAP.**
   4. The child with a TBI is not stable; therefore, the UAP should not transfer this client to the ICU.

3. 1. Immobilizing the child's leg is appropriate for Mr. Aaron; therefore, this would not warrant intervention by Ms. Laura.
   2. Mr. Aaron should explain the procedure to the 2-year-old using age-appropriate terms; therefore, this would not warrant intervention by Ms. Laura.
   3. The needle and syringe should be disposed of in the sharps container; therefore, this action does not warrant intervention.
   4. **Mr. Aaron should not recap the needle after administering the medication, so this warrants intervention by Ms. Laura. The syringe and needle should be disposed of in the sharps container.**

4. 1. Ms. Diane, the UAP, can document intake and output, and the child has a chronic illness; therefore, the child is stable. This task could be delegated safely.
   2. **The child with an acute exacerbation of IBD must be NPO; therefore, this task should not be delegated to Ms. Diane. This cannot be delegated by Ms. Ruth.**
   3. Ms. Diane can elevate this child's leg and it is appropriate to elevate the leg to help decrease edema. This task could be delegated safely.
   4. Ms. Diane can take laboratory specimens to the laboratory.

5. 1. Ms. Laura should suspect this child has otitis media and would not have to assign Ms. Polly to this child. A less experienced emergency department nurse could care for this client.
   2. **Ms. Laura should suspect this child is experiencing an acute exacerbation of reactive airway disease and assign Ms. Polly to this child. This child is in a potentially life-threatening situation.**
   3. Ms. Laura should suspect this child has a urinary tract infection, which is not a life-threatening situation. Ms. Laura should think about possible sexual abuse but the most experienced nurse would not need to care for this child.
   4. Ms. Laura should suspect the child has pneumonia, which is not a life-threatening situation; therefore, the most experienced nurse does not need to be assigned to this child.

6. 1. The child's temperature should be reduced by receiving an antipyretic medication such as Tylenol, but it is not the first intervention Ms. Laura should implement.
   2. **Ms. Laura should suspect bacterial meningitis and place the child in isolation until definitive diagnosis is made. Ms. Laura must protect the child but also all the other clients, visitors, and staff in the emergency department. This intervention must be implemented first.**
   3. The child will need to receive a lumbar puncture for definitive diagnosis of bacterial meningitis, but it is not the first intervention. Protecting others from this very contagious disease by placing the child in isolation is the priority.
   4. Notifying the infection control nurse is an important intervention, but not priority over protecting other individuals in the emergency department.

7. 1. The mother should call 911 so that immediate medical treatment can be given to the child.
 2. This is an appropriate question to ask to determine appropriate treatment, but the first thing Mr. Aaron should do is to have direct contact with Poison Control to determine the medical treatment for the child.
 3. Syrup of ipecac is no longer recommended because vomiting may cause more damage to the child, or lead to aspiration pneumonia.
 4. **Contacting Poison Control is the first intervention. Poison Control will be able to provide Mr. Aaron with the correct instructions to give to the mother to help dilute this poison and remove it from the daughter's body.**

8. 1. The object should not be removed until surgery. Removing the object can cause more damage and possible hemorrhaging.
 2. The child's medical history and allergies should be determined, but it is not Ms. Laura's first intervention.
 3. **Ms. Laura should first stabilize the pencil in place so further damage will not take place. The left eye should be patched to prevent eye movement. If the uninjured eye moves, the injured eye will also move involuntarily, possibly causing more damage.**
 4. The child's vital signs and pulse oximeter reading should be assessed but not prior to stabilizing the injury.

9. 1. **The best response on the Glasgow Coma Scale is 15, so a score of 12 indicates neurological deterioration and requires notifying the neurologist first. Mr. Aaron cannot implement any independent nursing interventions to help the child.**

 2. Mr. Aaron should document the findings in the chart, but first should notify the neurologist since this indicates a deteriorating condition. To select this option the data in the stem must be expected or normal for the client.
 3. Mr. Aaron should continue to assess the client's Glasgow Coma Scale, but not prior to notifying the neurologist.
 4. Placing the child in the high-Fowler's position will not help increased intracranial pressure; therefore, Mr. Aaron should not implement this intervention.

10. 1. Ms. Laura should suspect acute epiglottis, which is a potential medical emergency and should not be assigned to an inexperienced nurse.
 2. Ms. Laura should suspect this child will be having emergency abdominal surgery and should not assign the child to an inexperienced nurse.
 3. **This child is stable and will need an x-ray; therefore, an inexperienced nurse could care for this client.**
 4. Ms. Laura should realize this child may be hospitalized and should assign this child to a more experienced nurse.

11. 1. **The child is stable and Ms. Michelle can escort the child to the car. This task can be delegated by Ms. Ruth.**
 2. This is assessment and Ms. Ruth cannot delegate assessment, teaching, evaluation, medications, or an unstable client to a UAP.
 3. This is teaching and Ms. Ruth cannot delegate teaching.
 4. The UAP may be able to assist the HCP with this task, but of the four options the test taker should select the least invasive, and/or the task that will require the least amount of nursing knowledge.

Mental Health Management

13

Be nice to people on your way up because you meet them on your way down.

—Jimmy Durante

1. The nurse in the outpatient psychiatric unit is returning phone calls. Which client should the psychiatric nurse call first?
   1. The female client diagnosed with histrionic personality disorder who needs to talk to the nurse about something very important.
   2. The male client diagnosed with schizophrenia who is hearing voices telling him to hurt his mother.
   3. The male client diagnosed with major depression whose wife called and said he was talking about killing himself.
   4. The client diagnosed with bipolar disorder who is manic and has not slept for the last 2 days.

2. The nurse is caring for children in a psychiatric unit. Which client requires immediate intervention by the psychiatric nurse?
   1. The 10-year-old child diagnosed with oppositional defiant disorder who refuses to follow the directions of the mental health worker (MHW).
   2. The 5-year-old child diagnosed with pervasive developmental disorder who refuses to talk to the nurse and will not make eye contact.
   3. The 7-year-old child diagnosed with conduct disorder who is throwing furniture against the wall in the day room.
   4. The 8-year-old mentally retarded child who is sitting on the playground and eating dirt and sand.

3. The male client diagnosed with major depression is returning to the psychiatric unit from a weekend pass with his family. Which intervention should the nurse implement first?
   1. Ask the wife for her opinion of how the visit went.
   2. Determine whether the client took his medication.
   3. Ask the client for his opinion of how the visit went.
   4. Check the client for sharps or dangerous objects.

4. The client on the psychiatric unit is yelling at other clients, throwing furniture, and threatening the staff members. The charge nurse determines the client is at imminent risk for harming the staff/clients and instructs the staff to place the client in seclusion. Which intervention should the charge nurse implement first?
   1. Document the client's behavior in the nurse's notes.
   2. Instruct the MHWs to clean up the day room area.
   3. Obtain a restraint/seclusion order from the HCP.
   4. Ensure that none of the other clients were injured.

5. A woman comes to the emergency department (ED) and tells the triage nurse she was raped by two men. The woman is crying and disheveled, and has bruises on her face. Which action should the triage nurse implement first?
   1. Ask the client whether she wants the police department notified.
   2. Notify a Sexual Assault Nurse Examiner (SANE) to see the client.
   3. Request an ED nurse to take the client to a room and assess for injuries.
   4. Assist the client to complete the emergency department admission form.

6. The nurse is working in an outpatient mental health clinic and returning phone calls. Which client should the psychiatric nurse call first?
   1. The client diagnosed with agoraphobia who is calling to cancel the clinic appointment.
   2. The client diagnosed with a somatoform disorder who has numbness in both legs.
   3. The client diagnosed with hypochondriasis who is afraid she may have breast cancer.
   4. The client diagnosed with post-traumatic stress disorder (PTSD) who is threatening his wife.

7. The psychiatric nurse is working in an outpatient mental health clinic. Which client should the nurse intervene with first?
   1. The client who had a baby 2 months ago and who is sitting alone and looks dejected.
   2. The client whose wife just died and who wants to go to heaven to be with her.
   3. The client whose mother brought her to the clinic because the mother thinks the client is anorexic.
   4. The client who is rocking compulsively back and forth in a chair by the window.

8. The emergency department nurse is assessing a female client who has a laceration on the forehead and a black eye. The nurse asks the man who is with the client to please leave the room. The man refuses to leave the room. Which action should the nurse take first?
   1. Tell the man the client needs to go to the x-ray department.
   2. Notify hospital security and have the man removed from the room.
   3. Explain that the man must leave the room while the nurse checks the client.
   4. Give the client a brochure with information about a woman's shelter.

9. The charge nurse received laboratory data for clients in the psychiatric unit. Which client data warrants notifying the psychiatric healthcare provider?
   1. The client on lithium (Eskalith) whose serum lithium level is 1.0 mEq/L.
   2. The client on clozapine (Clozaril) whose white blood cell count is 13,000.
   3. The client on alprazolam (Xanax) whose potassium level is 3.7 mEq/L.
   4. The client on quetiapine (Seroquel) whose glucose level is 128 mg/dL.

10. The client diagnosed with a panic attack disorder in the busy day room of a psychiatric unit becomes anxious, starts to hyperventilate and tremble, and is diaphoretic. Which intervention should the nurse implement first?
   1. Administer the benzodiazepine alprazolam (Xanax).
   2. Discuss what caused the client to have a panic attack.
   3. Escort the client from the day room to a quiet area.
   4. Instruct the unlicensed assistive personnel (UAP) to take the client's vital signs.

11. The client diagnosed with a somatization disorder is complaining of vomiting, having diarrhea, and having a fever. Which intervention should the nurse implement first?
   1. Assess the client's anxiety level on a scale of 1 to 10.
   2. Check the client's vital signs.
   3. Discuss problem-solving techniques.
   4. Notify the client's healthcare provider.

12. Which nursing intervention is priority for the client diagnosed with anorexia who is admitted to an inpatient psychiatric unit?
   1. Obtain the client's weight.
   2. Assess the client's laboratory values.
   3. Discuss family issues and health concerns.
   4. Teach the client about selective serotonin reuptake inhibitors.

13. Which client should the psychiatric clinic nurse assess first?
    1. The client with long-term alcoholism who wants to stop drinking.
    2. The client who is a cocaine abuser who is having chest discomfort.
    3. The client with obsessive-compulsive disorder who won't quit washing his hands.
    4. The client who thinks she was given "the date rape drug" and was raped last night.

14. The client diagnosed with schizophrenia is being seen by the psychiatric clinic nurse
    for the initial visit. Which intervention should the nurse implement first?
    1. Develop a trusting nurse/client relationship.
    2. Determine the client's knowledge of medication.
    3. Assess the client's support systems.
    4. Allow the client to vent their feelings.

15. The client diagnosed with hypochondriasis is angry and yells at the psychiatric clinic
    nurse, "No one believes I am sick! Not my family, not my doctor, and not you."
    Which statement is the nurse's best response?
    1. "Have you discussed your feelings with your family?"
    2. "I am sure your doctor believes you are sick."
    3. "I can see you are upset. Sit down and let's talk."
    4. "We cannot find any physiological reason for your illness."

16. The clinical manager assigned the psychiatric nurse a client diagnosed with major de-
    pression who attempted suicide and is being discharged tomorrow. Which discharge
    instruction by the psychiatric nurse would warrant intervention by the clinical manager?
    1. The nurse provides the client with phone numbers to call if needing assistance.
    2. The nurse makes the client a follow-up appointment in the psychiatric clinic.
    3. The nurse gives the client a prescription for a 1-month supply of antidepressants.
    4. The nurse tells the client not to take any over-the-counter medications.

17. The charge nurse is caring for clients in an acute care psychiatric unit. Which client
    would be most appropriate for the charge nurse to assign to the licensed practical
    nurse (LPN)?
    1. The client diagnosed with dementia who is confused and disoriented.
    2. The client diagnosed with schizophrenia who is experiencing tardive dyskinesia.
    3. The client diagnosed with bipolar disorder who has a lithium level of 2.0 mEq/L.
    4. The client diagnosed with chronic alcoholism who is experiencing delirium
       tremens.

18. Which task would be inappropriate for the psychiatric charge nurse to delegate to the
    mental health worker (MHW)?
    1. Instruct the MHW to escort the client to the multidisciplinary team meeting.
    2. Ask the MHW to stay in the day room and watch the clients.
    3. Tell the MHW to take care of the client on a 1-to-1 suicide watch.
    4. Request the MHW to draw blood for a serum carbamazepine (Tegretol) level.

19. The male client in the psychiatric unit asks the MHW to mail a letter to his family for
    him. Which action would warrant intervention by the psychiatric nurse?
    1. The MHW tells the client to place the letter in the mailbox.
    2. The MHW informs the client he cannot send mail to his family.
    3. The MHW takes the letter and places it in the unit mailbox.
    4. The MHW reports the client mailed a letter at the team meeting.

20. The male client admitted to the medical unit after a motor vehicle accident (MVA)
    admits using heroin. The unlicensed assistive personnel (UAP) tells the nurse the
    client is really agitated and anxious, and has slurred speech. Which intervention
    should the nurse implement first?
    1. Assess the client for heroin withdrawal.
    2. Ask the UAP to take the client's vital signs.
    3. Notify the client's healthcare provider.
    4. Administer chlordiazepoxide (Librium), an antianxiety medication.

21. Which task would be most appropriate for the psychiatric nurse to delegate to the mental health worker (MHW)?
    1. Request the MHW to take the client with lithium toxicity to the emergency room.
    2. Have the MHW sit with a client diagnosed with bulimia for 1 hour after the meal.
    3. Encourage the MHW to teach the client how to express his or her anger in a positive way.
    4. Ask the MHW to sit with the client while the client talks to his mother on the telephone.

22. The psychiatric charge nurse is making shift assignments for the admission unit. The staff includes one registered nurse (RN), two licensed practical nurses (LPNs), four mental health workers (MHWs), and a unit secretary. Which task would be most appropriate to assign to the LPNs?
    1. Update the clients' individualized care plans.
    2. Stay in the lobby area and watch the clients.
    3. Administer routine medications to the clients.
    4. Transcribe the admission orders for a client.

23. The mental health worker (MHW) has tried to calm down the client on the psychiatric unit who is angry and attempting to fight with another client. The nurse observes the MHW "taking down" the client to the floor. Which intervention should the nurse implement?
    1. Assist the MHW with the "take down" of the client.
    2. Call the hospital security to come and assist the MHW.
    3. Document the client "take down" in the nurse's notes.
    4. Remove the other clients from the day room area.

24. The mental health worker (MHW) reports to the psychiatric nurse that two clients were kissing each other while watching the movie in the lobby area. Which action should the nurse implement?
    1. Tell the MHW to tell the clients not to kiss each other again.
    2. Discuss the inappropriate behavior at the weekly team meeting.
    3. Transfer one of the clients to another psychiatric unit.
    4. Talk to the clients about kissing each other in the lobby area.

25. The nurse is caring for clients in the psychiatric unit. Which task would be most appropriate for the nurse to delegate to the mental health worker (MHW)?
    1. Instruct the MHW to walk with the client who is agitated and anxious.
    2. Ask the MHW to clean up the floor where the client has urinated.
    3. Tell the MHW to phone the HCP to obtain a PRN medication order.
    4. Request the MHW to explain seizure precautions to another staff member.

26. Which behavior by the mental health worker (MHW) is an example of assault requiring immediate intervention by the psychiatric nurse?
    1. The MHW injures a client who is forcibly being put in the "quiet" room.
    2. The MHW refuses to let the client come into the day room until putting on socks.
    3. The MHW escorts the client to the anger management class in another building.
    4. The MHW threatened to forcibly remove the client who is refusing to get out of the bed.

27. The charge nurse has assigned the licensed practical nurse (LPN) to administer medications to the clients on an inpatient psychiatric unit. Which client should the LPN force to take the prescribed medications?
    1. The client with bipolar disorder who has been declared incompetent in a court of law.
    2. The client with major depression who voluntarily admitted herself to the unit.
    3. The client with paranoid schizophrenia who was involuntarily admitted to the unit.
    4. The client with a borderline personality who has legal charges pending in the court.

28. Which client should the psychiatric charge nurse assign to the nurse from the surgical unit who was assigned to the psychiatric unit for the shift?
    1. The client diagnosed with schizophrenia who is hallucinating and delusional.
    2. The client with bipolar disorder who is manic and aggressive toward staff and clients.
    3. The client who is diagnosed with chronic depression and will not talk to anyone.
    4. The client with schizophrenia and an Axis 2 antisocial personality.

29. The psychiatric nurse assigned the mental health worker (MHW) to stay with a client 1-to-1 due to high risk for suicide. Which behavior by the MHW warrants intervention by the nurse?
    1. The MHW stays with the client while in the bathroom.
    2. The MHW provides the client with plastic utensils for breakfast.
    3. The MHW stays outside the room during the client's group therapy.
    4. The MHW watches the client walking outside from the porch area.

30. Which statement by the mental health worker (MHW) warrants intervention by the psychiatric nurse?
    1. "I assisted the client with dressing and hygiene this morning."
    2. "I am going to the team meeting for the next hour."
    3. "I gave the client with heart burn some Maalox."
    4. "I am going to play cards with some clients in the day room."

31. The nurse on the substance abuse unit is administering medications. For which client would the nurse question administering the medication?
    1. The client admitted for alcohol detoxification who is receiving lorazepam (Ativan) and has an apical pulse of 110.
    2. The client admitted for heroin addiction who is receiving methadone (Methadose) and has a respiratory rate of 22.
    3. The client admitted for opioid withdrawal who is receiving clonidine (Catapres) and has a blood pressure (BP) of 88/60.
    4. The client diagnosed with Wernicke-Korsakoff syndrome receiving intravenous thiamine (vitamin B_1) who has an oral temperature of 96.8°F.

32. The psychiatric nurse overhears a mental health worker (MHW) telling a client diagnosed with schizophrenia, "You cannot use the phone while you are here on the unit." Which action should the psychiatric nurse take?
    1. Praise the MHW for providing correct information to the client.
    2. Tell the MHW this is not correct information in front of the client.
    3. Explain to the MHW that the client does not lose any rights.
    4. Discuss this situation at the weekly multidisciplinary team meeting.

33. The client diagnosed with bipolar disorder is admitted to the psychiatric unit in an acute manic state. The nurse needs to complete the admission assessment, but the client is restless, very energetic, and agitated. Which intervention should the nurse implement?
    1. In a very firm voice, ask the client to sit down.
    2. Administer lithium (Eskalith), an antimania medication.
    3. Ask questions while walking and pacing with the client.
    4. Do not complete the admission assessment at this time.

34. The client in the psychiatric setting tells the nurse, "There were so many people at the team meeting; I am not sure what the psychiatric social worker is supposed to do for me." Which statement is the psychiatric nurse's best response?
    1. "The social worker evaluates the effectiveness of the client's medication."
    2. "This person provides activities that promote constructive use of leisure time."
    3. "The social worker will assist you in keeping your job or help you find a new one."
    4. "This person works with your family and community and makes referrals if needed."

35. The male client diagnosed with paranoid schizophrenia is yelling, talking to himself, and blocking the view of the television. The other clients in the day room are becoming angry. Which action should the nurse take first?
1. Obtain a restraint order from the HCP.
2. Escort the other clients from the day room.
3. Administer an intramuscular (IM) antipsychotic medication.
4. Approach the client calmly along with two mental health workers (MHWs).

36. A young child, Joey, was admitted to the pediatric unit with a fractured jaw, bruises, and multiple cigarette burns to the arms. The mother reported the father hurt the child. A man comes to the nurse's station saying, "I am Joey's father; can you tell me how he is doing?" Which statement is the nurse's best response?
1. "Your son has a fractured jaw and some bruises but he is doing fine."
2. "I am sorry I cannot give you any information about your son."
3. "You should go talk to your wife about your son's condition."
4. "The social worker can discuss your son's condition with you."

37. During an interview, the female client tells the psychiatric nurse in a mental health clinic, "Sometimes I feel like life is not worth living. I am going to kill myself." Which interventions should the nurse implement? **Select all that apply.**
1. Make a no-suicide contract with the client.
2. Place the client on a 1-to-1 supervision.
3. Ask the client whether she has a plan.
4. Commit the client to the psychiatric unit.
5. Assess the client's support system.

38. The psychiatric nurse is caring for clients on a closed unit. Which client would warrant immediate intervention by the nurse?
1. The client who refuses to attend the anger management class.
2. The client who is requesting to go outside to smoke a cigarette.
3. The client who is nauseated and has vomited twice.
4. The client who has her menses and has abdominal cramping.

39. The clinical manager wants to reward the staff on the psychiatric unit for having no tardies or absences for 1 month. Which action would be most appropriate for the clinical manager?
1. Provide pizza, drinks, and dessert for all the shifts.
2. Post a thank you note on the board in the employee lounge.
3. Individually acknowledge this accomplishment with the staff.
4. Place official documentation in each staff's employee file.

40. The nurse is working in an outpatient psychiatric clinic. The male client tells the nurse, "I am going to kill my wife if she files for divorce. I know I can't live without her." Which action should the nurse implement?
1. Take no action because this is confidential information.
2. Document the statement in the client's nurse's notes.
3. Inform the client's psychiatric healthcare provider (HCP) of the comment.
4. Encourage the client to talk to his wife about the divorce.

41. Which interventions should the inpatient psychiatric nurse implement for the client experiencing sleepwalking? **Select all that apply.**
1. Encourage the client to exercise prior to going to bed.
2. Place the client on elopement precautions.
3. Instruct to client to drink decaffeinated beverages.
4. Place an alarm on the bed activated when client gets up.
5. Tell the MHW to be on a 1-to-1 watch during the night.

42. The nurse is discussing the grieving process with the client. Which stages are included in Kübler-Ross's stages of grief? Rank in the correct order.
    1. Acceptance.
    2. Bargaining.
    3. Denial.
    4. Anger.
    5. Depression.

43. The nurse is in the middle/working phase of the nurse/client relationship. Which statement is a task in the orientation phase?
    1. Identify the client's strengths and weaknesses.
    2. Help the client identify problem-solving techniques.
    3. Evaluate the client's experience while in the group.
    4. Establish the rules for how the meetings will be conducted.

44. Which situation requires priority intervention on an inpatient psychiatric unit?
    1. A client is threatening to throw the television at another client.
    2. A male client wants to use the phone to call his spouse.
    3. A client sitting in a chair is delusional and hallucinating.
    4. A client has refused to eat anything for the last 2 days.

45. The client with long-term alcoholism asks the nurse, "How does Alcoholics Anonymous help me quit drinking?" Which statements are the nurse's best responses? **Select all that apply.**
    1. "AA has sponsors whom you can contact if you want to take a drink."
    2. "AA discusses medications used to help prevent drinking alcohol."
    3. "AA is a support group of alcoholics who have successfully quit drinking."
    4. "AA helps you realize the power you have over your addiction to alcohol."
    5. "AA has professional guest speakers to address addictive personalities."

46. The client diagnosed with bipolar disorder and who is prescribed lithium, an antimania medication, is admitted to the psychiatric unit in an acute manic state. Which intervention should the nurse implement first?
    1. Have the laboratory draw a STAT serum lithium level.
    2. Evaluate what behavior prompted the psychiatric admission.
    3. Assess and treat the client's physiological needs.
    4. Administer a STAT dose of lithium to the client.

47. The psychiatric unit staff is upset about the new female charge nurse who just sits in her office all day. One of the staff members informs the clinical manager about the situation. Which statement by the clinical manager indicates a laissez-faire leadership style?
    1. "I will schedule a meeting to discuss the concerns of the charge nurse."
    2. "I hired the new charge nurse and she is doing what I told her to do."
    3. "You and the staff really should take care of this situation on your own."
    4. "I will talk to the charge nurse about your concerns and get back to you."

48. The mental health worker (MHW) reports that one of the nurses threatened to force-feed the male client diagnosed with schizophrenia if the client did not eat the meal on the lunch tray. Which action should the charge nurse take first?
    1. Tell the MHW that this intervention is part of the client's care plan.
    2. Request the nurse to come to the office and discuss the MHW's allegation.
    3. Ask the client what happened between him and the nurse during lunch.
    4. Ask the MHW to write down the situation to submit to the head nurse.

49. The client diagnosed with paranoid schizophrenia is imminently aggressive and is dangerous to himself, the other clients, and the psychiatric staff members. The client is placed in a seclusion room. Which interventions should the psychiatric nurse implement? **Select all that apply.**
    1. Assess the client every 2 hours for side effects of medication.
    2. Tell the client what behavior will prompt the release from seclusion.
    3. Do not notify the client's family of the initiation of seclusion.
    4. Explain that the client will be in the seclusion room for 24 hours.
    5. Instruct the MHW to check the client every 10 to 15 minutes.

50. The psychiatric nurse overhears a mental health worker (MHW) arguing with a client diagnosed with paranoid schizophrenia. Which action should the nurse implement?
    1. Ask the MHW to go to the nurse's station.
    2. Tell the MHW to quit arguing with the client.
    3. Notify the clinical manager of the psychiatric unit.
    4. Report this behavior to the client abuse committee.

51. Which client should the psychiatric nurse working in a mental health clinic refer to the psychiatric social worker?
    1. The client who was raped and wants help to be able to get on with her life.
    2. The client who is scheduled for the first electroconvulsive therapy treatment.
    3. The client who reports having difficulty going to work every day.
    4. The client who is unable to buy the prescribed antipsychotic medications.

52. The psychiatric nurse has taken 15 minutes extra for the lunch break two times in the last week. Which action should the female clinical manager implement?
    1. Take no action and continue to watch the nurse's behavior.
    2. Document the behavior in writing and place in the nurse's file.
    3. Tell the nurse to check in and out with her when taking lunch.
    4. Talk to the nurse informally about taking 45 minutes for lunch.

53. The client diagnosed with Alzheimer's disease is on a special unit for clients with cognitive disorders. Which assessment data would warrant immediate intervention by the psychiatric nurse?
    1. The client does not know his or her name, date, or place.
    2. The client is unable to dress himself or herself without assistance.
    3. The client is difficult to arouse from sleep.
    4. The client needs assistance when eating a meal.

54. The mother of a client recently diagnosed with schizophrenia says to the nurse, "I was afraid of my son. Will he be all right?" Which response by the psychiatric nurse supports the ethical principal of veracity?
    1. "I can see your fear; you are concerned your son will not be all right."
    2. "If your son takes medication, the symptoms can be controlled."
    3. "Why were you afraid of your son? Did you think he would hurt you?"
    4. "Schizophrenia is a mental illness and your son will not be all right."

55. The nurse is caring for clients in an outpatient psychiatric clinic. Which client would the nurse discuss with the healthcare provider?
    1. The client diagnosed with bipolar disorder who is receiving carbamazepine (Tegretol), an anticonvulsant.
    2. The client diagnosed with schizophrenia who reports taking the antacid Maalox daily for heartburn.
    3. The client diagnosed with major depression who is receiving isoniazid (INH), an antituberculosis medication.
    4. The client diagnosed with anorexia nervosa who is receiving amitriptyline (Elavil), a tricyclic antidepressant.

56. The client in the psychiatric unit tells the nurse, "Someone just put a bomb under the couch in the lobby." Which action should the nurse implement first?
  1. Look under the couch for a bomb.
  2. Implement the bomb scare protocol.
  3. Have the staff evacuate the unit.
  4. Tell the client there is no bomb.

57. The new nurse on the psychiatric unit tells the charge nurse, "I don't like how the shift report is given." Which statement is the charge nurse's best response?
  1. "Since you're new I think you should try it our way before making any comments."
  2. "We have been doing the shift report this way since I started working here more than 5 years ago."
  3. "Have you discussed your concerns about the shift report with the other nurses?"
  4. "I would be happy to listen to any ideas you have on how to give the shift report."

58. The client on the psychiatric unit tells the nurse, "I am so bored. I hate just sitting on the unit doing nothing." Which intervention should the nurse implement?
  1. Explain that with time the client will be able to go to the activity area.
  2. Allow the client to vent feelings of being bored on the unit.
  3. Notify the psychiatric recreational therapist about the client's concerns.
  4. Tell the client that there is nothing that can be done about being bored.

59. The head nurse in a psychiatric unit in the county emergency department is assigning clients to the staff nurses. Which client should be assigned to the most experienced nurse?
  1. The client who is crying and upset because she was raped.
  2. The client diagnosed with bipolar disorder who is agitated.
  3. The client who was found wandering the streets in a daze.
  4. The client diagnosed with schizophrenia who is hallucinating.

60. The client diagnosed with anorexia is refusing to eat and is less than 20% of ideal body weight (IBW) for her height and structure. The client has not eaten anything since admission 2 days ago. Which action should the nurse implement?
  1. Notify the psychiatrist to request a court order to feed the client.
  2. Take no action because the client has the right to refuse treatment.
  3. Discharge the client because she is not complying with the treatment.
  4. Physically restrain the client and insert a nasogastric tube for feeding.

61. The client on a psychiatric involuntary admission is threatening to run away from the unit. Which intervention should the nurse implement first?
  1. Notify the police department of the client's threats.
  2. Place the unit on high alert for unauthorized departure.
  3. Talk to the client about the threat of running away.
  4. Have the client sign out against medical advice (AMA).

62. The nurse answers the client's phone in the lobby area and the person asks, "May I speak to Mr. Jones?" Which action should the nurse implement?
  1. Ask the caller who is asking for Mr. Jones.
  2. Tell the caller Mr. Jones cannot have phone calls.
  3. Request the caller to give the access code for information.
  4. Find Mr. Jones and tell him he has a phone call.

63. The client seeing the psychiatric nurse in the mental health clinic tells the nurse, "If I tell you something very important, will you promise not to tell anyone?" Which statement is the nurse's best response?
  1. "I promise I will not tell anyone if you don't want me to."
  2. "If it affects your care I will have to tell someone who can help."
  3. "If you don't want me to tell anyone, then please don't tell me."
  4. "Why do you not want me to tell anyone if it is so important?"

64. Which situation would warrant immediate intervention by the charge nurse on the psychiatric unit after receiving the a.m. shift report?
1. The client diagnosed with paranoid schizophrenia who is delusional.
2. The p.m. shift licensed practical nurse (LPN) called in to say he or she would not be able to work today.
3. The male mental health worker (MHW) reports losing his unit key and identification card.
4. The unit secretary has HCP's orders that need to be co-signed.

65. The client enters a mental health clinic with a gun and is threatening to kill the nurse who told his wife to leave him. Which action should the nurse implement first?
1. Instruct a staff member to call the local police department.
2. Evacuate the clients and staff to a safe and secure place.
3. Encourage the client to talk about his feelings of anger.
4. Calmly and firmly ask the man to put the gun down on the floor.

66. The charge nurse of the psychiatric unit is making assignments. Which clients should be assigned to the medical-surgical nurse who is working in the psychiatric unit for the day? **Select all that apply.**
1. The client diagnosed with depression who has attempted suicide four times and now is refusing to go to therapy.
2. The client diagnosed with bipolar disease who has diabetes and requires blood glucose monitoring.
3. The female client diagnosed with dissociative identity disorder (DID) who is complaining that she is being falsely imprisoned.
4. The client diagnosed with schizophrenia who is blocking the screen of the television and refuses to move so other clients can watch the television.
5. The client diagnosed with major depression who started taking anti-depressant medication 2 days ago and who wants to remain in bed.

67. The outpatient clinic psychiatric nurse is preparing to assist the healthcare provider to perform electroconvulsive therapy. Rank in order of performance the nursing interventions to be implemented.
1. Attach the electrodes to the client.
2. Check the client's name and date of birth against the chart/orders.
3. Start an intravenous line and run at a keep open rate.
4. Determine that the client has not eaten or had any liquids since midnight.
5. Notify the healthcare provider to begin the procedure.

68. The psychiatric nurse is reviewing client lab values. Which of the following data requires immediate intervention by the nurse?

Client A.

Client: A. N. Allergies: None		
Diagnosis: Bipolar Disease **Medical Records Number:** 123456		
Laboratory Test	**Client Value**	**Normal Value**
Lithium Level	1.2	0.5–1.3 mEq/L

Client B.

Client: D.C. Allergies: Dilantin		
Diagnosis: Mania **Medical Records Number:** 109875		
Laboratory Test	**Client Value**	**Normal Value**
Valporic Acid Level	98	40–100 mcg/L

Client C.

Client: J.M. Allergies : NKDA		
Diagnosis: Schizophrenia **Medical Records Number:** 245689		
Laboratory Test	**Client Value**	**Normal Value**
White Blood Cell Count	2.68	5.0–10.0 (10^3)

Client D.

Client: S.R. Allergies: Penicillin		
Diagnosis: Acute Psychosis **Medical Records Number:** 874521		
Laboratory Test	**Client Value**	**Normal Value**
Potassium	4.68	4.5–5.5 mEq/L
Sodium	139	135–150 mEq/L
Chloride	102	96–106 mEq/L

1. Client A.
2. Client B.
3. Client C.
4. Client D.

69. The charge nurse responds to an emergency situation on the psychiatric unit in which the male client is angry, yelling, and attempting to hit other clients and the staff. Which interventions should the nurse implement? **Select all that apply.**
   1. Notify the operator to initiate a call for emergency responders to assist.
   2. Tell the client to sit down and be quiet or he will lose privileges.
   3. Have the mental health worker escort the other clients to their rooms.
   4. Make sure that the staff speaks loudly and directly to the client.
   5. Request the unit secretary to stand by the locked doors to allow emergency responders on the unit.

70. The psychiatric nurse is assessing the Abnormal Involuntary Movement Scale (AIMS) for clients on antipsychotic medications. Which client's scores require immediate intervention?

ABNORMAL INVOLUNTARY MOVEMENT SCALE (AIMS)		
Adapted		
PT Initials: _____ Gender: _____ Date: _____ Interviewer: _____		
MOVEMENT RATINGS: (Circle One)		
0 = None 1 = Minimal, may be extreme of normal 2 = Mild 3 = Moderate 4 = Severe		
Note: #10 0 = no awareness 1 = aware, no distress 2 = aware, mild distress 3 = aware, moderate distress 4 = aware, severe distress		
Facial & Oral Movements	**1. Muscles of facial expression** (e.g., movement of forehead, eyebrows, periorbital area, cheeks; include frowning, blinking, smiling, grimacing)	0 1 2 3 4
	2. Lips and perioral area (e.g., puckering, pouting, smacking)	0 1 2 3 4
	3. Jaw (e.g., biting, clenching, chewing, mouth opening, lateral movement)	0 1 2 3 4
	4. Tongue (Rate only increase in movement both in and out of mouth, NOT inability to sustain movement.)	0 1 2 3 4
Extremity Movements	**5. Upper body** (arms, wrists, hands, fingers) (e.g., include **choreic movements** [rapid, objectively purposeless, irregular, spontaneous], **athetoid movements** [slow irregular, complex, serpentine]). Do NOT include tremor (repetitive, regular, and rhythmic)	0 1 2 3 4
	6. Lower body (legs, knees, ankles, toes) (e.g., lateral knee movement, foot tapping, and heel dropping, foot squirming, inversion and eversion of foot.)	0 1 2 3 4
Trunk Movements	**7. Neck, shoulders, hips**	0 1 2 3 4
Global Judgments	**8. Severity of abnormal movements**	0 1 2 3 4
	9. Incapacitation due to abnormal movements	0 1 2 3 4
	10. Client's awareness of abnormal movements Rate only client's report. See note above.	0 1 2 3 4
Dental Status	**11. Current problem with teeth and/or dentures**	Yes = 1 No = 0
	12. Does client usually wear dentures?	Yes = 1 No = 0
	SCORE	

1. The client who scored a 6 on the scale.
2. The client who scored a 10 on the scale.
3. The client who scored a 15 on the scale.
4. The client who scored a 24 on the scale.

MENTAL HEALTH CLINICAL SCENARIO

Mr. Allan is the nurse manager in an outpatient mental health clinic. Mr. Allen has two RNs, Ms. Belinda and Ms. Marguerite, along with two LVNs, Mr. Benjamin and Ms. Jan, and two mental health workers (MHWs) who are unlicensed assistive personnel in the psychiatric arena, Ms. Mary Beth and Ms. Brenda. There are two receptionists at the front desk.

1. Mr. Allan is triaging and returning phone calls. Which client should Mr. Allan call first?
   1. The client diagnosed with a narcissistic personality disorder who needs to see the psychiatrist today.
   2. The client with schizophrenia who is hearing voices telling him to hurt his wife.
   3. The client with major depression who is refusing to get out of bed and go to work.
   4. The client with bipolar disorder who is manic and has sold the family car for cash.

2. Ms. Belinda is working in at the triage desk. Which client should Ms. Belinda intervene with first?
   1. The client who had a baby 2 months ago and thinks she has postpartum depression.
   2. The client who told the receptionist he wants to kill himself and has a gun in the car.
   3. The woman who thinks her mother has Alzheimer's disease because her mother is confused.
   4. The client who has been washing his hands in the bathroom for almost 20 minutes.

3. Mr. Allan is reviewing laboratory data for clients seen in the clinic. Which of the following client data warrants notifying the psychiatric healthcare provider?
   1. The client on lithium (Eskalith) whose serum lithium level is 2.0 mEq/L.
   2. The client on clozapine (Clozaril) whose white blood cell count is 10,000.
   3. The client on alprazolam (Xanax) whose potassium level is 3.7 mEq/L.
   4. The client on divalproex sodium (Depakote) who has a depakote serum level of 60 µg/mL.

4. Mr. Allan is working in the mental health clinic and returns a telephone call to a male client who says that "voices are telling me to hurt myself, now." Which intervention should Mr. Allan implement first?
   1. Call 911 and tell the paramedics the client is a danger to himself and/or others.
   2. Ask the client if he has taken his medication this morning.
   3. Notify the healthcare provider of the client's statement.
   4. Keep the client on the telephone to discuss the voices he is hearing.

5. The client diagnosed with a panic attack disorder in the clinic waiting room becomes anxious, starts to hyperventilate and tremble, and is diaphoretic. After removing the client from the day room which intervention should Ms. Marguerite implement next?
   1. Administer the benzodiazepine alprazolam (Xanax).
   2. Allow the client to verbalize feelings of anxiety.
   3. Encourage to the client to take slow, deep breaths.
   4. Instruct MHW to obtain the client's pulse oximetry reading.

6. Which client would be most appropriate for Mr. Allan to assign to Mr. Benjamin, the LPN, in the psychiatric clinic?
   1. The client diagnosed with dementia who is confused and disoriented.
   2. The client with schizophrenia who is experiencing extrapyramidal side effects.
   3. The client diagnosed with bipolar disorder who is pacing up and down the hallway.
   4. The client with anorexia nervosa who is hypotensive and complaining of dizziness.

7. Which task is inappropriate for Mr. Allan to delegate to the MHW?
   1. Instruct the MHW to observe the client who is exhibiting compulsive behavior.
   2. Ask the MHW to stay in the waiting room and watch the clients.
   3. Tell the MHW to sit with the client who reports being suicidal.
   4. Request the MHW to draw blood for a serum lithium level.

8. The client diagnosed with paranoid schizophrenia is yelling, talking to himself, and blocking the view of the television. The other clients in the waiting room are becoming angry. Which action should Mr. Allan implement first?
   1. Place the client in a quiet room.
   2. Escort the other clients from the day room.
   3. Request the receptionist to call 911.
   4. Approach the client calmly along with Mr. Benjamin.

9. Mr. Allan observes Ms. Brenda, the MHW, arguing with a client in the waiting room. Mr. Allan requests Ms. Brenda to go to his office immediately. Which action should Mr. Allan implement first?
   1. Ask the client what caused the argument.
   2. Discuss the behavior with Ms. Brenda.
   3. Document Ms. Brenda's behavior in writing.
   4. Terminate Ms. Brenda immediately.

10. Ms. Belinda has been late to work three times in the last week. Mr. Allan talks to Ms. Belinda and finds out Ms. Belinda has to take the bus to work until her car is fixed, which should be completed in 1 week. Which action should Mr. Allan implement?
   1. Ask Ms. Marguerite to give Ms. Brenda a ride to work until the car is fixed.
   2. Document the behavior in writing and place in Ms. Brenda's file.
   3. Tell Ms. Belinda if she is late again she will be placed on administrative leave.
   4. Do not take any action at this time since Ms. Belinda has an excellent attendance record.

ANSWERS AND RATIONALES

The correct answer number and rationale for why it is the correct answer are given in **boldface type**. Rationales for why the other possible answer options are incorrect also are given, but they are not in boldface type.

1. 1. The client with a histrionic personality has excessive emotionality and seeks attention. Her saying "something important" must be understood within this context and would not warrant calling this client first.
2. **The nurse should contact this client first because the client realizes the voices are telling him to hurt his mother. The nurse should inform this client to come to the clinic immediately, and he should be admitted to a psychiatric unit.**
3. Because the wife called the clinic, the client is being watched and should be safe from killing himself. The nurse should call this client immediately but not before a client who made the phone call himself and who may be alone and hearing voices.
4. The nurse should expect the client who is manic not to be sleeping; therefore, this is expected behavior. The nurse should call this client immediately but not before the client who is hearing voices telling him to hurt his mother.

Content – Mental Health: *Category of Health Alteration* – Mental Health: *Integrated Processes* – *Nursing Process: Assessment:* *Client Needs* – *Physiological Integrity: Reduction of Risk Potential:* *Cognitive Level* – *Analysis*

2. 1. Oppositional defiant disorder consists of a pattern of uncooperative, defiant, and hostile behavior toward authority figures. Not following the MHW's directions would be expected behavior in a child diagnosed with this disorder and would not require immediate intervention by the nurse.
2. Refusal to talk and/or make eye contact is a sign of autism, the best known of the pervasive developmental disorders; therefore, this client would not require immediate intervention by the nurse.
3. **The child with conduct disorder is aggressive to people and animals, bullies and threatens others, destroys property, and sets fires. Throwing furniture could endanger the child or other clients. This behavior warrants immediate intervention.**
4. Eating dirt and sand is pica, or the ingestion of non-nutritive substances such as paint, hair, cloth, leaves, sand, clay, or soil. It is commonly

seen in mentally retarded children, but it is not life threatening unless a medical complication such as a bowel obstruction, infection, or a toxic condition (e.g., lead poisoning) occurs. This behavior would not require immediate intervention.

Content – Mental Health: *Category of Health Alteration* – Mental Health: *Integrated Processes* – *Nursing Process: Analysis:* *Client Needs* – *Psychosocial Integrity:* *Cognitive Level* – *Synthesis*

MAKING NURSING DECISIONS: **When deciding which client to assess first, the test taker should determine whether the signs/symptoms the client is exhibiting are normal for the client's situation. After eliminating the expected options, the test taker should determine which situation is more life threatening.**

3. 1. The nurse should discuss how the visit went, but it is not the first intervention.
2. The nurse should make sure the client took his medications during the weekend pass, but it is not the first intervention.
3. The client should discuss how the visit went, but it is not the first intervention.
4. **The nurse's first intervention should be to ensure the client's safety by checking to make sure the client has no sharps or dangerous objects that he could use to hurt himself, since he is diagnosed with major depression.**

Content – Mental Health: *Category of Health Alteration* – Mental Health: *Integrated Processes* – *Nursing Process: Implementation:* *Client Needs* – *Safe and Effective Care Environment: Management of Care:* *Cognitive Level* – *Application*

4. 1. The nurse must document the client's behavior that prompted the need for seclusion, but it is not the first intervention.
2. The day room area should be cleaned up, but it is not the nurse's first intervention.
3. **The use of restraints and seclusion requires an HCP's order every 24 hours. The nurse must obtain this order first after placing the client in the seclusion room. The nurse can place the client in seclusion for the safety of the client/staff/other clients, but the nurse must then immediately obtain a HCP's order.**
4. The charge nurse should make sure the other clients are not injured, but the first intervention is to put the client who is acting out into seclusion, safely and legally.

Content – *Mental Health:* **Category of Health Alteration** – *Mental Health:* **Integrated Processes** – *Nursing Process: Implementation:* **Client Needs** – *Safe and Effective Care Environment: Safety and Infection Control:* **Cognitive Level** – *Application*

5. 1. The client may or may not want the police notified, but this is not the triage nurse's first intervention. The triage nurse should first care for the client.
   2. The SANE nurse is a nurse who is specialized in caring for clients who have been raped. The SANE nurse is able to spend time with the client, is knowledgeable of legal issues, and would be an appropriate intervention, but it is not the triage nurse's first intervention.
   3. **The triage nurse's first intervention is to address the client's physiological needs, which means to assess for any type of trauma or injury.**
   4. The client can complete the admission form while in the room; the triage nurse's first intervention should be to care for the client, not paperwork.

Content – *Mental Health:* **Category of Health Alteration** – *Mental Health:* **Integrated Processes** – *Nursing Process: Implementation:* **Client Needs** – *Physiological Integrity: Physiological Adaptation:* **Cognitive Level** – *Application*

MAKING NURSING DECISIONS: When the question asks which intervention to implement first, the test taker should determine whether any of the options concern the physiological needs of the client and then apply Maslow's Hierarchy of Needs to find the correct answer. Remember: Physiological needs take priority over all other needs.

6. 1. The client with agoraphobia is afraid to leave the house; therefore, canceling a clinic appointment would be expected of this client. The nurse would not need to return this client's phone call first.
   2. The client with a somatoform disorder has physical symptoms without a physiological cause; therefore, complaining of numbness in the legs is expected behavior. The nurse would not need to return this client's phone call first.
   3. The client with hypochondriasis is preoccupied with the fear that one has or will get a serious disease; fearing breast cancer is then expected behavior. The nurse would not need to return this client's phone call first.
   4. **Post-traumatic stress disorder is an illness that occurs to someone who has experienced a traumatic event. The client feels a numbing of general responsiveness but has outbursts of anger. The nurse should return this call first and assess the situation**

to determine whether the client should be seen in the clinic.

Content – *Mental Health:* **Category of Health Alteration** – *Mental Health:* **Integrated Processes** – *Nursing Process: Assessment:* **Client Needs** – *Safe and Effective Care Environment: Safety and Infection Control:* **Cognitive Level** – *Analysis*

MAKING NURSING DECISIONS: When deciding which client to assess first, the test taker should determine whether the signs/symptoms the client is exhibiting are normal or expected for the client situation. After eliminating the expected options, the test taker should determine which situation is more life threatening.

7. 1. The client who is depressed would be expected to look dejected; therefore, the nurse would not need to assess this client first.
   2. **This client who says he wants to go to heaven to be with his wife may be suicidal and should be assessed first to see whether he has a plan.**
   3. This client needs to be assessed for anorexia but not before a client who may be suicidal.
   4. The nurse should not interrupt a client who is acting compulsively. The nurse should wait until the client finishes the behavior before talking to the client.

Content – *Mental Health:* **Category of Health Alteration** – *Mental Health:* **Integrated Processes** – *Nursing Process: Implementation:* **Client Needs** – *Psychosocial Integrity:* **Cognitive Level** – *Application*

8. 1. **The nurse needs to remove the man from the room so that the nurse can talk to the client and discuss probable abuse. Taking the client to the x-ray department may not arouse suspicion in the man and may allow the client to discuss the situation.**
   2. This may be needed, but it is not the first intervention. This action may cause the man to get angrier in the emergency department, or it may cause more problems for the woman if she goes home with him.
   3. The nurse could demand the man leave the room, but this action may cause the man's anger to escalate; therefore, the first intervention is to remove the client from the room.
   4. The nurse should not allow the man to see the nurse discussing a woman's shelter with the client or providing a client with a brochure. This could cause further anger in the man, especially if the woman goes home with the man.

Content – *Mental Health:* **Category of Health Alteration** – *Mental Health:* **Integrated Processes** – *Nursing Process: Implementation:* **Client Needs** – *Safe and Effective Care Environment: Safety and Infection Control:* **Cognitive Level** – *Application*

9. 1. The therapeutic serum level for lithium is 0.6 to 1.5 mEq/L. Because the client's 1.0 mEq/L level is within normal limits, the charge nurse would not need to notify the psychiatric HCP.
   2. **The WBC count is elevated, which may indicate that the client is experiencing agranulocytosis, a life-threatening complication of clozapine. This laboratory data would warrant notifying the psychiatric healthcare provider.**
   3. The client's serum potassium level is within normal limits; therefore, this laboratory information does not warrant notifying the psychiatric healthcare provider.
   4. This glucose level is slightly elevated but would not warrant notifying the psychiatric healthcare provider.

   Content – Mental Health: **Category of Health Alteration** – Mental Health: **Integrated Processes** – Nursing Process: Evaluation: **Client Needs** – Safe and Effective Care Environment: Management of Care: **Cognitive Level** – Synthesis

10. 1. This is an appropriate medication for an anxiety attack, but it will take at least 15 to 30 minutes for the medication to treat the physiological signs/symptoms. Therefore, this is not the first intervention.
   2. The nurse should discuss the panic attack and what prompted it, but it is not the nurse's first intervention.
   3. **The first intervention is to remove the client from the busy day room to a quiet area to help decrease the anxiety attack.**
   4. The client's vital signs should be taken, but this is not the nurse's first intervention.

   Content – Mental Health: **Category of Health Alteration** – Mental Health: **Integrated Processes** – Nursing Process: Implementation: **Client Needs** – Psychosocial Integrity: **Cognitive Level** – Application

11. 1. The nurse should assess the client's anxiety level but not prior to ruling out a physiological reason for the client's complaints.
   2. **The nurse should first determine if the client's vital signs are abnormal, which rules out any physiological reason for the client's complaints.**
   3. The nurse should discuss techniques to address increased anxiety level, but a physiological cause of these symptoms should be ruled out first.
   4. The client's HCP will need to be notified if the complaints are secondary to a physiological reason, but would not if the vital signs are within normal limits.

   Content – Mental Health: **Category of Health Alteration** – Mental Health: **Integrated**

Processes – Nursing Process: Assessment: **Client Needs** – Physiological Integrity: Reduction of Risk Potential: **Cognitive Level** – Analysis

MAKING NURSING DECISIONS: If the question asks the nurse, "Which intervention to implement first?" then the test taker should apply the nursing process. The psychiatric nurse must first assess to determine if the client has a physiological problem; since option A and B are assessment interventions then the test taker should select physiological assessment over psychosocial assessment.

12. 1. The nurse should assess the client's weight, but it is not a priority over assessing laboratory values, which may be life threatening, especially potassium level.
   2. **The client's laboratory values are priority because these reflect long-term effects of anorexia and possible life-threatening values that must be corrected immediately, especially potassium.**
   3. This is an appropriate intervention, but physiological needs are priority over problem-solving.
   4. A teaching intervention is not priority over a physiological need.

   Content – Mental Health: **Category of Health Alteration** – Mental Health: **Integrated Processes** – Nursing Process: Implementation: **Client Needs** – Physiological Integrity: Reduction of Risk Potential: **Cognitive Level** – Analysis

MAKING NURSING DECISIONS: When a question asks, "Which intervention should the nurse implement first?" the test taker should use the nursing process to determine the correct answer. If the client is not in distress then the nurse should assess. If two options address assessment, select the intervention that addresses a life-threatening complication.

13. 1. This client needs to be assessed but not prior to the client with chest discomfort. If the client exhibited signs of alcohol withdrawal then this client would have a physiological need.
   2. **Cocaine causes vasoconstriction of the coronary arteries and can lead to life-threatening cardiovascular problems; therefore, this client should be seen first.**
   3. The client who is performing compulsive behavior should not be interrupted but be allowed to finish the behavior.
   4. This client is not exhibiting physiological complications; therefore, this client should not be assessed first.

   Content – Mental Health: **Category of Health Alteration** – Mental Health: **Integrated Processes** – Nursing Process: Assessment: **Client Needs** – Physiological

*Integrity: Reduction of Risk Potential: **Cognitive Level** – Analysis*

MAKING NURSING DECISIONS: The test taker should first determine if the signs/symptoms are normal or expected for the client situation. If there are two or more clients exhibiting unexpected signs/symptoms, then select the client who is exhibiting life-threatening signs/symptoms, needs more assessment, or would warrant notifying the healthcare provider.

14. 1. **If the nurse does not establish the foundation for a trusting nurse/client relationship, then the nurse will not be effective in caring for this client. This is the first nursing intervention.**
2. Medication is a vital part of the treatment for schizophrenia, but on the initial visit a trusting relationship is priority.
3. Support systems are an important part of the client's treatment in the community but the client must be able to trust the nurse when sharing information.
4. Ventilating feelings about disease, his or her situation, and life is vital to the treatment of a client with schizophrenia, but the client must be able to trust the nurse when sharing feelings.

*Content – Mental Health: **Category of Health Alteration** – Mental Health: **Integrated Processes** – Nursing Process: Implementation: **Client Needs** – Safe and Effective Care Environment: Management of Care: **Cognitive Level** – Application*

MAKING NURSING DECISIONS: In mental health nursing, the foundation for all nursing care is having a trusting nurse/client relationship. All the options are possible or plausible for the nurse to implement, but there is only one correct answer.

15. 1. The psychiatric nurse should address the client's feelings, not the feelings of family members.
2. This comment does not address the client's feelings, and the nurse should not talk about what the doctor believes or doesn't believe.
3. **The nurse must first calm the client, assess the situation, and ensure a therapeutic nurse/client relationship. This response addresses all these issues.**
4. This response will more than likely further antagonize the client and is not a therapeutic response.

*Content – Mental Health: **Category of Health Alteration** – Mental Health: **Integrated Processes** – Nursing Process: Implementation: **Client Needs** – Psychosocial Integrity: **Cognitive Level** – Application*

MAKING NURSING DECISIONS: The psychiatric nurse's responsibility is to deescalate the client's anger. Being empathetic and allowing the client to verbalize feelings is the nurse's priority intervention.

16. 1. Providing phone numbers for the client and family is an intervention that the nurse should discuss with the client and would not warrant intervention by the clinical manager.
2. Follow-up appointments are important for the client after being discharged from a psychiatric facility; therefore, this instruction would not warrant intervention by the clinical manager.
3. **The client should be given a 7-day supply of antidepressants because safety of the client is priority. As antidepressant medications become more effective, the client is at a higher risk for suicide; therefore, the nurse should ensure that the client cannot take an overdose of medication. This instruction warrants intervention by the clinical manager.**
4. The client should not take any OTC medications without talking to the HCP or pharmacist. This instruction would not warrant intervention by the clinical manager.

*Content – Mental Health: **Category of Health Alteration** – Mental Health: **Integrated Processes** – Nursing Process: Analysis: **Client Needs** – Physiological Integrity: Physiological Adaptation: **Cognitive Level** – Synthesis*

17. 1. **The client diagnosed with dementia would be expected to have confusion and disorientation; therefore, the LPN could be assigned this client. This client is not experiencing any potentially life-threatening complication of dementia.**
2. The client is experiencing tardive dyskinesia, a potentially life-threatening complication of antipsychotic medication. An experienced RN should be assigned to this client.
3. The therapeutic serum level for lithium is 0.6 to 1.5 mEq/L. The client's level is toxic, and an experienced RN should care for the client.
4. This client is experiencing a potentially life-threatening complication of alcohol withdrawal. An experienced RN should be assigned to this client.

*Content – Mental Health: **Category of Health Alteration** – Mental Health: **Integrated Processes** – Nursing Process: Planning: **Client Needs** – Safe and Effective Care Environment: Management of Care: **Cognitive Level** – Synthesis*

ANSWERS

MAKING NURSING DECISIONS: The test taker must determine which client is the most stable, which makes this an "except" question. Three clients are either unstable or have potentially life-threatening conditions.

18. 1. Clients are allowed, encouraged, and expected to participate in the multidisciplinary team meeting. This is an appropriate task to delegate to the MHW.
    2. One of the MHW's primary responsibilities is to watch clients in the day room area. This is an appropriate task to delegate.
    3. The MHW can remain with a client who is on 1-to-1 suicide watch. This is an appropriate nursing task to delegate.
    4. **The MHW does not draw blood, and this would be an inappropriate task to delegate. The laboratory technician draws the client's blood work.**
    Content – *Mental Health:* **Category of Health Alteration** – *Mental Health:* **Integrated Processes** – *Nursing Process: Planning:* **Client Needs** – *Safe and Effective Care Environment: Management of Care:* **Cognitive Level** – *Synthesis*

19. 1. Telling the client to place the letter in the mailbox is empowering the client to take responsibility. This action would not warrant intervention by the nurse.
    2. **The nurse should explain to the MHW that mental health clients retain all of the civil rights afforded to all persons, except the right to leave the hospital in the case of involuntary commitments. The client has the right to mail and receive letters.**
    3. Mailing the client's letter is an appropriate action to take; therefore, this would not warrant intervention by the nurse.
    4. Reporting the client mailed a letter to his family at the team meeting may or may not be pertinent to the client's care, but this action would not warrant intervention by the nurse.
    Content – *Mental Health:* **Category of Health Alteration** – *Mental Health:* **Integrated Processes** – *Nursing Process: Implementation:* **Client Needs** – *Psychosocial Integrity:* **Cognitive Level** – *Comprehension*

20. 1. **Whenever the nurse is given information that indicates a complication or is potentially life threatening, the nurse must first assess the client.**
    2. The client is unstable; therefore, the nurse should not instruct the UAP to take the client's vital signs.
    3. The nurse should not notify the healthcare provider before assessing the client.
    4. Librium is a medication used for alcohol withdrawal, not for heroin withdrawal.

Content – *Substance Abuse:* **Category of Health Alteration** – *Mental Health:* **Integrated Processes** – *Nursing Process: Implementation:* **Client Needs** – *Physiological Integrity: Reduction of Risk Potential:* **Cognitive Level** – *Application*

MAKING NURSING DECISIONS: If the test taker wants to select "notify the HCP" as the correct answer, the test taker must examine the other three options. If information in any of the other options is data the HCP would need to make a decision, then the test taker should eliminate the "notify the HCP" option.

21. 1. The client with lithium toxicity is unstable, and the nurse should not delegate this task to an MHW.
    2. **Having someone stay with the client after a meal will prevent the client from inducing vomiting and could be delegated to an MHW. The client diagnosed with bulimia needs someone there to prevent vomiting, which is a sign of this mental health problem.**
    3. The nurse should not delegate teaching. Helping the client with anger management would be the responsibility of the nurse or possibly the therapy department.
    4. The client has a right to talk to his mother on the phone without someone listening.
    Content – *Mental Health:* **Category of Health Alteration** – *Mental Health:* **Integrated Processes** – *Nursing Process: Planning:* **Client Needs** – *Safe and Effective Care Environment: Management of Care:* **Cognitive Level** – *Synthesis*

22. 1. The RN should be assigned to update the individualized care plans.
    2. The MHWs should be assigned to watch the clients in the day area.
    3. **The LPNs' scope of practice allows the administration of medication. This is an appropriate assignment.**
    4. The LPNs can transcribe an HCP's orders, but the unit secretary can also transcribe orders, which the RN/LPN can co-sign. This would not be the most appropriate assignment for the LPNs.
    Content – *Mental Health:* **Category of Health Alteration** – *Mental Health:* **Integrated Processes** – *Nursing Process: Planning:* **Client Needs** – *Safe and Effective Care Environment: Management of Care:* **Cognitive Level** – *Synthesis*

23. 1. **All psychiatric staff members are taught how to "take down" a client physically if the client is a danger to him- or herself or to others. The nurse should assist the MHW in subduing the client so that no one is injured.**

2. The psychiatric staff members are trained to deal with clients who are angry and aggressive; there is no need to contact hospital security.
3. The nurse can document the occurrence, but because the nurse observed the "take down," the nurse should assist the MHW. The psychiatric staff members have to be able to depend on each other no matter what the situation.
4. The nurse can have other staff members remove clients from the day room area; the psychiatric nurse should help the MHW with the "take down."

Content – Mental Health: **Category of Health Alteration** – Mental Health: **Integrated Processes** – Nursing Process: Implementation: **Client Needs** – Safe and Effective Care Environment: Management of Care: **Cognitive Level** – Application

24. 1. The nurse should address the behavior with the clients and not delegate this task to the MHW. This inappropriate behavior needs further investigation to determine whether it is consensual or under duress.
2. The inappropriate behavior should be addressed immediately with both clients.
3. If the behavior does not stop, one of the clients may need to be transferred to another unit, but this is not the appropriate action at this time.
4. **The nurse needs to talk to the clients to determine whether the kissing was consensual or under duress. Either way, the behavior is inappropriate, and the clients should be told there is no kissing or sexual activity allowed between clients while they are hospitalized on the psychiatric unit.**

Content – Mental Health: **Category of Health Alteration** – Mental Health: **Integrated Processes** – Nursing Process: Implementation: **Client Needs** – Psychosocial Integrity: **Cognitive Level** – Application

25. 1. **The MHW could walk with the client who is agitated. This may help decrease the client's agitation and anxiety.**
2. The nurse should not assign a task that is the responsibility of another staff member. The housekeeping or custodial department should be assigned to clean the floor.
3. The MHW cannot take or transcribe phone orders from a HCP. This must be done by a licensed nurse.
4. The nurse cannot delegate teaching to an MHW. The nurse should explain seizure precautions to staff members.

Content – Management of Care: **Category of Health Alteration** – Mental Health: **Integrated Processes** – Nursing Process: Planning: **Client Needs** – Safe and

Effective Care Environment: Management of Care: **Cognitive Level** – Synthesis

MAKING NURSING DECISIONS: The nurse cannot delegate assessment, evaluation, teaching, administering medications, or the care of an unstable client to a UAP.

26. 1. This is an example of battery, which is the touching of a client without consent.
2. This is an example of false imprisonment, which is the deliberate and unauthorized confinement of a person within fixed limits by the use of verbal or physical means.
3. This is an appropriate action by the MHW, which would not require immediate intervention.
4. **This is an example of assault, which is an act that results in a person's genuine fear and apprehension that he or she will be touched without consent.**

Content – Mental Health: **Category of Health Alteration** – Mental Health: **Integrated Processes** – Nursing Process: Analysis: **Client Needs** – Safe and Effective Care Environment: Safety and Infection Control: **Cognitive Level** – Comprehension

MAKING NURSING DECISIONS: The nurse is responsible to ensure all clients' legal rights are maintained, even when on a locked psychiatric unit.

27. 1. **When an individual is declared incompetent in a court, a guardian makes decisions for the client. The client loses the right to refuse medication.**
2. Unless a mental health court orders the client to receive medication, the LVN cannot force the client to take the medication. This client voluntarily admitted herself to the unit.
3. Unless a mental health court orders the client to receive the medication, the LPN cannot force a client to take it, even if the client was involuntarily admitted to the unit.
4. Charges pending in court do not remove the client's rights to refuse to take medication.

Content – Legal: **Category of Health Alteration** – Mental Health: **Integrated Processes** – Nursing Process: Planning: **Client Needs** – Safe and Effective Care Environment: Safety and Infection Control: **Cognitive Level** – Synthesis

MAKING NURSING DECISIONS: The charge nurse must be knowledgeable of the client's rights in the mental health–nursing arena. The two options addressing a court of law should be included as possible correct options since the word "force" is in the stem of the question.

28. 1. The more experienced psychiatric nurse should be assigned the client who is actively hallucinating and delusional.
    2. The client who is aggressive should be assigned to a more experienced psychiatric nurse since this is a safety issue.
    3. **The client who is chronically depressed should be assigned to the surgical nurse who is being floated to the psychiatric unit. The client is not identified as suicidal in the option.**
    4. The client with a Cluster B personality disorder (antisocial) is manipulative and tends to split staff, so this client should be assigned to a more experienced psychiatric nurse.
    Content – *Mental Health:* **Category of Health Alteration** – *Mental Health:* **Integrated Processes** – *Nursing Process: Planning:* **Client Needs** – *Safe and Effective Care Environment: Management of Care:* **Cognitive Level** – *Synthesis*

MAKING NURSING DECISIONS: The test taker should select the client who is most stable and would require the least amount of psychiatric nursing knowledge. The primary concern on the psychiatric unit is safety to the client and others, on which client assignments must be based.

29. 1. A client on a 1-to-1 watch must not be left alone for any reason and the MHW should be within arm's length at all times.
    2. The client should not be allowed steel utensils while on suicide watch, so plastic utensils are appropriate.
    3. As long as the client is with a member of the staff, the client can attend group therapy.
    4. **The MHW should be beside the client (within arm's length), not observing the client from the porch.**
    Content – *Mental Health:* **Category of Health Alteration** – *Mental Health:* **Integrated Processes** – *Nursing Process: Implementation:* **Client Needs** – *Safe and Effective Care Environment: Management of Care:* **Cognitive Level** – *Application*

MAKING NURSING DECISIONS: The nurse is responsible for supervising any task delegated to an MHW, who is an unlicensed assistive personnel in mental health nursing.

30. 1. The MHW can assist the client with activities of daily living.
    2. The MHW worker is a vital part of the mental health team and is included in team meetings to discuss the client's psychiatric care.
    3. **The MHW cannot administer medication; therefore, this comment warrants intervention.**

4. The MHW should stay in the day room to maintain safety for the clients, so this comment does not warrant intervention.
    Content – *Mental Health:* **Category of Health Alteration** – *Mental Health:* **Integrated Processes** – *Nursing Process: Implementation:* **Client Needs** – *Safe and Effective Care Environment: Management of Care:* **Cognitive Level** – *Application*

MAKING NURSING DECISIONS: The MHW is an unlicensed assistive personnel. The nurse cannot delegate assessment, teaching, evaluation, medication administration, or an unstable client to a UAP.

31. 1. Lorazepam is used to prevent delirium tremens, and an elevated pulse would not warrant questioning the administration of this medication.
    2. Methadone is prescribed to prevent withdrawal symptoms from heroin addiction, and an increased respiratory rate would not warrant questioning the administration of this medication.
    3. **Clonidine is administered primarily to treat hypertension but is also used to reduce the symptoms of withdrawal from opioids, nicotine, and alcohol. The nurse would question administering this medication because of the client's low blood pressure, no matter why it is being prescribed.**
    4. Thiamine is used to diminish Wernicke-Korsakoff encephalopathy, which is characterized by confusion, memory loss, and loss of cranial nerve function resulting from chronic alcohol abuse. The nurse would not question giving this medication to a client with Wernicke-Korsakoff syndrome, and a subnormal temperature would not warrant questioning administering this medication.
    Content – *Substance Abuse:* **Category of Health Alteration** – *Drug Administration:* **Integrated Processes** – *Nursing Process: Assessment:* **Client Needs** – *Physiological Integrity: Pharmacological and Parenteral Therapies:* **Cognitive Level** – *Analysis*

32. 1. This is not correct information; therefore, the nurse should not praise the MHW.
    2. The psychiatric nurse should not correct the MHW in front of the client because it will compromise the MHW's authority with the client.
    3. **The nurse should explain to the MHW that the mental health client retains all of the civil rights afforded to all persons, except the right to leave the hospital in the case of involuntary commitments. The client may have phone calls restricted if that is included in the care plan—for**

example, if the client is calling and threatening the president.

4. This situation does not need to be discussed at the weekly team meeting. The psychiatric nurse can discuss this on a one-on-one basis with the MHW.

Content – Mental Health: *Category of Health Alteration* – Mental Health: *Integrated Processes* – Nursing Process: Implementation: *Client Needs* – Safe and Effective Care Environment: Management of Care: *Cognitive Level* – Application

33. 1. The client has a chemical imbalance in the brain, and a firm voice will not be effective in getting the client to sit down. The client cannot sit still.
2. This is the medication of choice, but it takes up to 3 weeks to become therapeutic; therefore, this intervention would not help the nurse complete the admission assessment.
3. **Walking or pacing with the client will allow the client to work off energy and may decrease restlessness and agitation. The nurse should implement this intervention to obtain information for the admission assessment.**
4. The nurse must obtain an admission assessment; therefore, the nurse should walk and pace with the client while attempting to obtain the priority admission assessment.

Content – Mental Health: *Category of Health Alteration* – Mental Health: *Integrated Processes* – Nursing Process: Implementation: *Client Needs* – Physiological Integrity: Reduction of Risk Potential: *Cognitive Level* – Analysis

34. 1. Evaluating the effectiveness of a client's medication is primarily the role of the psychiatric nurse, psychologist, and psychiatrist, not the social worker.
2. The recreational therapist helps the client to balance work and play in his or her life and provides activities that promote constructive use of leisure or unstructured time.
3. The vocational therapist helps the client with job-seeking or job-retention skills as well as with the pursuit of further education if needed and desired.
4. **According to the NSCBN referrals area content on the NCLEX-RN® test blueprint, the psychiatric social worker may conduct therapy and often has the primary responsibility for working with families, for community support, and for referrals.**

Content – Mental Health: *Category of Health Alteration* – Mental Health: *Integrated Processes* – Nursing Process: Implementation: *Client Needs* – Psychosocial Integrity: *Cognitive Level* – Application

35. 1. The first intervention should be to talk to the client and remove him from the day room to the least restrictive environment. Restraining the client is the most restrictive environment.
2. The nurse should first attempt to talk to the client and remove the client from the day room area, not try to remove all the other clients.
3. The client will probably need a PRN medication to calm the behavior, but it is not the nurse's first intervention. An intramuscular medication takes at least 30 minutes to become effective.
4. **The first intervention is to approach the client calmly and attempt to remove him from the day room. Staff members should not approach the agitated client alone, but should be accompanied by other personnel.**

Content – Mental Health: *Category of Health Alteration* – Mental Health: *Integrated Processes* – Nursing Process: Implementation: *Client Needs* – Safe and Effective Care Environment: Management of Care: *Cognitive Level* – Application

36. 1. This child has been abused, and until Child Protective Services has been notified, the nurse should not share any information with the child's father.
2. **The Health Insurance Portability and Accountability Act (HIPAA) considers parents the "personal representative" of the minor child with the right to information. However, there are exceptions to this rule, including when the provider reasonably believes that the minor may be a victim of abuse or neglect by the parents/guardians. This statement is the nurse's best response.**
3. Because the mother is accusing the father of the abuse, this is not an appropriate response.
4. The social worker must adhere to HIPAA regulations; therefore, referring the father to the social worker will not help the father find out how his son is doing.

Content – Child Health: *Category of Health Alteration* – Mental Health: *Integrated Processes* – Nursing Process: Implementation: *Client Needs* – Psychosocial Integrity: *Cognitive Level* – Comprehension

MAKING NURSING DECISIONS: The nurse is responsible for knowing and complying with local, state, and federal standards of care.

37. 1, 3, and 5 are correct.
1. **A no-suicide contract is one of the first interventions the nurse implements with the client. It states that if the client feels**

suicidal, he or she will talk to someone and will not take action on the thoughts.

2. This is the most stringent form of supervision in which one staff person per shift is assigned to be no greater than one arm's length away from the client. This would be implemented in an inpatient psychiatric unit, not an outpatient clinic.

3. **The nurse should ask the client whether she has a plan. The more the specific the plan is, the more seriously the statement should be taken.**

4. The nurse cannot commit to a psychiatric unit every client with thoughts of killing him- or herself. The nurse must assess the lethality, the absolute possibility, and the available support systems prior to committing a client to the psychiatric unit. After the nurse requests an emergency commitment, the client must be evaluated by a psychiatrist.

5. **The nurse should assess the client's support system and the type of help each person or group can give the client, such as hotlines, church groups, and self-help groups, as well as family members.**

Content – *Mental Health:* **Category of Health Alteration** – *Mental Health:* **Integrated Processes** – *Nursing Process: Implementation:* **Client Needs** – *Psychosocial Integrity:* **Cognitive Level** – *Analysis*

38. 1. This client should be instructed to go to the anger management class, but this does not warrant immediate intervention.

2. The mental health worker (MHW) could escort the client outside to smoke, but this does not warrant immediate intervention by the nurse.

3. **This client who is nauseated and has vomited has a physiological problem that should be assessed by the nurse immediately. This client warrants immediate intervention.**

4. A client who has her menses, or "period," may experience abdominal cramping and would need to be assessed, but not before the client who has vomited twice.

Content – *Mental Health:* **Category of Health Alteration** – *Mental Health:* **Integrated Processes** – *Nursing Process: Assessment:* **Client Needs** – *Physiological Integrity: Reduction of Risk Potential:* **Cognitive Level** – *Synthesis*

39. 1. **Because the clinical manager wants to reward the unit for no absences or tardies, the manager must reward all shifts, so providing a thank you meal to all shifts would be most appropriate. This allows all the staff members to celebrate the unit accomplishment.**

2. A thank you note is a nice action, but knowing the clinical manager took the time to arrange for the meal means a lot to staff members. The meal could encourage the staff to try and do the same the next month.

3. Individually telling the staff "job well done" is a possible action to take, but for the clinical manager to take the time to arrange for the meal on all shifts is above and beyond just saying thank you to each individual staff member.

4. Having no absences or tardies for 1 month for an individual employee is the expected behavior. The fact the entire unit had no absences/tardies is what is being acknowledged.

Content – *Management:* **Category of Health Alteration** – *Mental Health:* **Integrated Processes** – *Nursing Process: Implementation:* **Client Needs** – *Safe and Effective Care Environment: Management of Care:* **Cognitive Level** – *Application*

40. 1. The nurse must take action to protect the wife.

2. The statement can be documented, but this is not the appropriate action for the nurse to implement.

3. **Mental health clinicians have a duty to warn identifiable third parties of threats made by a person even if these threats were discussed during a therapy session (*Tarasoff v. Regents of the University of California*, 1976). The nurse should notify the client's psychiatric HCP so that the wife can be notified of the threat.**

4. The nurse should not encourage this behavior because it could cause serious harm to the wife.

Content – *Mental Health:* **Category of Health Alteration** – *Mental Health:* **Integrated Processes** – *Nursing Process: Implementation:* **Client Needs** – *Safe and Effective Care Environment: Safety and Infection Control:* **Cognitive Level** – *Application*

41. **3 and 4 are correct.**

1. Exercise often causes the client to have trouble sleeping. This intervention is not appropriate.

2. Elopement precautions are implemented for clients who are at risk for leaving the facility; therefore, this is not appropriate.

3. **Caffeinated beverages are stimulants; therefore, this is an appropriate intervention.**

4. **An alarm on the bed would help ensure safety for the client because the nurse will know immediately when the client leaves the bed.**

5. Watches known as 1-to-1 are for clients who are suicidal; therefore, this is not an appropriate intervention.

*Content – Mental Health: **Category of Health
Alteration** – Mental Health: **Integrated Processes** –
Nursing Process: Implementation: **Client Needs** – Safe
and Effective Care Environment: Management of Care:
Cognitive Level – Analysis*

MAKING NURSING DECISIONS: The test taker
must select one or more interventions for "select
all that apply" questions. The test taker should
read each option and determine if it is an
appropriate intervention.

42. Correct Answer: 3, 4, 2, 5, 1
    3. Denial.
    4. Anger.
    2. Bargaining.
    5. Depression.
    1. Acceptance.
    *Content – Mental Health: **Category of Health
    Alteration** – Mental Health: **Integrated Processes** –
    Caring: **Client Needs** – Psychosocial Integrity: **Cognitive
    Level** – Comprehension*

MAKING NURSING DECISIONS: This is a
knowledge-based question but the test taker
must remember many facts that must be applied
when taking the NCLEX-RN® examination.
This information is the basis for many questions
addressing the grieving process. The nurse
must know these in the correct order, and the
appropriate interventions for each stage of grief.

43. 1. Identifying strengths and weaknesses is
       included in the orientation phase.
    2. **Identifying problem-solving techniques is
       part of the working phase.**
    3. Evaluating the client's experience is part of
       the termination phase.
    4. Establishing the rules for the meetings is part
       of the orientation phase.
    *Content – Mental Health: **Category of Health
    Alteration** – Mental Health: **Integrated Processes** –
    Caring: **Client Needs** – Psychosocial Integrity: **Cognitive
    Level** – Comprehension*

MAKING NURSING DECISIONS: If the test taker is
not familiar with the phases of group dynamics,
then the word "middle" may give the test taker
an idea of what may be the goals of this part of
group dynamics. Evaluation is usually done at
the end.

44. 1. **On the inpatient psychiatric unit, the
       priority is maintaining safety for the
       clients and staff.**
    2. Contacting family members is not priority
       over safety.
    3. **Safety is priority over a client who is
       exhibiting behavior common to an
       inpatient psychiatric unit.**

4. This client needs to be assessed but not
   eating for 2 days is not a safety issue for the
   inpatient psychiatric unit.
*Content – Mental Health: **Category of Health
Alteration** – Mental Health: **Integrated Processes** –
Nursing Process: Implementation: **Client Needs** – Safe
and Effective Care Environment: Safety and Infection
Control: **Cognitive Level** – Synthesis*

MAKING NURSING DECISIONS: When answering
questions in mental health nursing the test taker
should identify safety as a priority intervention
in any situation. All of these situations require
intervention but safety is priority.

45. 1 and 3 are correct.
    1. **Each member of AA has a sponsor who
       has successfully quit drinking and is a
       support to a new member trying to stop
       drinking.**
    2. AA does not discuss medications used to help
       prevent drinking alcohol.
    3. **AA is a support group made up of recov-
       ering alcoholics who help others to stop
       drinking based on the 12-step approach.**
    4. AA helps an alcoholic realize he/she is
       helpless over his or her addiction. He/she
       has no power over the addiction.
    5. Recovering alcoholics speak at the meetings,
       not professional guest speakers.
    *Content – Substance Abuse: **Category of Health
    Alteration** – Mental Health: **Integrated Processes** –
    Nursing Process: Implementation: **Client Needs** –
    Health Promotion and Maintenance: **Cognitive
    Level** – Comprehension*

MAKING NURSING DECISIONS: "Select all that
apply" questions require the test taker to select
more than one option. The test taker must select
all correct options to get the question correct.
This is an alternate type of question on the
NCLEX-RN®.

46. 1. The nurse should determine the lithium
       level, but it is not the first intervention the
       nurse should implement.
    2. The nurse should assess the behavior that
       prompted the admission, but this is not the
       first intervention.
    3. **The nurse should first assess the client's
       physiological needs because the client
       in the manic state may not have slept,
       bathed, or had anything to eat for days.
       The client's physiological needs are
       priority.**
    4. Lithium takes 2 to 3 weeks to become thera-
       peutic; therefore, a STAT dose of lithium
       orally will not help the client's manic state.
       This is not the nurse's first intervention.

*Content – Mental Health: **Category of Health Alteration** – Mental Health: **Integrated Processes** – Nursing Process: Implementation: **Client Needs** – Physiological Integrity: Reduction of Risk Potential: **Cognitive Level** – Application*

47. 1. A democratic manager is people oriented and emphasizes efficient group functioning. The environment is open and communication flows both ways, which includes having meetings to discuss concerns.
2. This statement is that of an autocratic manager who uses an authoritarian approach to direct the activities of others.
3. **This statement is that of a laissez-faire manager who maintains a permissive climate with little direction or control. Instructing the staff to handle the situation on their own does not support the staff.**
4. This statement is taking control of the situation; therefore, this is not a statement indicating a laissez-faire manager.

*Content – Management: **Category of Health Alteration** – Mental Health: **Integrated Processes** – Nursing Process: Implementation: **Client Needs** – Safe and Effective Care Environment: Management of Care: **Cognitive Level** – Comprehension*

48. 1. Unless the client is anorexic and there is a court order, the nurse cannot force-feed a client.
2. **This is client abuse, and the charge nurse must investigate the allegation immediately with the nurse. If the allegations are true, they should be documented in writing and reported to the client abuse committee.**
3. The charge nurse should not ask the client about the situation first. The nurse and MHW should be involved in the investigation of the allegation. Then, if needed, the client can be asked about the situation.
4. The charge nurse should investigate the allegations first and then, if needed, have the MHW write down the situation.

*Content – Mental Health: **Category of Health Alteration** – Mental Health: **Integrated Processes** – Nursing Process: Implementation: **Client Needs** – Safe and Effective Care Environment: Management of Care: **Cognitive Level** – Application*

49. 1, 2, and 5 are correct.
1. **The nurse should assess the client for any injury, side effects of medication, and general well-being every 2 to 4 hours.**
2. **As soon as possible, the nurse must inform the client of what behavior will allow the client to be released from the seclusion room.**

3. According to the Joint Commission Restraint and Seclusion Standards for Behavioral Health, the client's family is notified promptly of the initiation of restraint or seclusion.
4. The nurse's goal is to release the client as soon as possible from the seclusion room. When the client has calmed down and is able to verbalize feelings and concerns in a rational manner, the client should be released. The seclusion order must be renewed every 24 hours, but the client should not be kept for 24 hours unless absolutely necessary.
5. **Clients must be checked at least every 10 to 15 minutes in person and may be continuously monitored on video cameras.**

*Content – Mental Health: **Category of Health Alteration** – Mental Health: **Integrated Processes** – Nursing Process: Implementation: **Client Needs** – Safe and Effective Care Environment: Safety and Infection Control: **Cognitive Level** – Application*

50. 1. **The nurse should first separate the MHW from the client; therefore, asking the MHW to go to the nurse's station would be the first intervention.**
2. The nurse should not correct the MHW in front of the client and should not use the word "arguing"; therefore, this would not be an appropriate action.
3. The psychiatric nurse should handle this situation immediately. If this is a pattern of behavior of the MHW, then the clinical manager should be notified.
4. This behavior may or may not need to be reported to the client abuse committee, but if the nurse overhears the MHW and client arguing, the nurse should stop the behavior.

*Content – Management: **Category of Health Alteration** – Mental Health: **Integrated Processes** – Nursing Process: Implementation: **Client Needs** – Psychosocial Integrity: **Cognitive Level** – Application*

51. 1. The psychiatric social worker can refer clients, but the nurse should assess the client to see what type of help she wants.
2. The psychiatric social worker does not perform or participate in ECT treatment; therefore, this client should not be referred.
3. The nurse needs to assess the client to determine why the client is having difficulty going to work. For example, is it sedation secondary to medications?
4. **The psychiatric social worker can assist with financial arrangements, referrals, and nonphysiological concerns.**

*Content – Mental Health: **Category of Health Alteration** – Mental Health: **Integrated Processes** – Nursing Process: Planning: **Client Needs** – Safe and*

Effective Care Environment: Management of Care:
***Cognitive Level** – Application*

52. 1. Two times in 1 week is becoming a pattern of behavior. The clinical manager should talk informally to the nurse to find out what is going on.
2. This is only the second time the nurse has taken 45 minutes for lunch and does not warrant formal counseling. The clinical manager should assess the situation before formally documenting the behavior.
3. This is very punitive behavior for the psychiatric nurse. The clinical manager should talk to the nurse before taking this type of action.
4. **The clinical manager should talk to the nurse informally and find out what is going on. This behavior cannot continue, but it is not behavior that requires anything more than informally finding out why the nurse has been late.**

Content – *Management:* **Category of Health Alteration** – *Mental Health:* **Integrated Processes** – *Nursing Process: Implementation:* **Client Needs** – *Safe and Effective Care Environment: Management of Care:* **Cognitive Level** – *Application*

53. 1. The client diagnosed with Alzheimer's disease would be expected to be confused; therefore, this would not warrant immediate intervention.
2. The client diagnosed with Alzheimer's disease has difficulty completing simple routine activities of daily living. This would not warrant immediate intervention.
3. **The client diagnosed with Alzheimer's disease should not be difficult to arouse from sleep. This is not a typical symptom of this disease and would warrant immediate intervention from the nurse.**
4. The client diagnosed with Alzheimer's disease has difficulty completing simple routine activities of daily living. This would not warrant immediate intervention.

Content – *Mental Health:* **Category of Health Alteration** – *Mental Health:* **Integrated Processes** – *Nursing Process: Evaluation:* **Client Needs** – *Physiological Integrity: Reduction of Risk Potential:* **Cognitive Level** – *Synthesis*

54. 1. This is a therapeutic response that helps the client to vent feelings, but this statement does not support the ethical principle of veracity.
2. **Veracity is the ethical principle "to tell the truth." The truth is that schizophrenia is a thought disorder caused by a chemical imbalance of the brain. Antipsychotic medication can control the client's hallucinations and delusions.**

3. This is interviewing the client, and this statement does not support the ethical principle of veracity.
4. Schizophrenia is a mental illness, but if the client takes the antipsychotic medication, the client may be able to work, get married, and live a productive life. This is a false statement.

Content – *Nursing Ethics:* **Category of Health Alteration** – *Mental Health:* **Integrated Processes** – *Nursing Process: Implementation:* **Client Needs** – *Psychosocial Integrity:* **Cognitive Level** – *Application*

55. 1. Tegretol is a medication that is often prescribed for clients diagnosed with bipolar disorder even though it is classified as an anticonvulsant. Many times, a medication with a different classification is prescribed for another disease process.
2. **Antacids neutralize gastric acid and may reduce the effects of antipsychotic medications and lead to medication failure. The client diagnosed with schizophrenia would be on an antipsychotic medication; therefore, the nurse should discuss this client with the psychiatric HCP.**
3. The client receiving antitubercular medications must receive them to prevent resistant strains of tuberculosis and protect the community. The nurse would not need to discuss this client with the HCP.
4. Elavil has shown efficacy in promoting weight gain in clients with anorexia nervosa; therefore, the nurse would not discuss this medication with the HCP.

Content – *Mental Health:* **Category of Health Alteration** – *Mental Health:* **Integrated Processes** – *Nursing Process: Assessment:* **Client Needs** – *Physiological Integrity: Pharmacological and Parenteral Therapies:* **Cognitive Level** – *Analysis*

56. 1. **The nurse must know the bomb scare policy of the facility, and in many cases the nurse looks for the bomb but does not touch it if it is found. In some instances, the nurse should not attempt to look for a bomb, but because the client is on a psychiatric unit, the nurse should look for a suspicious-looking object before notifying the bomb squad and evacuating the clients.**
2. The nurse would implement the bomb scare protocol if there was a bomb or suspicious-looking bag, but the nurse should first investigate the comment because the client is on a psychiatric unit.
3. The nurse would evacuate the clients if a bomb or suspicious-looking bag was under the couch. The nurse should have the clients leave the lobby area, but not the unit.

4. Just because the client is in a psychiatric unit does not mean that someone did or did not put a bomb under the couch. The nurse should look under the couch and take appropriate action.

Content – Mental Health: **Category of Health Alteration** *– Mental Health:* **Integrated Processes** *– Nursing Process: Implementation:* **Client Needs** *– Safe and Effective Care Environment: Safety and Infection Control:* **Cognitive Level** *– Application*

57. 1. The response is closed and does not allow the new nurse to voice her opinion and be part of the team.
2. The charge nurse should be open to change. Just because something has been done the same way for years does not mean it can't be done another way.
3. The charge nurse should not make the new nurse talk to the other nurses just because she doesn't like the way shift report is done.
4. **The best response is to allow the new nurse to share any new ideas with the charge nurse. The charge nurse could then talk to the other staff members and take the change to the clinical manager to determine whether the change should be instituted.**

Content – Management: **Category of Health Alteration** *– Mental Health:* **Integrated Processes** *– Nursing Process: Implementation:* **Client Needs** *– Safe and Effective Care Environment: Management of Care:* **Cognitive Level** *– Application*

58. 1. The client may eventually be able to go to the activity area, but while the client is confined to the unit, the nurse should refer the client to a recreational therapist to be provided with activities to alleviate boredom.
2. Allowing the client to vent feelings will not help alleviate the client's boredom on the unit.
3. **According to the NCLEX-RN® test blueprint, the nurse must be knowledgeable of the multidisciplinary team. The recreational therapist helps the client to balance work and play in his or her life and provides activities that promote constructive use of leisure or unstructured time.**
4. The nurse should acknowledge the client's concern and contact the recreational therapist.

Content – Mental Health: **Category of Health Alteration** *– Mental Health:* **Integrated Processes** *– Nursing Process: Implementation:* **Client Needs** *– Psychosocial Integrity:* **Cognitive Level** *– Application*

59. 1. A client who was raped would be expected to be upset and crying. This client would not require the most experienced nurse.

2. The client who is diagnosed with bipolar disorder would be agitated in the manic state. This client would not require the most experience nurse.
3. **The client who was found wandering in a daze has no diagnosis and requires an in-depth assessment. This client should be assigned to the most experienced nurse.**
4. The client diagnosed with schizophrenia would have hallucinations if not taking antipsychotic medication. The client would not require the most experienced nurse.

Content – Mental Health: **Category of Health Alteration** *– Mental Health:* **Integrated Processes** *– Nursing Process: Planning:* **Client Needs** *– Safe and Effective Care Environment: Management of Care:* **Cognitive Level** *– Synthesis*

60. 1. **When a person is admitted to a psychiatric unit, the client does not lose any rights. The client has a right to refuse treatment, but if the client is a danger to herself, then the psychiatric team must go to court and obtain an order to force-feed the client. This could be with nasogastric tube feedings or total parenteral nutrition.**
2. The client has a right to refuse treatment, but if the client is a danger to herself, then the psychiatric team must intervene. If the client does not eat, the client will die.
3. If the client is discharged and dies, the psychiatric team will be responsible. If a person is mentally ill, the psychiatric team must protect the client.
4. This is against the client's rights. The nurse cannot restrain a client without a court order.

Content – Mental Health: **Category of Health Alteration** *– Mental Health:* **Integrated Processes** *– Nursing Process: Implementation:* **Client Needs** *– Physiological Integrity: Reduction of Risk Potential:* **Cognitive Level** *– Application*

61. 1. The nurse would notify the police department if the client ran away from the unit.
2. **The nurse's first intervention is to place the unit on high alert, which includes putting signs on the exit doors warning all people coming in and out that there is a client threatening to leave the unit.**
3. The nurse should talk to the client, but the first intervention is to prevent the client from making good on the threat of running away.
4. The client who is on an involuntary admission loses the right to sign out of the psychiatric unit against medical advice (AMA).

Content – Mental Health: **Category of Health Alteration** *– Mental Health:* **Integrated**

*Processes – Nursing Process: Implementation: **Client Needs** – Safe and Effective Care Environment: Safety and Infection Control: **Cognitive Level** – Application*

62. 1. The nurse does not have a right to ask the caller for his or her name. Mr. Jones has a right to telephone calls.
    2. Mr. Jones retains all his civil rights when admitted to a psychiatric unit unless phone restriction is part of the individualized care plan.
    3. The access code for client information is requested when the caller is asking questions about the client. It is not used when the caller wants to talk directly to the client.
    4. **The nurse should find Mr. Jones and tell him he has a phone call. The client cannot have rights restricted unless it is a part of the client's individualized care plan. For example, the client may not be able to use the phone if he or she is calling 911 and making false reports.**
    *Content – Mental Health: **Category of Health Alteration** – Mental Health: **Integrated Processes** – Nursing Process: Implementation: **Client Needs** – Physiological Integrity: Basic Care and Comfort: **Cognitive Level** – Application*

63. 1. The psychiatric nurse should not make promises he or she cannot keep. If the information must be shared with the healthcare team, then the nurse will have to break a promise to the client. This will destroy the nurse-client relationship.
    2. **This is the nurse's best response. The nurse is being honest with the client but will keep the information confidential if it does not affect the client's care.**
    3. The client may need to share information that is pertinent to the client's care and should not tell the client he or she cannot talk to the nurse.
    4. Asking the client why may put the client on the defensive and he or she would not share the information.
    *Content – Mental Health: **Category of Health Alteration** – Mental Health: **Integrated Processes** – Nursing Process: Implementation: **Client Needs** – Psychosocial Integrity: **Cognitive Level** – Application*

64. 1. The client diagnosed with schizophrenia would be expected to be delusional; therefore, this situation would not warrant immediate intervention.
    2. The charge nurse has the entire shift to arrange for another nurse to cover the LPN; therefore, this situation does not warrant immediate intervention.
    3. **The loss of a unit key is priority because the nurse must determine when the MHW**

last had the key and determine whether it may be lost on the psychiatric unit. If a client finds the key, then the unit is no longer secure.
    4. The signing of the HCP's orders is important, but it does not warrant immediate intervention.
    *Content – Mental Health: **Category of Health Alteration** – Mental Health: **Integrated Processes** – Nursing Process: Implementation: **Client Needs** – Safe and Effective Care Environment: Management of Care: **Cognitive Level** – Analysis*

65. 1. The local police department needs to be called, but the nurse must first talk to the man and attempt to diffuse the situation. This action tries to ensure safety for the man, the other clients, and the staff.
    2. Ensuring safety of the other clients and staff is important, but the nurse should first attempt to make contact with the man.
    3. The nurse should not encourage the client to talk about his feelings until the gun is removed. The anger may cause the client to shoot an innocent person accidentally or on purpose.
    4. **The nurse should first try to talk to the client and diffuse the situation. This action is attempting to ensure the safety of the man, the other clients, and the staff.**
    *Content – Mental Health: **Category of Health Alteration** – Mental Health: **Integrated Processes** – Nursing Process: Implementation: **Client Needs** – Safe and Effective Care Environment: Safety and Infection Control: **Cognitive Level** – Application*

66. 2 and 5 are correct.
    1. This client requires the care of a nurse who can make attempts to get him/her to participate in therapy.
    2. **The client with diabetes can be monitored by the medical-surgical nurse. The option does not state that any unusual situations are occurring with the client's diagnosed illness. The client wishes to remain in bed and the medications have not had enough time in the client's body to make him or her a suicide risk.**
    3. Dissociative Identity Disorder (DID) is formally known as Multiple Personality Disorder (MPD). This client may be experiencing a different personality; an experienced psychiatric nurse should assess this situation.
    4. This client is creating a disturbance in the day room by blocking the television and may be at risk from the other clients. This client needs intervention by an experienced psychiatric nurse to diffuse the situation.

5. A client with major depression who has started anti-depressant medications 2 days ago could be cared for by the medical-surgical nurse. It is expected that this client has not received medication therapy long enough to make a difference in the depression. The medication requires 2 to 3 weeks of administration before showing effectiveness.

*Content – Mental Health: **Category of Health Alteration** – Mental Health: **Integrated Processes** – Nursing Process: Planning: **Client Needs** – Safe and Effective Care Environment: Management of Care: **Cognitive Level** – Synthesis*

MAKING NURSING DECISIONS: The test taker must evaluate each option individually and make a determination based solely on the facts included in the option to select correct or incorrect in a "select all that apply" question. One option does not rule out another option. The test taker must decide if the medical-surgical nurse has the knowledge required to care for the client.

67. Correct Answer: 2, 4, 3, 1, 5
    2. Part of the National Patient Safety Goals is implementing two identifiers when the client is to receive a procedure. The nurse must do this to determine that it is the correct client and the correct procedure.
    4. The client should have been NPO for several hours prior to the procedure for safety reasons. If the client were to vomit during the procedure then aspiration might occur.
    3. The client will require an intravenous line for medication administration and emergency reasons.
    1. The electric impulses will be administered via electrodes.
    5. The healthcare provider is not notified to begin the procedure until the nurse is sure that all the required pre-procedure steps are complete.

*Content – Mental Health: **Category of Health Alteration** – Mental Health: **Integrated Processes** – Nursing Process: Implementation: **Client Needs** – Safe and Effective Care Environment: Safety and Infection Control: **Cognitive Level** – Analysis*

MAKING NURSING DECISIONS: The test taker should mentally place him- or herself in the procedure area and identify which steps he/she would be required to complete. Some steps such as identifying the correct client should be first after washing the nurse's hands.

68. 1. This lab value is within normal range.
    2. This lab value is within normal range.

3. This client has schizophrenia and also has a low white blood cell count. Many clients diagnosed with schizophrenia are placed on atypical antipsychotic agents such as clozapine (Clozaril); these medications can cause agranulocytosis. This places the client at risk for a life-threatening infection. The nurse should hold the dose of any atypical antipsychotic medications and notify the healthcare provider of the result.
4. This lab value is within normal range.

*Content – Mental Health: **Category of Health Alteration** – Mental Health: **Integrated Processes** – Nursing Process: Evaluation: **Client Needs** – Physiological Integrity: Reduction of Risk Potential: **Cognitive Level** – Analysis*

MAKING NURSING DECISIONS: The test taker must be aware of complications that occur as a result of treatments for particular diseases. However, the lab data in this question have only one abnormal result. If the test taker is unsure, then the abnormal result should be chosen.

69. 1, 3, and 5 are correct.
    1. Psychiatric units have emergency codes to request assistance for a "take down" procedure when a client is deemed uncontrollable; the charge nurse should request this assistance.
    2. The client is in an excited state, so telling him that he will lose privileges is useless at this time.
    3. The other clients should be removed from possible harm.
    4. The staff should speak in a calm, soft tone to assist the client in regaining composure.
    5. The psychiatric unit is a locked unit. When the notification is made for assistance, someone must open the door so the emergency responders can enter the unit.

*Content – Mental Health: **Category of Health Alteration** – Mental Health: **Integrated Processes** – Nursing Process: Implementation: **Client Needs** – Safe and Effective Care Environment: Safety and Infection Control: **Cognitive Level** – Application*

MAKING NURSING DECISIONS: The test taker must decide on each option individually and cannot make a decision based on any other option in "select all that apply" questions. A "take down" procedure requires that safety is a major consideration for the client and staff.

70. 1. This client has some beginnings of tardive dyskinesia but can continue the antipsychotic medications.
    2. This client has some moderate signs of tardive dyskinesia but can continue the antipsychotic medications.

3. This client has some tardive dyskinesia but can continue the antipsychotic medications with frequent monitoring of the AIMS test. At a score of 20 or above the medications must be discontinued.

4. **This client is exhibiting severe abnormal behavior and the antipsychotic medication should be discontinued. The AIMS test was devised to detect extrapyramidal symptoms. If continued the client will have permanent tardive dyskinesia from the medications.**

***Content** – Mental Health:* **Category of Health Alteration** – *Mental Health:* **Integrated Processes** – *Nursing Process: Evaluation:* **Client Needs** – *Physiological Integrity, Reduction of Risk Potential:* **Cognitive Level** – *Synthesis*

MAKING NURSING DECISIONS: This question can be answered from the chart by recognizing that the higher the number, the more serious the side effects of the medications will be.

CLINICAL SCENARIO ANSWERS AND RATIONALES

The correct answer number and rationale for why it is the correct answer are given in **boldface type**. Rationales for why the other possible answer options are incorrect also are given, but they are not in boldface type.

1. 1. Narcissistic personality disorder (NPD) is a personality disorder in which the client is described as being excessively preoccupied with issues of personal adequacy, power, prestige, and vanity.
   2. **The nurse should contact this client first because the client realizes the voices are telling him to hurt his wife. The nurse should inform this client to come to the clinic immediately, and he should be admitted to a psychiatric unit.**
   3. The nurse should call this client but refusing to get out of the bed is not priority over the client who is hearing voices and may hurt his wife.
   4. The nurse should expect the client who is manic to make poor decisions such as selling a car. The nurse should call this client but the client is not a danger to self or others so the phone call does not need to be returned first.

2. 1. This client needs to be assessed but not prior to a client who is suicidal.
   2. **This client who is suicidal and has a gun in the car should be assessed first to see whether he has a plan to use the gun. This client needs to be assessed first.**
   3. This client needs to be assessed for Alzheimer's disease but not before a client who may be suicidal.
   4. The nurse should not interrupt a client who is acting compulsively. The nurse should wait until the client finishes the behavior before talking to the client.

3. 1. **The therapeutic serum level for lithium is 0.6 to 1.5 mEq/L. Because the client's level is 2.0 mEq/L, Mr. Allan should notify the client's psychiatric healthcare provider.**
   2. The WBC count is within normal limits (5,000 to 10,000), so Mr. Allan would not need to notify the psychiatric HCP. An elevated WBC count may indicate the client is experiencing agranulocytosis, a life-threatening complication of clozapine.
   3. The client's serum potassium level is within normal limits; therefore, this laboratory information does not warrant notifying the psychiatric healthcare provider.

4. A serum depakote level between 50 and 125 μg/mL is within normal limits, so Mr. Allan does not need to notify the client's psychiatric healthcare provider.

4. 1. **The client is a risk to himself and the EMS should be notified to go to the client and make sure that no harm comes to the client. The client is not in the outpatient clinic with the nurse; therefore, the EMS should be notified to go to the client before the client harms himself.**
   2. This is an assessment question but not the first intervention. The first intervention is to arrange for help to get to the client as soon as possible.
   3. The HCP will be notified but it is not the first intervention.
   4. Mr. Allan should remain on the telephone to try to keep the client occupied until the paramedics arrive on the scene.

5. 1. This is an appropriate medication for an anxiety attack, but it will take at least 15 to 30 minutes for the medication to treat the physiological signs/symptoms. Therefore, this is not the first intervention.
   2. Allowing the client to vent feelings is an appropriate intervention, but not the first intervention since the client is hyperventilating.
   3. **The first intervention is to address the client's physical discomfort, which is hyperventilating; therefore, encouraging the client to take slow, deep breaths is the next intervention for Ms. Marguerite.**
   4. The client's pulse oximetry reading can be obtained, but it will not address the client's hyperventilating; therefore, it is not the nurse's first intervention.

6. 1. **The client diagnosed with dementia would be expected to have confusion and disorientation; therefore, the LVN could be assigned this client. This client is not experiencing any potentially life-threatening complication of dementia.**
   2. Extrapyramidal side effects are a complication of antipsychotic medication. A more experienced RN should be assigned to this client.
   3. The client who is pacing up and down the hallway is exhibiting the manic behavior of bipolar disorder. This client needs further assessment and should be assigned to a registered nurse.

4. This client is experiencing potentially life-threatening complications of anorexia and needs further assessment, so he should be assigned to a registered nurse.

7. 1. The client who is exhibiting compulsive behavior should be observed, but the MHW should not attempt to stop the client's behavior. This is an appropriate task to delegate to the MHW.
   2. An MHW can sit in the waiting room and watch the clients. This is an appropriate nursing task to delegate.
   3. The MHW can sit with a client who is suicidal even though the client may be unstable. The MHW just has to be within an arm's length of the suicidal client. This is an appropriate nursing task to delegate.
   4. **The MHW does not draw blood, and this would be an inappropriate task to delegate. The laboratory technician draws the client's blood work.**

8. 1. The first intervention should be to approach the client calmly. Placing the client in a quiet room may be appropriate depending on the behavior of the client, but it is not the first intervention.
   2. The nurse should first attempt to talk to the client and remove the client from the day room area, not try to remove all the other clients.
   3. Calling 911 may be an appropriate intervention, but it is not the first intervention Mr. Allan should implement. Talking to the client is the first intervention.
   4. **The first intervention is to approach the client calmly and attempt to remove him from the day room. Staff members should not approach the agitated client alone, but should be accompanied by other personnel.**

9. 1. Mr. Allan should talk to the client but not to discuss the argument. Mr. Allan should diffuse the situation and calm the client, not interview the client to determine what happened. That should be discussed with Ms. Brenda.
   2. **Mr. Allan should discuss the behavior with Ms. Brenda, then take appropriate disciplinary action. Psychiatric staff members cannot argue with clients.**
   3. Mr. Allan needs to document Ms. Brenda's behavior, but Mr. Allan should discuss the situation with Ms. Brenda before taking any other action.
   4. Ms. Brenda's behavior may warrant termination, but the first action of Mr. Allan is to discuss the behavior with Ms. Brenda.

10. 1. Mr. Allan should not involve other employees in Ms. Brenda's situation. A clinical manager should allow Ms. Brenda to resolve the problem.
    2. Since Ms. Belinda has a reason for being late and the car will be fixed in a week, the behavior does not need to be documented and placed in her file.
    3. This is very punitive behavior for Mr. Allan to take, since she is having car trouble and riding the bus to get to work.
    4. **Mr. Allan needs to work with the employees, and being understanding of situations is an attribute of an effective clinical manager. Ms. Belinda has a valid reason for being late and since she has an excellent attendance record. Mr. Allan should be understanding and work with Ms. Belinda.**

Case Studies: Care of Clients in Various Settings 14

MEDICAL NURSING CASE STUDY

Ms. Teresa is the staff nurse on a medical unit assigned to care for the following clients during the 7a to 7p shift.

(A) Mr. Brody, a 42-year-old African American male, diagnosed with abdominal pain, etiology unknown.

(B) Ms. White, a 60-year-old Asian female, admitted with a diagnosis of bacterial pneumonia.

(C) Mr. Gonzales, a 48-year-old Hispanic male, diagnosed with chest pain rule out myocardial infarction.

(D) Ms. Smith, a 24-year-old Caucasian female, diagnosed with diabetic ketoacidosis.

(E) Mr. George, a 38-year-old white male, diagnosed with renal calculi.

Based on the information provided determine the order in which the clients should be seen and the reasoning behind the nurse's decision.

1) _____

_____

2) _____

_____

3) _____

_____

4) _____

_____

5) _____

_____

Ms. Teresa has received the shift report and will care for her assigned clients. Answer the questions below.

Mr. Brody is scheduled for an endoscopy this morning. He is scheduled to receive an intravenous proton-pump inhibitor and an oral ACE inhibitor. List at least four interventions Ms. Teresa should implement when preparing Mr. Brody for this diagnostic test.

1) _____

2) _____

3) _____

4) _____

1. Identify at least six assessment interventions Ms. Teresa should implement when completing the morning shift assessment for Ms. White, who is diagnosed with bacterial pneumonia.

   1) _____

   2) _____

   3) _____

   4) _____

   5) _____

   6) _____

2. Ms. Teresa is preparing to administer a loop diuretic to Ms. Gonzales. Identify five interventions Ms. Teresa should implement when administering this medication.

   1) _____

   2) _____

   3) _____

   4) _____

   5) _____

3. Ms. Teresa is preparing to administer 30 units of 70/30 insulin to Ms. Smith. Identify five interventions Ms. Teresa should implement when caring for this client.

   1) _____

   2) _____

   3) _____

   4) _____

   5) _____

4. The unlicensed assistive personnel informs Ms. Teresa that Mr. George is complaining of severe pain. Identify seven interventions Ms. Teresa should implement when administering intravenous narcotic pain medication to Mr. George.

   1) _____

   2) _____

   3) _____

   4) _____

   5) _____

   6) _____

   7) _____

5. Ms. Teresa has delegated a.m. care for Ms. Smith. Which nursing tasks can the UAP implement for Ms. Smith? **Select all that apply.**
   ✓ Assist Ms. Smith to the shower.
   ✓ Change the linens on the bed.
   ✓ Cut Ms. Smith's toenails.
   ✓ Wash Ms. Smith's hair.
   ✓ Rub and massage Ms. Smith's lower extremities.
   ✓ Feed Ms. Smith the breakfast meal.

6. Mr. Brody has a nasogastric tube. Identify five assessment interventions Ms. Teresa should implement when completing Mr. Brody's shift assessment.

   1) _____

   2) _____

   3) _____

   4) _____

   5) _____

7. Which diagnostic test should Ms. Teresa check to determine whether Mr. Gonzales has had a myocardial infarction?

   _____

8. Mr. George has just passed a renal stone. Which action should Ms. Teresa implement?

   _____

9. Ms. Smith is being discharged home. List five discharge instructions Ms. Teresa should discuss when implementing diabetic teaching.

   1) _____

   2) _____

   3) _____

   4) _____

   5) _____

10. The laboratory determined Mr. George had an oxalate renal calculi. The HCP ordered a low oxalate diet. Identify five interventions Ms. Teresa should discuss with Mr. George.

    1) _____

    2) _____

    3) _____

    4) _____

    5) _____

11. Mr. Gonzales did not have a myocardial infarction. He was diagnosed with angina. List five interventions Ms. Teresa should discuss with Mr. Gonzales.

    1) _____

    2) _____

    3) _____

    4) _____

    5) _____

12. Mr. Brody has just returned from the endoscopy. List three interventions Ms. Teresa should implement.

    1) _____

    2) _____

    3) _____

13. The UAP tells Ms. Teresa that Ms. Smith is complaining of being jittery, feels nervous, and has a headache. List three interventions Ms. Teresa should implement.

    1) _____

    2) _____

    3) _____

14. Ms. White is having shortness of breath. List five interventions Ms. Teresa should implement.

    1) _____

    2) _____

    3) _____

    4) _____

    5) _____

CASE STUDIES

CRITICAL CARE NURSING CASE STUDY

The nurses are caring for clients in the critical care unit in a community hospital. Answer the following questions.

1. Ms. Paula is caring for the client on the ventilator with an endotracheal intubation. List 10 interventions Ms. Paula should implement for the ventilator care.

1) _____
2) _____
3) _____
4) _____
5) _____
6) _____
7) _____
8) _____
9) _____
10) _____

2. Ms. Debbie is caring for the client who may be developing disseminated intravascular coagulation (DIC). List five nursing interventions and medical interventions the nurse should implement when caring for this client.

1) _____
2) _____
3) _____
4) _____
5) _____

3. Ms. Gail is caring for the client who may be developing acute respiratory distress syndrome (ARDS). List five nursing interventions and medical interventions the nurse should implement when caring for this client.

1) _____
2) _____
3) _____
4) _____
5) _____

4. Ms. Teresa is caring for a client diagnosed with C-6 spinal cord injury (SCI) in the critical care unit. List five nursing interventions and medical interventions the nurse should implement when caring for this client.

1) _____
2) _____
3) _____
4) _____
5) _____

5. Mr. Ben is caring for a client with a traumatic brain injury in the critical care unit. List five nursing interventions and medical interventions the nurse should implement when caring for this client.

   1) _____

   2) _____

   3) _____

   4) _____

   5) _____

6. Ms. Belinda is caring for a client admitted from the emergency department with diagnosis of rule out myocardial infarction. As the client moves from the stretcher to the CCU, he starts complaining of chest pain. List seven nursing interventions and medical interventions the nurse should implement when caring for this client.

   1) _____

   2) _____

   3) _____

   4) _____

   5) _____

   6) _____

   7) _____

7. Ms. Belinda monitors the client with the acute myocardial infarction for complications. List five complications Ms. Belinda is monitoring for.

   1) _____

   2) _____

   3) _____

   4) _____

   5) _____

8. Ms. Teresa is caring for a client whose telemetry shows ventricular fibrillation. List five interventions Ms. Teresa should implement.

   1) _____

   2) _____

   3) _____

   4) _____

   5) _____

9. Ms. Paula is caring for a client on a ventilator in the critical care unit. The client is a risk for numerous complications and special problems. List five problems with three interventions each.

Problem 1: _____

  1) _____

  2) _____

  3) _____

Problem 2: _____

  1) _____

  2) _____

  3) _____

Problem 3: _____

  1) _____

  2) _____

  3) _____

Problem 4: _____

  1) _____

  2) _____

  3) _____

Problem 5: _____

  1) _____

  2) _____

  3) _____

OUTPATIENT NURSING CASE STUDY

Ms. Judy is caring for clients in a free outpatient clinic. Answer the following questions.

1. Ms. Judy requests a variety of laboratory and diagnostic tests for the clients coming to the outpatient clinic. Identify which laboratory/diagnostic test Ms. Judy should order with the client's complaint.

Client Complaint

_____ 1. "I am having burning upon urination."

_____ 2. "I have been having Charlie horses or leg cramps in my calves." Client takes diuretics.

_____ 3. "I am taking Coumadin, an anticoagulant, every day."

_____ 4. "I am having pain in my right lower abdomen and I have a low-grade fever."

_____ 5. "I am having burning in my chest after I eat, especially if I lie down after I eat."

_____ 6. "I have type 2 diabetes and have been taking my medication as directed for the last 3 months."

_____ 7. "I am weak all the time since I became a vegetarian. My family tells me I am pale and I don't have any energy."

_____ 8. "I have been a type 2 diabetic for 20 years and I think I may have diabetic nephropathy."

_____ 9. "The last doctor I saw told me I might have a peripheral nerve disease and needed a test but I can't remember the name of the test."

_____ 10. "I think I have myasthenia gravis, like my sister. Could you please give me the test to diagnose MG?"

_____ 11. "I am hot all the time, I have problems holding my pen when I write, and I am breathing faster."

_____ 12. "I think I may have been exposed to syphilis."

_____ 13. "I am receiving chemotherapy and have noticed bleeding after I brush my teeth and when I blow my nose."

_____ 14. "I have been on a heart healthy diet for over 6 months since my heart attack."

_____ 15. "My wife says I am having trouble hearing but I don't think so."

_____ 16. "I think I am allergic to dust or mold because my nose gets stuffy, I sneeze all the time, and sometimes I break out in a rash."

Laboratory/Diagnostic Test

a. upper gastrointestinal endoscopy

b. serum iron level

c. serum potassium level

d. serum creatinine level

e. International Normalized Ratio (INR)

f. Thyroid function tests

g. platelet count

h. clean-catch or midstream urinary specimen

i. cholesterol level

j. Scratch test

k. Tensilon test

l. audiometry

m. electromyography (EMG)

n. RPR (rapid plasma regain) and VDRL

o. glycosylated hemoglobin A_{1c}

p. white blood cell count

CASE STUDIES

2. Ms. Judy is talking to a male client about the diagnostic test of endoscopy. Identify the teaching interventions Ms. Judy should include when explaining the procedure to the client.

_____

_____

_____

_____

_____

3. Ms. Judy is explaining the diagnostic procedure of colonoscopy to a female client. Identify the teaching interventions Ms. Judy should include when explaining the procedure to the client.

_____

_____

_____

_____

_____

4. Ms. Judy must obtain a throat specimen for a client who has possible strep throat. List in order the 10 interventions Ms. Judy should implement to perform this procedure correctly.

1) _____

2) _____

3) _____

4) _____

5) _____

6) _____

7) _____

8) _____

9) _____

10) _____

5. Ms. Judy is caring for a client who has a sprained right ankle. List the interventions Ms. Judy should discuss with the client prior to discharging the client home.

_____

_____

_____

_____

_____

6. The client diagnosed with a cold asks Ms. Judy, "Why won't my doctor give me some antibiotics when I feel so bad? What can I do for this cold?" Explain why the HCP will not write an antibiotic prescription for the client's cold; then list five interventions Ms. Judy should recommend to the client to help with the cold symptoms.

Explanation: _____

_____

1) _____

2) _____

3) _____

4) _____

5) _____

7. Ms. Judy has noticed many of the clients coming to the outpatient clinic are taking herbs. She is developing a chart with some of the most common herbs and why clients take them. Identify which herb is taken for which medical condition.

Medical Condition

_____ **1)** Helps relieve stomachaches, nausea, and diarrhea.

_____ **2)** Helps with increasing memory and treating Alzheimer's disease.

_____ **3)** Helps treat first-degree burns, wound healing, sunburn, radiation-induced skin reactions, genital herpes, psoriasis.

_____ **4)** Helps treat colds.

_____ **5)** Recommended by HCP for treatment of benign prostatic hypertrophy.

_____ **6)** Used to treat liver diseases, including hepatitis, fatty liver, cirrhosis, and liver protection.

_____ **7)** Used to treat atherosclerosis, hypertension, and peripheral vascular diseases.

_____ **8)** Used to treat depression.

_____ **9)** Helps relieve headaches and decrease anxiety.

_____ **10)** Used to treat urinary and bladder infections.

Herb

a. aloe vera gel—topical

b. saw palmetto

c. ginkgo biloba

d. garlic

e. Echinacea

f. lavender

g. cranberries

h. ginger

i. milk thistle

j. St. John's wort

8. Ms. Judy is discussing the American Cancer Society health promotion screenings for adult clients at a community meeting. She has requested participants to ask questions concerning screenings. Answer the clients' questions.

Question 1: "What should I do to determine if I have breast cancer?"

_____

_____

_____

_____

Question 2: "What is recommended for detecting colon or rectal cancer?"

_____

_____

_____

_____

Question 3: "What are the recommendations for detecting cervical cancer?"

_____

_____

_____

_____

Question 4: "What should be done to detect prostate cancer?"

_____

_____

_____

_____

Question 5: "What can I tell my son about screening for testicular cancer?"

_____

_____

_____

_____

HOME HEALTH CASE STUDY

Ms. Teresa is caring for the following clients in the Angel Home Healthcare Agency.

1. Ms. Teresa is caring for a female client who needs the indwelling urinary catheter changed. List the procedure (in the correct order) for inserting an indwelling urinary catheter.

_____

_____

_____

_____

_____

2. Ms. Teresa is caring for a client who has a right sided subclavian dressing. List the procedure (in the correct order) for changing and cleaning the subclavian insertion site.

_____

_____

_____

_____

_____

3. Ms. Teresa is caring for a client who needs a daily wet to dry dressing for an abdominal wound. The wet to dry dressing is done daily to mechanically debride the abdominal wound. List the procedure (in the correct order) for performing wound care.

_____

_____

_____

_____

_____

4. Ms. Teresa must collect a midstream urine specimen on a male client. List the procedure (in the correct order) for collecting a midstream urine specimen.

_____

_____

_____

_____

_____

5. Ms. Teresa must administer a tap water enema to a client. List the procedure (in the correct order) for administering a tap water enema.

_____

_____

_____

_____

_____

6. Ms. Teresa will be teaching the home health aide how to perform a colostomy irrigation for the client with a sigmoid colostomy. List the procedure (in the correct order) for performing a colostomy irrigation.

_____

_____

_____

_____

_____

CASE STUDIES

7. Ms. Teresa must draw an International Normalized Ratio (INR) for the client who is taking warfarin (Coumadin) daily. List the procedure (in the correct order) for drawing venous blood.

_____

_____

_____

_____

_____

_____

8. Ms. Teresa must insert the nasogastric tube for the client receiving tube feedings for 1 month. List the procedure (in the correct order) for inserting a nasogastric tube.

_____

_____

_____

_____

_____

_____

9. Ms. Teresa must teach the client how to administer 20 units of 70/30 insulin to the client. List the procedure (in the correct order) for administering subcutaneous insulin in the abdomen.

_____

_____

_____

_____

_____

_____

10. Ms. Teresa must teach the client's significant other how to transfer the client from the bed to the chair. List the procedure (in the correct order) for transferring the client from the bed to the chair.

_____

_____

_____

_____

_____

MENTAL HEALTH NURSING CASE STUDY

Mr. Aaron is the charge nurse on an inpatient psychiatric unit. He is orienting new nurses to the psychiatric unit, the client's admission process, nursing documentation, and care of the client with a mental illness.

1. Mr. Aaron explains the importance of identifying defense mechanisms. Match the defense mechanism with the description and example of defense mechanism.

Description and Example of Defense Mechanism

1) Burying a painful feeling or thought from awareness, though it may resurface in symbolic form. Sometimes considered a basis of other defense mechanisms. EX: The client remembers his/her father's funeral.

2) Not accepting reality because it is too painful. EX: The client is arrested for drunk driving several times but doesn't believe he/she has a problem with alcohol.

3) Reverting to an older, less mature way of handling stresses and feelings. EX: The client and significant other get into an argument so the client stomps off into another room and pouts.

4) Attributing unacceptable thoughts or feelings to someone or something else. EX: The client gets really mad at her husband but screams he's the one mad at the client.

5) Everything in the world is seen as all good or all bad with nothing in between. EX: The client thinks her boyfriend is absolutely worthless because he forgot a lunch date with the client.

6) Attempting to avoid a painful thought or feeling by objectifying and emotionally detaching oneself from the feeling. EX: Acting aloof and indifferent toward someone when the client really dislikes the person.

7) Channeling a feeling or thought from its actual source to something or someone else. EX: When the client gets mad at her sister, the client breaks her drinking glass by throwing it against the wall.

8) Adopting beliefs, attitudes, and feelings contrary to what the client really believes. EX: The female client says she is angry but she really is not.

9) Justifying one's behaviors and motivations by substituting "good," acceptable reasons for these real motivations. EX: The client always studies hard for tests and knows a lot of people who cheat so it's not a big deal the client cheated this time.

10) Handling one's own pain by helping others. EX: After the client's wife dies, he keeps himself busy by volunteering at the local church.

Name of Defense Mechanism

a. Splitting

b. Reaction formation

c. Undoing

d. Repression

e. Humor

f. Projection

g. Suppression

h. Rationalization

i. Denial

j. Sublimation

k. Regression

l. Isolation of Affect

m. Altruism

n. Displacement

continued

     11) Focusing on funny aspects of a painful situation. EX: A person's treatment for cancer makes him lose his hair so he makes jokes about being bald.

     12) Redirecting unacceptable, instinctual drives into personally and socially acceptable channels. EX: Intense rage redirected in the form of participation in sports such as boxing or football.

     13) The effort to hide and control unacceptable thoughts or feelings. EX: The client is attracted to someone but says she really doesn't like the person at all.

     14) Trying to reverse or "undo" a thought or feeling by performing an action that signifies an opposite feeling than originally thought or felt. EX: The client has feelings of dislike for someone but buys them a gift.

2. Mr. Aaron explains the nurses will be responsible for leading groups on the unit such as medication, symptom management, anger management, and self-care groups. Identify and discuss the three phases of the group work.

    1) _____

    2) _____

    3) _____

3. Mr. Aaron is admitting Mr. Chandler, a 27-year-old client, diagnosed with paranoid schizophrenia to the inpatient psychiatric unit. Identify three signs/symptoms Nurse Aaron would expect Mr. Chandler to exhibit.

    1) _____

    2) _____

    3) _____

4. Later in the shift, Mr. Aaron is admitting Ms. Smith, 33-year-old client, diagnosed with bipolar disorder, severe mania, to the unit. List six signs/symptoms Mr. Aaron would expect Ms. Smith to exhibit.

    1) _____

    2) _____

    3) _____

    4) _____

    5) _____

    6) _____

5. Mr. Aaron is having a very busy shift and is admitting Mrs. Jones, a 44-year-old client who is diagnosed with major depression. List six signs/symptoms Mr. Aaron would expect Mrs. Jones to exhibit.

    1) _____

    2) _____

    3) _____

    4) _____

    5) _____

    6) _____

6. Mrs. Jones, diagnosed with major depression, tells Mr. Aaron, "I am tired of living. I just need to die and everyone will be better off." Discuss how Mr. Aaron should evaluate Mrs. Jones suicidal intent and suicide risk.

_____

_____

_____

_____

7. Mr. Aaron is caring for Ms. Smith, diagnosed with severe mania. List five nursing interventions Mr. Aaron should implement when caring for Ms. Smith.

1) _____

2) _____

3) _____

4) _____

5) _____

8. Mr. Aaron is caring for Mr. Chandler, diagnosed with paranoid schizophrenia. Mr. Chandler is having active hallucinations and thinks he is God. List five nursing interventions Mr. Aaron should implement when caring for Mr. Chandler.

1) _____

2) _____

3) _____

4) _____

5) _____

9. Mr. Aaron determines Mr. Jones is having alcohol withdrawal and arranges for him to be transferred to the acute care hospital. List five nursing interventions for the client experiencing alcohol withdrawal.

1) _____

2) _____

3) _____

4) _____

5) _____

10. Mr. Aaron is discussing the client's diagnosis with one of the new nurses who is orienting to the unit. Mr. Aaron asks the nurse to identify the five axes. List the five axes on the psychiatric diagnosis.

1) _____

2) _____

3) _____

4) _____

5) _____

MATERNAL-CHILD CASE STUDY

Ms. Ann is working in the newborn nursery, Ms. Laura is working in the labor and delivery unit, and Ms. Courtney is working in the postpartum unit.

1. Ms. Ann is assessing the newborn for reflexes. Identify five reflexes and how to elicit the response from the newborn.

   1) _____

   2) _____

   3) _____

   4) _____

   5) _____

2. Ms. Laura is assessing the newborn to determine an Apgar score. Identify the five assessment interventions used to determine the newborn's Apgar score.

   1) _____

   2) _____

   3) _____

   4) _____

   5) _____

3. Ms. Ann is assessing a 2-hour-old newborn. Identify the assessment interventions Ms. Ann should implement. Do not list what is normal; list only the components of the physical assessment.

   _____

   _____

   _____

   _____

4. Ms. Courtney is caring for clients in the postpartum unit. She is assessing for postpartum complications. Match the complications with the signs/symptoms.

Signs/Symptoms

_____ **1)** The mother is light-headed, syncopal, hypotensive, and tachycardiac, and has oliguria.

_____ **2)** The mother has fever, uterine tenderness, and foul-smelling lochia.

_____ **3)** The mother is sad, weeping, irritable, anxious, and confused.

_____ **4)** The mother has dark bleeding with clots and there is a noncontracted, boggy uterine fundus.

_____ **5)** The mother has a sudden rise in uterine fundal height, indicating the formation of clots inside the uterine cavity.

_____ **6)** The mother is complaining of severe, sharp perineal pain and swelling in the perineal wall.

_____ **7)** The mother is exhibiting bizarre behavior and has disorganization of thought, hallucinations, and delusions.

_____ **8)** The mother has pain and has a fever along with localized tenderness, swelling, and redness of the left leg.

_____ **9)** The mother has marked breast engorgement, acute breast pain, tenderness, and fever and chills.

Complication

a. Postpartum depression

b. Uterine atony

c. Thrombophlebitis

d. Retained placental fragments in the uterus

e. Endometritis

f. Mastitis

g. Postpartum psychosis

h. Hematoma

i. Postpartum hemorrhage

5. Ms. Laura is teaching parents in a child preparation class about labor and delivery. Define the stages of labor.

_____

_____

_____

_____

6. Ms. Courtney is performing discharge teaching to the mother. List five interventions Ms. Courtney should discuss with the mother.

1) _____

2) _____

3) _____

4) _____

5) _____

ANSWERS TO CASE STUDIES

MEDICAL NURSING CASE STUDY ANSWERS

Determining the order to see the clients

The first client to be seen by the nurse should be the client who has unexpected or abnormal data. If all of the clients are apparently stable, then the client who has the greatest risk for a complication should be seen first. In this scenario:

1) (C) Mr. Gonzales, diagnosed with chest pain rule out myocardial infarction should be seen first. Chest pain associated with lack of oxygen reaching the cardiac muscle is a high risk for a complication.

2) (D) Ms. Smith, diagnosed with diabetic ketoacidosis, should be seen next to determine blood glucose levels and whether insulin replacement therapy is needed.

3) (A) Mr. Brody or (E) Mr. George can be seen next since both have issues with pain; pain does not kill but should be addressed to make sure that neither is experiencing pain at this time.

4) (A) Mr. Brody or (E) Mr. George can be seen next since both have issues with pain; pain does not kill but should be addressed to make sure that neither is experiencing pain at this time.

5) (B) Ms. White, diagnosed with bacterial pneumonia, should be seen last. Ms. White has been in the facility long enough for the nurse to receive a report. This client should have received at least the first dose of antibiotic by this time.

1. 1) Ensure the client is NPO.
   2) Hold the client's oral medication.
   3) Administer the intravenous medication.
   4) Make sure the informed consent form is signed.

2. 1) Assess the client's breath sounds.
   2) Assess the client's respiratory rate.
   3) Assess the extremities for capillary refill time.
   4) Assess for buccal or circumoral cyanosis.
   5) Assess level of consciousness.
   6) Assess pulse oximeter reading.
   7) Assess the client for productive/non-productive cough.

3. 1) Check the client's serum potassium level.
   2) Question the medication if the client's B/P is less than 90/60.
   3) Question the medication if the client is dehydrated.
   4) Check the client's intake and output.
   5) Assess the client for signs/symptoms of hypokalemia.

4. 1) Check the client's glucose level.
   2) Check to determine if the client is NPO.
   3) Ensure the client eats breakfast to cover the regular insulin.
   4) Ensure the client eats lunch to cover the intermediate insulin.
   5) Administer the medication in the client's abdomen.
   6) Assess the client for hypoglycemia throughout the shift.

5. 1) Assess the client's pain on a scale of 1 to 10.
   2) Rule out any complications prior to administering pain medication (assess urine for blood; strain the client's urine).
   3) Check the medication administration record (MAR) to determine the last time Mr. George received pain medication.
   4) Sign out narcotic medication from the medication delivery system (PIXYS).
   5) Check MAR against client's ID band.
   6) Determine if pain medication is compatible with primary IV.
   7) Check patency of client's IV site.
   8) Push intravenous pain medication slowly over 5 minutes.
   9) Assess client's respiratory rate.
   10) Document on MAR and in nurse's notes.
   11) Implement safety issues, bed low position, side rails up, call light within reach.

6. The following should not be delegated:
   - **Cut Ms. Smith's toenails.** UAPs and nurses should not cut a client's toenails, especially a client who has diabetes. This presents an opportunity for the client to develop an infection and possibly lose the foot.
   - **Rub and massage Ms. Smith's lower extremities.** Nurses and UAPs do not massage the lower extremities because of the risk for dislodging a clot in the extremity.
   - **Feed Ms. Smith the breakfast meal.** The UAP should not feed a client who is 24 and can feed herself. The client should be encouraged to be independent.

7. 1) Assess bowel sounds in all four quadrants.
   2) Assess abdomen for firmness and tenderness.
   3) Assess last bowel movement.
   4) Determine type of bowel movement (soft, hard, dark color).
   5) Assess N/G tube output (coffee ground, green bile).
   6) Assess amount of N/G tube output.
   7) Determine if N/G tube is on low intermittent suction.
   8) Assess the client's nare for irritation.

8. Assess cardiac enzymes including troponin, CPK-MB.

9. 1) Put the calculi (stone) in a sterile lab cup.
   2) Label the cup and send to laboratory.

10. Ms. Teresa should not make assumptions about what Ms. Smith knows:
    1) Ensure client knows how to take insulin injections, correct way and time.
    2) Ensure client knows how to treat hypoglycemia.
    3) Ensure client knows how to treat hyperglycemia and when to call the HCP.
    4) Ensure client knows how to count carbohydrates.
    5) Ensure client knows importance of daily exercise.
    6) Ensure client knows how to assess and care for feet.
    7) Ensure client knows sick day rules.

11. 1) Refer to a dietician.
    2) Provide Mr. George with written handouts.
    3) Limit oxalate to 40 to 50 mg each day.
    4) Drink 8 to 12 cups of fluid each day.

    5) The body may turn extra vitamin C into oxalate. Avoid high doses of vitamin C supplements (more than 2,000 mg of vitamin C per day).
    6) Oxalate is found in many foods. Limit foods such as soy cheese, soy milk, soy yogurt, cereal (bran or high fiber), fruitcake, pretzels, wheat bran, wheat germ, whole wheat bread, whole wheat flour, dark or "robust" beer, black tea, chocolate milk, cocoa, instant coffee, and hot chocolate.

12. 1) Discuss use of sublingual nitroglycerin (NTG): take one every 5 minutes; if no pain relief, get to the emergency department (do not drive), keep NTG in dark bottle, medication should burn under tongue.
    2) Instruct Mr. Gonzales to stop any activity if chest pain occurs; then take NTG as above.
    3) Discuss a low-fat, low-cholesterol (no fried foods; instead, boil, bake, and grill meats).
    4) Discuss the importance of walking daily for 30 minutes.
    5) Discuss the importance of not smoking or being around secondhand smoke.
    6) Discuss the need to eat small, frequent meals and avoid large meals.

13. 1) Determine Mr. Brody's gag reflex has returned prior to giving PO fluids or food.
    2) Assess the client for any abdominal bleeding.
    3) Administer Mr. Brody's a.m. medications.
    4) Give Mr. Brody water and breakfast or lunch meal.

14. 1) Check Ms. Smith's blood glucometer reading.
    2) Give Ms. Smith a glass of orange juice.
    3) Give Ms. Smith a complex carbohydrate after feeling better such as graham crackers, peanut butter crackers, or cheese and crackers.
    4) Ensure Ms. Smith stays in bed.

15. 1) Elevate the head of Ms. White's bed.
    2) Administer or increase oxygen via nasal cannula.
    3) Notify the respiratory therapist.
    4) Stay with Ms. White and attempt to calm her.
    5) Request client to take slow, deep breaths.
    6) Assess Ms. White's bilateral lung sounds.

CRITICAL CARE NURSING CASE STUDY ANSWERS

1. 1) Check ventilator settings with prescribed settings.
    - Tidal volume
    - Rate
    - Positive-end-expiratory pressure (PEEP)
    - FIO_2 (oxygen concentration)
    - Mode of ventilation—control, assist-control, intermittent mandatory (IMV), synchronized intermittent mandatory ventilation (SIMV), pressure support ventilation (PSV)
   2) Check ET tube placement.
   3) Maintain proper cuff inflation.
   4) Check all ventilator connections.
   5) Have manual resuscitative bag at bedside (ambu bag).
   6) Ensure all ventilator alarms are on and answered promptly.
   7) Empty condensed water from water traps.
   8) Assess client's respiratory status, pulse oximeter, arterial blood gases.
   9) Complete respiratory assessment (lung sounds, LOC, etc.).
   10) Assess client's reaction to muscle-paralyzing agents.
   11) Ensure upper extremity restraints are on properly and assess for neurovascular compromise.
   12) Suction with end-line suction as needed.
   13) Collaborate with respiratory therapist.

2. 1) Assess for pallor, petechiae, purpura, oozing blood, hematomas, and occult hemorrhage.
   2) Assess PT/PTT (prolonged); fibrinogen and platelets (reduced).
   3) Administer blood products: platelets, cryoprecipitate, fresh frozen plasma.
   4) Administer heparin or low-molecular-weight heparin.
   5) Avoid IV and IM injections.
   6) Use soft-bristle toothbrush.
   7) Use electric razor.
   8) Protect from trauma that may cause bleeding.

3. 1) Administer high liter oxygen and monitor pulse oximeter/arterial blood gases.
   2) If pulse oximeter readings/ABG results continue to drop while client is receiving supplemental oxygen, it is ARDS.
   3) Prepare to place client on ventilator (only treatment) along with treating underlying cause.

   4) See question 1 for care of the client on the ventilator.
   5) Some clients respond positively to being placed in the prone position.
   6) Address nutritional needs.
   7) Assess client's respiratory status.

4. 1) Assess for spinal shock (decreased reflexes, loss of sensation, flaccid paralysis).
   2) Assess for neurogenic shock (hypotension and bradycardia).
   3) Assess for respiratory status since C-6 and ascending paralysis.
   4) Maintain bowel and bladder integrity.
   5) Address immobility issues of the client (pneumonia, pressure ulcers, DVTs, contractures).
   6) Maintain appropriate temperature of environment.

5. 1) Frequent neurological assessment using the Glasgow Coma Scale.
   2) Assess for increased intracranial pressure (ICP).
   3) Monitor respiratory status.
   4) Place client with head of bed up 30° or greater, to promote venous drainage.
   5) Limit suction passes to <15 seconds, to prevent increased ICP.
   6) Keep client normothermia.
   7) Decrease environmental stimuli.
   8) Assess for raccoon eyes, rhinorrhea, Battle's sign with otorrhea, halo or ring sign.

6. 1) Ensure patent airway.
   2) Administer pain medication, including nitroglycerin sublingual and intravenous morphine.
   3) Administer oxygen via nasal cannula or non-rebreather mask, and monitor pulse oximetry.
   4) Obtain 12-lead EKG.
   5) Monitor ECG telemetry readings.
   6) Monitor cardiac isoenzymes, including troponin, CPK-MB.
   7) Prepare to administer thrombolytic therapy, if appropriate.
   8) Provide reassurance and emotional support to client and family.
   9) Perform cardiovascular assessment frequently.
   10) Bed rest and activity limitation for 12 to 24 hours, with gradual increase of activity.

7. 1) 80% of the clients have dysrhythmias.
   2) Heart failure.
   3) Cardiogenic shock.
   4) Papillary muscle dysfunction.
   5) Ventricular aneurysm.
   6) Pericarditis.
   7) Thromboembolism.

8. 1) Shout, shake client, and check for carotid pulse.
   2) Call a code.
   3) Start CPR/Advanced Cardiac Life Support (ACLS).
   4) Defibrillate at 360 joules.
   5) Administer epinephrine IVP.
   6) Administer lidocaine or amiodorone IVP.

9. Problem 1: Nutritional problems
   1) What to feed, when to feed, how to feed (route of administration).
   2) Collaborate with registered dietician.
   3) Enteral or parenteral nutrition.
   Problem 2: Anxiety
   1) Encourage client to calmly verbalize concerns and ask questions.
   2) Include client and family in all teaching; explain purpose of equipment and procedures.
   3) Administer anti-anxiety medications cautiously.
   Problem 3: Inability to communicate
   1) Use alternate methods of communication (picture boards, magic slates).
   2) Use hand gestures; have client use eye blinks for yes/no questions.
   3) Assess client for non-verbal communication.

Problem 4: Intensive care psychosis (sensory-perceptual problems)
1) Identify and address factors that may precipitate delirium.
2) Use clocks and calendars in the ICU to help orient to time.
3) Limit noise in ICU, such as monitoring how many equipment alarms are going off, no paging.
Problem 5: Sleep disturbances
1) Attempt to structure sleep, by creating a wake cycle: cluster activities, schedule rest periods.
2) Dim lights at night, and open curtains during the day.
3) Administer sleep medications, if needed.
Problem 6: Pain
1) Assess client's pain on 1 to 10 scale.
2) Rule out any complications secondary to pain that require medical interventions.
3) Keep client comfortable.
Problem 7: Include family/significant other in all aspect of client care
1) Share pertinent information with family.
2) Allow family to be involved in decision making.
3) Ms. Paula should discuss what to expect when visiting clients in ICU, such as machines, noise.
4) Least restrictive visiting hours.

OUTPATIENT NURSING CASE STUDY ANSWERS

1. **1)** h
   2) c
   3) e
   4) p
   5) a
   6) o
   7) b
   8) d
   9) m
   10) k
   11) f
   12) n
   13) g
   14) i
   15) l
   16) j

2. **1)** Tell the client an informed consent form must be signed for this procedure.
   2) Explain the client cannot eat or drink anything 8 hours prior to the procedure.
   3) Tell the client an IV will be started and he will be sedated during the procedure.
   4) Inform the client he will not remember the procedure when he wakes up.
   5) Tell the client the nurse will be taking vital signs every 15 to 30 minutes after the procedure.
   6) Explain the client's gag reflex will have to be intact prior to any food or drink being given, usually 2 to 4 hours.
   7) Tell the client the throat should not be painful but may experience some discomfort.
   8) When the client can drink without vomiting, the client will be discharged from outpatient clinic.
   9) Instruct the client to contact HCP if any bleeding, pain, or vomiting.

3. **1)** The client will sign informed consent form.
   2) A bowel preparation will be prescribed by the HCP the day before the procedure—which could be Golytely, Fleet's enema—and the bowel must be free of feces prior to the procedure.
   3) The client will be on a clear liquid diet 24 hours prior to the procedure and NPO 8 hours prior to the procedure (no red fluids).
   4) Explain that an IV will be started and the client will be sedated during the procedure and should not remember anything.

   5) Client will be positioned in a knee-chest position with the anal area exposed.
   6) A sigmoidoscope will be attached to suction machine and the HCP will insert the scope into rectum.
   7) After the procedure, client will be placed in a comfortable position.
   8) The nurse will assess the client's bowel sounds, vital signs, and the anal area for bleeding.
   9) The client will be able to go home if no complications.
   10) Instruct the client to report any rectal bleeding, any dizziness or light-headedness (signs of blood loss), and any abdominal pain.
   11) Explain to the client she can eat as needed and encourage the client to rest for a few days.

4. **1)** Explain the procedure to the client and gather the needed equipment.
   2) Perform hand hygiene and don non-sterile gloves.
   3) Position the client in the high-Fowler's position.
   4) Remove the sterile applicator from the culture tube by rotating the cap to break seal.
   5) Instruct the client to tilt head back and open mouth.
   6) Use tongue depressor (if desired) to depress tongue.
   7) Swab the back of the throat along the tonsillar area from left to right.
   8) Remove the applicator stick and place in the specimen tube.
   9) Insert the stick into the tube until the swab is saturated with culture medium and the cap reaches black dot.
   10) Label specimen tube and send to laboratory.

5. **1)** Tell the client to remember the acronym "RICE"—rest, ice, compression, and elevation.
   2) Rest prevents further injury and avoids stress on the injured ankle. The client should wear a brace or splint provided by the HCP.
   3) Teach the client how to use crutches so no weight can be placed on the right ankle.
   4) Tell the client to apply ice to the injury to help decrease pain and edema.
   5) Instruct client not to apply ice directly to the skin; use a towel between the ice and the skin and apply ice for 20 minutes at a time,

allowing at least 30 minutes to elapse between applications.

6) Apply a compression to support and help prevent inflammation.

7) Show the client or significant other how to apply an ACE bandage by making a figure 8 wrap.

8) Inform the client not to apply it too tightly; toes should not be cold, turn blue, or tingle.

9) Explain elevation helps the body absorb fluid that has leaked into the tissue.

10) Tell the client to elevate the right foot above the level of the heart.

11) Recommend the client use ibuprofen for pain, and take the medication every 4 hours with food; the client can alternate Tylenol to help control pain.

12) Instruct the client to return to outpatient clinic or emergency department if pain is not relieved by ibuprofen/Tylenol, foot becomes numb, the client is unable to move the toes, or they are cold to the touch, or if edema has not decreased in 48 hours.

6. Explanation: Antibiotics are not prescribed for the "common cold" because antibiotics treat bacterial infections and the common cold is caused by a virus.

1) Explain the cold symptoms will usually last about 1 or 2 weeks.

2) Recommend the client drink water, juice, and clear broth, which will help loosen congestion and prevent dehydration.

3) Recommend the client not drink alcohol, coffee, or caffeinated sodas, which will increase possibility of dehydration.

4) Recommend salt water gargle to help relieve scratchy throat—1/2 teaspoon salt in 8 ounces of warm water.

5) Recommend saline nasal drops and sprays for nasal stuffiness and congestion.

6) Zinc products are recommended for a cold and can be purchased over the counter.

7) Recommend chicken noodle soup, which may have anti-inflammatory and mucous-thinning effects which makes the client feel better.

8) Explain there are numerous over-the-counter cold and cough medications; however, they will not prevent a cold or shorten the duration of a cold. Some OTC medication may cause complications; for example, Tylenol can cause liver dysfunction, and many cause drowsiness so the client should not operate machinery or drive a car.

7. 1) h
   2) c
   3) a
   4) e
   5) b
   6) i
   7) d
   8) k
   9) f
   10) g

8. Question 1: The American Cancer Society Web site recommends the following for detecting breast cancer:

• Yearly mammograms are recommended starting at age 40 and continuing for as long as a woman is in good health.

• Clinical breast exam (CBE) is recommended about every 3 years for women in their 20s and 30s and every year for women 40 and over.

• Women should know how their breasts normally look and feel and report any breast change promptly to their healthcare provider. Breast self-exam (BSE) is an option for women starting in their 20s.

Question 2: The American Cancer Society recommends the following beginning at age 50; both men and women should follow one of these testing schedules:

• Tests that find polyps and cancer
  • Flexible sigmoidoscopy every 5 years, or
  • Colonoscopy every 10 years, or
  • Double-contrast barium enema every 5 years, or
  • CT colonography (virtual colonoscopy) every 5 years

• Tests that primarily find cancer
  • Yearly fecal occult blood test (gFOBT), or
  • Yearly fecal immunochemical test (FIT) every year, or
  • Stool DNA test (sDNA), interval uncertain

Question 3: The American Cancer Society recommends the following to screen for cervical cancer:

• All women should begin cervical cancer screening about 3 years after they begin having vaginal intercourse, but no later than 21 years old. Screening should be done every year with the regular Pap test or every 2 years using the newer, liquid-based Pap test.

• Beginning at age 30, women who have had three normal Pap test results in a row may get screened every 2 to 3 years. Women older than 30 may also get screened every 3 years with either the conventional or liquid-based Pap test, plus the human papillomavirus (HPV) test.

- Women 70 years of age or older who have had three or more normal Pap tests in a row and no abnormal Pap test results in the last 10 years may choose to stop having Pap tests.
- Women who have had a total hysterectomy (removal of the uterus and cervix) may also choose to stop having Pap tests, unless the surgery was done as a treatment for cervical cancer or pre-cancer. Women who have had a hysterectomy without removal of the cervix should continue to have Pap tests.

Question 4: The American Cancer Society recommends men make an informed decision with their doctor about whether to be tested for prostate cancer. Research has not yet proved the potential benefits of testing outweigh the harms of testing and treatment. The American Cancer Society believes men should not be tested without learning about what is known and not known about the risks and possible benefits of testing and treatment.

Starting at age 50, talk to your doctor about the pros and cons of testing so you can decide if testing is the right choice for you. If you are African American or have a father or brother who had prostate cancer before age 65, you should have this talk with your doctor starting at age 45. If you decide to be tested, you should have the PSA blood test with or without a rectal exam.

Question 5: There is no standard or routine screening test for testicular cancer. Teach the client to perform self-testicular exams monthly to feel for lumps in the testes. This cancer is often found accidently by the client.

HOME HEALTH CASE STUDY ANSWERS

1. 1) Perform hand hygiene and provide privacy for the client.
    2) Explain the procedure to the client and ensure all equipment is within reach.
    3) Open sterile catheter set package.
    4) Place sterile absorbent pad under the client's buttocks.
    5) Don sterile gloves from package on dominant hand.
    6) Remove sterile articles from tray and arrange on sterile field.
    7) Pour antiseptic solution over cotton balls or open swabs with stick end up.
    8) Lubricate end of catheter, replace in sterile sleeve, and place between the client's legs on sterile field.
    [NOTE: It is controversial to check inflation of balloon—follow hospital policy.]
    9) Cleanse the client's urinary meatus, separate the client's labia and keep separated during procedure.
    10) Use sterile gloved hand with forceps (cotton balls) or swabs to cleanse meatus; one downward stroke only and discard in non-sterile area or bag; repeat 3 or 4 times.
    11) Using sterile gloved hand insert lubricated catheter 2 inches or until urine enters tube.
    12) Inject entire contents of prefilled syringe (10 mL) into side arm of the catheter.
    13) Retract the catheter until resistance is felt.
    [NOTE: If client experiences pain, deflate balloon and insert further and reinflate.]

2. 1) Perform hand hygiene, don non-sterile gloves, and provide privacy for the client.
    2) Explain procedure to the client and ensure all equipment is within reach.
    3) Carefully remove old dressing, noting drainage and appearance of needle insertion site.
    4) Inspect site for redness, edema, inflammation, tenderness, and exudate (notify HCP if any signs of infection).
    5) Inspect catheter and hub for intactness and remove non-sterile gloves.
    6) Apply sterile gloves.
    7) Clean insertion site with material included in the dressing kit, cleanse inside to outside in a circular motion to maintain sterile technique, and cleanse about a 3-cm area.
    8) Allow area to dry and cover with transparent dressing; note the date and time of the dressing change.

    9) Secure tubing to client's clothing.
    10) Dispose of soiled dressing and equipment in separate trash bag.

3. 1) Perform hand hygiene and provide privacy for client.
    2) Explain procedure to client and ensure all equipment is within reach.
    3) Cuff the top of disposable waterproof bag and place in reach of work area.
    4) Don non-sterile gloves and place waterproof pad under client.
    5) Remove old dressing, and do not apply water if dressing is adhering to the wound. Inform the client of possible discomfort or pre-medicate 30 minutes prior to procedure if needed.
    6) Assess the drainage of dressing and dispose in the waterproof bag and remove non-sterile gloves.
    7) Prepare sterile dressing supplies; pour prescribed solution over non-mesh gauze.
    8) Don sterile gloves.
    9) Assess the wound color, character of drainage, presence of type of sutures, and presence of any drainage.
    10) Cleanse wound from least to most contaminated area.
    11) Apply fine mesh gauze into wound in a single layer; be sure to crunch gauze.
    12) Apply dry sterile 4x4 gauze over wet gauze.
    13) Cover with ABD pad and secure firmly to abdomen with tape.
    14) Remove sterile gloves and put old dressing and equipment in separate trash bag.

4. 1) Perform hand hygiene and provide privacy for client.
    2) Explain procedure to the client and ensure all equipment is within reach.
    3) Open specimen container and place cap sterile inside service up; do not touch inside of container.
    4) Give client antiseptic wipe and instruct the client to hold penis with one hand; using a circular motion, cleanse area with antiseptic wipe from center outside.
    5) Tell the client to urinate into commode then place sterile container under urine stream and collect 30 to 60 mL of urine in the cup.
    6) Remove specimen container before flow of urine stops and before releasing the penis.
    7) Replace specimen cap on the cup, and cleanse urine from external surface of container.

8) Discard gloves and wash hands.

9) Label specimen container with the client's name and pertinent data.

5. 1) Perform hand hygiene, provide privacy for the client, and place protection (towels) under the client.

2) Explain the procedure to the client, ensure all equipment is within reach, and determine if the client can make it to the bathroom or obtain a bed pan.

3) Fill water container with 750 to 1,000 mL of lukewarm solution.

4) Prime the tubing with water.

5) Hang the enema bag on IV pole at bedside 18 inches above the rectum.

6) Don non-sterile gloves.

7) Place client on left side in Sims position.

8) Lubricate tip of tubing with water-soluble lubricant.

9) Gently spread buttocks; instruct the client to take slow breaths, and insert tubing 3 to 4 inches.

10) Open regulating clamp and allow solution to flow slowly.

11) Hold tubing in place and instruct client to take slow, deep breaths.

12) After solution has infused, gently remove tubing.

13) Instruct the client to hold fluid for at least 10 to 15 minutes or as long as possible.

14) Place the client on commode or on bed pan and provide privacy until the client has expelled total volume of enema.

6. 1) Instruct the home health aide to perform hand hygiene and provide privacy for the client.

2) Tell the home health aide to explain the procedure to the client and ensure all equipment is within reach but the client does not have to wear gloves when performing irrigation.

Teach the home health aide the following and perform with the client so aide can better understand the procedure:

3) Position the client on a chair in front of the toilet.

4) Remove used pouch gently and dispose of in separate trash bag.

5) Apply irrigation sleeve over stoma and allow the end to be in the commode water.

6) Fill irrigation bag with 1,000 mL of tap water and clear tubing of air.

7) Hang irrigation bag no higher than shoulder height.

8) Lubricate tube tip and hold snuggly against stoma opening (do not force cone into stoma) and start inflow of water.

9) Allow water to flow in over 5 to 10 minutes; if cramping starts, stop the flow until cramping stops; encourage the client to take deep breaths.

10) After fluid has entered colostomy, clamp tubing and wait 15 minutes to prevent sudden backflow of water from stoma.

11) Allow 15 minutes for initial evacuation of stool from colostomy, then dry tip of sleeve and clamp irrigation sleeve and leave in place for 30 minutes to allow more stool to be evacuated.

12) Encourage the client to ambulate while sleeve is on.

13) After 30 minutes, unclamp sleeve, empty fecal content, and remove the sleeve and rinse with liquid cleanser and cool water; hang sleeve to dry.

14) Rinse stoma site with water, note if any rash or irritation around stoma (contact HCP if needed); stoma should be pink and moist. If dark purple or dry, contact HCP.

15) Apply new colostomy pouch over stoma.

7. 1) Perform hand hygiene and don non-sterile gloves.

2) Explain procedure to the client and ensure all equipment is within reach.

3) Place arm straight in dependent position and place towel under arm.

4) Place tourniquet 4 to 6 inches above client's elbow; instruct client to open and close hand.

5) Cleanse antecubital fossa with antimicrobial wipe starting at vein site and cleanse in circular motion and let dry.

6) Hold skin taut and insert needle with bevel up at 30° angle.

7) Lower needle toward skin and thread needle along path of vein.

8) When blood is obtained, pull syringe plunger back gently and then transfer blood to appropriate tube. For vacutainer system, insert blood collection tube into plastic holder while holding plastic adapter steady.

9) Fill syringe to desired amount.

10) Remove needle from vein; cover venipuncture site with a sterile sponge to stop bleeding.

8. 1) Perform hand hygiene and don non-sterile gloves.

2) Explain procedure to the client and ensure all equipment is within reach.

3) Elevate the client's head of bed.

4) Ask the client if nose has been fractured or has a deviated septum. Check for nares patency.

5) Place towel on chest and provide emesis basin.

6) Measure N/G tube from tip of the client's nose to earlobe to xiphoid process then mark tube.

7) Coil end of N/G tube over fingers.

8) Lubricate end of tube with water-soluble lubricant.

9) Have client slightly extend head, then insert tube through nostril to back of throat.

10) Ask the client to flex head forward.

11) Have the client sip water while inserting tube until predetermined mark is reached.

12) Aspirate gastric contents to determine correct tube placement.

9. 1) Teach the client to pull plunger down to 20 units of air.

2) Insert air into 70/30 bottle in upright position.

3) Flip bottle to downward position and withdraw 20 units of 70/30 insulin.

4) Have the client expose abdomen and identify an area 2 inches from umbilicus (belly button) and instruct to rotate sites (right side to left side).

5) Instruct the client to hold syringe like a dart between the thumb and forefinger.

6) Insert needle into skin at a 45° or 90° angle. client does not have to cleanse skin.

7) Slowly insert 70/30 insulin (client does not have to aspirate for blood).

8) Remove needle and apply a swab to injection site.

9) Discard needle safely so no one else can use needle (plastic milk carton).

10. 1) Instruct significant other to place chair with arms at side of bed.

2) Assist the client to dangle legs on side of bed until stable.

3) Ensure the client has nonslip shoes on.

4) Have the client scoot to side of bed, and instruct significant other how to place gait belt on client, if necessary.

5) Instruct significant other to place his or her foot closest to chair between the client's feet.

6) Rock the client and on the count of three assist client to standing position.

7) Grasp gait belt and pivot the client to chair.

8) Instruct the client to place hands on the arms of and slowly lower the client into the chair.

9) Tell the client to scoot back in the chair so the client's back is flush with back of the chair.

MENTAL HEALTH NURSING CASE STUDY ANSWERS

1. 1) d
   2) i
   3) l
   4) f
   5) a
   6) m
   7) o
   8) b
   9) h
   10) n
   11) e
   12) k
   13) g
   14) c

2. 1) Initial phase—usually the first one or two meetings in which the client's anxiety is high; during these meetings address the reason for the group and group rules, and establish a trusting relationship with the nurse leader along with appropriate interactions with group members.
   2) Working phase—these are meetings in which problems are identified, clients begin problem solving, and the group develops a sense of "we-ness"; these meetings allow the clients to accomplish goals.
   3) Termination phase—this is usually the last one or two meetings; the clients should evaluate the group experience; some clients may be anxious about ending the group, but others may be glad to disband the group.

3. 1) Hallucinations (auditory and visual).
   2) Delusions.
   3) Disorganized speech.
   4) Disorganized behavior.

4. 1) Flight of ideas.
   2) Continuous activity, and does not respect boundaries.
   3) Sexually acting out.
   4) Talkative and pressured speech.
   5) Easily distracted.
   6) Bizarre dress and grooming.
   7) Agitated or explosive.
   8) Delusions of grandeur.

5. 1) Loss of pleasure in life.
   2) Change in appetite that may cause weight loss or gain.
   3) Inability to sleep.
   4) Listless, no energy, or easily fatigued.
   5) Feelings of hopelessness or worthlessness.
   6) Inability to concentrate or think clearly.
   7) May have suicidal tendencies.

6. First, Mr. Aaron must ask Mrs. Jones directly if she is thinking of killing herself.

   Second, if Mrs. Jones says yes then Mr. Aaron must ask is she has a plan (the more specific the plan, the more serious the threat).

   Third, see if Mrs. Jones has the method available (such as sleeping pills, a gun).

   Mr. Aaron should determine if Mrs. Jones has ever attempted suicide before; this is a risk factor for attempting suicide.

7. 1) Set limits on intrusive behavior and help the client respect boundaries.
   2) Be calm, non-judgmental, and do not get "feelings" hurt.
   3) Encourage the client to walk, throw basketball, and tear rags—any type of physical activity.
   4) Discourage the client from playing competitive games such as cards, ping pong.
   5) Do not argue or become defensive with the client interpreting the nurse as being intrusive.
   6) Administer anti-mania medication (which will take up to 3 weeks to be effective).

8. 1) Do not fight Mr. Chandler's delusion.
   2) Use distraction and involve client in reality-based topics.
   3) Ask Mr. Chandler what the hallucinations are saying.
   4) Mr. Aaron must take action if Mr. Chandler is having command hallucinations (which may cause harm to self or others).
   5) Do not pretend to understand what Mr. Chandler is saying.
   6) Give short, simple directions.
   7) Orient the client by using unit orientation board (has date, month, season, and next holiday).

9. 1) Assess Mr. Jones for delirium tremens (seizure activity).
   2) Administer benzodiazepines (anti-anxiety) medications to prevent seizures, e.g., chlordiazepoxide (Librium), diazepam (Valium), clonazepam (Klonopin).
   3) Provide high-protein diet.
   4) Increase client's oral fluid intake.
   5) Monitor intravenous fluids, which may include vitamins (known as "banana boat").
   6) Keep environmental stimuli to a minimum.
   7) Monitor Mr. Jones's vital signs.

10. 1) Axis I—psychiatric diagnosis.
    2) Axis II—personality disorder.
    3) Axis III—medical or physical problems.
    4) Axis IV—psychological issues affecting the client such as being homeless or jobless, having no family, is divorced.
    5) Axis V—Global Assessment Functioning (GAF) tool; the higher the number (1–100), the more apt it will be that the client can live independently.

MATERNAL-CHILD CASE STUDY ANSWERS

1. 1) Moro reflex (startle reflex) is initiated by pulling the infant up from the floor and then releasing the infant: the legs and head extend while the arms jerk up and out with the palms up and thumbs flexed. Shortly afterward the arms are brought together and the hands clench into fists, and the infant cries loudly. The reflex normally disappears by 3 to 4 months of age.

   2) Walking (stepping reflex) is elicited when the soles of the feet touch a flat surface. The infant will attempt to "walk" by placing one foot in front of the other. This reflex disappears at 6 weeks due to an increased ratio of leg weight to strength.

   3) Rooting reflex is elicited when the infant's cheek or mouth searches for the object by moving his head in steadily decreasing arcs until the object is found. After becoming used to responding in this way (if breastfed, approximately 3 weeks after birth), the infant will move directly to the object without searching.

   4) Sucking reflex is elicited by the roof of the infant's mouth and the infant will suddenly start to suck, simulating the way the infant naturally eats.

   5) Tonic-neck reflex, known as asymmetric tonic-neck reflex or "fencing posture," is initiated when the child's head is turned to the side. The arm on that side will straighten and the opposite arm will bend (sometimes the motion will be very subtle or slight).

   6) Palmar grasp reflex is elicited when an object is placed in the infant's hand and strokes the palm. The fingers will close and the infant will grasp it; the grip is strong but unpredictable. Although it may be able to support the infant's weight, he or she may also release the grip suddenly and without warning.

   7) Plantar reflex is a normal reflex that involves plantar flexion of the foot in which toes move away from the shin, and curl down.

   8) Babinski's sign is initiated when the foot is stroked and there is dorsiflexion of the foot (foot angles toward the shin, big toe curls up).

2. For an Apgar score, a newborn is assessed at 1 minute and 5 minutes and each area can have a score of 0, 1, or 2, with 10 points as the maximum. A total score of 10 means a baby is in the best possible condition; Apgar scores of 3 or less often mean a baby needs immediate attention and care. However, only 1.4% of babies have Apgar scores less than 7 at 5 minutes after birth.

Sign	Score = 0	Score = 1	Score = 2
Heart Rate	Absent	Below 100 per minute	Above 100 per minute
Respiratory Effort	Absent	Weak, irregular, or gasping	Good, crying
Muscle Tone	Flaccid	Some flexion of arms and legs	Well flexed, or active movements of extremities
Reflex/Irritability	No response	Grimace or weak cry	Good cry
Color	Blue all over, or pale	Body pink, hands and feet blue	Pink all over

3. Assess the general health including sleep, feeding, elimination, cry, alertness, respiration, temperature, and apical pulse. A complete newborn screening includes movement, muscle tone, symmetry, and also assesses for jaundice, hydration, and umbilicus.

4. 1) i
   2) e
   3) a
   4) b
   5) d
   6) h
   7) g
   8) c
   9) g

5. Stage 1—latent phase—this is the first phase and is the longest and least intense; contractions become more frequent, helping the cervix to dilate so the baby can pass through the birth canal; the cervix will dilate approximately 3 or 4 centimeters and efface.

   Stage 1—active phase—the cervix dilates from 4 to 7 centimeters; the mother may feel intense pain or pressure in the back or abdomen during each contraction; she may feel the urge to push or bear down but must wait until the cervix is completely dilated.

   Stage 1—transition phase—the cervix fully dilates to 10 centimeters; contractions are very strong, painful, and frequent, coming every 3 to 4 minutes and lasting from 60 to 90 seconds. Stage 1 is complete when the cervix is fully dilated and effaced.

   Stage 2—this stage begins when the cervix is completely opened; the doctor will instruct the mother to push; the force of contractions will propel the baby through the birth canal; the fontanels on the baby's head allow it to fit through the narrow canal; the baby's head crowns when the widest part of it reaches the vaginal opening; pushing helps to deliver the baby's shoulders and body.

   Stage 3—this is the final stage of labor after the baby has been delivered; the placenta is delivered.

6. 1) Hygiene—shower and wash hair at any time, change pads frequently and cleanse with warm water using peri-bottle at every change, wipe from front to back, and do not douche or use internal tampons for 4 to 6 weeks. Perineal stitches are absorbable and do not need to be removed. Take a sitz bath three times a day and use perineal wipes on your perineum or hemorrhoids.

   2) Constipation—avoid constipation by eating a well-balanced diet including fruits and vegetables and drink plenty of fluids. Stool softeners or mild laxatives may be used.

   3) Exercise/rest—take frequent rest periods, especially when the baby is sleeping, avoid lifting anything heavier than the baby for 3 to 4 weeks, and do not start vigorous exercises until approved by your provider. Perineal exercises can be started when at home.

   4) Call the physician immediately if your temperature is above 100°F; you experience severe cramping or abdominal pains with chills and fever; have heavy bleeding and/or pass large blood clots; have foul-smelling vaginal discharge; have increased tenderness, redness, drainage, or separation of stitches; have pain, burning, or difficulty urinating.

   5) It is normal to feel tired or overwhelmed or have "postpartum blues" after going home; this is because of the many physical, hormonal, and emotional changes that occur after delivery. If these feelings continue for more than a few days, notify your provider.

QUESTIONS

1. The new graduate working on a medical unit night shift is concerned that the charge nurse is drinking alcohol on duty. On more than one occasion, the new graduate has smelled alcohol when the charge nurse returns from a break. Which action should the new graduate nurse implement first?
   1. Confront the charge nurse with the suspicions.
   2. Talk with the night supervisor about the concerns.
   3. Ignore the situation unless the nurse cannot do her job.
   4. Ask to speak to the nurse educator about the problem.

2. The charge nurse observes two unlicensed assistive personnel (UAPs) arguing in the hallway. Which action should the nurse implement first in this situation?
   1. Tell the manager to check on the UAPs.
   2. Instruct the UAPs to stop arguing in the hallway.
   3. Have the UAPs go to a private room to talk.
   4. Mediate the dispute between the UAPs.

3. The graduate nurse is working with an unlicensed assistive personnel (UAP) who has been an employee of the hospital for 12 years. However, tasks delegated to the UAP by the graduate nurse are frequently not completed. Which action should the graduate nurse take first?
   1. Tell the charge nurse the UAP will not do tasks as delegated by the nurse.
   2. Write up a counseling record with objective data and give it to the manager.
   3. Complete the delegated tasks and do nothing about the insubordination.
   4. Address the UAP to discuss why the tasks are not being done as requested.

4. The primary nurse informs the shift manager one of the unlicensed assistive personnel (UAPs) is falsifying vital signs. Which action should the shift manager implement first?
   1. Notify the unit manager of the potential situation of falsifying vital signs.
   2. Take the assigned client's vital signs and compare with the UAP's results.
   3. Talk to the UAP about the primary nurse's allegation.
   4. Complete a counseling record and place in the UAP's file.

5. The nurse hung the wrong intravenous antibiotic for the postoperative client. Which intervention should the nurse implement first?
   1. Assess the client for any adverse reactions.
   2. Complete the incident or adverse occurrence report.
   3. Administer the correct intravenous antibiotic medication.
   4. Notify the client's healthcare provider.

6. The nurse, a licensed practical nurse (LPN), and an unlicensed assistive personnel (UAP) are caring for clients in a critical care unit. Which task would be most appropriate for the nurse to assign/delegate?
   1. Instruct the UAP to obtain the client's serum glucose level.
   2. Request the LPN to change the central line dressing.
   3. Ask the LPN to bathe the client and change the bed linens.
   4. Tell the UAP to obtain urine output for the 12-hour shift.

7. Which task should the critical care nurse delegate to the unlicensed assistive personnel (UAP)?
   1. Check the pulse oximeter reading for the client on a ventilator.
   2. Take the client's sterile urine specimen to the laboratory.
   3. Obtain the vital signs for the client in an Addisonian crisis.
   4. Assist the HCP with performing a paracentesis at the bedside.

8. Which situation would prompt the healthcare team to utilize the client's advance directive when needing to make decisions for the client?
   1. The client with a head injury who is exhibiting decerebrate posturing.
   2. The client with a C-6 spinal cord injury (SCI) who is on a ventilator.
   3. The client in chronic renal disease who is being placed on dialysis.
   4. The client diagnosed with terminal cancer who is mentally retarded.

9. The nurse is caring for clients on a skilled nursing unit. Which task should not be delegated to the unlicensed assistive personnel (UAP)?
   1. Instruct the UAP to apply sequential compression devices to the client on strict bed rest.
   2. Ask the UAP to assist the radiology tech to perform a STAT portable chest x-ray.
   3. Request the UAP to prepare the client for a wound debridement at the bedside.
   4. Tell the UAP to obtain the intakes and outputs (I&Os) for all the clients on the unit.

10. The nurse is assigned to a quality improvement committee to decide on a quality improvement project for the unit. Which issue should the nurse discuss at the committee meetings?
    1. Systems that make it difficult for the nurses to do their job.
    2. How unhappy the nurses are with their current pay scale.
    3. Collective bargaining activity at a nearby hospital.
    4. The number of medication errors committed by an individual nurse.

11. The clinic manager is discussing osteoporosis with the clinic staff. Which activity is an example of a secondary nursing intervention when discussing osteoporosis?
    1. Obtain a bone density evaluation test on a female client older than 50.
    2. Perform a spinal screening examination on all female clients.
    3. Encourage the client to walk 30 minutes daily on a hard surface.
    4. Discuss risk factors for developing osteoporosis.

12. The female home health (HH) aide calls the office and reports pain after feeling a pulling in her back when she was transferring the client from the bed to the wheel-chair. Which priority action should the HH nurse tell the HH aide?
    1. Explain how to perform isometric exercises.
    2. Instruct her to go to the local emergency room.
    3. Tell her to complete an occurrence report.
    4. Recommend that she apply an ice pack to the back.

13. The female client with osteoarthritis is 6 weeks postoperative for open reduction and internal fixation of the right hip. The home health (HH) aide tells the HH nurse the client will not get in the shower in the morning because she "hurts all over." Which action would be most appropriate by the HH nurse?
    1. Tell the HH aide to allow the client to stay in bed until the pain goes away.
    2. Instruct the HH aide to get the client up to a chair and give her a bath.
    3. Explain to the HH aide the client should get up and take a warm shower.
    4. Arrange an appointment for the client to visit her healthcare provider.

14. The home health (HH) nurse is discussing the care of a client with the female HH aide. Which task should the HH nurse delegate to the HH aide?
  1. Instruct her to assist the client with a shower.
  2. Ask her to prepare the breakfast meal for the client.
  3. Request her to take the client to an HCP's appointment.
  4. Tell her to show the client how to use a glucometer.

15. The unlicensed assistive personnel (UAP) is preparing to provide postmortem care to a client with a questionable diagnosis of anthrax. Which instruction is priority for the nurse to provide to the UAP?
  1. The UAP is not at risk for contracting an illness.
  2. The UAP should wear a mask, gown, and gloves.
  3. The UAP may skip performing postmortem care.
  4. Ask whether the UAP is pregnant before she enters the client's room.

16. The client on a medical unit died of a communicable disease. Which information should the nurse provide to the mortuary workers?
  1. No information can be released to the mortuary service.
  2. The nurse should tell the funeral home the client's diagnosis.
  3. Ask the family for permission to talk with the mortician.
  4. Refer the funeral home to the HCP for information.

17. The new graduate nurse is assigned to work with an unlicensed assistive personnel (UAP) to provide care for a group of clients. Which action by the nurse is the best method to evaluate whether delegated care is being provided?
  1. Check with the clients to see whether they are satisfied.
  2. Ask the charge nurse whether the UAP is qualified.
  3. Make rounds to see that the clients are being turned.
  4. Watch the UAP perform all the delegated tasks.

18. The charge nurse is making assignments on a pediatric unit. Which client should be assigned to the licensed practical nurse (LPN)?
  1. The 6-year-old client diagnosed with sickle cell crisis.
  2. The 8-year-old client diagnosed with biliary atresia.
  3. The 10-year-old client diagnosed with anaphylaxis.
  4. The 11-year-old client diagnosed with pneumonia.

19. The nurse is caring for the following clients on a medical unit. Which client should the nurse assess first?
  1. The client with disseminated intravascular coagulation (DIC) who has blood oozing from the intravenous site.
  2. The client with benign prostatic hypertrophy (BPH) who is complaining of terminal dribbling and inability to empty bladder.
  3. The client with renal calculi who is complaining of severe flank pain and has hematuria.
  4. The client with Addison's disease who has bronze skin pigmentation and hypoglycemia.

20. The charge nurse is making assignments in the day surgery center. Which client should be assigned to the most experienced nurse?
  1. The client who had surgery for an inguinal hernia and who is being prepared for discharge.
  2. The client who is in the preoperative area and who is scheduled for laparoscopic cholecystectomy.
  3. The client who has completed scheduled chemotherapy treatment and who is receiving two units of blood.
  4. The client who has end-stage renal disease and who has had an arteriovenous fistula created.

21. The charge nurse of a critical care unit is making assignments for the night shift. Which client should be assigned to the graduate nurse who has just completed an internship?
    1. The client diagnosed with a head injury resulting from a motor vehicle accident (MVA) whose Glasgow Coma Scale score is 13.
    2. The client diagnosed with inflammatory bowel disease (IBD) who has severe diarrhea and has a serum K+ level of 3.2 mEq/L.
    3. The client diagnosed with Addison's disease who is lethargic and has a BP of 80/45, P of 124, and R rate of 28.
    4. The client diagnosed with hyperthyroidism who has undergone a thyroidectomy and has a positive Trousseau's sign.

22. The nurse on a medical unit has just received the evening shift report. Which client should the nurse assess first?
    1. The client diagnosed with a deep vein thrombosis (DVT) who has a heparin drip infusion and a PTT of 92.
    2. The client diagnosed with pneumonia who has an oral temperature of 100.2°F.
    3. The client diagnosed with cystitis who complains of burning on urination.
    4. The client diagnosed with pancreatitis who complains of pain that is an 8.

23. The 75-year-old client has undergone an open cholecystectomy for cholelithiasis 2 days ago and has a t-tube drain in place. Which intervention should the nurse delegate to the unlicensed assistive personnel (UAP)? **Select all that apply.**
    1. Explain the procedure for using the patient-controlled analgesia (PCA) pump.
    2. Check the client's abdominal dressing for drainage.
    3. Take and record the client's vital signs.
    4. Empty the client's indwelling catheter bag at the end of the shift.
    5. Assist the client to ambulate in the hallway three to four times a day.

24. The surgical unit has a low census and is overstaffed. Which staff member should the house supervisor notify first and request to stay home?
    1. The nurse who has the most vacation time.
    2. The nurse who requested to be off.
    3. The nurse who has the least experience on the unit.
    4. The nurse who has called in sick the previous 2 days.

25. The nurse and the unlicensed assistive personnel (UAP) are caring for residents in a long-term care facility. Which task should the nurse delegate to the UAP?
    1. Apply a sterile dressing to a Stage IV pressure wound.
    2. Check the blood glucose level of a resident who is weak and shaky.
    3. Document the amount of food the residents ate after a meal.
    4. Teach the residents how to play different types of bingo.

26. The director of nurses in a long-term care facility observes the licensed practical nurse (LPN) charge nurse explaining to an unlicensed assistive personnel (UAP) how to calculate the amount of food a resident has eaten from the food tray. Which action should the director of nurses implement?
    1. Ask the charge nurse to teach all the other UAPs.
    2. Encourage the nurse to continue to work with the UAP.
    3. Tell the charge nurse to discuss this in a private area.
    4. Give the UAP a better explanation of the procedure.

27. The wound care nurse in a long-term care facility asks the unlicensed assistive personnel (UAP) for assistance. Which task should not be delegated to the UAP?
    1. Apply the wound debriding paste to the wound.
    2. Keep the resident's heels off the surface of the bed.
    3. Turn the resident at least every 2 hours.
    4. Encourage the resident to drink a high-protein shake.

28. The older adult client becomes confused and wanders in the hallways. Which fall precaution intervention should the nurse implement first?
1. Place a Posey vest restraint on the client.
2. Move the client to a room near the station.
3. Ask the HCP for an antipsychotic medication.
4. Raise all four side rails on the client's bed.

29. The clinic nurse is caring for a client diagnosed with osteoarthritis. The client tells the nurse, "I am having problems getting in and out of my bathtub." Which intervention should the clinic nurse implement first?
1. Determine whether the client has grab bars in the bathroom.
2. Encourage the client to take a shower instead of a bath.
3. Initiate a referral to a physical therapist for the client.
4. Discuss whether the client takes nonsteroidal anti-inflammatory drugs (NSAIDs).

30. The employee health nurse has cared for six clients who have similar complaints. The clients have a fever, nausea, vomiting, and diarrhea. Which action should the nurse implement first after assessing the clients?
1. Have another employee drive the clients home.
2. Notify the public health department immediately.
3. Send the clients to the emergency department.
4. Obtain stool specimens from the clients.

31. The clinic nurse is caring for clients in a pediatric clinic. Which client should the nurse assess first?
1. The 4-year-old child who fell and is complaining of left leg pain.
2. The 3-year-old child who is drooling and does not want to swallow.
3. The 8-year-old child who has complained of a headache for 2 days.
4. The 10-year-old child who is thirsty all the time and has lost weight.

32. Which statement is an example of community-oriented, population-focused nursing?
1. The nurse cares for an older adult client who had a kidney transplant and who lives in the community.
2. The nurse develops an educational program for the type 2 diabetics in the community.
3. The nurse refers a client with Cushing's syndrome to the registered dietician.
4. The nurse provides the client chronic renal disease with pamphlets.

33. The home health (HH) agency director of nursing is making assignments for the nurses. Which client should be assigned to the HH nurse new to HH nursing?
1. The client diagnosed with AIDS who is dyspneic and confused.
2. The client who does not have the money to get prescriptions filled.
3. The client with full-thickness burns on the arm who needs a dressing change.
4. The client complaining of pain who is diagnosed with diabetic neuropathy.

34. The home health (HH) nurse along with an HH aide is caring for a client who is 3 weeks postoperative for open reduction and internal fixation of a right hip fracture. Which task would be appropriate for the nurse to delegate to the aide?
1. Instruct the HH aide to palpate the right pedal pulse.
2. Ask the HH aide to change the right hip dressing.
3. Tell the HH aide to elevate the right leg on two pillows.
4. Request the HH aide to mop the client's bedroom floor.

35. The charge nurse has received laboratory data for clients in the medical department. Which client would require intervention by the charge nurse?
1. The client diagnosed with a myocardial infarction (MI) who has an elevated troponin level.
2. The client receiving the IV anticoagulant heparin who has a partial thromboplastin time (PTT) of 68 seconds.
3. The client diagnosed with end-stage liver failure who has an elevated ammonia level.
4. The client receiving the anticonvulsant phenytoin (Dilantin) who has levels of 24 mg/dL.

36. Which client would most benefit from acupuncture, a traditional Chinese medicine considered complementary alternative medicine?
1. The client who is diagnosed with deep vein thrombosis.
2. The client who is diagnosed with Alzheimer's disease.
3. The client diagnosed with reactive airway disease.
4. The client diagnosed with osteoarthritis.

37. The home health (HH) nurse notes the 88-year-old female client is unable to cook for herself and mainly eats frozen foods and sandwiches. Which intervention should the nurse implement?
1. Discuss the situation with the client's family.
2. Refer the client to the HH occupational therapist.
3. Request the HH aide to cook all the client's meals.
4. Contact the community's Meals on Wheels.

38. Which legal intervention should the nurse implement on the initial visit when admitting a client to the home healthcare agency?
1. Discuss the professional boundary-crossing policy with the client.
2. Provide the client with a copy of the NAHC Bill of Rights.
3. Tell the client how many visits the client will have while on service.
4. Explain that the client must be homebound to be eligible for home healthcare.

39. The unlicensed assistive personnel (UAP) accidentally pulled the client's chest tube out while assisting the client to the bedside commode (BSC). Which intervention should the nurse implement first?
1. Securely tape petroleum gauze over the insertion site.
2. Instruct the UAP how to move a client with a chest tube.
3. Assess the client's respirations and lung sounds.
4. Obtain a chest tube and a chest tube insertion tray.

40. The nurse and licensed practical nurse (LPN) have been assigned to care for clients on a pediatric unit. Which nursing task should be assigned to the LPN?
1. Administer PO medications to a client diagnosed with gastroenteritis.
2. Take the routine vital signs for all the clients on the pediatric unit.
3. Transcribe the HCP's orders into the computer.
4. Assess the urinary output of a client diagnosed with nephrotic syndrome.

41. The hospital will be implementing a new medication administration record (MAR) for documenting medication administration. Which action should the clinical manager take first when implementing the new MAR?
1. Discuss the new MAR with each nurse individually.
2. Schedule meetings on all shifts to discuss the new MAR.
3. Require the nurse to read a handout explaining the new MAR.
4. Ask the nurses to watch a video explaining the new MAR.

42. Which client warrants immediate intervention from the nurse on the medical unit?
1. The client diagnosed with an abdominal aortic aneurysm who has an audible bruit.
2. The client with adult respiratory distress syndrome (ARDS) who has bilateral crackles.
3. The client diagnosed with bacterial meningitis who has nucal rigidity and neck pain.
4. The client with Crohn's disease who has right lower abdominal pain and has diarrhea.

43. Which assessment data warrants immediate intervention by the nurse for the client diagnosed with chronic kidney disease (CKD) who is on peritoneal dialysis?
1. The client's serum creatinine level is 2.4 mg/dL.
2. The client's abdomen is soft to touch and nontender.
3. The dialysate being removed from the abdomen is cloudy.
4. The dialysate instilled was 1,500 mL and removed was 2,100 mL.

44. The nurse is taking a history on a client in a women's clinic when the client tells the nurse, "I have been trying to get pregnant for 3 years." Which question is the nurse's best response?
1. "How many attempts have you made to get pregnant?"
2. "What have you tried to help you get pregnant?"
3. "Does your insurance cover infertility treatments?"
4. "Have you considered adoption as an option?"

45. The nurse working at the county hospital is admitting a client who is Rh-negative to the labor and delivery unit. The client is gravida 2, para 0. Which assessment data is most important for the nurse to assess?
1. Why the client did not have a viable baby with the first pregnancy.
2. If the mother received a Rhogam injection after the last pregnancy.
3. The period of time between the client's pregnancies.
4. When the mother terminated the previous pregnancy.

46. The unconscious 4-year-old child with bruises covering the torso in varying stages of healing is brought to the emergency department by paramedics. The nurse notes small burn marks on the child's genitalia. Which actions should the nurse implement? **Select all that apply.**
1. Notify Child Protective Services.
2. Ask the parent how the child was injured.
3. Perform a thorough examination for more injuries.
4. Tell the parents that the police have been called.
5. Prepare the child for skull x-rays and a CT scan.

47. The 24-month-old toddler is admitted to the pediatric unit with vomiting and diarrhea. Which interventions should the nurse implement? Rank in order of performance.
1. Teach the parent about weighing diapers to determine output status.
2. Show the parent the call light and explain safety regimens.
3. Assess the toddler's tissue turgor.
4. Place the appropriate size diapers in the room.
5. Take the toddler's vital signs.

48. The nurse has received the shift report. Which client should the nurse assess first?
1. The client diagnosed with a deep vein thrombosis (DVT) who complains of a feeling of doom.
2. The client diagnosed with gallbladder ulcer disease who refuses to eat the food served.
3. The client diagnosed with pancreatitis who wants the nasogastric tube removed.
4. The client diagnosed with osteoarthritis who is complaining of stiff joints.

49. The nurse and the unlicensed assistive personnel (UAP) are caring for clients on a pediatric unit. Which task should the nurse delegate to the UAP?
1. Sit with the 6-year-old client while the parent goes outside to smoke.
2. Stay with the 4-year-old client during scheduled play therapy sessions.
3. Position the 2-year-old client for the postural drainage therapy.
4. Weigh the diaper of the 6-month-old client who is on intake and output (I&O).

50. The home health nurse is planning his rounds for the day. Which client should the nurse plan to see first?
1. The 56-year-old client diagnosed with multiple sclerosis who is complaining of a cough.
2. The 78-year-old client diagnosed with congestive heart failure (CHF) who reports losing 3 pounds.
3. The 42-year-old client diagnosed with an L-5 spinal cord injury who has developed a Stage 4 pressure ulcer.
4. The 80-year-old client diagnosed with a cerebrovascular accident (CVA) who has right-sided paralysis.

51. The nurse is preparing to perform a sterile dressing change on a client with full-thickness burns on the right leg. Which intervention should the nurse implement first?
  1. Pre-medicate the client with a narcotic analgesic.
  2. Prepare the equipment and bandages at the bedside.
  3. Remove the old dressing with non-sterile gloves.
  4. Place a sterile glove on the dominant hand.

52. The physical therapist has notified the unit secretary that the client will be ambulated in 45 minutes. After receiving notification from the unit secretary, which task should the charge nurse delegate to the unlicensed assistive personnel (UAP)?
  1. Administer a pain medication 30 minutes before therapy.
  2. Give the client a washcloth to wash his or her face before walking.
  3. Check to make sure the client has been offered the use of the bathroom.
  4. Find a walker that is the correct height for the client to use.

53. The volunteer on a medical unit tells the nurse that one of the clients on the unit is her neighbor and asks about the client's condition. Which information should the nurse discuss with the volunteer?
  1. Determine how well she knows the client before talking with the volunteer.
  2. Tell the volunteer the client's condition in layperson's terms.
  3. Ask the client if it is all right to talk with the volunteer.
  4. Explain that client information is on a need-to-know basis only.

54. The medical unit is governed by a system of shared governance. Which statement best describes an advantage of this system?
  1. It guarantees that unions will not be able to come into the hospital.
  2. It makes the manager responsible for sharing information with the staff.
  3. It involves staff nurses in the decision-making process of the unit.
  4. It is a system used to represent the nurses in labor disputes.

55. The visitor on a medical unit is shouting and making threats about harming the staff because of perceived poor care his loved one has received. Which statement is the nurse's best initial response?
  1. "If you don't stop shouting, I will have to call security."
  2. "I hear that you are frustrated. Can we discuss the issues calmly?"
  3. "Sir, you are disrupting the unit. Calm down or leave the hospital."
  4. "This type of behavior is uncalled for and will not resolve anything."

56. The experienced nurse has recently taken a position on a medical unit in a community hospital, but after 1 week on the job, he finds that the staffing is not what was discussed during his employment interview. Which approach would be most appropriate for the nurse to take when attempting to resolve the issue?
  1. Immediately give a 2-week notice and find a different job.
  2. Discuss the situation with the manager who interviewed him.
  3. Talk with the other employees about the staffing situation.
  4. Tell the charge nurse the staffing is not what was explained to him.

57. The nurse is preparing to administer the client's first intravenous antibiotic. Prioritize the nurse's actions from first (1) to last (5).
  1. Check the healthcare provider's order in the chart.
  2. Determine if the client has any known allergies.
  3. Hang the secondary IV piggyback higher than the primary IV.
  4. Set the intravenous pump at the correct rate.
  5. Determine if the antibiotic is compatible with the primary IV.

58. At 0830, the day shift nurse is preparing to administer medications to the client. Which action should the nurse take first?

Client's Name:	Account Number: 123456	Allergies: NKDA	
Height: 62 inches	**Weight:** 105 pounds		
Date | **Medication**	**2301–0700**	**0701–1500**	**1501–2300**
Lanoxin (digoxin) 0.125 mg PO every day		0900	
Lasix (furosemide) 40 mg PO BID		0900	1600
Zantac (ranitidine) 150 mg in 250 mL NS IV continuous infusion every 24 hours	0300 NN@ 11 mL/hr		
Vancomycin 850 mg IVPB every 24 hours		1200	1800
Signature/Initials	**Day Nurse RN DN**	**Night Nurse RN NN**	

1. Check the client's armband against the medication administration record (MAR).
2. Assess the client's IV site for redness and patency.
3. Ask for the client's date of birth.
4. Determine the client's last K– level.

59. A major disaster has been called, and the charge nurse on a medical unit must recommend to the medical discharge officer on rounds which clients to discharge. Which client should not be discharged?
1. The client diagnosed with chronic angina pectoris who has been on new medication for 2 days.
2. The client diagnosed with deep vein thrombosis (DVT) who has had heparin discontinued and has been on warfarin (Coumadin) for 4 days.
3. The client with an infected leg wound who is receiving vancomycin IVPB every 24 hours for methicillin-resistant *Staphylococcus aureus* (MRSA) infection.
4. The client diagnosed with COPD who has the following arterial blood gas (ABG) levels: pH, 7.34; P_{CO_2}, 55; H_{CO_3}, 28; Pa_{O_2}, 89.

60. The nurse has been named in a lawsuit concerning the care provided. Which action should the nurse take first?
1. Consult with the hospital's attorney.
2. Review the client's chart.
3. Purchase personal liability insurance.
4. Discuss the case with the supervisor.

61. The nurse has accepted the position of clinical manager for a medical-surgical unit. Which role is an important aspect of this management position?
1. Evaluate the job performance of the staff.
2. Be the sole decision maker for the unit.
3. Take responsibility for the staff nurse's actions.
4. Attend the medical staff meetings.

62. The charge nurse notices that one of the staff takes frequent breaks, has unpredictable mood swings, and often volunteers to care for clients who require narcotics. Which priority action should the charge nurse implement regarding this employee?
1. Discuss the nurse's actions with the unit manager.
2. Confront the nurse about the behavior.
3. Do not allow the nurse to take breaks alone.
4. Prepare an occurrence report on the employee.

63. A male HCP frequently tells jokes with sexual overtones at the nursing station. Which action should the female charge nurse implement?
1. Tell the HCP that the jokes are inappropriate and offensive.
2. Report the behavior to the medical staff committee.
3. Discuss the problem with the chief nursing officer.
4. Call a Code Purple and have the nurses surround the HCP.

64. The night shift nurse is caring for clients on the surgical unit. Which client situation would warrant immediate notification of the surgeon?
1. The client who is 2 days postoperative for bowel resection and who refuses to turn, cough, and deep breathe.
2. The client who is 5 hours postoperative for abdominal hysterectomy who reported feeling a "pop" and then her pain went away.
3. The client who is 2 hours postoperative for TKR and who has 400 mL in the cell-saver collection device.
4. The client who is 1 day postoperative for bilateral thyroidectomy and who has a negative Chvostek sign.

65. Which client should the nurse in the post-anesthesia care unit (PACU) assess first?
1. The client who received general anesthesia who is complaining of a sore throat.
2. The client who had right knee surgery and has a pulse oximeter reading of 90%.
3. The client who received epidural surgery and has a palpable 2+ dorsalis pedal pulse.
4. The client who had abdominal surgery and has green bile draining from the N/G tube.

66. The client with a below-the-knee amputation (BKA) has a large amount of bright red blood on the residual limb dressing and the nurse suspects an arterial bleed. Which intervention should the nurse implement first?
1. Increase the client's intravenous rate.
2. Assess the client's vital signs.
3. Apply a tourniquet above the amputation.
4. Notify the client's healthcare provider.

67. The client who had surgery on the right elbow has no right radial pulse and the fingers are cold, the client complains of tingling, and she cannot move the fingers of the right hand. Which intervention should the nurse implement first?
1. Document the findings in the client's chart.
2. Elevate the client's right hand.
3. Assess the radial pulse with the Doppler.
4. Notify the client's healthcare provider.

68. The HCP writes an order for the client with a fractured right hip to ambulate with a walker four times per day. Which action should the nurse implement?
1. Tell the unlicensed assistive personnel (UAP) to ambulate the client with the walker.
2. Request a referral to the physical therapy department.
3. Obtain a walker that is appropriate for the client's height.
4. Notify the social worker of the HCP's order for a walker.

69. Which task would be most appropriate for the nurse to delegate to the unlicensed assistive personnel (UAP) working on a surgical unit?
1. Escort the client to the smoking area outside.
2. Obtain vital signs on a newly admitted client.
3. Administer a feeding to the client with a gastrostomy tube.
4. Check the toes of a client who just had a cast application.

70. The licensed practical nurse (LPN) is working in a surgical rehabilitation unit. Which nursing task would be most appropriate for the LPN to implement?
1. Bathe the client who is incontinent of urine.
2. Document the amount of food the client eats.
3. Conduct the afternoon bingo game in the lobby.
4. Perform routine dressing changes on assigned clients.

71. The unlicensed assistive personnel (UAP) is changing a full sharps container in the client's room. Which action should the nurse implement?
1. Tell the UAP she cannot change the sharps container.
2. Explain the housekeeping department changes the sharps containers.
3. Praise the UAP for taking the initiative to change the sharps container.
4. Report the behavior to the clinical manager on the unit.

72. The unlicensed assistive personnel (UAP) tells the nurse the client who is 5 hours postoperative for an L-3/L-4 laminectomy is complaining of feeling numbness in both feet. Which intervention should the nurse implement?
1. Ask the UAP to take the client's vital signs.
2. Request the UAP to log roll the client to the right side.
3. Complete the neurovascular assessment on the client's legs.
4. Contact the physical therapist to check the client.

73. The ED nurse is requesting a bed in the intensive care unit (ICU). The ICU charge nurse must request a transfer of one client from the ICU to the surgical unit to make room for the client coming into the ICU from the ED. Which client should the ICU charge nurse request to transfer to the surgical unit?
1. The client diagnosed with flail chest who has just come from the operating room with a right-sided chest tube.
2. The client diagnosed with acute diverticulitis who is 1 day postoperative for creation of a sigmoid colostomy.
3. The client who is 1 day postoperative for total hip replacement (THR) whose incisional dressing is dry and intact.
4. The client who is 2 days postoperative for repair of a fractured femur and who has had a fat embolism.

74. A terrible storm causes the electricity to go out in the hospital and the emergency generator lights come on. Which action should the charge nurse implement?
1. Request all family members to leave the hospital as soon as possible.
2. Instruct the staff to plug critical electrical equipment into the red outlets.
3. Have the unlicensed assistive personnel (UAP) place a portable flashlight on each bedside table.
4. Contact the maintenance department to determine how long the electricity will be out.

75. The HCP is angry and yelling in the nurse's station because the client's laboratory data are not available. Which action should the charge nurse implement first?
1. Contact the laboratory for the client's results.
2. Ask the HCP to step into the nurse's office.
3. Tell the HCP to discuss the issue with the laboratory.
4. Report the HCP's behavior to the chief nursing officer.

76. The staff nurse is concerned about possible increasing infection rates among clients with peripherally inserted central catheters (PICCs). The nurse has noticed several clients with problems in the last few months. Which action would be appropriate for the staff nurse to implement first?
1. Discuss the infections with the chief nursing officer.
2. Contact the infection control nurse to discuss the problem.
3. Assume the employee health nurse is monitoring the situation.
4. Volunteer to be on an ad hoc committee to research the infection rate.

77. The charge nurse on the 30-bed surgical unit has been told to send one staff member to the medical unit. The surgical unit is full, with multiple clients who require custodial care. Which staff member would be most appropriate to send to the medical unit?
1. Send the unlicensed assistive personnel (UAP) who has worked on the surgical unit for 5 years.
2. Send the RN who has worked in the hospital for 8 years in a variety of areas.
3. Send the licensed practical nurse (LPN) who has 3 years of experience, which includes 6 months on the medical unit.
4. Send the new graduate nurse who is orienting to the surgical unit.

78. The nurse educator is discussing fire safety with new employees. List in order of performance the following actions the nurse should teach to ensure the safety of clients and employees in the case of fire on the unit.
    1. Extinguish.
    2. Rescue.
    3. Confine.
    4. Alert.

79. The client tells the nurse, "I am having surgery on my right knee." However, the operative permit is for surgery on the left knee. Which action should the nurse implement first?
    1. Notify the operating room team.
    2. Initiate the time-out procedure.
    3. Clarify the correct extremity with the client.
    4. Call the surgeon to discuss the discrepancy.

80. The older adult client fell and fractured her left femur. The nurse finds the client crying, and she tells the nurse, "I don't want to go to the nursing home but my son says I have to." Which response would be most appropriate by the nurse?
    1. "Let me call a meeting of the healthcare team and your son."
    2. "Has the social worker talked to you about this already?"
    3. "Why are you so upset about going to the nursing home?"
    4. "I can see you are upset. Would you like to talk about it?"

81. The client is confused and pulling at the IV and indwelling catheter. Which order from the HCP should the nurse clarify concerning restraining the client?
    1. Restrain the client's wrists, as needed.
    2. Offer the client fluids every 2 hours.
    3. Apply a hand mitt to the arm opposite the IV site for 12 hours.
    4. Check circulation of the restrained limb every 2 hours.

82. The charge nurse on a 20-bed surgical unit has one RN, two licensed practical nurses (LPNs), and two unlicensed assistive personnel (UAPs) for a 12-hour shift. Which task would be an inappropriate delegation of assignments?
    1. The RN will perform the shift assessments.
    2. The LPN should administer all IVP medications.
    3. The UAP will complete all a.m. care.
    4. The RN will monitor laboratory values.

83. The head nurse is completing the yearly performance evaluation on a nurse. Which data regarding the nurse's performance should be included in the evaluation?
    1. The number of times the nurse has been tardy.
    2. The attitude of the nurse at the client's bedside.
    3. The thank you notes the nurse received from clients.
    4. The chart audits of the clients for whom the nurse cared.

84. The nurse is discharging the 72-year-old client who is 5 days postoperative for repair of a fractured hip with comorbid medical conditions. At this time, which referral would be the most appropriate for the nurse to make for this client?
    1. To a home healthcare agency.
    2. To a senior citizen center.
    3. To a rehabilitation facility.
    4. To an outpatient physical therapist.

85. The nurse is caring for clients on a 12-bed intermediate care surgical unit. Which task should the nurse implement first?
    1. Reinsert the nasogastric tube for the client who has pulled it out.
    2. Complete the preoperative checklist for the client scheduled for surgery.
    3. Instruct the client who is being discharged home about colostomy care.
    4. Change the client's surgical dressing that has a 20 cm area of drainage.

86. The nurse is preparing to administer medications to clients on a surgical unit. Which medication should the nurse question administering?
    1. The antiplatelet clopidogrel (Plavix) to a client scheduled for surgery.
    2. The anticoagulant enoxaparin (Lovenox) to a client who had a TKR.
    3. The sliding scale insulin Humalog to a client who had a Whipple procedure.
    4. The aminoglycoside vancomycin to a client allergic to the antibiotic penicillin.

87. The nurse is caring for clients on a surgical intensive care unit. Which client should the nurse assess first?
    1. The client who is 4 hours postoperative for abdominal surgery who is complaining of abdominal pain and has hypoactive bowel sounds.
    2. The client who is 1 day postoperative for total hip replacement (THR) who has voided 550 mL of clear amber urine in the last 8 hours.
    3. The client who is 8 hours postoperative for open cholecystectomy who has a T-tube draining green bile.
    4. The client who is 12 hours postoperative for total knee replacement (TKR) who is complaining of numbness and tingling in the foot.

88. Which situation should the charge nurse in the critical care unit address first after receiving the shift report?
    1. Talk to the family member who is irate over his loved one's nursing care.
    2. Complete the 90-day probationary evaluation for a new ICU graduate intern.
    3. Call the laboratory concerning the type and crossmatch for a client who needs blood.
    4. Arrange for a client to be transferred to the telemetry step-down unit.

89. The nurse in the critical care unit of a medical center answers the phone and the person says, "There is a bomb in the hospital kitchen." Which action should the nurse take?
    1. Notify the kitchen that there is a bomb.
    2. Call the operator to trace the phone call.
    3. Notify the hospital security department.
    4. Call the local police department.

90. The critical care unit is having problems with staff members clocking in late and clocking out early from the shift. Which statement by the charge nurse indicates he has a democratic leadership style?
    1. "You cannot clock out 1 minute before your shift is complete."
    2. "As long as your work is done you can clock out any time you want."
    3. "We are going to have a meeting to discuss the clocking in procedure."
    4. "The clinical manager will take care of anyone who clocks out early."

91. The nurse in the burn unit is preparing to perform a wound dressing change at the bedside. Which interventions should the nurse implement? Rank in order of priority.
    1. Obtain the needed supplies for the procedure.
    2. Explain the procedure to the client.
    3. Remove the old dressing with non-sterile gloves.
    4. Medicate the client with narcotic analgesics.
    5. Assess the client's burned area.

92. Which client should the charge nurse of a long-term care facility see first after receiving shift report?
    1. The client who is unhappy about being placed in a long-term care facility.
    2. The client who wants to have the HCP to order a nightly glass of wine.
    3. The client who is upset because the call light was not answered for 30 minutes.
    4. The client whose son is being discharged from the hospital after heart surgery.

93. The male client in a long-term care facility complains that the staff does not listen to his complaints unless a family member also complains. Which action should the director of nurses implement?
    1. Call a staff meeting and tell the staff to listen to the resident when he talks to them.
    2. Determine who neglected to listen to the resident and place the staff member on leave.
    3. Ignore the situation because a resident in long-term care cannot determine his needs.
    4. Talk with the resident about his concerns and then initiate a plan of action.

94. The newly admitted client in a long-term care facility stays in the room and refuses to participate in client activities. Which statement is a priority for the nurse to discuss with the client?
    1. "You have to get out of this room or you will never make friends here at the home."
    2. "It is not so bad living here; you are lucky that we care about what happens to you."
    3. "You seem sad; would you like to talk about how you are feeling about being here?"
    4. "The activities director can arrange for someone to come and visit you in your room."

95. The charge nurse overhears two unlicensed assistive personnel (UAPs) discussing a client in the hallway. Which action should the charge nurse implement first?
    1. Remind the UAPs that clients should not be discussed in a public area.
    2. Tell the unit manager that the UAPs might have been overheard.
    3. Have the UAPs review policies on client confidentiality and HIPAA.
    4. Find some nursing tasks the UAPs can be performing at this time.

96. The family member of a client in a long-term care facility is unhappy with the care being provided for the loved one. Which person would be most appropriate to investigate the complaint and report the findings during a client care conference?
    1. The ombudsperson for the facility.
    2. The social worker for the facility.
    3. The family member who is unhappy.
    4. The director of nurses.

97. The 65-year-old client is being discharged from the hospital following major abdominal surgery and is unable to drive. Which referral should the nurse make to ensure continuity of care?
    1. A church that can provide transportation.
    2. A home health agency.
    3. An outpatient clinic.
    4. The healthcare provider's office.

98. The nurse in an assisted living facility notes that the male client has several new bruises on both of his arms and hands. Which intervention should the nurse implement first?
    1. File an elder abuse report with the Department of Human Services.
    2. Ask the client whether he has fallen and hurt himself during the night.
    3. Check the medication administration record (MAR) to determine which medications the client is receiving.
    4. Notify the client's family of the bruises so they are not surprised on their visit.

99. The resident in a long-term care facility tells the nurse, "I think my family just put me here to die because they think I am too much trouble." Which statement is the nurse's best response?
    1. "Can you tell me more about how you feel since your family placed you here?"
    2. "Your family did what they felt was best for your safety."
    3. "Why would you think that about your family? They care for you."
    4. "Tell me, how much trouble were you when you were at home?"

100. The admitting nurse is subpoenaed to give testimony in a case in which the client fell from the bed and fractured the left hip. The nurse initiated fall precautions on admission but was not on duty when the client fell. Which issue should the nurse be prepared to testify about the incident?
1. What preceded the client's fall from the bed.
2. The extent of injuries the client sustained.
3. The client's mental status before the incident.
4. The facility's policy covering falls prevention.

101. The charge nurse must notify a staff member to stay home because of low census. The unit currently has 35 clients who all have at least one IV and multiple IV medications. The unit is staffed with two RNs, three licensed practical nurses (LPNs), and three unlicensed assistive personnel (UAPs). Which nurse should be notified to stay home?
1. The least experienced RN.
2. The most experienced LPN.
3. The UAP who asked to be requested off.
4. The UAP who was hired 4 weeks ago.

102. The charge nurse in an extended care facility notes an elderly male resident holding hands with an elderly female resident. Which intervention should the charge nurse implement?
1. Do nothing, because this is a natural human need.
2. Notify the family of the residents about the situation.
3. Separate the residents for all activities.
4. Call a care plan meeting with other staff members.

103. The chief nursing officer (CNO) of an extended care facility is attending shift report with two charge nurses, and an argument about a resident's care ensues. Which action should the CNO implement first?
1. Ask the two charge nurses to stop arguing and go to a private area.
2. Listen to both sides of the argument and then implement a plan of care.
3. Ask the family to join the discussion before deciding how to implement care.
4. Tell the nurses to stop arguing and continue to give report.

104. Which action by the nurse is a violation of the Joint Commission's Patient Safety Goals?
1. The surgery nurse calls a time-out when a discrepancy is noted on the surgical permit.
2. The unit nurse asks the client for his or her date of birth before administering medications.
3. The nurse educator gives the orientee the answers to the quiz covering the IV pumps.
4. The admitting nurse initiates the facility's fall prevention program on an older adult client.

105. The community health nurse is triaging victims at a bus accident. Which client would the nurse categorize as red, priority 1?
1. The client with head trauma whose pupils are fixed and dilated.
2. The client with compound fractures of the tibia and fibula.
3. The client with a sprained right wrist with a 1-inch laceration.
4. The client with a piece of metal embedded in the right eye.

106. The clinic nurse is reviewing the laboratory data of clients seen in the clinic the previous day. Which client requires immediate intervention by the nurse?
1. The client whose white blood cell (WBC) count is 9.5 mm^3.
2. The client whose cholesterol level is 230 mg/dL.
3. The client whose calcium level is 10.4 mg/dL.
4. The client whose International Normalized Ratio (INR) is 3.8.

107. The community health nurse is triaging victims at the scene of a building collapse. Which intervention should the nurse implement first?
1. Discuss the disaster situation with the media.
2. Write the client's name clearly in the disaster log.
3. Place disaster tags securely on the victims.
4. Identify an area for family members to wait.

108. Which statement best describes the role of the parish nurse?
1. The parish nurse practices holistic healthcare within a faith community.
2. The parish nurse cares for clients in a religious-based hospital.
3. The parish nurse practices nursing in a parish clinic.
4. The parish nurse is a licensed practical nurse (LPN) who cares for clients in the home.

109. The IIII aide calls the HH nurse to report that the client has a reddened area on the sacral area. Which intervention should the nurse implement first?
1. Notify the client's healthcare provider.
2. Visit the client to assess the reddened area.
3. Document the finding in the client's chart.
4. Refer the client to the wound care nurse.

110. The 32-year-old male client with a traumatic right above-the-elbow amputation tells the home health (HH) nurse he is worried about supporting his family and finding employment since he can't be a mechanic anymore. Which intervention should the nurse implement?
1. Contact the HH agency's occupational therapist.
2. Refer the client to the state rehabilitation commission.
3. Ask the HH agency's social worker about disability.
4. Suggest he talk to his wife about his concerns.

111. The labor and delivery nurse has assisted in the delivery of a 37-week fetal demise. Which intervention should the nurse implement?
1. Remove the baby from the delivery area quickly.
2. Tell the father to arrange to take the infant home.
3. Wrap the infant in a towel and place it aside.
4. Obtain a lock of the infant's hair for the parents.

112. The newborn nursery nurse has received report. Which client should the nurse assess first?
1. The 2-hour-old infant who has nasal flaring and is grunting.
2. The 6-hour-old infant who has not passed meconium stool.
3. The 12-hour-old infant who refuses to latch onto the breast.
4. The 24-hour-old infant who has a positive startle reflex.

113. The psychiatric clinic nurse is returning telephone calls. Which telephone call should the nurse return first?
1. The female client who reports being slapped by her husband when he got drunk last night.
2. The male client who reports he is tired of living, since his wife just left him because he lost his job.
3. The female client diagnosed with anorexia who reports she does not think she can stand to eat today.
4. The male client diagnosed with Parkinson's disease who reports his hands are shaking more than yesterday.

114. The psychiatric nurse and mental health worker (MHW) on a psychiatric unit are caring for a group of clients. Which nursing task should the nurse delegate to the MHW?
1. Take the school-aged children to the on-campus classroom.
2. Lead a group therapy session on behavior control.
3. Explain the purpose of recreation therapy to the client.
4. Give a bipolar client a bed bath and shampoo the hair.

115. The 36-year-old client in the women's health clinic is being prescribed birth control pills. Which information is important for the nurse to teach the client? Select all that apply.
1. Do not smoke while taking birth control pills.
2. Take one pill at the same time every day.
3. If a birth control pill is missed, do not double up.
4. Stop taking the pill if breakthrough bleeding occurs.
5. There can be interactions with other medications.

116. The nurse is caring for a female client 3 days post–knee replacement surgery when the client complains of vaginal itching. The medication administration report (MAR) indicates the client has been receiving the antacid calcium carbonate (Maalox), the antibiotic ceftriaxone (Rocephin), and the anticoagulant enoxaparin (Lovenox). Which priority intervention should the nurse implement?
1. Request the dietary department to send yogurt on each tray.
2. Explain to the client this is the result of the antibiotic therapy.
3. Notify the HCP on rounds of the client's vaginal itching.
4. Ask the client whether she is having unprotected sexual activity.

117. The nurse manager of the maternal-child department is developing the budget for the next fiscal year. Which statement best explains the first step of the budgetary process?
1. Ask the staff for input about needed equipment.
2. Assess any new department project for costs.
3. Review the department's current year budget.
4. Explain the new budget requirements to the staff.

118. The nurse on the psychiatric unit observes one client shove another client. Which intervention should the nurse implement first?
1. Discuss the aggressive behavior with the client.
2. Document the occurrence in the client's chart.
3. Approach the client with another staff member.
4. Instruct the client to go to the unit's quiet room.

119. The client in the operating room states, "I don't think I will have this surgery after all." Which intervention should the nurse implement first?
1. Have the surgeon speak with the client.
2. Ask the client to discuss the concerns.
3. Continue to prep the client for surgery.
4. Immediately stop the surgical procedure.

120. Which data indicates therapy has been effective for the client diagnosed with bipolar disorder?
1. The client only has four episodes of mania in 6 months.
2. The client goes to work every day for 9 months.
3. The client wears a nightgown to the day room for therapy.
4. The client has had three motor vehicle accidents.

ANSWERS AND RATIONALES

The correct answer number and rationale for why it is the correct answer are given in **boldface type**. Rationales for why the other possible answer options are incorrect also are given, but they are not in boldface type.

1. 1. The new graduate must work under this charge nurse; confronting the nurse would not resolve the issue because the nurse can choose to ignore the new graduate. Someone in authority over the charge nurse must address this situation with the nurse.
  2. **The night supervisor or the unit manager has the authority to require the charge nurse to submit to drug screening. In this case, the supervisor on duty should handle the situation.**
  3. The new graduate is bound by the nursing practice acts to report potentially unsafe behavior regardless of the position the nurse holds.
  4. The nurse educator would not be in a position of authority over the charge nurse.
  Content – Management of Care: **Category of Health Alteration** *– Management of Care:* **Integrated Processes** *– Nursing Process: Implementation:* **Client Needs** *– Safe and Effective Care Environment: Management of Care:* **Cognitive Level** *– Application*

2. 1. The nurse should stop the behavior from occurring in a public place. The charge nurse can discuss the issue with the UAPs and determine whether the manager should be notified.
  2. **The first action is to stop the argument from occurring in a public place. The charge nurse should not discuss the UAPs' behavior in public.**
  3. The second action is to have the UAPs go to a private area before resuming the conversation.
  4. The charge nurse may need to mediate the disagreement; this would be the third step.
  Content – Management of Care: **Category of Health Alteration** *– Management of Care:* **Integrated Processes** *– Nursing Process: Implementation:* **Client Needs** *– Safe and Effective Care Environment: Management of Care:* **Cognitive Level** *– Application*

3. 1. The graduate nurse should handle the situation directly with the UAP first before notifying the charge nurse.
  2. This may need to be completed, but not prior to directly discussing the behavior with the UAP.
  3. The graduate nurse must address the insubordination with the UAP, not just complete the tasks that are the responsibility of the UAP.

  4. **The graduate nurse must discuss the insubordination directly with the UAP first. The nurse must give objective data as to when and where the UAP did not follow through with the completion of assigned tasks.**
  Content – Management of Care: **Category of Health Alteration** *– Management of Care:* **Integrated Processes** *– Nursing Process: Implementation:* **Client Needs** *– Safe and Effective Care Environment: Management of Care:* **Cognitive Level** *– Application*

4. 1. This should not be implemented until verification of the allegation is complete, and the shift manager has discussed the situation with the UAP.
  2. **The shift manager should have objective data prior to confronting the UAP about the allegation of falsifying vital signs; therefore, the shift manager should take the client's vital signs and compare them with the UAP's results before taking any other action.**
  3. The shift manager should not confront the UAP until objective data are obtained to support the allegation.
  4. Written documentation should be the last action when resolving staff issues.
  Content – Management of Care: **Category of Health Alteration** *– Management of Care:* **Integrated Processes** *– Nursing Process: Implementation:* **Client Needs** *– Safe and Effective Care Environment: Management of Care:* **Cognitive Level** *– Synthesis*

5. 1. **The nurse should first assess the client prior to taking any other action to determine if the client is experiencing any untoward reaction.**
  2. An incident report must be completed by the nurse but not prior to taking care of the client.
  3. The nurse should administer the correct medication but not prior to assessing the client.
  4. The client's HCP must be notified, but the nurse should be able to provide the HCP with pertinent client information, so this is not the first intervention.
  Content – Medical/Surgical: **Category of Health Alteration** *– Medication Administration:* **Integrated Processes** *– Nursing Process: Implementation:* **Client Needs** *– Safe and Effective Care Environment: Management of Care:* **Cognitive Level** *– Application*

6. 1. The serum blood glucose level requires a venipuncture, which is not within the scope of the UAP's expertise. The laboratory technician would be responsible for obtaining a venipuncture.

2. This is a sterile dressing change and requires assessing the insertion site for infection; therefore, this would not be the most appropriate task to assign to the LPN.

3. The nurse should ask the UAP to bathe the client and change bed linens because this is a task the UAP can perform. The LPN could be assigned higher-level tasks.

4. The UAP can add up the urine output for the 12-hour shift; however, the nurse is responsible for evaluating whether the urine output is what is expected for the client.

Content – Medical/Surgical: **Category of Health Alteration** *– Management of Care:* **Integrated Processes –** *Nursing Process: Planning:* **Client Needs** *– Safe and Effective Care Environment: Management of Care:* **Cognitive Level** *– Synthesis*

7. 1. The client on the ventilator is unstable; therefore, the nurse should not delegate any tasks to the UAP.

2. The UAP can take specimens to the laboratory; these are not medications and they are not vital to the client.

3. The client in an Addisonian crisis is unstable; therefore, the nurse should not delegate any tasks to the UAP.

4. The UAP cannot assist the HCP with an invasive procedure at the bedside.

Content – Medical/Surgical: **Integrated Processes –** *Nursing Process: Planning:* **Client Needs** *– Safe and Effective Care Environment: Management of Care:* **Cognitive Level** *– Synthesis*

8. **1. The client must have lost decision-making capacity because of a condition that is not reversible or must be in a condition that is specified under state law, such as a terminal, persistent vegetative state, irreversible coma, or as specified in the advance directive. A client who is exhibiting decerebrate posturing is unconscious and unable to make decisions.**

2. The client on a ventilator has not lost the ability to make healthcare decisions. The nurse can communicate by asking the client to blink his or her eyes to yes/no questions.

3. The client receiving dialysis is alert and does not lose the ability to make decisions; therefore, the advance directive should not be consulted to make decisions for the client.

4. Mental retardation does not mean the client cannot make decisions for him- or herself unless the client has a legal guardian who has a durable power of attorney for healthcare. If

the client has a legal guardian, then the client cannot complete an advance directive.

Content – Medical/Surgical: **Integrated Processes –** *Nursing Process: Assessment:* **Client Needs** *– Psychosocial Integrity:* **Cognitive Level** *– Analysis*

9. 1. The UAP can apply sequential compression devices to the client on strict bed rest.

2. The UAP can assist with a portable STAT chest x-ray, as long as it is not a female UAP who is pregnant.

3. The client will need to be pre-medicated for a wound debridement; therefore, this task cannot be delegated to the UAP.

4. The UAP can obtain intake and output for clients.

Content – Medical/Surgical: Integrated Process: Nursing Process: Planning: **Client Needs** *– Safe and Effective Care Environment: Management of Care:* **Cognitive Level** *– Synthesis*

10. **1. A quality improvement project looks at the way tasks are performed and attempts to see whether the system can be improved. A medication delivery system in which it takes a long time for the nurse to receive a STAT or "now" medication is an example of a system that needs improvement, and should be addressed by a quality improvement committee.**

2. Financial reimbursement of the staff is a management issue, not a quality improvement issue.

3. Collective bargaining is an administrative issue, not a quality improvement issue.

4. The number of medication errors committed by a nurse is a management-to-nurse issue and does not involve a systems issue, unless several nurses have committed the same error because the system is not functioning properly.

Content – Medical/Surgical: **Integrated Processes –** *Nursing Process: Implementation:* **Client Needs** *– Safe and Effective Care Environment: Management of Care:* **Cognitive Level** *– Application*

11. **1. A secondary nursing intervention includes screening for early detection. The bone density evaluation will determine the density of the bone and is diagnostic for osteoporosis.**

2. Spinal screening examinations are performed on adolescents to detect scoliosis. This is a secondary nursing intervention, but not to detect osteoporosis.

3. Teaching the client is a primary nursing intervention. This is an appropriate intervention to help prevent osteoporosis, but it is not a secondary intervention.

4. Discussing risk factors is an appropriate intervention, but it is not a secondary nursing intervention.

Content – Medical/Surgical: **Category of Health Alteration** *– Musculoskeletal:* **Integrated Processes** *– Nursing Process: Planning:* **Client Needs** *– Physiological Integrity: Reduction of Risk Potential:* **Cognitive Level** *– Synthesis*

12. 1. Isometric exercises such as weight lifting increase muscle mass. The HH nurse should not instruct the HH aide to do this type of exercises.

2. The HH aide may go to the emergency department, but the HH nurse should address the aide's back pain. Many times, the person with back pain does not need to be seen in the emergency room.

3. An occurrence report explaining the situation is important documentation and should be completed. It provides the staff member with the required documentation to begin a workers' compensation case for payment of medical bills. However, the HH nurse on the phone should help decrease the HH aide's pain, not worry about paperwork.

4. **The HH aide is in pain, and applying ice to the back will help decrease pain and inflammation. The HH nurse should be concerned about a coworker's pain. Remember: Ice for acute pain and heat for chronic pain.**

Content – Medical/Surgical: **Category of Health Alteration** *– Musculoskeletal:* **Integrated Processes** *– Nursing Process: Implementation:* **Client Needs** *– Physiological Integrity: Reduction of Risk Potential:* **Cognitive Level** *– Application*

13. 1. Allowing the client to stay in bed is inappropriate because a client with osteoarthritis should be encouraged to move, which will decrease the pain.

2. A bath at the bedside does not require as much movement from the client as getting up and walking to the shower. This is not an appropriate action for a client with osteoarthritis.

3. **Movement and warm or hot water will help decrease the pain; the worst thing the client can do is not to move. The HH aide should encourage the client to get up and take a warm shower or bath.**

4. Osteoarthritis is a chronic condition, and the HCP could not do anything to keep the client from "hurting all over."

Content – Medical/Surgical: **Category of Health Alteration** *– Musculoskeletal:* **Integrated Processes** *– Nursing Process: Implementation:* **Client Needs** *– Physiological Integrity: Basic Care and Comfort:* **Cognitive Level** *– Application*

14. 1. **The HH aide's responsibility is to care for the client's personal needs, which includes assisting with a.m. care.**

2. The HH aide is not responsible for cooking the client's meals.

3. The HH aide is not responsible for taking the client to appointments. This also presents an insurance problem, because the client would be riding in the HH aide's car.

4. Even in the home, the HH nurse should not delegate teaching.

Content – Medical/Surgical: **Category of Health Alteration** *– Management of Care:* **Integrated Processes** *– Nursing Process: Planning:* **Client Needs** *– Safe and Effective Care Environment: Management of Care:* **Cognitive Level** *– Synthesis*

15. 1. The UAP may be at risk of contacting the illness.

2. **The UAP should wear appropriate personal protective equipment when providing any type of care.**

3. The UAP should not be told to skip performing assigned tasks.

4. The fetus is not affected by anthrax.

Content – Medical/Surgical: **Category of Health Alteration** *– Respiratory:* **Integrated Processes** *– Nursing Process: Planning:* **Client Needs** *– Safe and Effective Care Environment: Safety and Infection Control:* **Cognitive Level** *– Synthesis*

16. 1. The mortuary service is considered part of the healthcare team in this case. The personnel in the funeral home should be made aware of the client's diagnosis.

2. **The mortuary service is considered part of the healthcare team. In this case, the personnel in the funeral home should be made aware of the client's diagnosis.**

3. The nurse does not need to ask the family for permission to protect the funeral home workers.

4. The nurse, not the HCP, releases the body to the funeral home.

Content – Medical/Surgical: **Category of Health Alteration** *– Communicable Disease:* **Integrated Processes** *– Nursing Process: Implementation:* **Client Needs** *– Safe and Effective Care Environment: Safety and Infection Control:* **Cognitive Level** *– Application*

17. 1. The clients would not understand the importance of the specific tasks. Clients will tell the nurse whether the UAP is pleasant when in the room but not whether the delegated tasks have been completed.

2. The nurse retains responsibility for the delegated tasks. The charge nurse may be able to tell the nurse that the UAP has been checked

off as being competent to perform the care but would not know whether the care was actually provided.

3. **The nurse retains responsibility for the care. Making rounds to see that the care has been provided is the best method to evaluate the care.**

4. The nurse would not have time to complete his or her own work if the nurse watched the UAP perform all of the UAP's work.

Content – Medical/Surgical: ***Category of Health Alteration*** *– Management of Care:* ***Integrated Processes*** *– Nursing Process: Implementation:* ***Client Needs*** *– Safe and Effective Care Environment: Safety and Infection Control:* ***Cognitive Level*** *– Application*

18. 1. A client in a crisis should be assigned to the registered nurse (RN).
2. Biliary atresia involves liver failure, involving multiple body systems. This client should be assigned to the RN.
3. Anaphylaxis is an emergency situation. The client should be assigned to the RN.
4. **The LPN can administer routine medications and care for clients who have no life-threatening conditions.**

Content – Medical/Surgical: ***Category of Health Alteration*** *– Management of Care:* ***Integrated Processes*** *– Nursing Process: Planning:* ***Client Needs*** *– Safe and Effective Care Environment: Safety and Infection Control:* ***Cognitive Level*** *– Synthesis*

19. 1. The nurse would expect the client with DIC to be oozing blood; therefore, the nurse should not need to assess this client first.
2. The nurse would expect the client with BPH to have urinary signs and symptoms such as terminal dribbling, so the nurse should not need to assess this client first.
3. **The nurse would not expect the client with renal calculi to have blood in the urine (hematuria) and the pain should not be severe; therefore, this client should be assessed to determine if the client is having complications.**
4. The nurse would expect the client with Addison's disease to have a bronze pigmentation and hypoglycemia; therefore, the nurse should not need to assess this client first.

Content – Medical/Surgical: ***Category of Health Alteration*** *– Genitourinary:* ***Integrated Processes*** *– Nursing Process: Assessment:* ***Client Needs*** *– Safe and Effective Care Environment: Management of Care:* ***Cognitive Level*** *– Analysis*

20. 1. **The most experienced nurse should be assigned to the client who requires teaching and evaluation of knowledge for home healthcare, because the client is in the surgery center for less than 1 day.**

2. A routine preoperative client does not require the most experienced nurse.
3. Any nurse can administer and monitor blood transfusion to the client.
4. Although the creation of an arteriovenous fistula requires assessment and teaching on the part of the most experienced nurse, this client is not being discharged home at this time.

Content – Medical/Surgical: ***Category of Health Alteration*** *– Management of Care:* ***Integrated Processes*** *– Nursing Process: Planning:* ***Client Needs*** *– Safe and Effective Care Environment: Management of Care:* ***Cognitive Level*** *– Synthesis*

21. 1. **The Glasgow Coma Scale ranges from 0 to 15, with 15 indicating the client's neurological status is intact. A Glasgow Coma Scale score of 13 indicates the client is stable and would be the most appropriate client to assign to the graduate nurse.**
2. This client's K+ level is low, and the client is at risk for developing cardiac dysrhythmias; therefore, the client should be assigned to a more experienced nurse.
3. This client has a low blood pressure and evidence of tachycardia and could possibly go into an Addisonian crisis, which is a potentially life-threatening condition. A more experienced nurse should be assigned to this client.
4. A positive Trousseau sign indicates the client is hypocalcemic and is experiencing a complication of the surgery; therefore, this client should be assigned to a more experienced nurse.

Content – Medical/Surgical: ***Category of Health Alteration*** *– Neurological:* ***Integrated Processes*** *– Nursing Process: Nursing Process: Planning:* ***Client Needs*** *– Safe and Effective Care Environment: Management of Care:* ***Cognitive Level*** *– Synthesis*

22. 1. **The therapeutic PTT level should be 1½ to 2 times the control. Most controls average 36 seconds, so the therapeutic levels of heparin would place the control between 54 and 72. With a PTT of 92, the client is at risk for bleeding, and the heparin drip should be held. The nurse should assess this client first.**
2. A client diagnosed with pneumonia would be expected to have a fever. This client can be seen after the client diagnosed with a DVT.
3. Cystitis is inflammation of the urinary bladder, and burning on urination is an expected symptom.
4. Pancreatitis is a very painful condition. Pain is a priority but not over the potential for hemorrhage.

Content – Medical/Surgical: **Category of Health Alteration** *– Management of Care:* **Integrated Processes** *– Nursing Process: Planning:* **Client Needs –** *Safe and Effective Care Environment: Management of Care:* **Cognitive Level** *– Synthesis*

23. **3, 4, and 5 are correct.**
    1. Teaching is the responsibility of the nurse and cannot be delegated to a UAP.
    2. The word "check" indicates a step in the assessment process, and the nurse cannot delegate assessing to a UAP.
    3. **The client is 2 days postoperative and vital signs should be stable, so the UAP can take vital signs. The nurse must make sure the UAP knows when to immediately notify him/her of vital signs not within the guidelines the nurse provides to the UAP.**
    4. **This action does not require judgment on the part of the UAP: it does not require assessing, teaching, or evaluating. This can be delegated to the UAP.**
    5. **A client who is 2 days postoperative should be ambulating frequently. The UAP can perform this task.**

    Content – Medical/Surgical: **Category of Health Alteration** *– Management of Care:* **Integrated Processes** *– Nursing Process: Planning:* **Client Needs –** *Safe and Effective Care Environment, Management of Care:* **Cognitive Level** *– Synthesis*

24. 1. Staff members will not stay if forced to always use their paid time off for the hospital's convenience.
    2. **This nurse wants to take time off. Therefore, it is the best option to let the nurse desiring to be off from work to take time off if all other situations are equal.**
    3. The nurse will not gain experience if always requested not to come to work, and presumably this nurse would not have benefit time to pay for the time out of work.
    4. This nurse could be allowed to stay home only if the nurse is still ill.

    Content – Medical/Surgical: **Category of Health Alteration** *– Management of Care:* **Integrated Processes** *– Nursing Process: Planning:* **Client Needs –** *Safe and Effective Care Environment: Management of Care:* **Cognitive Level** *– Synthesis*

25. 1. A nurse, not the UAP, should perform sterile dressing changes.
    2. This client is unstable, and a nurse should perform this task.
    3. **The UAP can check to see the amount of food the residents consumed and document the information.**
    4. This is the job of the activity director and volunteers working with the activities department. Staffing is limited in any nursing area; the UAP should be assigned a nursing task.

Content – Medical/Surgical: **Category of Health Alteration** *– Management of Care:* **Integrated Processes** *– Nursing Process: Planning:* **Client Needs –** *Safe and Effective Care Environment: Management of Care:* **Cognitive Level** *– Synthesis*

26. 1. The charge nurse is not the nurse educator but is responsible for the UAPs working under him or her. This is adding additional duties to the charge nurse.
    2. **The director of nurses should encourage responsible behavior on the part of all staff. The charge nurse is performing a part of the responsibility of the charge nurse and should be encouraged to work with the UAP.**
    3. Because this is not a private conversation about a client, there is no reason for the charge nurse to be told to go to a private area. The charge nurse is not reprimanding the UAP.
    4. The director of nurses should not interfere with a "better explanation." This could intimidate the charge nurse and make it difficult for the charge nurse to perform his or her duties.

    Content – Medical/Surgical: **Category of Health Alteration** *– Management of Care:* **Integrated Processes** *– Nursing Process: Implementation:* **Client Needs –** *Safe and Effective Care Environment: Management of Care:* **Cognitive Level** *– Application*

27. 1. **Wound debriding formulations are medications, and a UAP cannot administer medications.**
    2. The UAP can position the resident so that pressure is not placed on the resident's heels.
    3. The UAP can turn the resident.
    4. The UAP can give the resident a protein shake to drink.

    Content – Medical/Surgical: **Category of Health Alteration** *– Drug Administration:* **Integrated Processes** *– Nursing Process: Planning:* **Client Needs –** *Safe and Effective Care Environment: Management of Care:* **Cognitive Level** *– Synthesis*

28. 1. The nurse should implement the least restrictive measures to ensure client safety. Restraining a client is one of the last measures implemented.
    2. **Moving the client near the nursing station where the staff can closely observe the client is one of the first measures in most fall prevention policies.**
    3. This is considered medical restraints and is one of the last measures taken to prevent falls.
    4. Four side rails are considered a restraint. Research has shown that having four side rails up does not prevent falls and only gives the client farther to fall when the client climbs over the rails before falling to the floor.

*Content – Medical/Surgical: **Category of Health Alteration** – Safety: **Integrated Processes** – Nursing Process: Implementation: **Client Needs** – Safe and Effective Care Environment: Safety and Infection Control: **Cognitive Level** – Application*

29. 1. **The first intervention is for the nurse to ensure the client is safe in the home. Assessing for grab bars in the bathroom is addressing the safety of the client.**
    2. Taking a shower in a stall shower may be safer than getting in and out of a bathtub, but the nurse should first determine whether the client has grab bars and safety equipment even when taking a shower.
    3. According to the NCLEX-RN® test blueprint for management of care, the nurse must be knowledgeable of referrals. The physical therapist is able to help the client with transferring, ambulation, and other lower extremity difficulties and is an appropriate intervention, but it is not the nurse's first intervention. Safety is priority.
    4. NSAIDs are used to decrease the pain of osteoarthritis, but this intervention will not address safety issues for the client getting into and out of the bathtub.

*Content – Medical/Surgical: **Category of Health Alteration** – Safety: **Integrated Processes** – Nursing Process: Implementation: **Client Needs** – Safe and Effective Care Environment: Safety and Infection Control: **Cognitive Level** – Synthesis*

30. 1. The employee health nurse should keep the clients at the clinic or send them to the emergency department. The clients should be kept together until the cause of their illnesses is determined. If it is determined that the clients are stable and not contagious, they should be driven home.
    2. **The employee health nurse should be aware that six clients with the same signs/symptoms indicate a potential deliberate or accidental dispersal of toxic or infectious agents. The nurse must notify the public health department so that an investigation of the cause can be instituted and appropriate action to contain the cause can be taken.**
    3. As long as the clients are stable, the nurse should keep the clients in the employee health clinic. These clients should not be exposed to other clients and emergency department staff. If the clients must be transferred, decontamination procedures may need to be instituted.
    4. The client may need to provide stool specimens, but this would be done at the emergency department. Employee health clinics

do not have laboratory facilities to perform tests on stools.

*Content – Medical/Surgical: **Category of Health Alteration** – Infection Control: **Integrated Processes** – Nursing Process: Implementation: **Client Needs** – Safe Effective Care Environment: Safety and Infection Control: **Cognitive Level** – Application*

31. 1. This child needs an x-ray to rule out a fractured left leg, but this is not life threatening.
    2. **Drooling and not wanting to swallow are the cardinal signs of epiglottitis, which is potentially life threatening. This child should be assessed first. The nurse should not attempt to visualize the throat area and should allow the HCP to do this in case an emergency tracheostomy is required.**
    3. A child usually does not complain of a headache and this child should be assessed, but it is not life threatening.
    4. This client may have type 1 diabetes mellitus and should be assessed, but this is not life threatening at this time.

*Content – Medical/Surgical: **Category of Health Alteration** – Pediatrics: **Integrated Processes** – Nursing Process: Assessment: **Client Needs** – Safe and Effective Care Environment: Management of Care: **Cognitive Level** – Analysis*

32. 1. This is an example of community-based nursing where nurses care for a client living in the community.
    2. **Community-oriented, population-focused nursing practice involves the engagement of nursing in promoting and protecting the health of populations, not individuals in the community. Therefore, this is an example of community-oriented, population-focused nursing.**
    3. This is an example of community-based nursing where nurses care for a client living in the community.
    4. This is an example of community-based nursing where nurses care for a client living in the community.

*Content – Medical/Surgical: **Category of Health Alteration** – Community Health: **Integrated Processes** – Nursing Process: Planning: **Client Needs** – Safe and Effective Care Environment: Management of Care: **Cognitive Level** – Comprehension*

33. 1. Dyspnea and confusion are not expected in a client diagnosed with AIDS; therefore, this client would warrant a more experienced nurse to assess the reason for the complications.
    2. The client with financial problems should be assigned to a social worker, not to a nurse.
    3. A full-thickness (third-degree) burn is the most serious burn and requires excellent

assessment skills to determine whether complications are occurring. This client should be assigned to a more experienced nurse.

4. **The client diagnosed with diabetic neuropathy would be expected to have pain; therefore, this client could be assigned to a nurse new to home health nursing. The client is not exhibiting a complication or an unexpected sign/symptom.**

Content – Medical/Surgical: **Category of Health Alteration** – Endocrine: **Integrated Processes** – Nursing Process: Planning: **Client Needs** – Safe and Effective Care Environment: Management of Care: **Cognitive Level** – Synthesis

34. 1. The nurse cannot delegate assessment to the HH aide.

2. The HH aide cannot assess the incisional wound, and the wound should be assessed. The nurse cannot delegate assessment.

3. **The HH aide can place the right leg on two pillows. This task does not require assessment, teaching, or evaluating, and the client is stable.**

4. Mopping the floor is not part of the HH aide's responsibility. This is not an appropriate task to delegate.

Content – Medical/Surgical: **Category of Health Alteration** – Musculoskeletal: **Integrated Processes** – Nursing Process: Planning: **Client Needs** – Safe and Effective Care Environment: Management of Care: **Cognitive Level** – Synthesis

35. 1. The nurse would expect the client diagnosed with a myocardial infarction to have an elevated troponin level; thus, the nurse would not assess this client first.

2. Because the client's PTT of 68 seconds is 1.5 to 2 times the normal range, it is considered therapeutic and would not warrant the nurse's assessing this client first.

3. The nurse would expect a client with end-stage liver failure to have an elevated ammonia level.

4. **The therapeutic range for Dilantin is 10 to 20 mg/dL. This client's higher level warrants intervention because the serum level is above the therapeutic range.**

Content – Medical/Surgical: **Category of Health Alteration** – Laboratory Values: **Integrated Processes** – Nursing Process: Assessment: **Client Needs** – Physiological Integrity: Reduction of Risk Potential: **Cognitive Level** – Analysis

36. 1. This client would not benefit from acupuncture.

2. Mental health issues are not treated with acupuncture. They may be treated with herbal supplements.

3. The client with asthma must be treated with a medical regime.

4. **Acupuncture, the most common complementary therapy recommended by healthcare providers, would benefit a client with osteoarthritis.**

Content – Medical/Surgical: **Category of Health Alteration** – Complementary Alternative Medicine: **Integrated Processes** – Diagnosis: **Client Needs** – Physiological Integrity: Pharmacological and Parenteral Therapies: **Cognitive Level** – Analysis

37. 1. The nurse should not make the client dependent on family members to prepare meals. If the family were willing to do this, they would probably already be doing it.

2. The occupational therapist would teach the client how to cook, but this client is 88 years old and needs meals provided. Therefore, providing meals through Meals on Wheels is the most appropriate intervention.

3. The HH aide's duties do not include cooking all three meals for the client.

4. **Meals on Wheels delivers a hot, nutritionally balanced meal once a day on weekdays, usually at noon for older people who do not have assistance in the home for food preparation. This intervention would be most helpful to the client.**

Content – Medical/Surgical: **Integrated Processes** – Nursing Process: Implementation: **Client Needs** – Psychosocial Integrity: **Cognitive Level** – Application

38. 1. HH care agency employees are responsible for knowing and adhering to the professional boundary-crossing standards. The nurse should not discuss this with the client.

2. **Home healthcare agencies are required by law to address the concepts in the National Association for Home Care (NAHC) Bill of Rights with all home health clients on the initial visit. The agencies may also make additions to the NAHC's original Bill of Rights.**

3. The nurse should discuss this with the client, but it is not a legal intervention.

4. This is a true statement, but it is not a legal intervention. If the client is not homebound, he or she is not eligible for home healthcare.

Content – Legal: **Integrated Processes** – Nursing Process: Implementation: **Client Needs** – Safe and Effective Care Environment: Management of Care: **Cognitive Level** – Application

39. 1. **Taping petroleum gauze over the chest tube insertion site will prevent air from entering the pleural space. This is the first intervention.**

2. The nurse should make sure the UAP knows the correct method to assist a client with a chest tube, but the safety of the client is the first priority.

3. This is the second intervention the nurse should implement. Remember, if the client is in distress and the nurse can do something to relieve that distress, then the nurse should not assess first. The nurse should take action to take care of the client.

4. The nurse should obtain the necessary equipment for the HCP to reinsert the chest tube, but the priority intervention is to prevent air from entering the pleural space.

Content – Medical/Surgical: *Category of Health Alteration* – Respiratory: *Integrated Processes* – Nursing Process: Implementation: *Client Needs* – Physiological Integrity: Reduction of Risk Potential: *Cognitive Level* – Analysis

40. 1. **The LPN can administer routine medications.**
2. The UAP, not the LPN, should be assigned to take the routine vital signs.
3. The unit secretary, not an LPN, should be assigned to transcribe the HCP orders.
4. The RN, not the LPN, should assess the urinary output of the client. The RN should not delegate assessment.

Content – Management of Care: *Integrated Processes* – Nursing Process: Planning: *Client Needs* – Safe and Effective Care Environment: Management of Care: *Cognitive Level* – Synthesis

41. 1. The clinical manager may need to discuss the MAR with some nurses individually, but it is not the clinical manager's first intervention.
2. **The first intervention should be to arrange meetings to explain the new MAR and allow nurses to ask questions to clarify the new policy.**
3. The clinical manager can provide a written handout explaining the new MAR, but the first intervention should be small discussion groups.
4. A video is an excellent tool for explaining new procedures, but the first intervention should be small discussion groups so that all questions can be answered.

Content – Medical/Surgical: *Category of Health Alteration* – Drug Administration: *Integrated Processes* – Nursing Process: Planning: *Client Needs* – Safe and Effective Care Environment: Management of Care: *Cognitive Level* – Synthesis

42. 1. The nurse would expect the client with an abdominal aortic aneurysm to have an audible bruit; therefore, this client does not warrant immediate intervention.

2. The nurse would expect the client with ARDS to have respiratory signs/symptoms; therefore, this client does not warrant immediate intervention.

3. One of the signs/symptoms of bacterial meningitis is nucal rigidity; therefore, this client does not warrant immediate intervention.

4. **The client with Crohn's disease should be asymptomatic, so pain and diarrhea warrant intervention by the nurse. Pain could indicate a complication.**

Content – Medical/Surgical: *Category of Health Alteration* – Gastrointestinal: *Integrated Processes* – Nursing Process: Assessment: *Client Needs* – Physiological Integrity: Reduction of Risk Potential: *Cognitive Level* – Analysis

43. 1. The client with chronic kidney disease (CKD) would have an elevated creatinine level. The normal creatinine level is 0.7 to 1.8 mg/dL. The data would not warrant immediate intervention.

2. Peritonitis, inflammation of the peritoneum, is a serious complication that would result in a hard, rigid abdomen; therefore, a soft abdomen would not warrant immediate intervention.

3. **The dialysate return should be colorless or straw colored but should never be cloudy, which indicates an infection; therefore, the data warrant immediate intervention.**

4. Because the client has ESRD, fluid must be removed from the body, so the output should be more than the amount instilled; therefore, this indicates the peritoneal dialysis is effective and does not warrant intervention.

Content – Medical/Surgical: *Category of Health Alteration* – Genitourinary: *Integrated Processes* – Nursing Process: Assessment: *Client Needs* – Physiological Integrity: Reduction of Risk Potential: *Cognitive Level* – Analysis

44. 1. The nurse could ask this question, but the client has already told the nurse that 3 years have passed, so the client has tried approximately 36 times.

2. **This is the best question to assess the client. The nurse would not want to suggest an intervention that has been futile.**

3. Infertility treatments are very expensive, but the nurse should assess the client's attempts.

4. This question is not helpful for assessing the client or addressing the client's statement.

Content – Medical/Surgical: Category of Health Alteration – Family Planning: Integrated Processes – Nursing Process: Implementation: Client Needs – Physiological Integrity: Reduction of Risk Potential: Cognitive Level – Application

45. 1. The reason that the first pregnancy did not yield a viable infant is not relevant at this time. The relevant information is whether the mother received the Rhogam injection.

2. **The important information to assess is whether the client received the Rhogam injection within 72 hours of the loss of the first pregnancy. If the client did not receive the injection, the fetus is at risk for erythroblastosis fetalis (blue baby).**

3. This is not important information at this time.

4. This is not important information at this time.

Content – Medical/Surgical: Category of Health Alteration – Maternity: Integrated Processes – Nursing Process: Assessment: Client Needs – Physiological Integrity: Reduction of Risk Potential: Cognitive Level – Analysis

46. 1, 3, and 5 are correct.
1. **This child has injuries consistent with child abuse. Child Protective Services and the police should be notified.**

2. This could result in not being able to prosecute the perpetrator if the nurse is not trained in forensic medicine.

3. **The nurse should determine the full extent of the child's injuries.**

4. The nurse should not notify the parent of the potential involvement. The police are fully capable of doing this for themselves. The nurse could instigate an inflammatory situation with this action.

5. **The child needs x-ray studies to determine the extent of internal injuries.**

Content – Medical/Surgical: Category of Health Alteration – Musculoskeletal: Integrated Processes – Nursing Process: Implementation: Client Needs – Safe and Effective Care Environment: Management of Care: Cognitive Level – Application

47. Correct Answer: 5, 3, 2, 4, 1
5. **Taking the vital signs is part of the assessment and a beginning point for the nurse.**

3. **Since the child has been losing fluids, the nurse should assess tissue turgor to try and determine if fluid replacement by the parents has been effective.**

2. **The nurse should make sure that the parents do not leave the child alone in the room, making sure the parents are aware of any safety measures used to protect the** toddler from abduction, and how to call the nurse in case of need.

4. **The client will need diapers. They should be available to the parents so the diaper can be changed and the child will not develop skin irritation problems.**

1. **When the nurse provides the diapers, it is a good opportunity for the nurse to teach the parents about weighing the diapers before and after the child soils them.**

Content – Medical/Surgical: Category of Health Alteration – Gastrointestinal: Integrated Processes – Nursing Process: Implementation: Client Needs – Safe and Effective Care Environment: Management of Care: Cognitive Level – Synthesis

48. 1. **This client is exhibiting signs and symptoms of a potentially fatal complication of DVT—pulmonary embolism. The nurse should assess this client first.**

2. Refusing to eat hospital food should be discussed with the client, but the nurse could ask the unit secretary to have the dietitian see the client.

3. Clients diagnosed with pancreatitis have nasogastric tubes to rest the bowel. However, these tubes are typically uncomfortable. Regardless, the nurse should see this client after the client diagnosed with DVT has been assessed and appropriate interventions initiated. The nurse should discuss the importance of maintaining the tube with the client.

4. This is an expected symptom of osteoarthritis. This client does not need to be assessed first.

Content – Medical/Surgical: Category of Health Alteration – Respiratory: Integrated Processes – Nursing Process: Assessment: Client Needs – Safe and Effective Care Environment: Management of Care: Cognitive Level – Synthesis

49. 1. This is not an appropriate delegation. Taking the UAP from the floor to stay with a child so the parent can smoke is supporting a bad health habit.

2. The play therapist will stay with the client during the therapy.

3. The respiratory therapist will position the client for postural therapy.

4. **The UAP is capable of completing intake and output on clients. Weighing a diaper is the method of obtaining the output in an infant.**

Content – Pediatrics: Category of Health Alteration – Management of Care: Integrated Processes – Nursing Process: Planning: Client Needs – Safe and Effective Care Environment: Management of Care: Cognitive Level – Synthesis

50. 1. **This client may be developing a complication of immobility, one of which is pneumonia. The nurse should assess this client first.**
    2. Loss of weight in a client with CHF indicates the client is responding to therapy. This client does not need to be assessed first.
    3. Pressure ulcers are a chronic problem, which frequently occur in clients who are paralyzed. This client does not need to be assessed first.
    4. Paralysis is expected for a CVA. This client does not need to be assessed first.
    Content – Medical/Surgical: **Category of Health Alteration** *– Respiratory:* **Integrated Processes** *– Nursing Process: Assessment:* **Client Needs** *– Safe and Effective Care Environment: Management of Care:* **Cognitive Level** *– Synthesis*

51. 1. **The nurse should first medicate the client since this procedure is very painful for the client.**
    2. The nurse should prepare the equipment, but not prior to medicating the client. This should be done 30 minutes before procedure starts.
    3. The nurse should use non-sterile gloves to remove the old dressing but not prior to medicating the client.
    4. The nurse should don sterile gloves (can put one on dominant hand), but not prior to medicating client.
    Content – Medical/Surgical: **Category of Health Alteration** *– Integumentary:* **Integrated Processes** *– Nursing Process: Implementation:* **Client Needs** *– Physiological Integrity: Basic Care and Comfort:* **Cognitive Level** *– Application*

MAKING NURSING DECISIONS: When the question asks the nurse which intervention to implement first, it means all the options are plausible. The nurse should not select equipment first over taking care of the client's body (pain medication).

52. 1. Administering pain medication is the nurse's responsibility, not that of the UAP.
    2. A washcloth should be provided to the client before a meal, but not before ambulating with the physical therapist.
    3. **The client should be ready to work on therapy when the physical therapist arrives. The UAP should make sure the client has used the bathroom or has not been incontinent before the therapist arrives, thus making the most efficient use of the therapist's time.**
    4. Obtaining a walker that is the correct height for the client is the physical therapist's responsibility, not that of the UAP.
    Content – Medical: **Category of Health Alteration** *– Musculoskeletal:* **Integrated Processes** *– Nursing Process:*

Planning: **Client Needs** *– Physiological Integrity: Reduction of Risk Potential:* **Cognitive Level** *– Synthesis*

53. 1. The fact that the client is a neighbor of the volunteer has no bearing on whether or not the nurse can discuss a client's condition with the volunteer. The nurse should inform the volunteer that information obtained inadvertently is still confidential.
    2. The nurse cannot release the client's information in layperson's or medical terms; this is a violation of the Health Insurance Portability and Accountability Act (HIPAA). In many facilities, the client can give a "password" to individuals who can receive information about the client's condition.
    3. The nurse should not discuss the situation with the client. This would alert the client to potential breeches in confidentiality.
    4. **The nurse should remind the volunteer of the HIPAA and confidentiality rules that govern any information concerning clients in a healthcare setting.**
    Content – Legal: **Integrated Processes** *– Nursing Process: Implementation:* **Client Needs** *– Psychosocial Integrity:* **Cognitive Level** *– Application*

54. 1. Under shared governance, some nurses become so involved with the management of facilities that they are no longer eligible for representation by a bargaining agent (union), but there are no guarantees.
    2. The manager is responsible for disseminating information under a centralized system of organization.
    3. **Shared governance is an organizational framework in which the nurse has autonomy over his or her own practice. The nurse is given direct input into the working of the unit.**
    4. Shared governance is a system in which the nurse represents himself or herself.
    Content – Legal: **Integrated Processes** *– Nursing Process: Implementation:* **Client Needs** *– Safe and Effective Care Environment: Management of Care:* **Cognitive Level** *– Application*

55. 1. This might be the second statement for the nurse to make if the client does not calm down and discuss the problems with the nurse. Because it could escalate the anger, it should not be the first statement.
    2. **The nurse should remain calm and try to allow the client to vent his frustrations in a more acceptable manner. The nurse should repeat calmly in a low voice any instructions given to the client.**
    3. This statement will escalate the situation and could cause the visitor to lash out at the nurse.

4. This statement will escalate the situation and could cause the visitor to lash out at the nurse.

Content – *Mental Health:* **Integrated Processes** – *Nursing Process: Implementation:* **Client Needs** – *Safe and Effective Care Environment: Safety and Infection Control:* **Cognitive Level** – *Application*

56. 1. The nurse should leave if he determines that the staffing is not now or ever will be as it was relayed to him in the interview; however, there may be a temporary situation that can be resolved.
    2. **The nurse should give the manager a chance to discuss the situation before quitting. A temporary problem, such as illness, may be affecting staffing.**
    3. This action could cause the manager to think of the new nurse as a troublemaker.
    4. The nurse should not discuss this with the charge nurse because this may cause a rift between the charge nurse and the new nurse. The nurse should clarify the staffing situation with the unit manager.

    Content – *Management of Care:* **Integrated Processes:** *Nursing Process: Implementation:* **Client Needs** – *Safe and Effective Care Environment: Management of Care:* **Cognitive Level** – *Application*

57. Correct answer: 1, 5, 2, 3, 4
    1. **This is the first intervention the nurse should implement. Checking the HCP's order is priority.**
    5. **This is the second intervention; the nurse should not administer the antibiotic if it is not compatible with the primary IV.**
    2. **This is the third intervention the nurse should implement. Determining if the antibiotic is compatible is second, because client allergies won't be assessed if the medication is not compatible.**
    3. **This is the fourth intervention. The secondary piggyback (antibiotic) must be hung above the primary IV bag so the secondary piggyback will infuse.**
    4. **This is the fifth intervention. Ensuring the right rate is necessary prior to starting the infusion.**

    Content – *Medical/Surgical:* **Category of Health Alteration** – *Drug Administration:* **Integrated Processes** – *Nursing Process: Planning:* **Client Needs** – *Physiological Integrity: Pharmacological and Parenteral Therapies:* **Cognitive Level** – *Synthesis*

58. 1. Checking the client's armband is done prior to actually administering the medications, but it is not the first action for the nurse to take.
    2. The nurse should have assessed the client's IV site on first rounds. At this time, all medications to be administered are oral.

3. This is part of the two-identifier system of medication administration implemented to prevent medication errors, but it is not the first action for the nurse to take.
4. **The nurse should assess the client's last potassium (K+) level because hypokalemia (abnormally low K+ level) is the most common cause of dysrhythmias in clients receiving digoxin secondary to clients concurrently taking diuretics. Furosemide (Lasix) is a loop diuretic. The nurse should check for digoxin and K+ levels and apical pulse (AP) prior to administering digoxin.**

Content – *Medical/Surgical:* **Category of Health Alteration** – *Drug Administration:* **Integrated Processes** – *Nursing Process: Assessment:* **Client Needs** – *Physiological Integrity: Pharmacological and Parenteral Therapies:* **Cognitive Level** – *Analysis*

59. 1. This client has been on a medication to control the angina for 2 days and could be discharged.
    2. This client is currently completing the amount of care that would be provided in the hospital setting. The client can be taught to continue the Coumadin at home and return to the HCP's office for blood work, or a home health nurse can be assigned to go to the client's home and draw blood for the lab work.
    3. **Because resistant infections are very difficult to treat, this client should remain in the hospital for the required IVPB medication.**
    4. These blood gases are expected for a client diagnosed with COPD. This client could go home with oxygen and home health follow-up care.

    Content – *Medical/Surgical:* **Category of Health Alteration** – *Respiratory:* **Integrated Processes** – *Nursing Process: Assessment:* **Client Needs** – *Safe and Effective Care Environment: Management of Care:* **Cognitive Level** – *Analysis*

60. 1. The nurse may wish to consult the hospital's attorneys or retain an attorney of his or her own, but this is not the first action for the nurse.
    2. **The nurse should be familiar with the chart and the situation so that details can be remembered. This should be the nurse's first action.**
    3. It is too late to purchase liability insurance to cover the current situation. The nurse may wish to purchase insurance for any future litigation.
    4. The nurse should refrain from discussing the case with anyone who could be called as a witness or be named in the suit.

*Content – Legal: **Category of Health Alteration** – Management of Care: **Integrated Processes** – Nursing Process: Implementation: **Client Needs** – Safe and Effective Care Environment: Management of Care: **Cognitive Level** – Application*

61. 1. **One of the many jobs of a manager is to see that performance evaluations are completed on the staff.**
    2. The manager should receive input from many sources to make decisions. Some decisions are made for the manager by administration based on costs or any number of other reasons.
    3. The nurses retain responsibility for their own actions because they practice under the state's nursing practice act. The manager retains responsibility for the functioning of the unit.
    4. The nurse manager attends many meetings pertaining to nursing but attends medical committee meetings only when a nursing issue is being discussed.

    *Content – Management of Care: **Category of Health Alteration** – Management of Care: **Integrated Processes** – Nursing Process: Implementation: **Client Needs** – Safe and Effective Care Environment: Management of Care: **Cognitive Level** – Application*

62. 1. **Usually, the charge nurse should attempt to settle a conflict at the lowest level possible, in this case, confronting the nurse. However, the charge nurse does not have the authority to require a drug screen, which is the intervention needed in this situation. The nurse should notify the unit manager.**
    2. The charge nurse does not have the authority to force the nurse to submit to a drug screening, which is what this behavior suggests. Therefore, the charge nurse should not confront the staff nurse. The nurse should notify the supervisor.
    3. Nurses have the right to take breaks with or without their peers. The charge nurse cannot enforce this option.
    4. An occurrence report is not used for this type of situation. This is a management or a peer review issue. The nurse can go through the manager or a peer review committee.

    *Content – Management of Care: **Integrated Processes** – Nursing Process: Implementation: **Client Needs** – Safe and Effective Care Environment, Management of Care: **Cognitive Level** – Application*

63. 1. **Telling jokes with sexual innuendos creates a "hostile work environment" and should be addressed with the HCP. This is a courtesy to the HCP to allow him to correct the behavior without being embarrassed.**

2. If the behavior is not corrected, then the nurse should report the HCP to the manager or chief nursing officer (CNO). The manager or CNO may find it necessary to report the behavior to the medical staff committee or president.
3. The charge nurse should first report the behavior to the manager and then, if the problem is not resolved, to the CNO; in other words, follow the chain of command.
4. Some facilities have a code for staff to use when an HCP is acting out, but it is rarely, if ever, used.

*Content – Management of Care: **Integrated Processes** – Nursing Process: Implementation: **Client Needs** – Safe and Effective Care Environment: Management of Care: **Cognitive Level** – Application*

64. 1. The nurse would not need to notify the surgeon of the client's refusal because this is a situation the nurse should manage.
    2. **Feeling a "pop" after an abdominal hysterectomy may indicate possible wound dehiscence, which is a surgical emergency and requires the nurse to notify the surgeon via telephone.**
    3. This situation indicates that it is time for the nurse to reinfuse the lost blood.
    4. A negative Chvostek sign is normal and indicates the calcium level is within normal limits.

    *Content – Medical/Surgical: **Integrated Processes** – Assessment: **Client Needs** – Safe and Effective Care Environment: Management of Care: **Cognitive Level** – Analysis*

65. 1. The client who had an endotracheal tube would have a sore throat; therefore, the PACU nurse would not assess this client first.
    2. **A pulse oximeter reading of less than 93% indicates an oxygenation problem; therefore, this client should be assessed first.**
    3. Epidural surgery affects the lower extremities, so a palpable pedal pulse indicates a sufficient blood supply; this client should not be assessed first.
    4. Drainage of green bile from the nasogastric (N/G) tube is normal; therefore, this client should not be seen first.

    *Content – Medical/Surgical: **Category of Health Alteration** – Respiratory: **Integrated Processes** – Nursing Process: Assessment: **Client Needs** – Physiological Integrity: Reduction of Risk Potential: **Cognitive Level** – Analysis Processes*

66. 1. After assessing the client's vital signs the nurse may need to increase the client's intravenous rate but it is not the first intervention.
    2. The nurse should assess the client's vital signs but not prior to stopping the bleeding.

3. **The nurse should keep a large tourniquet at the client's bedside and should apply it when suspecting arterial bleeding; this is the nurse's first intervention.**

4. The nurse will need to notify the client's HCP but the nurse must first address the immediate concern, hemorrhaging.

*Content – Medical/Surgical: **Category of Health Alteration** – Musculoskeletal: **Integrated Processes** – Nursing Process: Implementation: **Client Needs** – Physiological Integrity: Reduction of Risk Potential: **Cognitive Level** – Application*

MAKING NURSING DECISIONS: When the question asks the test taker to identify the first intervention, it means one or more of the options are interventions a nurse could implement. The test taker can ask, "Is the client in distress?" If the client is in distress, do not assess.

67. 1. The nurse should always document the findings in the chart, but the first intervention is to get help since the client has neurovascular compromise.

2. Elevating the client's right hand will not help neurovascular compromise.

3. The Doppler can be used to assess the radial pulse, but this client is experiencing neurovascular compromise, which requires immediate medical intervention.

4. **The client is exhibiting severe neurovascular compromise, which indicates a surgical complication and requires notifying the surgeon immediately.**

*Content – Medical/Surgical: **Category of Health Alteration** – Musculoskeletal: **Integrated Processes** – Nursing Process: Implementation: **Client Needs** – Physiological Integrity: Reduction of Risk Potential: **Cognitive Level** – Application*

MAKING NURSING DECISIONS: The nurse must realize when the client is experiencing a surgical emergency that requires a medical intervention. The nurse should not select equipment, a Doppler, over the client's body.

68. 1. The first time a client ambulates after hip surgery should be with a physical therapist or a nurse qualified to evaluate the client's ability to ambulate safely with a walker. The UAP does not have these qualifications.

2. **According to the National Council of State Boards of Nursing (NCSBN), collaboration with interdisciplinary team members is part of the Management of Care. Physical therapy is responsible for management of the client's ability to move and transfer.**

3. The physical therapist will measure and obtain the correct walker for the client.

4. The social worker is not responsible for assisting the client to ambulate, but may assist the client on discharge in obtaining needed medical equipment in the home.

*Content – Medical/Surgical: **Category of Health Alteration** – Musculoskeletal: **Integrated Processes** – Nursing Process: Implementation: **Client Needs** – Physiological Integrity: Reduction of Risk Potential: **Cognitive Level** – Application*

69. 1. The UAP is being paid to assist the nurse to care for clients on the surgical unit, not take clients downstairs to smoke.

2. **The UAP can take vital signs on a newly admitted client.**

3. The client has a tube into the stomach via the abdominal wall that requires assessing the residual to determine whether the stomach is digesting the tube feeding. This task is not appropriate to delegate to the UAP.

4. If the toes are cold, have a capillary refill time of more than 3 seconds, or are pale, the nurse must make a judgment as to the circulatory status of the foot; therefore, the nurse would not delegate this task.

*Content – Management of Care: **Integrated Processes** – Nursing Process: Planning: **Client Needs** – Safe and Effective Care Environment: Management of Care: **Cognitive Level** – Synthesis*

70. 1. The LPN can bathe a client, but this should be assigned to the UAP, thereby allowing the LPN to perform a higher-level task.

2. The LPN can document the amount of food the client eats, but this should be assigned to the UAP, thereby allowing the LPN to perform a higher-level task.

3. According to the NCLEX-RN® test plan, collaboration with interdisciplinary team members is part of the management of care. The activity director of the long-term care facility would be responsible for this activity.

4. **The LPN's scope of practice allows routine sterile procedures on the client who is stable, such as clients in a surgical rehabilitation facility.**

*Content – Management of Care: **Integrated Processes** – Nursing Process: Planning: **Client Needs** – Safe and Effective Care Environment, Management of Care: **Cognitive Level** – Synthesis*

71. 1. Any member of the staff can change the sharps container when it is full. There is an OSHA fine if the sharps containers are over the full line.

2. The housekeeping department can change the sharps container as well as any staff member.

3. **The nurse should reward appropriate behavior by the other healthcare members.**

Verbal praise is always appreciated by anyone.

4. The nurse could let the clinical manager know the UAP was emptying the sharps container but the best action is to directly praise the UAP.

Content – *Management of Care:* **Integrated Processes –** *Nursing Process: Implementation:* **Client Needs –** *Safe and Effective Care Environment: Safety and Infection Control:* **Cognitive Level –** *Application*

72. 1. The nurse should assess the client's neurovascular status when the UAP reports any abnormality.
2. The client should be repositioned by log rolling, but it is not appropriate when the client has a neurovascular compromise.
3. **The nurse should assess the client whenever receiving any information from another member of the healthcare team.**
4. The nurse should not request another member of the healthcare team to assess a client who is exhibiting a possible surgical complication.

Content – *Medical/Surgical:* **Category of Health Alteration –** *Musculoskeletal:* **Integrated Processes –** *Nursing Process: Implementation:* **Client Needs –** *Physiological Integrity: Reduction of Risk Potential:* **Cognitive Level –** *Application*

73. 1. The client who has just returned from surgery should not be transferred from the ICU because he or she may not be stable.
2. A sigmoid colostomy is a surgical procedure that causes major fluid shifts and has the potential for multiple complications; therefore, this client should not be transferred to the surgical unit.
3. **Although the client is only 1 day postoperative for a total hip replacement, it is an elective procedure, which indicates that the client was stable prior to the surgery. The incision is also dry and intact. Of the four clients, this client is the most stable and should be transferred to the surgical unit.**
4. A fat embolism is a potentially life-threatening complication of a fracture; therefore, this client should not be transferred from the ICU.

Content – *Medical/Surgical:* **Integrated Processes –** *Nursing Process: Planning:* **Client Needs –** *Safe and Effective Care Environment: Management of Care:* **Cognitive Level –** *Synthesis*

74. 1. Family members should be asked to stay in the client's room until the lights come back on. This helps ensure safety of the family members.
2. **During an electrical failure, the red outlets in the hospital run on the backup**

generator, and all IV pumps and necessary equipment should be plugged into these outlets.
3. The hospital may provide tap bells for contacting the hospital staff, but would not provide flashlights to all clients. The hospital staff would need the flashlights.
4. The charge nurse should not tie up the phone lines during an emergency situation; the phones may not even be working.

Content – *Management of Care:* **Integrated Processes –** *Nursing Process: Implementation:* **Client Needs –** *Safe and Effective Care Environment: Safety and Infection Control:* **Cognitive Level –** *Application*

75. 1. The charge nurse should contact the laboratory, but the first action should be to address the HCP's behavior in a private area.
2. **This is the charge nurse's first action because it will diffuse the HCP's anger. Inappropriate behavior at the nurse's station should not occur in an area where visitors, clients, or staff will observe the behavior.**
3. The HCP can call the laboratory and share his or her concerns, but it is not the first intervention.
4. The charge nurse has the option to report any HCP's inappropriate behavior, but the immediate situation must be dealt with first.

Content – *Management of Care:* **Integrated Processes –** *Nursing Process: Implementation:* **Client Needs –** *Physiological Integrity: Reduction of Risk Potential:* **Cognitive Level –** *Application*

76. 1. The staff nurse should go through the chain of command when wanting to investigate a problem.
2. **Possibly increasing infection rates among clients with PICCs falls within the infection control nurse's scope of practice, and the infection control nursing staff will have data from all units in the hospital.**
3. The nurse should follow through with investigating a potential problem, but this problem does not fall within the scope of practice of the employee health nurse.
4. The staff nurse should be a part of the solution to a problem. Volunteering is a good action to effect change, but it is not the first action. More information—which the infection control nurse can provide—is necessary first.

Content – *Medical/Surgical:* **Category of Health Alteration –** *Infectious Disease:* **Integrated Processes –** *Nursing Process: Implementation:* **Client Needs –** *Safe and Effective Care Environment: Safety and Infection Control:* **Cognitive Level –** *Application*

77. 1. Because there are multiple surgical clients requiring custodial care, the charge nurse

should not send an experienced UAP to the medical unit.

2. The charge nurse should not send the experienced RN to the medical unit because this nurse represents the strength of the staff.

3. **The LPN would be the most appropriate staff to send to the medical unit because the LPN has experience on the unit. His or her expertise is also not required to perform custodial care.**

4. A new orientee should not be sent to an unfamiliar area.

Content – Management of Care: **Integrated Processes –** *Nursing Process: Planning:* **Client Needs –** *Safe and Effective Care Environment: Management of Care:* **Cognitive Level –** *Synthesis*

78. **Correct Answer: 2, 4, 3, 1**
The nurse must remember the acronym RACE, which is a recognized national standard for fire safety in healthcare facilities.
2. **R is for rescue.**
4. **A is for alert.**
3. **C is for confine.**
1. **E is for extinguish.**

Content – Managment of Care: **Integrated Processes –** *Nursing Process: Implementation:* **Client Needs –** *Safe and Effective Care Environment: Safety and Infection Control:* **Cognitive Level –** *Application*

79. 1 The nurse should notify the operating room team, but according to the Joint Commission, the first intervention is to call a time-out, which stops the surgery until clarification is obtained.

2. **According to the Joint Commission, the first intervention is to call a time-out, which stops the surgery until clarification is obtained.**

3. The nurse should discuss this with the client but should first initiate the time-out procedure.

4. Calling the surgeon is a part of the time-out procedure, so the first intervention is to call the time-out.

Content – Medical/Surgical: **Category of Health Alteration –** *Musculoskeletal:* **Integrated Processes –** *Nursing Process: Implementation:* **Client Needs –** *Safe and Effective Care Environment: Management of Care:* **Cognitive Level –** *Application*

80. 1. The nurse should initiate a client care conference to discuss the client's feelings, but at this time the most appropriate response is to allow the client to begin the grieving process.

2. The nurse could notify the social worker about the client's situation, but the most appropriate response is to allow the client to begin the grieving process, which the client

often goes through when experiencing any type of loss. In this situation, the client is losing her independence and her home.

3. The client does not owe the nurse an explanation for "feelings."

4. **According to the NCLEX-RN® test plan, advocacy is part of Management of Care under Safe and Effective Care Environment client needs. Therapeutic communication involves being an advocate in this situation, because sometimes the nurse cannot prevent a perceived "bad" situation from occurring.**

Content – Medical/Surgical: **Category of Health Alteration –** *Musculoskeletal:* **Integrated Processes –** *Nursing Process: Implementation:* **Client Needs –** *Psychosocial Integrity:* **Cognitive Level –** *Application*

81. 1. **The client cannot be restrained as needed. The nurse must have documentation for the need and an HCP's specific order that includes reason for restraint and time limited to no more than 24 hours. This HCP order should be clarified.**

2. The client in restraints should be offered fluids at least every 2 hours.

3. Hand mitts are the least restrictive limb restraints and can be used to help prevent the client from pulling out lines.

4. The nurse must check to ensure that restrained limbs have adequate circulation at least every 2 hours.

Content – Medical/Surgical: **Category of Health Alteration –** *Mental Health:* **Integrated Processes –** *Nursing Process: Diagnosis:* **Client Needs –** *Safe and Effective Care Environment: Safety and Infection Control:* **Cognitive Level –** *Analysis*

82. 1. The RN is responsible for assessing clients; therefore, this is an appropriate assignment.

2. **The LPN may be allowed administer somc IVP medications in some facilities, but the word "all" makes this an inappropriate assignment. Many IVP medications are considered high risk, and only RNs should administer such IVP medications.**

3. This option has the word "all," but it is within the scope of the UAP to complete the a.m. care. The RN and LPN can perform a.m. care, but it should be assigned to the UAP.

4. The RN should monitor laboratory values because this requires interpretation, evaluation, and notification of the HCP in some instances.

Content – Medical/Surgical: **Category of Health Alteration –** *Drug Administration:* **Integrated Processes –** *Nursing Process: Planning:* **Client Needs –** *Safe and*

Effective Care Environment: Management of Care:
Cognitive Level – *Synthesis*

83. 1. Tardiness information is objective data obtained for all employees in the facility, but it does not specifically provide information about the nurse's performance.
    2. The attitude of the nurse is very subjective to evaluate and does not specifically provide information about the nurse's performance.
    3. Thank you notes from the clients are nice for the nurse to receive, but they are not taken into consideration during the evaluation process of the nurse.
    4. **The nurse's ability to document client care directly correlates with the nurse's performance; therefore, these data should be included in the yearly evaluation.**

    Content – *Management of Care:* **Integrated Processes** – *Nursing Process: Implementation:* **Client Needs** – *Safe and Effective Care Environment: Management of Care:* **Cognitive Level** – *Application*

84. 1. The home healthcare agency would not be the best referral because comorbid conditions increase the client's recovery time. The client at home does not have access to healthcare 24 hours a day.
    2. A senior citizen center may help the client's psychosocial needs but not the client's rehabilitation needs.
    3. **The rehabilitation facility will provide intensive therapy and address the comorbid conditions 24 hours a day. This will assist in the client's recovery.**
    4. An outpatient physical therapist does not have the education to address and care for the comorbid issues. The physical therapist is focused on the hip fracture only, and the client may have transportation problems going to an outpatient clinic.

    Content – *Medical/Surgical:* **Category of Health Alteration** – *Musculoskeletal:* **Integrated Processes** – *Nursing Process: Planning:* **Client Needs** – *Psychosocial Integrity:* **Cognitive Level** – *Synthesis*

85. 1. The nasogastric tube should be replaced, but this task will require more time and acquiring new equipment; therefore, it should not be done first.
    2. **The client scheduled for surgery is priority and must be ready when the OR calls; therefore, completing the preoperative checklist is the first task the nurse should implement. The preoperative checklist ensures the client's safety.**
    3. The client being discharged can wait until the safety needs of the client going to surgery have been addressed.

4. This is a minimal to moderate amount of drainage, which requires a dressing change, but not prior to making sure the client going to surgery is ready.

Content – *Medical/Surgical:* **Integrated Processes** – *Nursing Process: Implementation:* **Client Needs** – *Safe and Effective Care Environment: Management of Care:* **Cognitive Level** – *Application*

86. 1. **Antiplatelet medication will increase the client's bleeding time and should be held 5 days prior to surgery; therefore, this medication should be questioned.**
    2. A client with a TKR is at risk for developing deep vein thrombosis (DVT); therefore, an anticoagulant medication would not be questioned.
    3. The client with a Whipple procedure has had part of the pancreas removed and is placed on insulin; therefore, the nurse would not question administering Humalog.
    4. An aminoglycoside antibiotic is not in the penicillin family; therefore, the nurse would not question administering this medication.

    Content – *Medical/Surgical:* **Category of Health Alteration** – *Drug Administration:* **Integrated Processes** – *Nursing Process: Implementation:* **Client Needs** – *Physiological Integrity: Pharmacological and Parenteral Therapies:* **Cognitive Level** – *Application*

87. 1. A client who is 4 hours postoperative for abdominal surgery would be expected to have abdominal pain and hypoactive bowel sounds secondary to general anesthesia. This client would not be assessed first.
    2. This output indicates the client is voiding at least 30 mL an hour; therefore, the nurse would not assess this client first.
    3. The client with an open cholecystectomy frequently has a T-tube that would normally drain green bile. This client would not be assessed first.
    4. **The client is exhibiting signs of compromised circulation; therefore, the nurse should assess this client first. The nurse should assess for the 6 Ps: pain, pulse, paresthesia, paralysis, pallor, and polar (cold).**

    Content – *Medical/Surgical:* **Category of Health Alteration** – *Gastrointestinal:* **Integrated Processes** – *Nursing Process: Assessment:* **Client Needs** – *Physiological Integrity: Reduction of Risk Potential:* **Cognitive Level** – *Analysis*

88. 1. **This situation should be addressed first because the charge nurse is responsible for family/client complaints. If the family contacts the administration, the charge nurse must be aware of the situation.**

2. The evaluation needs to be completed, but it does not take priority over handling an irate family member.
3. The charge nurse could assign this task to another nurse or ward clerk. Dealing appropriately with an irate family member takes priority over calling the laboratory.
4. The charge nurse could assign this task to another nurse or ward clerk. Dealing appropriately with an irate family member takes priority over transferring a client.

Content – Management of Care: **Integrated Processes** *– Nursing Process: Implementation:* **Client Needs** *– Psychosocial Integrity:* **Cognitive Level** *– Application*

89. 1. Notifying the kitchen will only scare the kitchen personnel and will not alert the bomb squad as to the situation.
2. The operator would not be able to trace a phone call that has been disconnected.
3. **The chain of command in a hospital is to notify the security department, and they will institute the hospital procedure for the bomb threat.**
4. The nurse should not directly call the local police department because the hospital security department is responsible for implementing the procedure for a bomb scare.

Content – Management of Care: **Integrated Processes** *– Nursing Process: Implementation:* **Client Needs** *– Safe Effective Care Environment: Management of Care:* **Cognitive Level** *– Application*

90. 1. Autocratic managers use an authoritarian approach to direct the activities of others.
2. Laissez-faire managers maintain a permissive climate with little direction or control.
3. **A democratic manager is people oriented and emphasizes efficient group functioning. The environment is open and communication flows both ways, and this includes having meetings to discuss concerns.**
4. This statement reflects shirking of responsibility, thus letting someone else address the problem, and is not characteristic of a democratic manager.

Content – Management of Care: **Integrated Processes** *– Nursing Process: Evaluation:* **Client Needs** *– Safe and Effective Care Environment: Management of Care:* **Cognitive Level** *– Synthesis*

91. **Correct Answer: 2, 4, 1, 3, 5**
2. **The nurse should always explain the procedure to the client even if the client has had the procedure done before.**
4. **This procedure is very painful and the nurse should premedicate the client 30 minutes prior to performing wound care.**

1. **Obtaining the needed supplies can be done after premedicating the client since the nurse should wait 30 minutes after medicating the client.**
3. **The nurse should remove the old dressing.**
5. **The nurse should assess the burned area for signs of infection, viable tissue, or any eschar.**

Content – Medical/Surgical: **Category of Health Alteration** *– Integumentary:* **Integrated Processes** *– Nursing Process: Implementation:* **Client Needs** *– Safe and Effective Care Environment: Safety and Infection Control:* **Cognitive Level** *– Application*

MAKING NURSING DECISIONS: The test taker must rank the nursing interventions in order of priority.

92. 1. This client will require time to adjust to living in an extended care facility. This would be an expected reaction.
2. This client may or may not be allowed a glass of wine at night. Some long-term care facilities do allow the client to have a controlled amount of alcohol with an HCP order and the family supplying the alcohol, but this client is not priority.
3. **This client may or may not have a valid complaint. The nurse should investigate whether or not the complaint is true. Failure to answer a call light can result in the client's attempting to ambulate without assistance and could be a safety issue. The nurse should speak with this client first.**
4. The nurse is not in control of the client's son and his discharge, but if the son is being discharged, it can be assumed that the son is in a stable condition, and it is not a priority for the charge nurse to see this client.

Content – Management of Care: **Integrated Processes** *– Nursing Process: Assessment:* **Client Needs** *– Safe and Effective Care Environment: Management of Care:* **Cognitive Level** *– Analysis*

93. 1. The director of nurses must first understand the extent of the complaint. Telling staff to ignore preconceived ideas about older adult clients does not work. The director of nurses should have valid information to discuss with the staff.
2. The client has a general complaint, and so more than one staff member may have ignored the client's statements. Neglect was not mentioned in the stem of the question. Not treating the client with the dignity that the client deserves is implied.
3. This is a false statement. Some residents in a long-term care facility may not be able to

determine their needs, but this is not true of all residents.

4. **The director of nurses should discuss the resident's complaints with the resident and then determine a plan of action to remedy the situation.**

*Content – Management of Care: **Integrated Processes –** Nursing Process: Assessment: **Client Needs** – Safe and Effective Care Environment: Management of Care: **Cognitive Level** – Analysis*

94. 1. This may be a true statement, but this client is exhibiting symptoms of depression. The client may or may not wish to make friends at the facility.

2. This is not acknowledging the client's feelings.

3. **This client is exhibiting symptoms of depression. Therapeutic conversation is implemented to help the client vent feelings. This statement acknowledges the client's feeling and offers help.**

4. This action may get the client to interact with other people, but it does not acknowledge the client's feelings.

*Content – Medical/Surgical: **Category of Health Alteration** – Mental Health: **Integrated Processes –** Nursing Process: Evaluation: **Client Needs** – Psychosocial Integrity: **Cognitive Level** – Synthesis*

95. 1. **The charge nurse should remind the UAPs not to discuss confidential information in a public place. This is the first action.**

2. The charge nurse may need to inform the manager of the breach of confidentiality, but the first action is to stop the conversation.

3. The charge nurse and/or the manager may need to make sure the UAPs are familiar with confidentiality, but the conversation should be terminated first.

4. This might be a better activity for the UAPs, but the first action is to stop the conversation.

*Content – Legal: **Integrated Processes** – Nursing Process: Implementation: **Client Needs** – Safe and Effective Care Environment: Management of Care: **Cognitive Level** – Application*

96. 1. **An ombudsman is a representative appointed to receive and investigate complaints made by individuals of abuses or capricious acts. All Medicare and Medicaid long-term care facilities must have an ombudsman to act as a neutral party in matters of dispute with the facility. This is the best person to investigate a complaint.**

2. The social worker is employed by the facility and is not the best person to investigate the complaint.

3. The upset family member should attend the conference but should have the ombudsman investigate the complaint.

4. The director will be biased; the best person to investigate the validity of the complaint is the ombudsman

*Content – Legal: **Integrated Processes** – Nursing Process: Implementation: **Client Needs** – Psychosocial Integrity: **Cognitive Level** – Application*

97. 1. The nurse should not refer the client to a church or volunteer organization to ensure continuity of care. The organization's work may depend on unpaid individuals, and a volunteer may or may not be available to transport the client when needed.

2. **The nurse should refer the client to a home health agency for follow-up care. The nurse will go to the client's home to assess the client and perform dressing changes. The home health agency will also assess the client and the client's home for further needs.**

3. The client is unable to drive and would not be able to get to an outpatient clinic.

4. The client is unable to drive and would not be able to get to the HCP's office.

*Content – Medical/Surgical: **Category of Health Alteration** – Gastrointestinal: **Integrated Processes –** Nursing Process: Planning: **Client Needs** – Physiological Integrity: Physiological Adaptation: **Cognitive Level** – Synthesis*

98. 1. The nurse must assess the cause of the bruises before filing a report of abuse. The nurse would file a report of elder abuse only if it is determined that the client has been abused.

2. **The nurse should ask the client whether there is a reason for the bruises that the nurse should be aware of. This is the first intervention and can be done while the nurse is currently with the client.**

3. The nurse should check the client's MAR to see whether he is currently on a medication, such as warfarin (Coumadin) or a systemic steroid, that would increase the risk for bruising; however, this would be done after talking with the client because the bruising is "new," and bruising from the medications can take several days to weeks to develop.

4. The family may need to be notified but not until the nurse assesses the situation.

*Content – Management of Care: **Integrated Processes –** Nursing Process: Implementation: **Client Needs –** Safe and Effective Care Environment: Safety and Infection Control: **Cognitive Level** – Application*

99. 1. **The client is expressing negative feelings about being placed in the nursing home. Asking about the client's feelings is a therapeutic response that encourages the client to discuss his or her feelings.**
    2. This is not acknowledging the client's feelings and is nontherapeutic because it is a judgmental statement.
    3. The client does not owe the nurse an explanation. "Why" is never therapeutic.
    4. This is assuming the client is correct in being "trouble at home" and agreeing that the family would punish the client for being a problem.
    Content – Mental Health: ***Integrated Processes –*** *Nursing Process: Implementation:* ***Client Needs –*** *Psychosocial Integrity:* ***Cognitive Level –*** *Application*

100. 1. The nurse cannot testify to what preceded the client's fall because the nurse was not on duty at the time.
    2. The nurse was not on duty to assess the client's injuries, so any information about the injuries received from the fall would have to be hearsay or obtained from the chart.
    3. The nurse cannot testify to the client's mental status prior to the fall because the nurse was not on duty at the time.
    4. **The nurse initiated a policy that is designed to prevent falls from occurring. This is all the nurse can testify to.**
    Content – Legal: ***Integrated Processes –*** *Nursing Process: Diagnosis:* ***Client Needs –*** *Safe and Effective Care Environment: Management of Care:* ***Cognitive Level –*** *Knowledge*

101. 1. The registered nurse, experienced or not, can be assigned nursing duties of assessment, planning, teaching, and other duties that cannot be delegated or assigned. The charge nurse has only two RNs for 35 clients. This nurse should not be requested to stay home.
    2. An experienced LPN will be needed by the unit to care for the many IV lines and medications.
    3. **The UAP cannot administer medications or IVs and has requested to be allowed to stay home. This is the best staff member to request to stay home.**
    4. This UAP may be less experienced on the floor but has not worked long enough to receive any paid time off, and this could greatly affect the UAP's pay.
    Content – Management of Care: ***Integrated Processes –*** *Nursing Process: Planning:* ***Client Needs –*** *Safe and Effective Care Environment: Management of Care:* ***Cognitive Level –*** *Synthesis*

102. 1. **The charge nurse does not have a right to interfere with two consenting adults having a relationship. Doing nothing is the correct action for the charge nurse. If one of the residents involved is incapable of giving consent to a relationship, then the charge nurse would need to get involved.**
    2. Two consenting adults have a right to form a bond. The family does not have a right to interfere with the expression of a basic human need, to form an intimate relationship with another human being.
    3. The residents have the right to companionship. They should be allowed to participate in any activity that they wish, when they wish.
    4. This is a normal situation, and no care plan meeting is needed.
    Content – Management of Care: ***Integrated Processes –*** *Nursing Process: Implementation:* ***Client Needs –*** *Psychosocial Integrity:* ***Cognitive Level –*** *Application*

103. 1. The argument should already be in a private area because the argument ensued during report. Report should always be held in a confidential area.
    2. **The CNO should evaluate the concerns of each charge nurse and then make a decision as to a plan of care for the resident. The CNO is the next in command over the charge nurses in an extended care facility.**
    3. This argument does not involve the family. If, after listening to both sides, the CNO thinks there is a need for a family member's input, then the CNO could contact the family, but a decision should be made until this can occur.
    4. The nurses each have a concern over a resident. This situation should be resolved before continuing report.
    Content – Management of Care: ***Integrated Processes –*** *Nursing Process: Implementation:* ***Client Needs –*** *Safe and Effective Care Environment: Management of Care:* ***Cognitive Level –*** *Application*

104. 1. Calling a time-out when a discrepancy is noted on the surgical permit is an appropriate action to prevent an error during a surgical procedure.
    2. The Joint Commission requires two identifiers be utilized prior to administering medications. Most hospitals use the client's date of birth for the second identifier. This is an appropriate action to prevent an error during a medication administration.
    3. **A quiz during orientation is given to assess whether the new employee**

understands the information being taught. Giving the answers to the quiz completes the required documentation for the employee's files but does not ensure the new hire understands how to utilize the IV pump. This is a violation of the Patient Safety Goals.

4. Initiating a fall prevention program for an older adult client to prevent falls is an appropriate action to attempt to ensure client safety.

Content – Management of Care: **Integrated Processes –** *Nursing Process: Implementation:* **Client Needs –** *Safe and Effective Care Environment: Management of Care:* **Cognitive Level –** *Application*

105. 1. This client should be categorized as black, priority 4, which means the injury is extensive and chances of survival are unlikely even with definitive care. Clients should receive comfort measures and be separated from other casualties but not abandoned.

2. This client should be categorized as red, priority 1, which means the injury is life threatening but survivable with minimal intervention. These clients can deteriorate rapidly without treatment.

3. This client should be categorized as green, priority 3, which means the injury is minor and treatment can be delayed hours to days. These clients should be moved away from the main triage area.

4. The client should be categorized as a yellow, priority 2, which means the injury is significant and requires medical care but can wait hours without threat to life or limb. Clients in this category receive treatment only after immediate casualties are treated.

Content – Triage: **Integrated Processes –** *Nursing Process: Planning:* **Client Needs –** *Physiological Integrity: Reduction of Risk Potential:* **Cognitive Level –** *Synthesis*

106. 1. The normal white blood cell count is 5.0 to 10.0 mm³; therefore, this client does not require immediate intervention.

2. The client's cholesterol level is elevated, but this would not require immediate intervention by the nurse. An elevated cholesterol level is not life threatening and can be discussed at the client's next appointment.

3. The client's calcium level is within the normal range of 9.0 to 10.5 mg/dL; therefore, this client does not require an immediate intervention.

4. The therapeutic range for an INR is 2 to 3. This client is at risk for bleeding and

requires immediate intervention by the nurse. The nurse should call the client and instruct the client to stop taking warfarin (Coumadin), an anticoagulant.

Content – Medical/Surgical: **Integrated Processes –** *Nursing Process: Assessment:* **Client Needs –** *Physiological Integrity: Reduction of Risk Potential:* **Cognitive Level –** *Analysis*

107. 1. A spokesperson should address the media away from the victim care area as soon as possible. This could be a nurse in some situations, but it is not the priority intervention when triaging victims.

2. The disaster tag number and the client's name should be recorded in the disaster log book, but it is not the priority intervention. The disaster tag must be attached to the client prior to logging the client into the disaster log book.

3. Client tracking is a critical component of casualty management. Disaster tags, which include name, address, age, location, description of injuries, and treatments or medications administered, must be securely attached to the client.

4. Family and friends arriving at the disaster must be cared for by the disaster workers, but it is not the first intervention for the nurse who is triaging disaster victims.

Content – Triage: **Integrated Processes –** *Nursing Process: Implementation:* **Client Needs –** *Safe and Effective Care Environment: Safety and Infection Control:* **Cognitive Level –** *Application*

108. **1. Parish nursing emphasizes the relationship between spiritual faith and health. A parish nurse (PN) is a registered nurse with a minimum of 2 years' experience who works in a faith community to address health issues of its members as well as those in the broader community or neighborhood.**

2. The parish nurse works in the community, not in an acute care setting.

3. There is no such thing as a parish clinic.

4. The parish nurse can be an RN or an LPN.

Content – Community Health: **Integrated Processes –** *Nursing Process: Implementation:* **Client Needs –** *Safe and Effective Care Environment: Management of Care:* **Cognitive Level –** *Application*

109. 1. The client's HCP may need to be notified, but it is not the nurse's first intervention.

2. The nurse must first assess the reddened area to determine the stage of the pressure ulcer and what treatment should be recommended.

3. The reddened area should be documented in the chart, but this is not the first intervention.

4. The client may or may not need to be referred to a wound care nurse, but it is not the nurse's first intervention. If the reddened area is Stage 1 or 2, the wound care nurse probably would not be notified.

Content – Medical/Surgical: **Category of Health Alteration** *– Integumentary:* **Integrated Processes** *– Nursing Process: Implementation:* **Client Needs** *– Physiological Integrity: Reduction of Risk Potential:* **Cognitive Level** *– Application*

110. 1. The occupational therapist assists the client with activities of daily living, not with employment concerns.

2. The NCLEX-RN® test blueprint lists referrals under Management of Care. After a client has been injured and is unable to return to previous employment because of the injury, the rehabilitation commission of each state will help evaluate the client and determine whether the client is eligible to receive training or education for another occupation.

3. The client is not asking about disability but rather about employment. The nurse needs to refer the client to the appropriate agency.

4. The client should discuss his concerns with his wife, but the nurse should refer the client to an agency that can address his concerns about employment.

Content – Management of Care: **Category of Health Alteration** *– Musculoskeletal:* **Integrated Processes** *– Nursing Process: Implementation:* **Client Needs** *– Psychosocial Integrity:* **Cognitive Level** *– Application*

111. **1. The mother may want to see her infant before the body is removed from the room.**

2. The infant's body will be sent to a funeral home. The parents will not be allowed to take the body home.

3. The body should be treated with the dignity accorded to any human remains.

4. The nurse can present the parents with a lock of the infant's hair and a set of footprints. Giving the parents something of the infant helps with the grieving process.

Content – Caring: **Category of Health Alteration** *– Neonatal:* **Integrated Processes** *– Nursing Process: Implementation:* **Client Needs** *– Psychosocial Integrity:* **Cognitive Level** *– Application*

112. **1. Nasal flaring and grunting indicate the infant is in respiratory distress. The nurse should assess this infant first.**

2. The nurse would not worry about the infant not passing meconium until 20 to 24 hours

after birth. The nurse would not assess this infant first.

3. This situation requires teaching the mother and patience, but the infant is not in distress. The nurse would not assess this infant first.

4. This is normal for a newborn. The nurse would not assess this infant first.

Content – Medical/Surgical: **Category of Health Alteration** *– Pediatrics:* **Integrated Processes** *– Assessment:* **Client Needs** *– Physiological Integrity: Reduction of Risk Potential:* **Cognitive Level** *– Analysis*

113. 1. Because this client is reporting an incident that occurred hours ago and she is not in imminent danger, this client is not the first client the nurse should call.

2. The nurse should return this call first because the nurse must determine whether the client has a plan for suicide.

3. Not wanting to eat is part of the anorexia disease process. The nurse does not need to return this call first.

4. Hand trembling is part of the Parkinson's disease process. Control of the symptoms of Parkinson's disease is affected by several factors, including the amount of sleep the client had, fatigue, and the development of tolerance to the medications. Because this client is not at risk for suicide, he is not the first client for the nurse to see.

Content – Medical/Surgical: **Category of Health Alteration** *– Mental Health:* **Integrated Processes** *– Nursing Process: Assessment:* **Client Needs** *– Psychosocial Integrity:* **Cognitive Level** *– Analysis*

114. **1. Pediatric clients in a psychiatric facility must keep up with schoolwork. Clients must be escorted from one building to another. The MHW should be assigned to this task.**

2. The MHW is not qualified for this task to lead a group therapy session.

3. Explaining the purpose of recreation therapy is teaching, and teaching cannot be delegated to an MHW.

4. Clients in a psychiatric facility are expected to meet their own hygiene needs as part of assuming responsibility for themselves. This is not the best task to assign to the MHW.

Content – Medical/Surgical: **Category of Health Alteration** *– Mental Health:* **Integrated Processes** *– Nursing Process: Planning:* **Client Needs** *– Safe and Effective Care Environment, Management of Care:* **Cognitive Level** *– Synthesis*

115. 1, 2, and 5 are correct.

1. Smoking while taking birth control pills increases the risk of adverse reactions such as formation of blood clots.

2. **The client should take the pill at approximately the same time each day to maintain a blood level of the hormone.**

3. The client should be instructed to take a missed pill as soon as she realizes she missed the dose during the intervening 24 hours. However, if the client doesn't realize she missed the pill until the next day, she should not take two pills at that time.

4. Breakthrough bleeding may indicate a change in dose is needed, but the client should not stop taking the pill.

5. **There may be interactions with other medications. Many antibiotics interfere with the action of the birth control pill, and the client should use other contraceptive methods when on an antibiotic.**

*Content – Medical/Surgical: **Category of Health Alteration** – Drug Administration: **Integrated Processes** – Nursing Process: Planning: **Client Needs** – Physiological Integrity: Pharmacological and Parenteral Therapies: **Cognitive Level** – Synthesis*

116. 1. Vaginal itching while receiving antibiotics indicates that the good bacterial flora in the vagina is being destroyed. Yogurt contains these bacteria and can replace the needed bacteria. However, requesting the dietary department to send yogurt each day is not the priority intervention.

2. **The nurse should first explain to the client that this is a side effect of the antibiotic medication. Then, the nurse should notify the dietitian and HCP. The antibiotic therapy cannot be discontinued because of the need for antibiotic therapy after knee replacement surgery.**

3. The HCP should be notified of the vaginal itching, but it is not an emergency and can wait until the HCP makes rounds.

4. The client's sexual history is not a concern because the vaginal infection is secondary to the antibiotic therapy.

*Content – Medical/Surgical: **Category of Health Alteration** – Drug Administration: **Integrated Processes** – Nursing Process: Implementation: **Client Needs** – Physiological Integrity: Pharmacological and Parenteral Therapies: **Cognitive Level** – Application Processes*

117. 1. **The manager should ask for input into the budgetary needs from the staff, but an assessment of the current year's budget is the first step.**

2. An assessment of the costs of any new department projects should be done, but the first step is to assess the present budget.

3. **The first step in a budgetary process is to assess the current budget.**

4. Explaining the new budget to the staff is the last step in the process.

*Content – Management of Care: **Integrated Processes** – Nursing Process: Planning: **Client Needs** – Safe and Effective Care Environment: Management of Care: **Cognitive Level** – Synthesis*

118. 1. The nurse should confront the client with the behavior, but this is not the first intervention.

2. The nurse should document the behavior in the client's chart, but this is not the first intervention.

3. **The nurse should intervene to stop the behavior first before one of the clients is injured. Approaching the client with another staff member shows strength and provides the nurse with the ability to perform a safe "take down."**

4. The client should be told to return to the room, but stopping the behavior is the first intervention.

*Content – Medical/Surgical: **Category of Health Alteration** – Mental Health: **Integrated Processes** – Nursing Process: Implementation: **Client Needs** – Safe Effective Care Environment: Safety and Infection Control: **Cognitive Level** – Application*

119. 1. This surgeon should speak with the client, but the first intervention is to stop the procedure.

2. Asking the client to discuss concerns should be done, but the first intervention is to stop the procedure.

3. Continuing to prep the client for the surgery can be done, but is inappropriate when the client no longer is giving consent.

4. **Stopping the surgical procedure is the first intervention for the nurse to implement.**

*Content – Medical/Surgical: **Integrated Processes** – Nursing Process: Implementation: **Client Needs** – Physiological Integrity: Reduction of Risk Potential: **Cognitive Level** – Application*

120. 1. Four episodes of mania in 6 months do not indicate therapy has been effective.

2. **The ability to hold a job for 9 months indicates the client is responding to therapy.**

3. Wearing a nightgown to the day room does not indicate the client is responding to treatment.

4. Three motor vehicle accidents do not indicate the client is responding to treatment.

*Content – Medical/Surgical: **Category of Health Alteration** – Mental Health: **Integrated Processes** – Nursing Process: Evaluation: **Client Needs** – Psychosocial Integrity: **Cognitive Level** – Synthesis*

Normal Laboratory Values

These values are obtained from *Davis's Comprehensive Handbook of Laboratory and Diagnostic Tests with Nursing Implications*. Laboratory results may differ slightly depending on the resource manual or the laboratory normal values.

Arterial Blood Gas	Adult
pH	7.35 to 7.45
Pco_2	35 to 45 mm Hg
Hco_3	22 to 26 mEq/L
Pao_2	80 to 100 mm Hg
O_2 saturation	93% to 100%

Chemistry 7	Adult
Cholesterol	Less than 200 mg/dL
HDL	40 to 65 mg/dL
LDL	Less than 200 mg/dL
Creatinine	0.6 to 1.2 mg/dL
Glucose	60 to 110 mg/dL
Potassium	3.5 to 5.5 mEq/L
Sodium	135 to 145 mEq/L
Triglycerides	Less than 150 mg/dL
Blood urea nitrogen	10 to 31 mg/dL

Blood Count	Adult
Hematocrit (Hct)	Male: 43% to 49% Female: 38% to 44%
Hemoglobin (Hgb)	Male: 13.2 to 17.3 g/dL Female: 11.7 to 15.5 g/dL
Activated partial thromboplastin time (APTT)	25 to 35 seconds
Prothrombin time (PT)	10 to 13 seconds
Red blood cell count (RBC)	Male: 4.7 to 5.1 10^6 cells/mm^3 Female: 4.2 to 4.8 10^6 cells/mm^3
White blood cell count (WBC)	4.5 to 11.0 1,000/mm^3
Platelets	150 to 450 10^3/μL/mm^3
Erythrocyte sedimentation rate (ESR)	Male: 0 to 20 mm/hr Female: 0 to 30 mm/hr

Drug Levels	Adult
Digoxin (Lanoxin)	0.8 to 2.0 ng/mL
International Normalized Ratio (INR)	2 to 3 2.5 to 3.5 if the client has a mechanical heart valve
Lithium mEq/L	0.6 to 1.2 mEq/L
Phenytoin (Dilantin)	10 to 20 mcg/mL
Theophylline (Aminophyllin)	10 to 20 mcg/mL
Valproic acid (Depakote)	50 to 100 mcg/mL
Vancomycin trough level	10 to 20 mcg/mL
Vancomycin peak level	30 to 40 mcg/mL

Glossary of English Words Commonly Encountered on Nursing Examinations

Abnormality – defect, irregularity, anomaly, oddity

Absence – nonappearance, lack, nonattendance

Abundant – plentiful, rich, profuse

Accelerate – go faster, speed up, increase, hasten

Accumulate – build up, collect, gather

Accurate – precise, correct, exact

Achievement – accomplishment, success, reaching, attainment

Acknowledge – admit, recognize, accept, reply

Activate – start, turn on, stimulate

Adequate – sufficient, ample, plenty, enough

Angle – slant, approach, direction, point of view

Application – use, treatment, request, claim

Approximately – about, around, in the region of, more or less, roughly speaking

Arrange – position, place, organize, display

Associated – linked, related

Attention – notice, concentration, awareness, thought

Authority – power, right, influence, clout, expert

Avoid – keep away from, evade, let alone

Balanced – stable, neutral, steady, fair, impartial

Barrier – barricade, blockage, obstruction, obstacle

Best – most excellent, most important, greatest

Capable – able, competent, accomplished

Capacity – ability, capability, aptitude, role, power, size

Central – middle, mid, innermost, vital

Challenge – confront, dare, dispute, test, defy, face up to

Characteristic – trait, feature, attribute, quality, typical

Circular – round, spherical, globular

Collect – gather, assemble, amass, accumulate, bring together

Commitment – promise, vow, dedication, obligation, pledge, assurance

Commonly – usually, normally, frequently, generally, universally

Compare – contrast, evaluate, match up to, weigh or judge against

Compartment – section, part, cubicle, booth, stall

Complex – difficult, multifaceted, compound, multipart, intricate

Complexity – difficulty, intricacy, complication

Component – part, element, factor, section, constituent

Comprehensive – complete, inclusive, broad, thorough

Conceal – hide, cover up, obscure, mask, suppress, secrete

Conceptualize – to form an idea

Concern – worry, anxiety, fear, alarm, distress, unease, trepidation

Concisely – briefly, in a few words, succinctly

Conclude – make a judgment based on reason, finish

Confidence – self–assurance, certainty, poise, self–reliance

Congruent – matching, fitting, going together well

Consequence – result, effect, outcome, end result

Constituents – elements, component, parts that make up a whole

Contain – hold, enclose, surround, include, control, limit

Continual – repeated, constant, persistent, recurrent, frequent

Continuous – constant, incessant, nonstop, unremitting, permanent

Contribute – be a factor, add, give

Convene – assemble, call together, summon, organize, arrange

Convenience – expediency, handiness, ease

Coordinate – organize, direct, manage, bring together

Create – make, invent, establish, generate, produce, fashion, build, construct

Creative – imaginative, original, inspired, inventive, resourceful, productive, innovative

Critical – serious, grave, significant, dangerous, life threatening

Cue – signal, reminder, prompt, sign, indication

Curiosity – inquisitiveness, interest, nosiness, snooping

Damage – injure, harm, hurt, break, wound

Deduct – subtract, take away, remove, withhold

Deficient – lacking, wanting, underprovided, scarce, faulty

Defining – important, crucial, major, essential, significant, central

Defuse – resolve, calm, soothe, neutralize, rescue, mollify

Delay – hold up, wait, hinder, postpone, slow down, hesitate, linger

Demand – insist, claim, require, command, stipulate, ask

Describe – explain, tell, express, illustrate, depict, portray

Design – plan, invent, intend, aim, propose, devise

Desirable – wanted, pleasing, enviable, popular, sought after, attractive, advantageous

Detail – feature, aspect, element, factor, facet

Deteriorate – worsen, decline, weaken

Determine – decide, conclude, resolve, agree on

Dexterity – skillfulness, handiness, agility, deftness

Dignity – self–respect, self–esteem, decorum, formality, poise

Dimension – aspect, measurement

Diminish – reduce, lessen, weaken, detract, moderate

Discharge – release, dismiss, set free

Discontinue – stop, cease, halt, suspend, terminate, withdraw

Disorder – complaint, problem, confusion, chaos

Display – show, exhibit, demonstrate, present, put on view

Dispose – to get rid of, arrange, order, set out

Dissatisfaction – displeasure, discontent, unhappiness, disappointment

Distinguish – to separate and classify, recognize

Distract – divert, sidetrack, entertain

Distress – suffering, trouble, anguish, misery, agony, concern, sorrow

Distribute – deliver, spread out, hand out, issue, dispense

Disturbed – troubled, unstable, concerned, worried, distressed, anxious, uneasy

Diversional – serving to distract

Don – put on, dress oneself in

Dramatic – spectacular

Drape – cover, wrap, dress, swathe

Dysfunction – abnormal, impaired

Edge – perimeter, boundary, periphery, brink, border, rim

Effective – successful, useful, helpful, valuable

Efficient – not wasteful, effective, competent, resourceful, capable

Elasticity – stretch, spring, suppleness, flexibility

Eliminate – get rid of, eradicate, abolish, remove, purge

Embarrass – make uncomfortable, make self–conscious, humiliate, mortify

Emerge – appear, come, materialize, become known

Emphasize – call attention to, accentuate, stress, highlight

Ensure – make certain, guarantee

Environment – setting, surroundings, location, atmosphere, milieu, situation

Episode – event, incident, occurrence, experience

Essential – necessary, fundamental, vital, important, crucial, critical, indispensable

Etiology – assigned cause, origin

Exaggerate – overstate, inflate

Excel – to stand out, shine, surpass, outclass

Excessive – extreme, too much, unwarranted

Exertion – intense or prolonged physical effort

Exhibit – show signs of, reveal, display

Expand – get bigger, enlarge, spread out, increase, swell, inflate

Expect – wait for, anticipate, imagine

Expectation – hope, anticipation, belief, prospect, probability

Experience – knowledge, skill, occurrence, know–how

Expose – lay open, leave unprotected, allow to be seen, reveal, disclose, exhibit

External – outside, exterior, outer

Facilitate – make easy, make possible, help, assist

Factor – part, feature, reason, cause, think, issue

Focus – center, focal point, hub

Fragment – piece, portion, section, part, splinter, chip

Function – purpose, role, job, task

Furnish – supply, provide, give, deliver, equip

Further – additional, more, extra, added, supplementary

Generalize – to take a broad view, simplify, to make inferences from particulars

Generate – make, produce, create

Gentle – mild, calm, tender

Girth – circumference, bulk, weight

Highest – uppermost, maximum, peak, main

Hinder – hold back, delay, hamper, obstruct, impede

Humane – caring, kind, gentle, compassionate, benevolent, civilized

Ignore – pay no attention to, disregard, overlook, discount

Imbalance – unevenness, inequality, disparity

Immediate – insistent, urgent, direct

Impair – damage, harm, weaken

Implantation – to put in

Impotent – powerless, weak, incapable, ineffective, unable

Inadvertent – unintentional, chance, unplanned, accidental

Include – comprise, take in, contain

Indicate – point out, sign of, designate, specify, show

Ineffective – unproductive, unsuccessful, useless, vain, futile

Inevitable – predictable, to be expected, unavoidable, foreseeable

Influence – power, pressure, sway, manipulate, affect, effect

Initiate – start, begin, open, commence, instigate

Insert – put in, add, supplement, introduce

Inspect – look over, check, examine

Inspire – motivate, energize, encourage, enthuse

Institutionalize – to place in a facility for treatment

Integrate – put together, mix, add, combine, assimilate

Integrity – honesty

Interfere – get in the way, hinder, obstruct, impede, hamper

Interpret – explain the meaning of, to make understandable

Intervention – action, activity

Intolerance – bigotry, prejudice, narrow–mindedness

Involuntary – instinctive, reflex, unintentional, automatic, uncontrolled

Irreversible – permanent, irrevocable, irreparable, unalterable

Irritability – sensitivity to stimuli, fretful, quick excitability

Justify – explain in accordance with reason

Likely – probably, possible, expected

Liquefy – to change into or make more fluid

Logical – using reason

Longevity – long life

Lowest – inferior in rank

Maintain – continue, uphold, preserve, sustain, retain

Majority – the greater part of

Mention – talk about, refer to, state, cite, declare, point out

Minimal – least, smallest, nominal, negligible, token

Minimize – reduce, diminish, lessen, curtail, decrease to smallest possible

Mobilize – activate, organize, assemble, gather together, rally

Modify – change, adapt, adjust, revise, alter

Moist – slightly wet, damp

Multiple – many, numerous, several, various

Natural – normal, ordinary, unaffected

Negative – no, harmful, downbeat, pessimistic

Negotiate – bargain, talk, discuss, consult, cooperate, settle

Notice – become aware of, see, observe, discern, detect

Notify – inform, tell, alert, advise, warn, report

Nurture – care for, raise, rear, foster

Obsess – preoccupy, consume

Occupy – live in, inhabit, reside in, engage in

Occurrence – event, incident, happening

Odorous – scented, stinking, aromatic

Offensive – unpleasant, distasteful, nasty, disgusting

Opportunity – chance, prospect, break

Organize – put in order, arrange, sort out, categorize, classify

Origin – source, starting point, cause, beginning, derivation

Pace – speed

Parameter – limit, factor, limitation, issue

Participant – member, contributor, partaker, applicant

Perspective – viewpoint, view, perception

Position – place, location, point, spot, situation

Practice – do, carry out, perform, apply, follow

Precipitate – to cause to happen, to bring on, hasten, abrupt, sudden

Predetermine – fix or set beforehand

Predictable – expected, knowable

Preference – favorite, liking, first choice

Prepare – get ready, plan, make, train, arrange, organize

Prescribe – set down, stipulate, order, recommend, impose

Previous – earlier, prior, before, preceding

Primarily – first, above all, mainly, mostly, largely, principally, predominantly

Primary – first, main, basic, chief, most important, key, prime, major, crucial

Priority – main concern, giving first attention to, order of importance

Production – making, creation, construction, assembly

Profuse – a lot of, plentiful, copious, abundant, generous, prolific, bountiful

Prolong – extend, delay, put off, lengthen, draw out

Promote – encourage, support, endorse, sponsor

Proportion – ratio, amount, quantity, part of, percentage, section of

Provide – give, offer, supply, make available

Rationalize – explain, reason

Realistic – practical, sensible, reasonable

Receive – get, accept, take delivery of, obtain

Recognize – acknowledge, appreciate, identify, aware of

Recovery – healing, mending, improvement, recuperation, renewal

Reduce – decrease, lessen, ease, moderate, diminish

Reestablish – reinstate, restore, return, bring back

Regard – consider, look upon, relate to, respect

Regular – usual, normal, ordinary, standard, expected, conventional

Relative – comparative, family member

Relevance – importance of

Reluctant – unwilling, hesitant, disinclined, indisposed, adverse

Reminisce – to recall and review remembered experiences

Remove – take away, get rid of, eliminate, eradicate

Reposition – move, relocate, change position

Require – need, want, necessitate

Resist – oppose, defend against, keep from, refuse to go along with, defy

Resolution – decree, solution, decision, ruling, promise

Resolve – make up your mind, solve, determine, decide

Response – reply, answer, reaction, retort

Restore – reinstate, reestablish, bring back, return to, refurbish

Restrict – limit, confine, curb, control, contain, hold back, hamper

Retract – take back, draw in, withdraw, apologize

Reveal – make known, disclose, divulge, expose, tell, make public

Review – appraisal, reconsider, evaluation, assessment, examination, analysis

Ritual – custom, ceremony, formal procedure

Rotate – turn, go around, spin, swivel

Routine – usual, habit, custom, practice

Satisfaction – approval, fulfillment, pleasure, happiness

Satisfy – please, convince, fulfill, make happy, gratify

Secure – safe, protected, fixed firmly, sheltered, confident, obtain

Sequential – chronological, in order of occurrence

Significant – important, major, considerable, noteworthy, momentous

Slight – small, slim, minor, unimportant, insignificant, insult, snub

Source – basis, foundation, starting place, cause

Specific – exact, particular, detail, explicit, definite

Stable – steady, even, constant

Statistics – figures, data, information

Subtract – take away, deduct

Success – achievement, victory, accomplishment

Surround – enclose, encircle, contain

Suspect – think, believe, suppose, guess, deduce, infer, distrust, doubtful

Sustain – maintain, carry on, prolong, continue, nourish, suffer

Synonymous – same as, identical, equal, tantamount

Systemic – affecting the entire organism

Thorough – careful, detailed, methodical, systematic, meticulous, comprehensive, exhaustive

Tilt – tip, slant, slope, lean, angle, incline

Translucent – see–through, transparent, clear

Unique – one and only, sole, exclusive, distinctive

Universal – general, widespread, common, worldwide

Unoccupied – vacant, not busy, empty

Unrelated – unconnected, unlinked, distinct, dissimilar, irrelevant

Unresolved – unsettled, uncertain, unsolved, unclear, in doubt

Utilize – make use of, employ

Various – numerous, variety, range of, mixture of, assortment of

Verbalize – express, voice, speak, articulate

Verify – confirm, make sure, prove, attest to, validate, substantiate, corroborate, authenticate

Vigorous – forceful, strong, brisk, energetic

Volume – quantity, amount, size

Withdraw – remove, pull out, take out, extract

Index

X